T0350450

An Occupational Perspective of Health

THIRD EDITION

An Occupational Perspective of Health

THIRD EDITION

ANN A. WILCOCK, PhD, BAppScOT, GradDipPH, FCOT
SOUTH AUSTRALIA

CLARE HOCKING, PhD, MHSc(OT), AdvDipOT, DipOT
AUCKLAND UNIVERSITY OF TECHNOLOGY
AUCKLAND, NEW ZEALAND

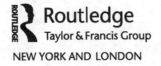

Routledge
Taylor & Francis Group

NEW YORK AND LONDON

Instructors: *An Occupational Perspective of Health, Third Edition Instructor's Manual* is also available. Don't miss this important companion to *An Occupational Perspective of Health, Third Edition.* To obtain the Instructor's Manual, please visit www.routledge.com/9781617110870

Dr. Ann A. Wilcock has no financial or proprietary interest in the materials presented herein.

Dr. Clare Hocking has no financial or proprietary interest in the materials presented herein.

First published in 2015 by SLACK Incorporated

Published 2024 by Routledge
605 Third Avenue, New York, NY 10017
4 Park Square, Milton Park, Abingdon, Oxon OX14 4RN

Routledge is an imprint of the Taylor & Francis Group, an informa business

Library of Congress Cataloging-in-Publication Data

Wilcock, Ann Allart, author.
 An occupational perspective of health / Ann A.Wilcock [and] Clare Hocking. -- Third edition.
  p. ; cm.
Includes bibliographical references and index.
ISBN 978-1-61711-087-0 (alk. paper)
I. Hocking, Clare, author. II. Title.
[DNLM: 1. Occupational Therapy. 2. Rehabilitation, Vocational. 3. Work--psychology. WB 555]
RM735.4
615.8'515--dc23
                         2014029389

ISBN: 9781617110870 (hbk)
ISBN: 9781003525233 (ebk)

DOI:10.4324/9781003525233

Contents

Contents

About the Authors

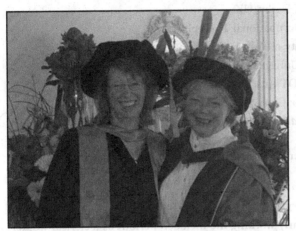

Ann A. Wilcock (née Ellison), PhD, BAppScOT, GradDipPh, FCOT, was born in the United Kingdom and was brought up in the Lake District. She graduated as an occupational therapist from the Derby School in 1961, and worked at Black Notley Hospital and Farnham Park Rehabilitation Centre before going to live in Australia in 1964. There she worked in large general hospitals in New South Wales and Tasmania in a variety of fields, including mental health, orthopedics, geriatric medicine, and neurology.

Figure. (Left) Clare Hocking. (Right) Ann Wilcock.

After many years as a practitioner, Ann moved into the academic sphere, eventually becoming Head of the School of Occupational Therapy at the University of South Australia, Adelaide, Australia, in 1987. Her graduate and doctoral studies have been in the field of public health at the University of Adelaide, Australia. Her formal academic career culminated in her appointment as Founding Professor of Occupational Science and Therapy at Deakin University, Victoria, Australia. Other appointments have included Doctoral Supervision at Auckland University of Technology, New Zealand; Visiting Professor at Brunel University, Uxbridge, England, UK; Adjunct Professor at Dalhousie University, Halifax, Nova Scotia, Canada; Charles Sturt University, Albury, Australia; and currently, the University of Canberra, Canberra, Australia.

Ann's research interests have spanned active aging; stroke; children's occupational potential; physiological influences on occupational performance; occupational balance; well-being; the effect of neurological disorder on the human need for occupation; population health; and the relationship between occupation, health, illness, occupational therapy, and public health. The highlight of her career has been encouraging the development of occupational science as an interdisciplinary and international force. She introduced occupational science to Australasia and in 1993 founded the *Journal of Occupational Science* and became the inaugural President of the International Society of Occupational Scientists (ISOS).

Ann co-authored *Help Yourselves—A Handbook for Hemiplegics and their Families* in 1966, was the sole author of *Occupational Therapy Approaches to Stroke* in 1986. As commissioned historian to the British College and Association of Occupational Therapists, she authored *Occupation for Health: A Journey from Self Health to Prescription* in 2001, and *Occupation for Health: A Journey from Prescription to Self Health* in 2002. The first and second editions of this text, *An Occupational Perspective of Health*, were published by SLACK Incorporated in 1998 and 2006, respectively.

As well as numerous chapters and articles, Ann has delivered keynote addresses at conferences in Australia, New Zealand, Canada, the United Kingdom, Sweden, Portugal, Japan, Thailand, Hong Kong, and the United States and at the World Federation of Occupational Therapists Congress in Montreal in 1998. She is the recipient of (or honored by) a range of prestigious awards internationally, which include the following:

- 2013 Establishment of the Ann Wilcock Prize, University of South Australia awarded for Academic Excellence
- 2012 Establishment of the Ann Wilcock Lecture, Australasian Occupational Science Symposia

- 2005 Honorary Professor of Deakin University, Victoria, Australia
- 2004 Honorary Fellow of Brunel University, London, England, UK
- Honorary Doctor of the University of Derby, UK
- Fellow of the British Association of Occupational Therapists
- Barbara Sexton Lectureship: University of Western Ontario, London, Ontario, Canada
- 2000 Thelma Cardwell Lectureship: University of Toronto, Canada
- 1999 The Silvia Docker Lectureship: OT Australia
- The Doris Sym Memorial Lectureship: Glasgow Caledonian University, Scotland, UK
- Inaugural Henry Nowic Trust *Occupation for Health* Lectureship: Charles Sturt University, Bathurst, Australia
- 1995 Wilma West Lectureship: University of Southern California, Los Angeles, California, USA

Clare Hocking, PhD, MHSc(OT), AdvDipOT, DipOT, was born and raised in New Zealand, sheltered by the hills of the Hutt Valley. Her early working life included periods as a clerical worker and time on the factory floor, inspecting components for telephone exchanges. Those experiences sharpened her sense of social justice, even before she knew that terminology.

Clare completed a Diploma in Occupational Therapy in 1982, then an Advanced Diploma in Occupational Therapy in 1989, both from the Central Institute of Technology in Heretaunga, New Zealand. In her first occupational therapy post in Christchurch, New Zealand, Clare gained experience in medical wards for older adults, long-stay wards for adults with profound musculoskeletal and neurological impairments, and with brief spells in hand therapy and burns wards. A move to Auckland, New Zealand in 1985 brought new opportunities running a vocational rehabilitation service for people recovering from traumatic brain injury, stroke, and multiple physical injuries, followed by a range of positions at one of Auckland's large psychiatric hospitals.

Gaining an Advanced Diploma opened the door to academia in the newly established occupational therapy program in Auckland in 1990. As an inaugural staff member, that involved a steep learning curve in lecturing, curriculum design, and student selection, as well as the demand for higher qualifications. Clare was fortunate to study occupational science under Ann Wilcock's tutelage. From there she took over the editorship of the *Journal of Occupational Science,* which Ann Wilcock had established, and Clare recruited Ann as her PhD supervisor. That pathway ultimately led to an appointment as New Zealand's first Professor of Occupational Science and Therapy in 2012.

Clare's early research was firmly grounded in occupational science, investigating the relationship between people and the things they make and use. That focus helped her form new insights into the identity issues associated with using assistive technologies, particularly wheelchairs and self-care equipment, and shed light on occupational therapy's move away from arts and crafts and toward mechanistic explanations of the therapeutic application of occupation for health. Supporting the growth of postgraduate education in New Zealand, Clare has subsequently supervised research in topics as diverse as living with motor neuron disease, the supervision of occupational therapists, the meaning of occupation, and how occupational therapists take up ideas from the professional literature.

Accordingly, Clare's extensive list of publications spans most of the English language occupational therapy journals and many key British and American texts. She has emerged as a critical voice within both occupational therapy and occupational science. Of note is her co-authorship of the World Federation of Occupational Therapists' *Minimum Standards for the Education of Occupational Therapists,* published in 2002. This ground breaking work positioned occupational science concepts as the basis of the profession's philosophy and practice. As co-chair of the Federation's International Advisory Group on Human Rights, Clare continues to influence the direction and focus of occupational therapy education. Also of note, she co-edited *Critical Perspectives on Occupational Science: Society, Inclusion, Participation* in 2012 with Gail Whiteford, the Pro-Vice Chancellor of Social Inclusion in Macquarie University in Sydney, Australia.

Clare has been an invited keynote speaker at events in Japan, Thailand, the US, Mexico, Britain, Australia, and South Africa. She has been honored with a range of prestigious appointments and awards in New Zealand and internationally which include the following:

- 2014 Adjunct Professor, Chiang Mai University, Thailand
- 2012 Visiting Scholar, Institute for Advanced Studies in Social Ethics, Salzburg, Austria
- 2011 Honorary Professor, Plymouth University, Plymouth, England, UK
- 2009 Adjunct Associate Professor, Charles Sturt University, Albury, Australia
- 2008 Ruth Zemke Lecture in Occupational Science, Society for the Study of Occupation: USA
- Occupational Science Visiting Scholar, Brenau University, Gainesville, Georgia, USA
- Visiting Scholar, Otago Polytechnic, Dunedin, New Zealand
- 2007 Sadie Philcox Lecture, University of Queensland, Brisbane, Australia
- Visiting Scholar, Canterbury Christ Church College, Canterbury, England, United Kingdom
- 2006 World Federation of Occupational Therapists Merit Award for exemplary service
- Visiting Scholar, Sør-Trøndelag University College, Trondheim, Norway
- 2003 Frances Rutherford Lectureship Award, New Zealand Association of Occupational Therapists

A number of activities have been identified as supportive of healing through fostering in children a sense of purpose, self-esteem, and identity. These include establishing daily routines such as going to school, preparing food, washing clothes, and working in the fields; providing children with the intellectual and emotional stimulation through structured group activities such as play, sports, drawing, drama, and storytelling; and providing the opportunity for expression, attachment, and trust that comes from a stable, caring, and nurturing relationship with adults.

The Impact of Armed Conflict on Child Development, United Nations[1]

The health enhancing properties ascribed to the occupations of children holds true for people of all ages

Preface

Like earlier editions, this book draws on historical and contemporary informants and international sources such as the United Nations (UN) and the World Health Organization (WHO) to offer critical commentary on understanding occupation as an important aspect of health. As explained in the Introduction and Purpose of this book, a holistic understanding of occupation as all that people do across the sleep-wake continuum is, at present, a poorly understood concern within health care. Instead, particular occupations or parts of what is understood in this text as occupation are considered in a reductionist fashion largely according to the interests of different disciplines.

Throughout the text, *occupation* is used to mean *all the things that people need, want or have to do across the sleep-wake continuum, individually and collectively*. People's occupational natures, needs, wants, and obligations are explored, as well as how they feel about what they do, how they relate to others through doing, and the growth, development, and enhancement potential of involvement. Those four aspects of occupation are conceptualized within the phrase "doing, being, belonging, and becoming." Occupation's connection with health is also considered from the perspective of sociopolitical and corporate organizations, as collectives of occupational beings whose activities affect individuals, families, communities, and nations, and have global ramifications.

This book addresses perspectives of population health founded on WHO policies and addresses them as focal points of each chapter. The chapters gradually uncover a different way to understand health in the light of how, what, with whom, and why people spend time and effort in "doing, being, belonging and becoming" through engagement in occupations. It explores the development and relationships between occupation, health, illness, health care, and the ideologies that surround them; the potential importance to population health of these relationships; and how these are or could be addressed by those who determine or influence the activities of others. Suggested approaches are complementary to and supportive of conventional medical practice, while addressing broader personal, social, economic, and environmental goals in line with WHO and population health in a changing world and a global economy. Occupational terminology is linked with that of global population health.

There are already many different ways to explain causal links between biology and determinants of health or illness. The body's cells can behave differently according to factors as various as people's social position, education, work, place of habitation, political situation, class, gender, ethnicity, social disadvantage, and marginalization.[2] While causal relationships are not precisely understood, behavioral, social, and biological causes of illness can work interactively, and the impact can be mediated by genetic structure, immunity, nutritional status, resilience, and ability to cope.[3]

This holistic view of occupation across a lifetime of days and nights holds a degree of similarity with the United Kingdom's notion of "lifeworld" that draws on Enlightenment philosophy. Like the conceptual basis for lifeworld, the occupational perspective taken here is based on the understanding that inequalities in health are both biological in origin and related to human activity; health outcomes capture the benefits and insults to health experienced on the journey through life; and occupations that lead to health inequities are avoidable, unfair, and unnecessary if the occupational causes can be altered. The perspective taken here concurs with the understanding that:

> The lifeworld is the locus of experience: social, psychological and physical. It is that social and emotional space which all of us uniquely inhabit. It is the world of the everyday; the world of the immediate experience and the aspects of life that we take for granted. It is where life is at its most meaningful and its most painful. ... Lifeworlds are the point at which stressors are moderated, mediated, or exacerbated. It is the point where insults are parried or where they have their noxious effects. It is the point where vulnerabilities translate

stressors into physical and emotional damage. It is where immunities – biological, physical or psychological – work their protective powers.[4]

Health outcomes can depend on the directions taken at every step of the occupation journey. Benefits and insults to health will differ, largely as a result of what people "do" across the continuum of daily lives. For example, they will differ for children at play or wrestling a living out of refuse dumps, for home-based child-carers, business executives, unemployed youths, hunter-gatherers, tradespeople, factory workers, subsistence farmers, asylum seekers, people with disabilities trying to live independently, or politicians. In terms of "doing," the lifeworld is where opportunities, barriers, difficulties, and disadvantages are experienced and dealt with; "being" is where uniquely personal emotions and feelings are played out as an expression of self; "belonging" is where the repetitive and routine nature of contact with others such as family, friends, and work or leisure colleagues happens; and "becoming" is where the ability or inability to change occupations occurs in advantageous or disadvantageous ways. Like lifeworlds, people's experiences of occupation may not be benign or cozy but cold, chronically difficult, and unforgiving where discrimination, disadvantage, marginalization, poverty, unemployment, bullying, or violence flourish.[5]

Addressing health from this different perspective is vital because the postmodern world does not have answers to the many health issues relating to what people "do," or fails to use those already uncovered. This leads to health inequities and occupational injustice. Addressing health inequalities that are about occupational injustice can be time consuming or difficult not in the least because they involve value judgements and have political implications.

In the Preface to the last edition, the unhealthy foundations and properties of occupations such as war, terrorism, rioting, ecological devastation, substance abuse, school absenteeism, unemployment, social welfare fraud, dependence on the state, over or under indulgence in food, family breakdown, suicide, aggression, and abuse were deplored. Such population driven and enacted occupations remain common news stories. Although such disorders appear most associated with the poor or disadvantaged, the affluent are not immune to occupation-based illnesses, and accounts of their consequences are on the increase. For example, recent reports of an emerging problem describe how addiction to the products of modern electronics has led to a growing number of people preferring to financially support that habit rather than essentials such as food.

For early homo species and creatures of all kinds, occupation was a lynch pin of health. Animals in the wild still remain able to live healthily through what they do as long as their environment is not changed too drastically. People are not so fortunate. Across the globe, natural environments and ways of life are so irreparably damaged that illness is a present reality for many and probable for most in the longer term. This negative background to people's experiences of health, in large part, can be blamed not only on what people have done or not done in the past but also on what people do currently, and in particular, what the pursuit of wealth by advanced countries and multinational corporations has led to.

While the glories of medical science and the struggles of a young environmental movement to right those wrongs are topics addressed almost daily in the world's news, the fact is that the occupational needs of people and how these relate to health or illness remain largely unexplored despite rules about "doing" being prescribed from the time, millennia ago, that people began to record their observations about the causes of health or illness. The rules survived until the advent of modern medicine, but their current equivalents are rarely applied in the present day except with regard to the taking of medication, rest, diet, and exercise.

The word *occupation* is most frequently used to refer to work for pay as it is understood in the present day and enacted in affluent or developed countries, but its meaning is much broader. As in millennia past, occupation provides the wherewithal of survival; the practical means of obtaining the requirements of life; the means to maintain health; the basis of growth and development; the nuts and bolts of social integration and cohesion; the means to dream; and the way to find enjoyment or meaning and to flourish or flounder at international, national, societal as well as individual levels. It is an ever changing and essential aspect of life; although it can be fragile in the face of occupational stress, deprivation, alienation and injustice as well as public policies that are themselves born of occupation, but largely unheeding of health or the greed and aggressiveness that may come about as a result of enactment.

Developing a health perspective centered on the total range of occupations across the sleep-wake continuum at individual and population levels is particularly difficult because occupation is such an integral part of every person's existence and of already accepted, but different, perspectives on life. To rethink issues from this divergent yet familiar focus requires scrutiny, analysis, and re-synthesis of current ideas despite them appearing to be true, unalterable, and inevitable. The prevailing reductionism of traditional scientific methods that are central within health research is a case in point.

Population-Based, Globally Focused Health Promotion

Recent initiatives toward positive health began to gather momentum with the emergence of what is known as the "New Public Health." This originated in the early 1970s when a WHO/United Children's Rights and Emergency Relief Organization Joint Committee on Health Policy debated alternative approaches to health care. The result was aimed at the provision of "basic health services" that had less emphasis on "sophisticated hospital-based services" but incorporated "disease prevention, curative medicine, and maternal and child health care."[6] Leading the push away from "medical high tech and top down disease campaigns" were E.J.R. Heyward, Deputy Executive of UNICEF, and his counterpart, Tejado de Rivero from the WHO. These men of foresight master-minded the International Conference on Primary Health Care held at Alma Ata in 1978. Black[6] describes how the current key ingredients of decentralization, participation, integration, maintenance, and sustainability grew from their questioning how:

> The strategy of 'basic services' to meet 'basic needs' ... passed into common development parlance. The idea of creating ownership and responsibility at the outer edge of service delivery and of engaging communities in their own development process remains operative today.[6]

The advent of primary health care led to initiatives to promote health and coincidentally reduce illness as the logical next step in the campaign, particularly with regards to maximizing advances in the developed world. In 1986, the first of several world conferences on health promotion was held in Ottawa, and directives from those provide ways to consider the maintenance and improvement of health from positive perspectives. Those and other directives from the WHO continue to stress the need for the re-orientation of all health professions toward the pursuit of health.

The new public health is also influenced by a postindustrial debate between the values of economic rationalism and social equality. Caught between medical science and the debate about social values, public health has largely failed to consider how basic human needs relate to health, unless the needs can be reduced to obvious physiological functioning or monetary terms. The idea of human needs is unfashionable and to a large extent ignored, being associated with "naturalistic fallacy,"[7] and out of step with the dominant notions of behaviorism and cultural relativism. This inhibits consideration of health from the point of view of "how a specimen" of any kind of organism, including people, "can be recognized as flourishing." This stance ignores many of the needs and potential of humans which are part of their hard-wired neuronal structure, and, even if needs are not identical with drives or a "motivational force instigated by a state of disequilibrium... neither are they disconnected from 'human nature." Doyal and Gough[8] maintain "to argue for such disconnection would be to identify humanity with no more than human reason and to bifurcate human existence from that of the rest of the animal world." It is fundamental to the line of reasoning here that health is related to the meeting of biological needs and potential and to learning "how nature intended human beings to live."[9] The simplicity and complexity of this concept is central to the occupational nature and needs of people.

It is important to recall that, currently, in postindustrialized societies, health care is dominated by medical science. This is based mainly on contemporary understanding of physiology, biochemistry, pathology, and biostatistics, and societal acceptance of modern technological, surgical, and pharmaceutical advances. Medical science values are so integral to postindustrial culture's thinking, it is difficult for those brought up in such a society to perceive health from another perspective, thus limiting the study of health to ideas, beliefs, and approaches that are valued, advocated, and deemed important by medical science. Even health professions that are different and distinct from medicine use medical science categories and theories, accept many medical science priorities, and are concerned with strategies to diagnose or analyze, reduce, or prevent illness resulting from physical, behavioral, or social factors. This emphasis leads to the major preoccupation in health research with uncovering the causes of illness and disease rather than the causes of health and wellness, notwithstanding the holistic philosophy of the "new public health" movement.[10] Recent interest in social determinants of health, health promotion, and wellness has also centered to a large extent on the prevention of illness, many people using the terms *prevention* and *health promotion* synonymously.

Even understanding about occupation has been directed in a reductionist way toward specific aspects such as "work," "exercise," and "eating." While those are very important aspects, seen separately and apart from a holistic framework that includes all doing, being, belonging, and becoming across the sleep-wake continuum ignores the interactive nature of both occupation and human health. Snapshots of understanding about what people do throughout their lives to meet economic, social, and personal needs are decontextualized. Such snapshots have effectively biased appreciation, exploration and action centered on occupation as a phenomenon of central importance in health. *An Occupational Perspective of Health, Third Edition*, brings such issues into focus by recognizing that the attainment of health and well-being can be largely achieved through the everyday occupations of life.

Ann A. Wilcock, PhD, BAppScOT, GradDipPH, FCOT

References

1. *The impact of armed conflict on child development.* United Nations. Available at: http://un.org/rights/impact.htm.

2. Braveman P. Health disparities and health equity: concepts and measurement. *Annu Rev Public Health.* 2006; 27:167-94.

3. National Institute for Health and Clinical Excellence: NICE. Appendix A Conceptual framework for the work of the Centre for Public Health Excellence (CPHE). Methods for the development of NICE public health guidance. 3rd edition. 26 September 2012.

4. Kelly M, Stewart E, Morgan A, Killoran A, Fischer A, Threlfall A, Bonnefoy J. A conceptual framework for public health: NICE's emerging approach. *Public Health.* 2009; 123(1): e18.

5. *UK NICE: A Conceptual Framework for Public Health.* 2008. http:/www.sciencedirect.com/science/article/pii/s0033350608002795#.

6. Black M. In Memory: E.J.R. (Dick) Heyward 1914-2005: Quiet architect of UNICEF and international systems. *UNICEF Staff News.* 2005; Issue 3: 25-32: 31.

7. Watts ED. Human needs. In: Kuper A, Kuper J, eds. *The Social Science Encyclopedia.* Rev ed. London, England: Routledge; 1989:367-368.

8. Doyal L, Gough I. *A Theory of Human Need.* London, England: Macmillan; 1991:35-36.

9. Coon CS. *The Hunting Peoples.* London, England: Jonathan Cape Ltd; 1972:393.

10. Ashton J, Seymour H. *The New Public Health: The Liverpool Experience.* Milton Keynes: Open University Press; 1988.

Introduction

This edition of *An Occupational Perspective of Health* continues the intention of the original publication and aims to encourage wide-ranging recognition of a holistic concept of occupation as a major contributor to all people's experiences of health, drawing on varied directives of the World Health Organization. The text explains the "what and why" rather than the "how" of the concept. Until there is improved interdisciplinary recognition and understanding of the 24-hour-a-day/lifetime nature of people's doing, it is premature to focus on the details of "how" to attain, maintain, or reclaim population health through occupation.

The common failure to appreciate occupation in holistic terms inclusive of all the things that people do in their lives across the sleep-wake continuum and the way they interact is caused by reductionism. This has resulted in a wide-ranging lack of understanding of occupation as a means to maintain and improve health and well-being and how it contributes to illness. Indeed, even at international and national levels, the role of occupation in terms of the physical, mental, and social health of both individuals and populations is so poorly understood that it is largely overlooked; not considered adequately in policy production, scrutiny, or enactment and seldom resourced except in terms of paid employment.

At present, reductionist ideas and practices across the specific frames of references of the many health-care disciplines dislocate what people do into fragments of specialization. Reductionism is compounded by differences between such professions in what is meant by the word *occupation*. This is even the case among those with a particular interest in what people "do," such as occupational therapists, time-use researchers, and occupational health or population health practitioners. All tend to concentrate on particular aspects such as self-care, work, exercise, sleep, or social activities rather than a total interactive picture. Furthermore, health practitioners usually experience restrictions in practice opportunities according to financial constraints, legislation, reductionist criteria, and prevailing traditions. Media interest further accentuates the importance of particular interventions without due understanding of, or reference to, the larger and perhaps less dramatic picture. It is therefore not surprising that the World Health Organization also uses the word *occupation* in a variety of ways, precluding an overarching holistic line of attack as discussed in this book.

Research Underlying the Text

Following the tradition of earlier editions, this book draws on critical text analysis to consider insights into the what, why, and how occupation relates to health using a research approach known as "history of ideas."[1] This approach enables a rounded glimpse of the relationship since human genesis. Ideas about both health and occupation have altered throughout time as environments and cultures evolved, but the connection is so fundamental that when a researcher starts to search for the connection, it cannot be overlooked. As Konrad Lorenz, an Austrian zoologist, explained animal and human behavior is the functional aspect "of a system owing its existence, as well as its special form, to a development process that has taken place in the history of the species, in the development of the individual and, in man, in cultural history."[2]

Histories of ideas aim to explain, associate, and correlate factors that, in present structures and reductionist ways of thinking, may appear unconnected. Arthur Lovejoy[1] developed the history of ideas approach in the 1920s to describe a form of research that reconsiders already known concepts from a different perspective so that new understandings emerge. He argued that this form of exploration is most useful if the history is concerned with widely held concepts that cross cultural boundaries, disciplines and thought such as justice, nature, and freedom.

A study of this kind is fairly unusual in the field of health and may appear to be "a strange combination of incongruences: general but detailed, straightforward but intricate, pragmatic but abstract,"[3] so the rigor of the research effort is easily overlooked. Furthermore, both health and occupation are core ideas fundamental to any time and place, taken for granted, and assumed to be largely unchangeable. That assumption proves to be far from the case as ideas about both have altered throughout history as environments and cultures evolved. Yet as Gergen,[4] a social psychologist, argued, the more usual methodologies for studying people can lead to inadequate and distorted findings because techniques frequently decontextualize and are atemporal, and deterministic.

The occupational theory of human nature that emerged from history of ideas research undertaken some 20 years ago is found in Chapter 4, as a foundation to the ever evolving relationship between health and occupation. It remains valid because biological characteristics, needs, and capacities guarantee that the human need and use of occupation is inbuilt and, like health, well-being and the prevention of illness are factors that transcend time. Consideration of those factors, in combination with modern, culture-concept approaches, continues to uncover the innate relationship between health and occupation.

This book outlines the association between health and occupation. Humans affected their health by what they did from the start of their existence, long before specialized caring for the health of others. Its history provides the context for this perspective in order to give due importance to the foundation and subsequent changes of the relationship throughout millennia; as specializations developed, the basic association between what people do and their health became increasingly overlooked.

The intensive research undertaken for the previous editions forms the core of the text and is supplemented by more recent research that supports the substance of this third edition, that like its forerunners, is based on the positive and negative relationships between health and occupation.

Occupational Science

This exploration both draws on and adds to studies that provide the ground swell of the fairly recently emerging academic discipline of *occupational science*. This science was in the first stages of development when research commenced on the first edition of this book. Developed during the 1980s and 1990s in the USA[5] and Australasia,[6,7] occupational science is the study of people as occupational beings. Originating within the discipline of occupational therapy, occupational science is conceived as multidisciplinary with the potential to provide legitimate and alternative means to consider central issues in life, as do psychology and sociology. Recognition of the need for a science of occupation is not entirely new. In the 17th century, philosopher and self-styled physician, John Locke (1632-1704), proposed that science as the means to explore, discover and understand the world included biology, ethics, and communication. He defined ethics in occupational terms as correctly applying personal action and skill to attain that which is "good and useful" and what people ought "to do, as a rational and voluntary agent for the attainment of any ends, especially happiness."[8] He anticipates 19th and early 20th century socialist reformers in Europe who recognized the value of human labor, and pragmatist philosophers in the United States such as William James who recognized the centrality of occupation to life. Perhaps it is not a coincidence that occupational science emerged from scholarship within occupational therapy, for as early as 1917 the American National Society for the Promotion of Occupational Therapy was formed with these objectives:

> *The advancement of occupation as a therapeutic measure; the study of the effect of occupation upon the human being; and the scientific dispensation of this knowledge.*[9]

There can be no gainsaying that the integrated complexities of occupation require rigorous investigation as a central aspect of living.[5] However, traditional experimental researchers would see the complexities of human characteristics and the variety of occupational environments as contaminants to research design.[10] Indeed, from the perspective of reductionist and contextually controlled studies, it is almost impossible to explore the complexities. However, to reduce people's engagement in occupation to component parts diminishes its study as is already the case when occupation is partitioned, named differently, and studied segmentally by diverse disciplines.

When the science emerged, development in many fields had illustrated a change of consciousness about the things that people do. There was for example, renewed interest in issues related to physical activity, paid employment, leisure pursuits, sports, education and early childhood learning as determinants of health. Unfortunately, such interest has not yet reached a stage that enables composite exploration to be the focus of large-scale multidisciplinary research nor has occupational science been adopted as the global and far-reaching discipline it has the potential to become. Notwithstanding the disappointment of the slow growth of the science, this third edition continues the discourse about the relationship between occupation and health according to:

1. How health has been, is, and can be conceptualized in occupational terms.

2. The role of occupation as "doing, being, belonging, and becoming" across the life-long, 24-hour sleep-wake continuum of human life, health, and survival.

3. Occupation as either a positive or negative influence on health.

4. How corporate, economic, and political occupations determine the occupational health or illness consequences for individuals.

5. The potential contribution of occupation-focused approaches to current WHO and global population health objectives.

6. Possible occupation for health focused actions that health practitioners might take at population levels.

Ann A. Wilcock, PhD, BAppScOT, GradDipPH, FCOT

References

1. Lovejoy AO. The study of the history of ideas. 1936. In: King P, ed. *The History of Ideas*. London, England: Croom Helm; 1983:179-194.

2. Lorenz K. *Civilized Man's Eight Deadly Sins*. Latzke M, trans. London, England: Methuen and Co Ltd; 1974:1.

3. Hamilton DB. The idea of history and the history of ideas. *Image: Journal of Nursing Scholarship*. 1993;25(1):45-48.

4. Gergen K. *Towards Transformation in Social Knowledge*. New York, NY: Springer-Verlag; 1982.

5. Yerxa EJ, Clark F, Frank G, et al. An introduction to occupational science: a foundation for occupational therapy in the 21st century. *Occupational Therapy in Health Care*. 1989;6(4):1-17.

6. Wilcock AA. 1989. *Is Occupational Science the Basis of Occupational Therapy?* 2nd South Australian Occupational Therapy Conference.

7. Wilcock AA. 1990. *Occupational Science*. World Federation of Occupational Therapists Congress, Melbourne.

8. Locke J. *An Essay Concerning Humane Understanding*. London: Printed for Tho, Basset, and sold by Edw. Mory at the sign of the Three Bibles in St Paul's Church-Yard; MDCXC (1690):361.

9. Dunton WR Jr. *Prescribing Occupational Therapy. 2nd ed.* Springfield, Ill: Charles C Thomas; 1928.

10. Yerxa EJ. A mind is a precious thing. *Australian Occupational Therapy Journal*. 1990;37(4):170-171.

Section I

Health and Illness

Theme 1

"Health is a state of complete physical, mental, and social well-being, not merely the absence of disease or infirmity."

WHO Definition of Health, 1946

DEFINING HEALTH

This introductory chapter will concentrate on how health is defined in the West, focusing on the World Health Organization (WHO) definition that provides the theme of this chapter. The focus will be on the complexities of trying to define it in a way that appears relevant to everyone. Health is a multifaceted subject differing according to cultural and spiritual beliefs, socially dominant and individual views, particular environments, and available health technologies. Ideas about what it is also differ according to who defines it, evolving and changing with scientific and societal developments. Definitions of health have also changed with the myriad opinions about the possible causes of illness as the array of health-related issues increase with medical understanding. However, concern has been expressed that "societies are letting technology define health for them" and some are worried by "the medicalization of everything organic and emotional."[1]

Although the idea of health is long standing, it appears that its current use as the principle descriptor of the state did not become common until the middle of the 20th century and the advent of the WHO. However, as early as the 5th Century BC, Pericles (c. 495-429 BC), a statesman considered partially responsible for the golden age of Ancient Greece,[2] was given credence for coining the first reported definition of health in the Western World, describing it as the "state of moral, mental and physical well-being that enables a person to face any crisis in life with the utmost grace and facility."[3] At approximately the same time, in the collection of medical treatises known

Wilcock AA, Hocking C.
An Occupational Perspective of Health, Third Edition (pp 2-31).
© 2015 Taylor & Francis Group.

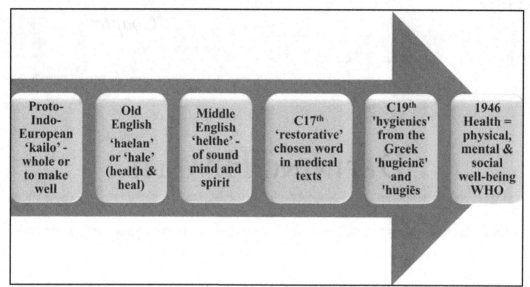

Figure 1-1. Origins and evolution of the word *health*.

as Corpus Hippocraticum, Hippocrates of Kos (c. 460–375 BC) advanced the idea of health being dependent on 4 humors concerned with body fluids— blood, phlegm, and yellow and black bile— but offered no actual definition. Derived from the Aristotelian doctrine explaining the nature of the earth known as *Stocheia*, the humoral theory of health was accepted in many parts of the world until recent advances in medicine over the past couple of centuries. Differing opinions about whether health is a broad issue that encompasses well-being, as in Pericles' definition, or a medical phenomenon directly related to physiology, as Hippocrates' work suggests, continues to this day.

The word health has not always been in common use as it is currently (Figure 1-1). In Old English, the word *haelan* or *hale* was derived from the Proto-Indo-European root "kailo," meaning "whole, uninjured, of good omen" and took on the added sense of "to make well." The words heal and health followed.[4,5] In Middle English, helthe came to mean of sound mind and spirit, but by the 17th century *restorative* was the preferred word in medical texts. This was replaced by hygienics toward the end of the 19th century, which was considered more scientific.[4] Hygienics was derived from the Greek words *hugieine* and *hugies*, meaning health and healthy, respectively, which stems from Hygeia, the name given to the Greek goddess who personified health.

The Health Organization, (prior to the WHO) a division of the League of Nations that was founded on January 10, 1920, used both health and hygiene. It was in June 1946 that the word *health* was adopted universally, after the WHO definition was created within a Preamble to the Constitution adopted by the International Health Conference held in New York. Signed in July by representatives of 61 States, it entered into force on April 7, 1948.[5] Throughout this text, that definition provides the background to all of the ideas that are discussed and many that are proposed as the way forward.

World Health Organization Definition of Health

The WHO's founding Constitution described health positively as "a state of complete physical, mental, and social well-being, not merely the absence of disease or infirmity."[5] Despite intense criticism, this definition has stood the test of time and emphasizes the importance of the promotion of health and the prevention of illness. Both aspects are fundamental to the improvement of population health across the globe and a central focus of the perspective taken here. It is important to compare it with other definitions to uncover some of the varied aspects of life that appear to be components of or important in the advancement of health. Further clarification of the WHO definition is provided later in the chapter because more extensive descriptions of population health have emerged in response to globalization over the past decades.

CRITIQUE, ALTERNATIVES, AND ADDITIONS

In the late 1950s and in the spirit of the WHO definition, René Dubos offered a broad humanistic explanation of health that critiqued the pursuit of technological fixes and addressed future expectations, as well as individual perspectives. He suggested that health and well-being are manifestations of the degree to which "the individual and the body maintain in readiness the resources required to meet the exigencies of the future."[6] A decade later, Maslow posited his hypothesis regarding the hierarchy of needs. This entwined physical, mental, and social health and well-being, with the postulate that basic physiological needs are primary, followed by needs for safety, love, esteem, and self-actualization.[7] Although not a specific definition of health, his theory has often been used as a means of interpreting the WHO's broad but less explicit description.

It has been suggested that the WHO definition is too idealized. Some critics, particularly during the mid-20th century, considered it too broad. Critique has been rife over the decades since its creation. For example, Callahan described it as "an irresistible straw man." Indeed, trying to "upset" it was the "aim of all players" and one of the "grandest games" available. His main complaint was that the "association of health and general well-being" lead to a "blurring of lines of responsibility between and among the professions, and between the medical profession and the political order" as social and health problems become one and the same. Although he recognized "more than a grain of truth in it" and the implication of "some intrinsic relationship between good of the body and good of the self," he believed that the definition of health should be limited to physical well-being.[8]

In his attempt to limit the responsibilities for health to the domain of medicine, Callahan[8] failed to sufficiently appreciate that health is the concern of everyone and that professions other than medicine have important roles in maintaining health. If this were not the case, a continuance of reductionism would prevail, the interactive nature of minds, bodies, communities and environment overlooked, and important connections would not be made. Indeed, current day segmentation and preoccupation with illness would be encouraged.

However, Callahan[8] is not alone in believing that the WHO focus is too broad and that definitions of health should be limited to matters responsive to interventions of medical science alone. For example, in medical dictionaries it is common to find definitions that are closely related to the absence of illness such as "the overall condition of an organism at a given time" and "soundness, especially of body or mind; freedom from disease or abnormality."[9] Some medical scientists suggest that the WHO definition is idealistic, unattainable, largely irrelevant, and difficult to measure[10,11] and that health cannot be achieved because it and disease are discreet and mutually exclusive entities.[12] In contrast, others suggest that "clinical definitions of health cannot provide a comprehensive framework for describing the condition,"[13] with some arguing that the focus is too narrow by seeming to exclude the spiritual and ethical dimensions of health.[14]

Almost contemporary with, but contrasting to, Callahan's view, Breslow, a Dean of Public Health, applauded the WHO change of focus from overcoming disease to achieving positive health. He understood the difficulty of absorbing the new concept for "those trained to approach health through pathology." To assist understanding, he describes how the Human Population Laboratory of Alameda County, California, began work on measuring health from the new positive point of view:

> *For an individual or a community, it appears possible to measure health status through questions that only individuals can answer about themselves, as in the Human Population*

Laboratory, and through testing by physical means the extent of functional reserves, as in multiphasic screening. Medicine would then focus on improving health in the sense of (i) moving people toward the favorable end of the health spectrum, as determined subjectively by responses to questions, and (ii) enhancing the bodily reserves, as determined by screening tests.[15]

It becomes clear that defining health as more than the absence of illness has many supporters and has elicited many ideas. For example, Kass provided a useful but simple version in which he describes health as a norm or a natural state of being in which the human organism works well as a whole.[16] Along similar lines, the archaeological viewpoint of Bush and Zvelebil offered a more detailed but useful way of thinking:

The human organism, and its surviving remains, is comprehended as a dynamic, histori-cal and adaptive system, reflecting the interaction between the biological organism and its environment during the individual's lifetime. Health is the biological and psychological condition of the individual, a state which can, at least in theory, be assessed by the incidence of insults and other abnormal symptoms ... Health is evaluated by cultural perceptions and parameters: ill-health and disease are culturally defined phenomena. In this non-biological sense, the definition of health can range from one of physical and mental well-being, with anything else being ill-health, to the other [of the] clinical presence of disease indicators or of the biological response to it with anything other considered healthy.[13]

Prior to World War II and the WHO definition of health, medical historian Sigerist[17] recog-nized health as a multidimensional concept inclusive of body, mind, and adjustment. Like others who followed, he recognized joyfulness and cheerfulness as indicators of health, along with being well-balanced and accepting of life's responsibilities. His view was possibly influenced by Johann Peter Frank who, as early as 1790, argued "that health and well-being could only be obtained where there was freedom from want and deprivation."[18] (Sigerist wrote an introduction for Frank's work when it was translated from the German version and republished in 1941).

More recently, of many other attempts by workers in a variety of fields, a description given by Greiner et al has an occupational bias:

Functioning is integral to health. There are physical, mental and social levels of function reflected in terms of performance and expectations. Loss of function may be a sign or symp-tom of a disease...a state of ill health.[19]

The authors describe how functional health patterns include activity-exercise, roles-relation-ships, sleep-rest, cognition-perception, self-perception-self-concept, and coping-stress tolerance.[19]

Debate continues and criticism still prevails. In a 2012 text for nurses, Sharma and Romas listed their dissatisfaction with the WHO definition, stating that health is a dynamic not a static state and the dimensions are inadequate; it is subjective, difficult to measure, and idealistic rather than realistic; it is a means not an end; and it lacks community orientation.[4] In a somewhat similar vein and in response to a 2005 WHO Bulletin editorial about "meaningful definitions" needing to call a "spade a spade,"[20] Awofeso appealed for a revision of the WHO definition.[21] Describing it as "uto-pian, inflexible, and unrealistic," he argued the descriptor "complete...makes it highly unlikely that anyone would be healthy for a reasonable period of time." Health and happiness, he reasoned, refer to separate experiences, "whose relationship is neither fixed nor constant."[21] His article drew on a 1997 article by Saracci, who defined health as "a condition of well-being free of disease or infirmity, and a basic and universal human right."[22] This links the "WHO's ideal to contemporary issues of human rights, equity and justice" and avoids use of the term "a state of complete physi-cal, mental, and social well-being" because that "corresponds more to happiness than to health."

In a December 2008 editorial in the *British Medical Journal*, Jadad and O'Grady called for a "global conversation" about how to define health, including comment from those who consider it impossible.[23] Although applauding the WHO definition that was created without the benefits of modern communication technology, they welcomed online offerings from those interested in either enhancing or replacing it. This led to a 2-day meeting in the Netherlands in December 2009 and a 2011 article from a group of distinguished health experts who concluded that the WHO definition is "no longer fit for purpose given the rise of chronic disease" and "may even be counter-productive."[24] They claimed that a major fault is the use of the word complete, which inadvertently furthers the "medicalization of society" because more issues can be regarded as health problems. Their proposed change of emphasis is "towards the ability to adapt and self manage in the face of social, physical and emotional challenges."[24] This emphasis should be a call to those interested in occupation as both a therapy and a means of population health.

A 2009 editorial in The *Lancet* continues the challenge: Health "is the ability to adapt" and not a "state of complete physical, mental, and social well-being" despite the relevance and power of the combination.[25] The threesome should be extended to include both the well-being of populations, because it is impossible to be "healthy in an unhealthy society," and "total planetary diversity," because people "do not exist in a vacuum." "Nor is it merely the absence of disease or infirmity" because new understandings illustrate that "even the most optimistic health advocate surely has to accept the impossibility of risk-free well-being."[25] Health and illness are not mutually exclusive and may coexist unless health is defined, in a restrictive way, as the absence of disease.[26,27] However, the absence of disease is, perhaps, the least controversial aspect of the definition for many medical scientists. Many relate to that belief. For example, four decades ago a French study found that a significant number of those sampled described health in that way.[28] Similarly, Audy described it as "potentially measurable by the individual's ability to rally from insults, whether chemical, physical, infectious, psychological or social."[29] Approximately 20 years later, Goodman defined it as "a function of the organism's ability to adjust to environmental constraints and stressors."[30]

The challenge of defining health and the debate among experts continues, and more of their past and present views will be discussed in the following sections; however, at this point it is useful to consider how health is defined by a broad cross-section of the population rather than experts. In 1990, Blaxter published the results of a survey of how 9,000 adults in the United Kingdom described health.[31] Surprisingly, 10% of respondents couldn't describe how it felt or its qualities, and even more interesting, couldn't think of anyone who was healthy. To describe their own health, 13% of those surveyed responded with "Absence of illness" and approximately 37% of them replied the same when describing the health of others. Some of those surveyed explained it as having a reserve to combat problems, behavior aimed at healthy lifestyle, physical fitness, social relationships, being able to function, psychosocial well-being, and energy and vitality. Women who defined health in terms of energy described it as "feeling like conquering the world, being keen and interested, lots of get-up-and-go, and properly alive." At times of absorbing interest, when physical, social, and mental capacities are able to meet the challenge, people are said to be able to resist disease and seem impervious to many problems and difficulties that beset them. The survey outcomes support the belief that views of health differ over the life course, have clear gender differences, and are, for most, a multidimensional concept. From Blaxter's findings, the idea of "a reserve to combat problems" appears to sit comfortably with the concept proposed by Huber et al about the "ability to adapt and self manage in the face of social, physical and emotional challenges."[24] In addition, like Saracci's[22] definition, the link between health and well-being is supported, so what is understood by those terms appears to be a key issue. In this text, the term health is understood to encompass and reflect the breadth of ideas apparent in Table 1-1 and discussed in this section of the chapter while remaining true to the spirit of the WHO definition.

Defining Wellness and Well-Being

Discussion will now turn to consideration of well-being and wellness. *Wellness* is a term closely aligned with well-being and most obviously opposite to illness, but appears to have been little used

Table 1-1
A SUMMARY OF SELECTED DEFINITIONS OF HEALTH

Reference	Definition
Frank J. 1790[18]	Health and well being can only be obtained where there was freedom from want and social deprivation.
WHO 1946-48[5]	A state of complete physical, mental, and social well-being, not merely the absence of disease or infirmity
Sigerist H. 1941[17]	A multidimensional concept of body, mind, and social adjustment, joyfulness, cheerfulness, well-balanced, accepting of life's responsibilities
Dubos R. 1959[6]	A manifestation of the degree to which the individual and the social body maintain in readiness the resources required to meet the exigencies of the future
Audy J. 1971[29]	Potentially measurable by the individual's ability to rally from insults, whether chemical, physical, infectious, psychological, or social
Kass L. 1981[16]	A norm or natural state of being in which the human organism works well as a whole
Blaxter M. 1990[31]	Views differ over life, between genders, a multidimensional concept, absence of illness, a reserve to combat problems, behavior aimed at healthy lifestyle, physical fitness, social relationships, being able to function, psychological well-being, energy, and vitality
Goodman A. 1991[30]	A function of the organism's ability to adjust to environmental constraints and stressors
Saracci R. 1997[22]	A condition of well being free of disease or infirmity and a basic and universal human right
Greiner P, Fain J, Edelman C. 2002[19]	Functioning is integral to health. There are physical, mental, and social levels of function reflected in terms of performance and expectations. Loss of function may be a sign or symptom of a disease ... a state of ill health.
The Lancet. 2009[25]	The ability to adapt
Huber et al. 2011[24]	Ability to adapt and self manage in the face of social, physical, and emotional challenges

at the time the WHO definition was conceived. However, there is a goodness of fit between it and the term *well-being*, so the definitions of both will be considered.

WELLNESS

Because the term *wellness* is often used interchangeably with well-being, it is useful to consider how it is defined. Like both health and well-being, it can be defined in a narrow way, such as "the condition of good physical and mental health, especially when maintained by proper diet, exercise, and habits,"[32] or as a multidimensional concept, such as in the definition given in 2006 by Smith et al relating to "the optimal state of health of individuals and groups":

> *There are two focal concerns: the realization of the fullest potential of an individual physically, psychologically, socially, spiritually, and economically, and the fulfilment of one's role expectations in the family, community, place of worship, workplace, and other settings.*[33]

The idea of wellness began an upward trek from the mid-20th century in America. Physician Halbert Dunn was largely responsible for furthering the concept. In 1954, he defined it as "an integrated method of functioning which is oriented toward maximizing the potential of which the individual is capable within the environment where he is functioning."[34] Inspired by Dunn's work, Don Ardell wrote extensively about wellness. He viewed wellness as a focused approach designed by individuals in pursuit of their personal highest level of health, and wellness lifestyles as "dynamic or ever-changing" as people altered throughout life.[35] His 1977 interpretation of a wellness lifestyle ranged from self-responsibility to environmental sensitivity. Contemporary with and complimentary to Ardell's[36] wide perspective of wellness, Howard[37] discussed balance, referring to work, play, and rest; to nutritional balance; to balance between use of physical, psychological, intellectual, and spiritual capacities; and to balance within the self, environment, and culture. The wellness health model assumes that every individual has innate capacities for healing, nurturing, self-reflection, taking risks, and making changes toward wellness; that all people are searching for answers about the life process, meaning, and purpose; and that health is also about individuals being able to live according to their beliefs.[38] Although some definitions are broad, most common are those confined to individual wellness, such as "the process and state of a quest for maximum human functioning that involves the body, mind, and spirit."[39]

Physician John Travis also pioneered the concept of wellness. Influenced by Dunn's 1961 High Level Wellness model,[40] Robbin's Health Risk Continuum,[41] and Maslow's Theory of Self Actualization,[42] he decided to concentrate on assisting people to improve health rather than treating illness. Opening the first Wellness Center in the United States in 1975, he explained:

> *High-level wellness involves giving good care to your physical self, using your mind constructively, expressing your emotions effectively, being creatively involved with those around you, and being concerned about your physical, psychological, and spiritual environments.*[43]

Travis grounded his ideas in open systems theory, which holds that a system continuously interacts with its environment. In that way, people can be considered as taking energy from their environment and returning it, after organizing and transforming it. Managing energy was a key to his approach. An online wellness program has been developed that is influenced by Travis' work and based on three key concepts that point to the following:

1. Wellness as a process, not a static state
2. Many degrees of wellness and of illness – to understand causal factors it is important to look below the surface
3. People are transformers of energy. The management of life processes, including illness, depends on how energy is managed.[44a]

In the continuum, the various levels of wellness and illness include lifestyle-behavioral factors, psychological-motivational factors, and spiritual being, transpersonal, philosophical, or metaphysical factors.[44a] Although the word wellness is not included in the WHO definition of health, the breadth and generality of ideas in Table 1-2 demonstrate that it is a multidimensional idea similar to the multidimensional concept of well-being. It adds a subtle, valuable, and, perhaps, more personal dimension. In this text, wellness is embraced by well-being that, in turn, is embraced by health.

WELL-BEING

In the thesaurus, the words often chosen to define well-being are *happiness, quality of life, comfort, security,* and *good fortune* rather than *health.* However, the idea that there are links between well-being and health has a long history going back at least two-and-a-half thousand years to ancient Greece.[2] In the Nicomachean Ethics, Aristotle included three dimensions of well-being (the material, the relational, and the affective/cognitive) when he discusses eudaimonia.[45] Although eudaimonia is most often explained as referring to happiness,[46] it encompasses ideas about the "proper conditions of a person's life, what we might more properly call 'well-being' or 'living well.'" It includes "a sense of material, psychological, and physical well-being over time,

Table 1-2

A COLLECTION OF WELLNESS DEFINITIONS

Reference	Definition
Dunn 1954[34]	An integrated method of functioning which is oriented toward maximizing the potential of which the individual is capable within the environment where he is functioning
Ardell 1977[35]	Lifestyle from self responsibility to environmental sensitivity
Ardell 1984[36]	A focused approach designed by individuals in pursuit of their personal highest level of health and lifestyles as "dynamic or ever changing" as people alter throughout life
Howard 1983[37]	Balance of work, play, and rest; nutritional balance; balance between use of physical, psychological, intellectual, and spiritual capacities; as well as within self, environment, and culture
Archer, Probert, & Gage 1987[39]	The process and state of a quest for maximum human functioning that involves the body, mind, and spirit
American Heritage Dictionary[32]	The condition of good physical and mental health, especially when maintained by proper diet, exercise, and habits
Myers, Sweeney, & Witmer 2000:252[44b] Myers & Sweeney 2005[44c]	A way of life oriented toward optimal health and well being, in which body, mind, and spirit are integrated by the individual to live life more fully within the human and natural community A dynamic process
Connolly & Myers, 2003[44d]	A holistic concept with physical, psychological, and spiritual components
Travis & Ryan, 2004[43]	High-level wellness involves giving good care to your physical self, using your mind constructively, expressing your emotions effectively, being creatively involved with those around you, and being concerned about your physical, psychological, and spiritual environments
Medilexicon 2006[44e]	A philosophy of life and personal hygiene, the full realization of one's physical and mental potential, as achieved through positive attitudes, fitness training, a diet low in fat and high in fiber, and the avoidance of unhealthful practices (smoking, drug and alcohol abuse, overeating)
WHO 2006[33]	The optimal state of individuals and groups, the realization of the fullest potential of an individual physically, psychologically, socially, spiritually and economically, and the fulfillment of one's role and expectations in the family, community, place of worship, workplace and other settings
East Carolina University 2007[44f]	Integration of mind, body, and spirit, achieve goals, find meaning and purpose in life, live life to the fullest, maximize personal potential in a variety of ways, continual learning, balance physical, intellectual, emotional, social, occupational, spiritual and environmental aspects of life
Gross, Boyd, & Cuddihy 2009[44g]	The active process through which individuals become aware of all aspects of the self and make choices toward a more healthy existence through balance and integration across multiple life dimensions
McKinley Health Center 2011[44h]	A state of optimal well-being oriented toward maximizing an individual's potential, a life-long process of moving towards enhancing physical, intellectual, emotional, social, spiritual and environmental well-being

for the fully happy life will include success for oneself, for one's immediate family, and for one's descendants."[46]

Since its appearance in the WHO definition, both the word itself and the concept of well-being have been subjected to popularization and critique. For example, in 1995, Seedhouse argued that well-being was "health promotion's red herring." He reasoned that authorities fail to offer a clear definition despite well-being frequently being health promotion's "ultimate goal." He summarized his views:

> Either: (a) "well-being" is an empty notion, or (b) "well-being" is an important and mean-ingful term which conveys meaning no other term conveys (and, given further research, will be shown to convey this meaning universally), or (c) "well-being" is "essentially con-tested"—its meaning and content fluctuates dependent on who is using it, and why they are using it.[47]

In a similar vein, Dinham agreed that a lack of consensus exists about how to recognize well-being, its composition, and its production, making it extremely difficult to use effectively except in general terms. "Well-being", he contends, has "joined 'community', 'participation' and 'empow-erment' as a kind of "hurrah" word that escapes meaning" and lacks definition in concept and practice.[48]

McAllister agreed that "well-being remains a contested concept, enjoying a wide variety of definitions,"[49] as did numerous others researchers.[50-56] Despite her reservations, McAllister deter-mined that whatever well-being is about, it is beyond the absence of illness or pathology and can be measured with both "subjective (self-assessed) and objective (ascribed) dimensions" at individual or societal levels. It "accounts for elements of life satisfaction that cannot be defined, explained, or primarily influenced by economic growth." McAllister also maintained that most researchers agreed about the spheres that comprise well-being: physical (health), emotional (personal stability and lack of depression), social (relationships), and material (income and wealth) well-being and development and activity (meaningful work and leisure).

Regardless of whether it can be adequately defined, the notion of well-being is apparent in policy documentation at national and international levels. For example, the Canada Well-Being Measurement Act was developed to inform Canada's citizens about the health and well-being of its people, communities and ecosystems.[57a] The Canada Well-Being Measurement Act's purpose is as follows:

> To develop and regularly publish measures to indicate the economic, social, and environ-mental well-being of people, communities, and ecosystems in Canada. Its key provisions require a standing committee of the House of Commons to receive input from the public through submissions and public hearings so that they can identify the broad societal values on which a set of indicators should be based.[57a]

In addition to reporting environmental issues related to pollution, resource depletion, and biodiversity, the Act addresses social issues that relate to a lack of opportunities to participate and failure to be able to account for nonmonetary aspects of well-being. Interestingly, the Act appears to accept that continual economic expansion may not lead to long-term well-being; that the funda-mental goal of communities is the well-being of both current and future generations; and that the meaning of well-being is worthy of continual debate, clarification, adjustment, and measurement based on more than monetary measures.

Another example is provided by a group within The Economic and Social Research Council (ESRC) that explores the effects of persistent poverty on well-being in developing countries (WeD). Over the past 5 years, this exploration has led to a definition of well-being as "a state of being with others, where human needs are met, where one can act meaningfully to pursue one's goals, and where one enjoys a satisfactory quality of life."[57b] With similar focus, *The African Report on Child Wellbeing 2011: Budgeting for Children* reported that "national budgets must reflect the impor-tance of children's rights and well-being to the future social, economic, and political health of a nation."[58] At the other end of the age spectrum, in America a comprehensive analysis compiled by the Federal Interagency Forum on Aging-Related Statistics found that, for many older Americans, the indications are that well-being is increasing. However, some groups are disproportionately disadvantaged, including women, minorities, and those with limited education.[59a]

Well-being has become such a popular concept that in March 2012 approximately 394,000,000 entries related to it were listed in a standard Google search of the World Wide Web. This suggests that to understand the numerous factors that impact health, there is a need to be aware of at least some of the many ways well-being has been considered in this context. Key points from a range of definitions are provided in Table 1-3.

Well-being has also been related to social supports, community cohesion, marital state, education, religious attitudes, beliefs, and activities.[60-65] In an ongoing project at Duke University, a Child Well-Being Index measures the trends of well-being over time and comprises several interrelated summary indices in 7 domains. These encompass physical, mental, and social criteria, including health, safety and behavioral concerns, emotional and spiritual well-being, social relationships with peers and family members, and place in the community.[66]

Once again, it is useful to consider how key concepts are defined by broad cross sections of populations. In 1985, Pybus and Thomson sampled 444 New Zealanders to uncover what, in their experience, was "being well." Answers included "being full of life," having "energy and interest," "feeling alive and vital," and being "able to do what I want to and enjoy it" and with "energy for things extra."[67] Similar ideas had emerged in Blaxter's study in Britain.[31] In a smaller Australian survey, 138 participants were asked to define their concept of well-being.[68] The 3 most common definitions related to having a sound mind, having a healthy body, and being happy. Ninety-five percent of participants agreed that they had felt what they would describe as well-being. The emotions they associated with it included happiness, peace, and confidence. The situations or environments they linked with the feeling concerned "relationships," "occupations," and "surroundings." Relationships are arguably the most often cited factor in sociopsychology research about well-being; however, in this study "occupations" was marginally the largest, totaling 60% of the responses. This was a composite of responses about work, leisure, rest, religious practices, selfless activity, self-care, and achievement. It did not take into account any occupations performed in conjunction with social relationships or spiritual (as opposed to religious) activities, so it could be that most of the sample identified some form of occupational behavior, situation, or environment as one of the circumstances associated with their experience of well-being.

Within the range of ideas in Table 1-3, the connection of well-being with lifestyles and occupations also appears strong. What can be described as occupational well-being results from more than paid employment, although there is a bias in that direction in a range of studies. For example, in the description given by Washington State University, occupational well-being is explained as:

> *...the degree of personal satisfaction and enrichment in our life through our occupation. Enhancing our occupational wellbeing may include finding a job that integrates and balances our skills and interests, or discovering a more satisfying way to incorporate our skills and interests into our current career. It also may encompass maintaining a suitable balance between work and other dimensions of our life.*[69]

Time-use is a term with a similar meaning to occupation that is popular among psychosocial researchers. Csikszentmihalyi found that when people are deeply involved in challenging and absorbing occupations well suited to their skills and capacities, they often experience a joyful state he called "flow."[70] In this state people feel "very significantly more happy, strong, satisfied, creative, and concentrated" than at other times and they sometimes experience a sense of timelessness. To many, that would be a good description of a state of well-being. Interestingly, Csikszentmihalyi[71] and Csikszentmihalyi and LeFevre[72] discovered that a typical employed adult in the United States experienced this phenomenon three times (54%) more often at work than in free time (17%). A more recent study explored the relationship between flow and happiness in an older population.[73]

Table 1-3

WELL-BEING: KEY WORDS AND PHRASES FROM DEFINITIONS

Reference	Definition
Sen 1999:285[59b]	The expansion of the "capabilities" of people to lead the kind of lives they value, and have reason to value
ICF, WHO 2001[59c]	A general term encompassing the total universe of human life domains including physical, mental, and social aspects (education, employment, environment, etc) that make up what can be called a "good life"
Ryan & Deci 2001:141-166[50]	Hedonic: pleasure attainment and pain avoidance Eudaimonic: meaning and self-realization: the degree to which a person is fully functioning
McAllister 2005:5[49]	Physical (health), emotional (personal stability and lack of depression), social (relationships), and material (income and wealth) development and activity (meaningful work and leisure)
Gough & McGregor 2007:6[59d]	What people are notionally able to do and to be, and what they have actually been able to do and to be
Bradshaw et al 2007:136[59e]	Actively creating well-being by balancing different factors, developing and making use of resources, and responding to stress
Angner 2008[59f]	"A life going well" in a variety of ways, including a person's good, benefit, advantage, interest, prudential value, welfare, happiness, eudaimonia, utility, quality of life, and who is thriving and flourishing
Diener 2009:11-58[59g]	Subjective well-being general evaluation of one's quality of life • A cognitive appraisal that one's life was good (life satisfaction) • Experiencing positive levels of pleasant emotions • Experiencing relatively low levels of negative moods
Camfield, Streuli, & Woodhead[59h]	A form of happiness: "a global assessment of a person's quality of life according to his own chosen criteria"
Barwais 2011[59i]	Clinical perspective: the "absence of negative conditions" Psychological perspective: The prevalence of particular characterisitics such as the active pursuit of well-being, a balance of attributes, positive effect or life satisfaction, pro behavior, multiple dimensions, and personal optimization
Gallup Healthways WBI[59j]	WHO reversed: Well being is a state of complete physical, mental, and social health and not merely the absence of disease or infirmity including physical health, emotional health, healthy behavior, work environment, access to basic necessities, and supportive environments
Research Group on WeD[57b]	A state of being with others, where human needs are met, where one can act meaningfully to pursue one's goals, and where one enjoys a satisfactory quality of life

Abbreviations: ICF, International Classification of Function; WBI, Well-being Index; WeD, Wellbeing in Developing Countries; WHO, World Health Organization.

The results demonstrate that the affective experiences of older adults have positive effect beyond a one-off flow experience.[73]

Part of the interest in the association between employment and well-being is the monetary factor. Numerous studies support the notion that there are connections between well-being and

Table 1-4	
MEASURES OF WELL-BEING ACROSS EMPLOYMENT GROUPS IN THE UNITED STATES OF AMERICA	
Occupation	*Overall Well-Being*
Business Owner	72.5
Professional	72.3
Manager/Executive	71.9
Farming/Forestry	69.0
Sales	68.1
Clerical	67.3
Construction	65.7
Installation	65.3
Service	64.9
Transportation	63.6
Manufacturing	63.5

Data from Gallup-Healthways Well-being Index, 2014.[77] Scores are based on respondents' answers to six categories of questions about work and life quality

income, financial status, and affluence or prosperity.[60,61,63,74-77] Indeed, prosperity is often one of the synonyms of well-being given in dictionaries and has more than an intuitive fit, as the opposite situation appears to prove: the experiences of people living in poverty in developing countries are obvious examples. Standardized mortality and morbidity statistics support the association of people with limited resources, wherever they live, experiencing poorer health, earlier death, and, it can be argued, less well-being.[78,79] For example, in the late 1980s it was found that children of unskilled workers in Britain were twice as likely to die in their first year of life than those of professional people.[80] This remained the case approximately 20 years later.[81] In both post-modern and developing economies, more affluent individuals are more easily able to meet the basic requirements for health and to make more use of health-promoting opportunities than poorer people. In addition, they experience little of the stress or worries attributed to poverty and the high social value accorded to money in the present day increases its potential effect on health status. However, affluence is only one factor in the well-being link to occupation and does not automatically lead to the experience of well-being.[82] Without other elements, such as adaptability and energy for life's activities, self-esteem, or social connectedness, prosperity can be a negative influence.

In the United States, large-scale, ongoing well-being research using telephone interview has led to the creation of the Gallup-Healthways Well-Being Index.[77] Beginning in 2008 to study people's well-being and their social, emotional, and physical health, the index correlates information about the prerequisites to health: Life Evaluation, Emotional Health, Physical Health, Healthy Behavior, Work Environment, and Basic Access to needs such as food, shelter, and safety. The size of the project makes it possible to obtain reliable data, but, from the perspective taken here, the results limit the occupation category to work or employment rather than all activities. Shellenbarger drew on the Well-Being Index (Table 1-4) to suggest that agreeable work that allows some control over the process and outcome that can be performed according to personal needs and promotes satisfaction and contentment for most people:

> In the broadest, most-comprehensive survey yet of how occupation affects happiness, business owners outrank 10 other occupational groups in overall well-being, based on the landmark survey of 100,826 working adults set for release today. Defined as self-employed store or factory owners, plumbers and so on, business owners surpassed 10 other occupational groups on a composite measure of six criteria of contentment, including emotional and physical health, job satisfaction, healthy behavior, access to basic needs, and self-reports of overall life quality.[83]

Not all people experience well-being for the same reasons. It is a complex rather than a clear or linear association. It appears that feelings of well-being can differ from person to person; that they can be as intangible and amorphous a concept as charm or style. Yet, despite its elusive quality, at times of absorbing interest, even when physical, social, and mental capacities are stretched to meet a challenge, people are said to be able to resist disease and seem impervious to many problems and difficulties that beset them because they are experiencing well-being.

The use of the word complete to describe well-being has been a concern for many researchers. Here, it is believed that aiming toward complete physical, mental, and social well-being represents the spirit of the definition rather than an absolute requirement. It is a fact that well-being can never be complete because it is always changing as situations and needs change, but aiming toward it and experiencing the feeling are vitally important to the health of all people. Similarly becoming through occupation, which is described in later chapters as a means of striving toward complete well-being, can never be attained or absolute. In a similar spirit, the WHO explained that:

> To reach a state of complete physical, mental and social well-being, an individual or group must be able to identify and to realize aspirations, to satisfy needs, and to change or cope with the environment. Health is, therefore, seen as a resource for everyday life, not the objective of living. Health is a positive concept emphasizing social and personal resources, as well as physical capacities.[11]

Physical, mental, and social well-being are interdependent and cannot exist alone. However, elements in their makeup need to be considered separately to appreciate the depth and extent of each, as well as links to engagement in occupation.

Physical Well-Being

Physical well-being is, perhaps, the aspect of health that has received the most attention and is the easiest to understand. Indeed, most people, when asked for a definition of health, talk about physical aspects of health. Physical well-being, like well-being itself, has attracted a variety of definitions, such as the following statement:

> Something a person can achieve by developing all health-related components of his/her lifestyle. Fitness reflects a person's cardiorespiratory endurance, muscular strength, flexibility, and body composition. Other contributors to physical well-being may include proper nutrition, bodyweight management, abstaining from drug abuse, avoiding alcohol abuse, responsible sexual behavior (sexual health), hygiene, and getting the right amount of sleep.[84]

In addition, physical well-being has also been described as occurring:

> When all internal and external body parts, organs, tissues and cells can function properly as they are supposed to function...perform their daily activities without restrictions...[and] for example, our ears can normally hear, our eyes have normal vision, our legs can walk, jump, run, and perform many other normal activities without problems.[85]

It has also been detailed as:

> Respecting your body's own uniqueness and diversity; engaging in practices that move you towards a higher level of health; improved cardiovascular capacity; improved flexibility;

improved strength; regular physical activity; knowledge about food and nutrition; knowledge about the body's anatomy and functions; knowledge of medical research involving the body and nutrition; medical self-care; appropriate use of the medical system; receiving appropriate health screenings; taking responsibility and care for minor illness; knowing when professional medical attention is needed; developing individual fitness plans; CPR/first aid training; avoiding tobacco, drugs, and excessive alcohol consumption; being able to monitor one's own vital signs whether perceived or measured; awareness of the body's true identity, depth of feelings, tension patterns, reactions, balance and harmony.[86]

Somewhat similar to the second of those detailed definitions, Doyal and Gough, describe physical health concisely as "optimizing life expectancy," as well as avoiding "serious physical disease and illness conceptualized in biomedical terms."[87]

Blaxter found that young people, and men in particular, associate health (and presumably physical well-being) with physical fitness, strength, energy, and athletic prowess and, in line with this, identify sports figures as their idea of health in others. Women tend to relate physical fitness and energy in terms of outward appearance and work-related activity rather than sports or particular leisure pursuits.[31] Small-scale studies performed with students tend to confirm Blaxter's findings that young people view physical fitness and well-being as synonymous and that there are differences in how men or women perceive it, often in accord with how health and well-being are reported in the media.[68] Other research has revealed that regular physical exercise is a vital aspect of well-being.[88] Carnall suggested that this is not surprising because the human body is designed for exercise. From the perspective taken here, the human body is designed not for exercise per se, but rather for a variety of occupations to meet the other requirements of survival, life, and health. By default, that includes exercise for pleasure or when necessary to hone particular skills or attributes.

Physical demands to meet survival requirements have decreased with the advent of technology in postindustrial societies, and the inherent biological mechanism has either been ignored or redirected into a fascination with all manner of sport and exercise. During the same period of time, there has been an apparent rise of interest in defeating disease and feeling well associated with a growth of alternative health services, such as acupuncture, reflexology, herbalism, homeopathy, naturopathy, massage, aromatherapy, and relaxation therapy for those unhappy with the extent of solutions provided by conventional medicine. Physical health and well-being has been "the basis for active living campaigns and the many nutrition drives that have swept the industrialized world. People are exposed to so much 'physical health' data these days that it is hard to decide what is relevant and what is not."[84]

Physical well-being is recognized as a feeling or mental state. It is experienced as pleasure in the exercise of body parts while "doing something" and in the relaxing after effects of activity. This is particularly so when function is challenged beyond the norm and the challenge is met; for many people, this is enhanced if the doing is shared with others. The extent of pleasure elicited can vary according to personal preference, mood, and skills. Maslow claimed that muscular people have to use their muscles to "feel good and to achieve the subjective feeling of harmonious, successful, uninhibited functioning."[7]

There is growing recognition that use of physical capacities has an effect on general well-being. For example, mental functioning benefits through increased blood supply to the brain and aerobic power and social interactions benefit through shared activity.[89,90] Examples of such recognition are provided by a review of the relationship between physical training and mental health in which Folkins and Sime[91] found evidence of a positive relationship between exercise, well-being, self-concept, and work ability; by Chamove's[92] study, which found that moderate physical exercise by people with psychiatric disorders decreased their depression, anxiety, disruptive, and psychotic behavior, increased self-concept and social well-being, and aided sleep and relaxation; by Morgan's[93] suggestion that nonspecific aspects of exercise, such as contact, may be instrumental in improved mental health and well-being; and by Oliver's[94] report that improved play and social interaction are benefits of physical education activity along with growth, fitness, agility, and coordination.

Mental Well-Being

In October 2011, the WHO defined mental health in a positive sense as:

A state of well-being in which every individual realizes his or her own potential, can cope with the normal stresses of life, can work productively and fruitfully, and is able to make a contribution to her or his community.[95]

However, it was recognized that differences in values across countries, cultures, classes, and genders might prevent global consensus.[95] Just as with people's occupations, what leads to well-being sometimes depends on geography, ethnic traditions, and, even, a moment in time. As Vaillant[96] suggested, although certain elements have a universal importance to mental health, any society's definition of it can have distinctive customs and variations. For example, what may be considered good in one place could have a particular slant in another, such as is it good for happiness or for survival; for the self or the social order; for creativity or simply fitting into an expected norm?[96]

The WHO definition makes it clear that occupation, encompassing all the things that people do, is a central issue in mental well-being.[95] Indeed, the effective functioning of individuals and communities is not only dependent on understanding that mental health is more than the absence of mental illness, but also linked to behavior and determined by multiple biological, psychological, social, socioeconomic, and environmental factors. In both the developed and developing world, evidence of the links between such diverse relationships is apparent when the opposite of well-being is examined. Greater risk of mental illness is associated with factors such as low income, limited education or work opportunities, lack of or stressful work, gender discrimination, poor housing, substance abuse, human rights violations, and feelings of insecurity and hopelessness.[27] Although many of those are closely related to poverty, some may also apply to the more affluent.

Over the past couple of decades, a WHO Collaborating Centre for Mental Health at the Frederiksborg General Hospital Psychiatric Research Unit has focused on the development of a mental well-being index known as the WHO-Five Well-being Index.[97-99] The WHO-Five covers positive mood, vitality, and general interests:

1. I have felt cheerful and in good spirits.
2. I have felt calm and relaxed.
3. I have felt active and vigorous.
4. I woke up feeling fresh and rested.
5. My daily life has been filled with things that interest me.[100]

At about the same time and in a somewhat similar nature, Myers et al described their five-point wellness model. Within sections for spirituality, work and leisure, friendship, love, and self-direction, were 12 subtasks that could be viewed as their definition of mental well-being: a sense of worth, sense of control, realistic beliefs, emotional awareness and coping, problem solving and creativity, a sense of humor, nutrition, exercise, self-care, stress management, gender identity, and cultural identity.[101] In addition, in their research into well-being in developing countries, WeD recognized a cognitive aspect of the subjective state, interpreted as satisfaction with the achievement of personally important goals.[102]

In her large-scale population study, Blaxter found that psychological fitness was a popular concept of health across all age groups and for both men and women when they described health for themselves rather than for others. Although it tended to be used more by women and those with better education, "health is a state of mind" and "health is a mental thing more than physical" were common statements among her research participants.[31]

With those descriptions in mind, it is possible to describe mental well-being as a term that encapsulates people's capacity to live full and creative lives and to deal with the inevitable challenges that can happen throughout life. It usually refers to the coping ability of well-working emotional, intellectual, and, sometimes, spiritual capacities. In combination, these capacities enable individuals to find meaning in their lives, interact effectively with others, be reflective, process and act on information, solve problems, develop skills for making decisions, clarify values and beliefs, cope with stress, and be flexible and adaptable to changes in life circumstances and demands. It also manifests in the ability to enjoy life, be adaptable, feel safe and secure, rebound from adversity, and achieve self-actualization and a sense of balance. All of these factors are important because "recognizing health as a state of balance including the self, others, and the environment helps communities and individuals understand how to seek its improvement."[27]

Mental well-being is described in these or similar terms in many popular texts addressing healthy living, such as Understanding Your Health.[103] According to this conception, although these varied capacities may not amount to well-being in themselves and the need to use them differs between people and at different life stages, they are seen as prerequisites to the experience of well-being.[104]

From Antonovsky's theory linking health with a sense of coherence comes the idea that one difference between who stays well and who does not is an individual's level of coping within his or her own boundaries. These boundaries, which enclose what is most important to each individual, may be narrow for some and broad for others. That is, "one need not necessarily feel that all of life is highly comprehensible, manageable, and meaningful in order to have a strong 'sense of coherence,'" but those with this sense will be able to cope better and to experience behavioral immunology and to experience mental well-being. It was in the 1980s that Antonovsky proposed the theory of salutogenesis (literally, the origin of health) as an alternative to a pathogenic approach that focuses on the origins of disease and system breakdown. Instead, he looked for factors such as coping, resilience, adaptation, social capital, and support that protect people from illness.[105]

Holistic models of mental health and well-being generally include concepts stemming from a range of disciplines, such as anthropology, sociology, medical science, population health and education, as well as from personality, social, clinical, developmental, and health psychology.[106,107] Indeed, psychologists have studied mental well-being over decades from various perspectives.[28,59g,108,109] For example, Strack et al[111] equated the concept of mental well-being with happiness, and Maslow equated it with full humanness.[112] The latter concept describes the highest level of personal development that enables individuals to recognize their potential and life roles and to fully use their personal strengths without selfishness.[112] Maslow stands in a tradition of humanist psychology, based on existentialism,[113] that extends from Burnham's[114] wholesome personality through Fromm's[115] productive character to Rogers'[116] descriptions of the fully functioning person.

This humanist tradition can be said to stem from the mental hygiene movement, founded in America in 1909, which was influential in the growth and development of mental health services of the first half of the century, including the birth of occupational therapy. The rhetoric of this approach became "equated with productiveness, social adjustment, and contentment—"the good life itself."[117] In turn, the mental hygiene movement can be seen to uphold the Renaissance tradition of human achievement and the ideals of the Age of Enlightenment. The central concept of such an approach is that well-being depends on the meeting of individual potential and is an important aspect of the perspective of population health discussed in this text. However, humanists have not, in a real sense, sought to integrate their perspective of mental well-being with physical and social well-being. Boddy, a nurse educator, claims that taken to extremes, considering the "achievement of one's goals" as the criterion for health is as focused and narrow as only considering physical factors.[118] However, she commended the approach as being "one of the few models that acknowledge the individuality of people and their creativity in defining their goals." The central concept of humanist approaches —that well-being depends on the meeting of individual potential—is also a central factor within the theory of humans as occupational beings, but coexists with the need to also meet communal, corporate, political, and environmental needs and potential.

Occupationally, mental well-being embraces the belief that the potential range of individuals' occupations will allow each of them to be creative and adventurous as they experience all human emotions, explore, and adapt appropriately and, without undue disruption, meet their life needs. If mental well-being is to be attained, occupations need to provide self-esteem, motivation, socialization, a sense of belonging, meaning, and purpose, as well as sufficient intellectual challenge to stimulate neuronal physiology and encourage efficient or enhanced problem solving, sensory integration, perception, attention, concentration, reflection, language, and memory. In addition, a balance of occupations between intellectual challenges, spiritual experiences, emotional highs and lows, and relaxation is required. This does not imply constant high-powered mental doing or feeling; rather, it implies that these should be interwoven with time for simply being, belonging, or becoming; that mental well-being will be enhanced if people choose their occupations so that they are able to: develop spiritual, cognitive, and emotive capacities; achieve a balanced combination of mental, physical, and social use; and experience meaning and a sense of timelessness.[119,120]

Social Well-Being

The WHO increased the debatable nature of its definition of health by including social well-being in addition to physical and mental well-being. The inclusion has enabled a valuable social model of health to emerge, although it is separated from the other two in many cases of health research and care. However, just as was the case in the 19th century with the genesis of public health, it is currently the social health problem of poverty that is the most critical in terms of global population health and requires the most attention if physical, mental, and social well-being are to be improved across the globe.

Throughout time, people have displayed a need to be part of cooperative social groups. Some theorists even argue that there is a correlation between the size of the neocortex and the size of social groups among primates, with humans having the largest brain relative to size and the largest and most complex societies.[121] Despite that, social well-being is less well researched, particularly in terms of conventional medicine, despite physical and mental well-being seeming to be dependent on its coexistence. Social well-being is defined in the Oxford Dictionary of Geography as:

> a state of affairs where the basic needs of the populace are met. This is a society where income levels are high enough to cover basic wants, where there is no poverty, where unemployment is insignificant, where there is easy access to social, medical, and educational services, and where everyone is treated with dignity and consideration.[122]

In 2003, the WHO, although not providing a definition per se, identified 10 important community factors of health, many of which reflect aspects of occupation.[123] The factors highlighted a need for policies to prevent people from "falling into long-term disadvantage or being affected by alcohol and other drugs" and identified the importance of the social and psychological environment, a good early childhood environment, the impact of work on health, employment and job security, friendships and social cohesion, social inclusion, access to supplies of healthy food for everyone, and healthy transport systems.[123] Since then, the WHO Commission on the Social Determinants of Health has continued, with extensive work internationally, and released an Interim Statement in 2007 entitled Achieving Health Equity: From Root Causes to Fair Outcomes.[124] This recognized a worldwide need to provide social policies addressing:

> housing, health and safety standards, family-friendly labour policies; active employment policies involving training and support; the provision of social safety nets, including those for income and nutrition; and the universal provision of good quality health, education, and other social services.[124]

Following a World Conference on Social Determinants of Health held in Rio de Janeiro in 2011, a call for global action provided, in many ways, a WHO definition of social health:

> We, Heads of Government, Ministers and government representatives, solemnly reaffirm our resolve to take action on social determinants of health to create vibrant, inclusive,

equitable, economically productive and healthy societies, and to overcome national, region-
al and global challenges to sustainable development. We offer our solid support for these
common objectives and our determination to achieve them.[125]

The statement makes it plain that social well-being cannot be defined without some mention of or inference about the interaction between the material, economic, political, social, and cultural contexts in which people live. Most definitions of well-being reflect particular aspects of that greater vision. For example, the ESRC Research Group on Wellbeing in Developing Countries noted that well-being is inclusive of social dimensions that offer people some degree of choice in pursuit of relationships or meaningful occupation.[102] People differ from one another in how they are able to act within society. Everyone has different social histories, living within different structures as part of different orders, and are enabled or limited by them. The group identifies that "universal human needs include health, autonomy, security, competence and relatedness, the satisfaction of which at a basic level enhances objective well-being everywhere" and "the denial of which generates harm in all circumstances."[102] With a focus on children, Bradshaw, Hoelscher and Richardson described social well-being by comparing opportunities in the 34 member countries of the OECD (Organisation for Economic Cooperation and Development) as,

the realisation of children's rights and the fulfilment of the opportunity for every child to
be all she or he can be in the light of a child's abilities, potential and skills." The degree to
which this is achieved can be measured in terms of positive child outcomes, whereas nega-
tive outcomes and deprivation point to the neglect of children's rights.[126]

In his 1986 Health Promotion Glossary, Nutbeam[10] argued that well-being in its entirety belongs within the broad context of the social model of health. In his later 1998 glossary, he provides the following definitions that relate to social well-being:

- Social Capital: This "represents the degree of social cohesion which exists in communities. It refers to the processes between people which establish networks, norms, and social trust, and facilitate co-ordination and co-operation for mutual benefit." The stronger the bonds and networks, the greater the likelihood of mutual benefit that, in turn, creates health.

- Social Networks: "Relations and links between individuals which may provide access to or mobilization of social support for health." In destabilizing circumstances, such as high unemployment or rapid urbanization, action to promote health and well-being might focus on the reestablishment of social networks.

- Social Support: "That assistance available to individuals and groups from within communities which can provide a buffer against adverse life events and living conditions, and can provide a positive resource for enhancing the quality of life."[127]

Empirical research supports the association of social well-being with other measures of health. Blaxter's[31] findings suggest "not only socioeconomic circumstances and the external environment, but also the individual's psychosocial environment carry rather more weight, as determinants of health, than healthy or unhealthy behaviors." In his study of the psychology of happiness, Argyle found that socially valued activities, such as those of a religious nature, and satisfying paid employment, have a positive correlation with both health and happiness. Relationships, such as marriage and others of a close, confiding, and supportive nature, enhance health by preserving the immune system and encouraging good health habits.[61]

In past decades, focus on and interest in social well-being has been apparent. For example, at a 1999 conference organized in London by the Office of Health Economics, attendees were advised that social policy is more important to health than medicines.[128] There is increased awareness of the impact of the physical environment and urban planning. Building healthy environments to encourage and support socially healthy communities has become a focus in many places across the world.[129] The more holistic notions of traditional Asian philosophies that recognize the relationship between well-being, spiritual, and social factors have also become increasingly acknowledged in Western countries. This acknowledgment is inclusive of understanding the connectedness of health and well-being with where and how people live, what they believe in, the amounts and types of activity they pursue, and the balance between rest, relaxation, and work.[130-132]

From an occupational perspective, social well-being is encouraged when the range of each individual's occupations and roles enables the maintenance and development of satisfying and stimulating social relationships between family members, with associates, and within the community in which they live. The same is true for communities when the maintenance and development of satisfying and mutually beneficial social relationships between nations and particular groups within them is sought, supported, and encouraged. Social well-being is dependent on shared, supporting, or complementary activity and, like physical and mental well-being, on a balance between doing, being, belonging, and becoming, and between social situations and time for quiet and reflection. Occupations that have the most obvious beneficial effects on health are those that people feel good about or that they know make others feel good, those that perhaps endow them with some kind of social status, and those that enable them freedom to effectively use personal capacities in combination with activities that are socially sanctioned, approved, and valued, even if only by a subculture.[133] It is this social well-being need that causes people to embrace the causes and occupations that may be unhealthy in other ways. Rioting and war-making are obvious current examples. Doyal and Gough go so far as to suggest that "to be denied the capacity for potentially successful social participation is to be denied one's humanity."[87]

Listed in Table 1-5 are topics addressed in various definitions and descriptions and deemed inclusive to the three categories of physical, mental, and social well-being. It is clear that physical, mental, and social well-being are complex in their own right. Perhaps it is not surprising that, when linked together, the complexity is increased to such an extent that dissention and division are rife in trying to come to agreement as to the best possible definition of health in its entirety. The past 20 years has seen the increased recognition of health as a global and localized public and/or personal issue, and the emergence of new definitions to address global population health.

Global Population Health

The WHO Primary Health Care report of the International Conference[134] held at Alma Ata in 1978 and the 1986 Ottawa Charter for Health Promotion[11] (Ottawa Charter) began the modern concern for and initiatives to improve population health across the globe. Those reports, as well as more recent ones in the same genre, stress the need for the reorientation of all health professions and a range of other professions and members of the population at large toward the pursuit of health. Although growing from a rich history of reform that marked its beginning, what is often described as the new public health, population health, or more recently, global health is so called to give prominence to the different approaches and methods that have been advocated since Alma Ata. These take a more comprehensive approach than previously taken to living conditions, lifestyles, and environments, drawing heavily on the WHO policies, such as the Ottawa Charter and the work that preceded the 2011 Rio Political Declaration on Social Determinants of Health.[125] Current initiatives also address ecological health issues, such as the economic and environmental effects of the depletion of the ozone layer, global warming, and uncontrolled water and air pollution.[109]

There is a lack of consensus about definitions. Some think the terms *public, population,* and *global* describe different aspects of health and others believe that the three terms are synonymous.[135-137] The term *public health* preceded population health that, in turn, preceded global health. The definitions overlap—the newer terms emerged as the ideas about health evolved and the world stage became smaller—but the intent of each is health for all. All terms are used in this text when referring to the health of populations across the globe. In addition, in this text, the "physical, mental, and social well-being clause" in the WHO definition of health is taken to refer to communities and the global population in all parts of the world whether asset rich or

Table 1-5

DEPENDENT ON ACCESS TO WORLD HEALTH ORGANIZATION PREREQUISITES FOR HEALTH INCLUDING FOOD, SHELTER, INCOME, PEACE, JUSTICE, EQUITY, SUSTAINABLE RESOURCES AND A STABLE ECOSYSTEM

Physical Well-Being	Mental Well-Being	Social Well-Being
Free of disease or infirmity Age-related fitness	Joy, love, and happiness	Freedom from want and social deprivation
Ability to rally from chemical, physical, or infectious insults	Ability to rally from psychological insults	Ability to rally from social insults
Sexual satisfaction	Friendship, esteem, relationships	Friendship, esteem, relationships
Good living and working conditions	Satisfying lifestyle, opportunity, continual learning	Education, equity
Timelessness/flow	Absorbing interest	Fulfillment of role expectations
Balance acitivity/diet	Consideration, dignity	Early childhood environment
Standard of living	Safety, security	Labor policies
Work, leisure, balanced activity, and rest	Finding spiritual meaning, relaxation	Culture permits realization of potential, share activity
Genetics, heredity	Reaching towards potential, making contributions to the community	Organizations, societies, communities, policies
Appropriate cardiorespiratory endurance	Access to psychological support	Access to medical services
Safe environment	Supportive environment	Interaction with environment
Avoidance of alcohol/substance abuse	Avoidance of alcohol/substance abuse	Few disparities between population groupings

poor, health affluent or deprived, as well as individuals, families, and groupings of people within particular spheres.

Almost 90 years ago, Winslow defined public health as:

> The science and art of preventing disease, prolonging life and promoting physical health and efficacy through organized community efforts for the sanitation of the environment, the control of communicable infections, the education of the individual in personal hygiene, the organization of medical and nursing services for the early diagnosis and preventive treatment of disease, and the development of social machinery which will ensure every individual in the community a standard of living adequate for the maintenance of health; so organizing these benefits in such a fashion as to enable every citizen to realize his birthright and longevity.[138]

A recent definition describes it as "the science and art of promoting health, preventing disease, and prolonging life through the organized efforts of society."[10] Historically, concepts of public health have been as broad as population and global health, except for the limitations of earlier times imposed by technology, geography, and a dominant biomedical paradigm. Following Alma Ata, the new public health gave prominence to solving major health concerns across populations. Particular attention was given to the overwhelming illness and disease problems faced by those in underdeveloped and less affluent countries that were in large part a result of social, political, and economic factors. New public health increasingly takes a comprehensive approach to living conditions and lifestyles, drawing heavily on the WHO policies to guide global, national, and local strategies. It also focuses on ecological, economic, and environmental determinants of health.[10] Green[1] argued that definitions need some consensus and concreteness to do the following:

- Measure the population health of large numbers of people.
- Monitor the trends in population health.
- Detect outbreaks of ill health.
- Trace causes or sources of outbreaks or epidemics.
- Evaluate progress and achievements of programs to protect or promote health.

The shift of nomenclature to population health is, in essence, a return to the historical roots of public health in "encompassing all the primary determinants of health in human populations."[139]

It was shortly after Alma Ata that the term *population health* began to be used as an alternative to public health, perhaps because it is more descriptive of an ever-widening domain of concern. The first formal use of the term was possibly when the Canadian Institute for Advanced Research, focusing on trying to understand the determinants of the health of populations, described it as a Population Health Program.[140,141a] Soon after, the Health Promotion and Programs Branch of Health Canada identified the overall goal of population health as the maintenance and improvement of the health of total populations, as well as lessening disparities between population groupings.[142] "Social, economic, and physical environments, personal health practices, individual capacity and coping skills, human biology, early childhood development, and health services" influence population health.[143] The term population health provides a "conceptual framework for thinking about why some populations are healthier than others."[144] In addition, it is a useful designation for policy developments, research agendas, and resource allocation. While some consider population health as a field of study of health determinants, others regard it as a concept of health.[141a]

Global health is the most recent term to be used. From 1948 to the end of the 20th Century, international health was the descriptor of approaches used by the WHO. Around the turn of the new century, perhaps in response to a "transformed international political context" or challenges to its dominant role, the WHO was reshaped as a "coordinator, strategic planner, and leader of global health initiatives."[145] Skolnik suggested that the term *global health* emerged as part of that historic process.[146] It certainly arose as technological advances facilitated easier collaboration between countries and as increasing awareness of shared responsibility for inequities grew across the world.[147] Kickbusch contended that it offered a fresh context, awareness, and strategic approach to international health issues. She offered five fundamental fields of action, health as a global public good, as a key component of global security, as a key factor of global governance of interdependence, as a responsible business practice and social responsibility, and as global citizenship,[148] describing the focus of global health as:

> the impact of global interdependence on the determinants of health, the transfer of health risks, and the policy response of countries, international organizations and the many other actors in the global health arena. Its goal is the equitable access to health in all regions of the globe.[149]

Among a growing number of definitions, Families USA offered their contribution to understanding global health as "health problems that transcend national borders" and "are of such magnitude that they have a global, political, and economic impact."[150] Similarly, Brown et al explained it as "the health of populations in a global context" that "transcends the perspectives and concerns of individual nations."[145] Koplan et al discussed global health as a fusion of population-based prevention and individual medical care and as a fashionable term provoking interest in academia, governments, foreign policy, and philanthropy. They called attention to "transnational health issues, determinants, and solutions"[151] and promote interdisciplinary collaboration. However, although it is frequently referenced, it is rarely defined. Arguing that global health differs from public health, Koplan et al defined it as "study, research, and practice that places a priority on

Table 1-6

A COLLECTION OF PUBLIC, POPULATION, AND GLOBAL HEALTH DEFINITIONS

Reference	Definition
Winslow 1920[138]	Public health: the science and art of preventing disease, prolonging life, and promoting health through the organized efforts and informed choices of societies, organizations, public and private, communities, and individuals
Nutbeam 1998[127]	Public health (Note: only very minor change from Winslow's "public health"): The science and art of promoting health, preventing disease, and prolonging life through the organized efforts of society
Health Canada 1998[142]	Population health: The maintenance and improvement of health of total populations as well as lessening disparities between population groupings
Kickbusch 2002[149]	Global health: The equitable access to health in all regions of the globe
Kindig and Stoddart 2003[141]	Population health: The health outcomes of a group of individuals, including the distribution of such outcomes within the group (combines definition with measurement of health outcomes and social distribution, determinants influencing outcomes and social policies influencing optimal balance of determinants)
Wanless 2004[141b]	Population health (Note: only very minor change from Winslow's "public health"): The art and science of preventing disease, prolonging life, and promoting health through organized efforts and informed choices of society, organizations public and private, communities, and individuals
Brown et al. 2006[145]	Global health: The health of populations in a global context that transcends the perspectives and concerns of individual nations
Global Health Initiative 2008[150]	Global health: Health problems that transcend national borders or have a global, political, and economic impact, are often emphasized.
MacFarlane et al. 2008[147]	Global health: Worldwide improvement of health, reduction of disparities, and protection against global threats that disregard national borders
Koplan et al. Lancet. 2009[151]	Global health: The area of study, research, and practice that places a priority on improving health and achieving equity in health for all people worldwide
Fried et al. Lancet. 2010[152]	Global health: The same as public health
Beaglehole and Bonita. 2010[153]	Global health: Collaborative international research and action

improving health and achieving equity in health for all people worldwide."[151] Later, Fried et al counter-argued that public and global health are one and the same, and that separation would be counter to crucial ideologies of global public health strategies that could realize optimum levels of population health.[152] In Table 1-6, a collection of public, population, and global health definitions are listed to illustrate differences and similarities of thought from 1920 to the present day.

The recommendations in the Ottawa Charter are central to the doctrines and directions of global population health.[11] It picks up on the broad intent obvious in the wording of the WHO definition of health, providing a list of prerequisites to achieve population health across the globe.[11] The list of requirements that are essential for health in modern times extends the WHO definition of health in fundamental terms. The prerequisites include peace, income, a stable ecosystem, sustainable resources, social justice and equity, as well as shelter, education, and food (Figure 1-2). All of the prerequisites require occupation in some form and will be discussed further throughout the book.

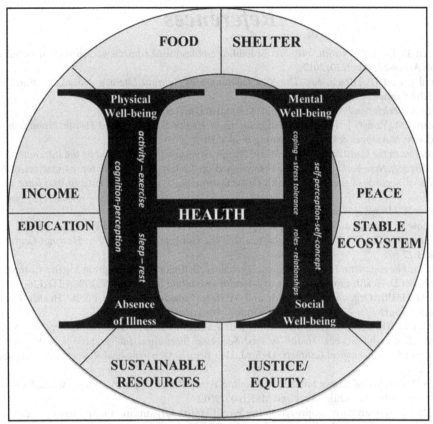

Figure 1-2. Well-being: key words and phrases from definitions.

Conclusion

Health is a state of complete physical, mental, and social well-being and not merely the absence of disease or infirmity.[5]

The 1946 definition of health provided by the WHO remains useful today because it allows for changes of direction taken by the Organization itself as decades pass and as health needs alter. Its generality encourages debate, investigation, and inclusion of wide ranging aspects. Its apparent simplicity masks the complexities and controversial nature of defining health, yet permits multidimensional concepts to be explored and theories developed from a range of perspectives that stem from ideas about absence of illness and physical, mental, and social well-being. This chapter has begun to uncover occupational perspectives of health already recognized by different professional groups, although not named as such, and framed in other ways. The multidimensional concept of people's occupational natures and needs and the theories that link these to health is the basis of the exploration that follows.

References

1. Green L. *Defining Health*. http://oxfordbibliographiesonline.com/view/.../obo-9780199756797-0132. xml. Accessed March 10, 2012.
2. Trefil J, Kett JF, Hirsch, eds. *The New Dictionary of Cultural Literacy*. 3rd ed. Boston: Houghton Mifflin Company; 2005.
3. Burn A. *Pericles and Athens*. London, UK: English University Press; 1956.
4. Sharma M, Romas J. *Theoretical Foundations of Health Education and Health Promotion*. 2nd ed. Sudbury, MA: Jones & Bartlett Learning Books; 2012.
5. *Preamble to the Constitution of the World Health Organization as adopted by the International Health Conference, New York, 19-22 June*, 1946; signed on 22 July 1946 by the representatives of 61 States (Official Records of the World Health Organization, no. 2, p. 100) and entered into force on 7 April 1948.
6. Dubos R. *Mirage of Health*. New York, NY: Harper & Row; 1959.
7. Maslow A. *Towards a Psychology of Being*. New York, NY: Van Nostrand Reinhold; 1962.
8. Callahan D. The WHO definition of 'health.' The Concept of Health. *The Hastings Center Studies*. 1973;1:77-87.
9. Health. *The American Heritage Medical Dictionary*. Bellmawr, NJ: Houghton Mifflin Company; 2007.
10. Nutbeam D. Health promotion glossary. *Health Promotion International*. 1986;1:113,126.
11. World Health Organization, Health and Welfare Canada, Canadian Public Health Association. *Ottawa Charter for Health Promotion*. Ottawa, Ontario, Canada 1986.
12. Wylie CM. The definition and measurement of health and disease. *Public Health Rep*. 1970;85:100-104.
13. Bush H, Zvelebil M, eds. *Health in Past Societies: Biocultural Interpretations of Human Skeletal Remains in Archeological Contexts*. Oxford, UK: British Archaeological Reports International Series 567; 1991.
14. Yach D. *Health and illness: the definition of the World Health Organization*. www. medizin-ethik.ch/ publik/health_illness.htm. Accessed March 05, 2012.
15. Breslow L. A quantitative approach to the World Health Organization definition of health: physical, mental and well-being. *Int J Epidemiol*. 1972;1:347-355.
16. Kass L. Regarding the end of medicine and the pursuit of health. *The Public Interest*. 1975; 40:11-42.
17. Sigerist H. *Medicine and Human Welfare*. New Haven, CT: Yale University Press; 1941.
18. Frank J. The people's misery, mother of diseases. An address delivered in 1790 translated from the Latin with an introduction by HE Sigerist. *Bulletin of the History of Medicine*. 1941;IX(1). Available at: http://www.deltaomega.org/documents/mother.pdf. Accessed May 18, 2014.
19. Greiner P, Fain J, Edelman C. Health defined: objectives for promotion and prevention. In: Edelman CL, Mandle CL, eds. *Health Promotion throughout the Lifespan*. 5th ed. St Louis, MO: Mosby; 2002:6.
20. Ustün B, Jakob R. Calling a spade a spade: meaningful definitions of health conditions. *Bull World Health Organ*. 2005;83:802.
21. Awofeso N. Re-defining 'health:' *Bull World Health Organ*. 2007. http://www.who.int/bulletin/bulletin_board/83/ustun11051/en/. Accessed May 16, 2014.
22. Saracci R. The World Health Organization needs to reconsider its definition of Health. *BMJ*. 1997;314:1409-1410.
23. Jadad AR, O'Grady L. How should health be defined? *BMJ*. 2008;337:a2900.
24. Huber M, Knottnerus JA, Green L, et al. How should we define health? *BMJ*. 2011;343:d4163.
25. What is health? The ability to adapt. *Lancet*. 2009;373:781.
26. Sartorius N, Andreoli V, Cassano G, et al, eds. *Anxiety: Psychobiological and Clinical Perspectives*. London: Taylor & Francis; 1990.
27. Herrman H, Saxena S, Moodie R, eds. *Promoting Mental Health Concepts. Emerging Evidence and Practice*. Geneva: World Health Organization; 2005:XVIII.
28. Herzlich C. *Health and Illness: A Psychological Analysis*. London, UK: Academic Press; 1973.
29. Audy J. Measurement and diagnosis of health. In: Shepard P, McKinley D, eds. *Environ/Mental*. Boston, MA: Houghton Mifflin; 1971; 140-162.
30. Goodman A. Health adaptation, and maladaptation in past societies. In: Bush H, Zvelebil M, eds. *Health in Past Societies*. Oxford, US: BAR international Series 567; 1991:31-38.
31. Blaxter M. *Health and Lifestyles*. London, UK: Tavistock/Routledge; 1990.

32. Wellness. *The American Heritage Dictionary of the English Language.* 4th ed. Houghton Mifflin Company. 2000. Updated in 2009. http://ahdictionary.com/. Accessed May 16, 2014.
33. Smith BJ, Tang KC, Nutbeam D. WHO health promotion glossary: new terms. *Health Promot Int.* 2006;21:340-345.
34. Dunn H. *High Level Wellness.* Arlington, VA: RW Beatty; 1954.
35. Ardell DB. *High Level Wellness: An Alternative to Doctors, Drugs and Disease.* Berkeley, CA.:Ten Speed Press; 1977.
36. Ardell DB. Perspectives on the history and future of wellness. *Wellness Perspectives: Journal of Individual Family and Community Wellness.* 1984;1:3-23.
37. Howard RB. Wellness: Obtainable goal or impossible dream. *Post Graduate Medicine.* 1983;73:15-19.
38. Dossey B, Guzzetta C. Wellness, values clarification and motivation. In: Dossey B, Keegan L, Kolkmeier L, Guzzetta C, eds. *Holistic Health Promotion. A Guide for Practice.* Rockville, MD: Aspen Publishers; 1989:69-70.
39. Archer J, Probert BS, Gage L. Attitudes towards wellness. *Journal of College Student Personnel.* 1987;28:311-317.
40. Dunn HL. *High Level Wellness.* 2nd ed. Arlington, VA: RW Beatty; 1961.
41. Alexander G. Health Risk Appraisal. *The International Electronic Journal of Health Education* (Special). 2000;3:133-137.
42. Maslow A. *Motivation and Personality.* 2nd ed. New York, NY: Harper & Row; 1970.
43. Travis JW, Ryan RS. *Wellness Index: A Self-Assessment of Health and Vitality: Celestial Arts.* 3rd ed. Berkeley, CA: Ten Speed Press; 2004.
44a. Wellpeople. *A New Vision of Wellness.* www.wellpeople.com/What_Is_Wellness.aspx. Accessed May 16, 2014.
44b. Myers JE, Sweeny TJ, Witmer JM. The wheel of wellness counseling for wellness: a holistic model for treatment planning. *Journal of Counseling and Development.* 2000;78:251-266.
44c. Myers JE, Sweeney TJ. *Counseling for Wellness: Theory, Research, and Practice.* American Counseling Assn. 2005.
44d. Connolly K, Myers J. Wellness and mattering: the role of holistic factors in job satisfaction. *Journal of Employment Counselling.* 2003;40(4):152-160.
44e. *Stedman's Medical Dictionary.* Lippincott Williams & Wilkins; 2006.
44f. East Carolina University. *What Is Wellness?* Campus Wellness Division. 2007. Available from: www. ecu.edu/cs-studentlife/campuswellness/what-is-wellness.cfm
44g. Goss H, Cuddihy T. Wellness as higher education curriculum: a comprehensive framework for health education and promotion. *Creating Active Futures.* 2009: 319.
44h. Mckinley Health Center. *Wellness.* University of Illinois, 2011. Available at: www.mckinley.illinois. edu/. Accessed May 29, 2012.
45. Aristotle. *Nicomachean Ethics.* Translated by W. D. Ross. 350BC. The Internet Classics Archive. http:// classics.mit.edu/Aristotle/nicomachaen.html
46. Johnston I. *Lecture on Aristotle's Nicomachaean Ethics.* Malaspina College. November 1997. Available at: http://records.viu.ca/~johnstoi/introser/aristot.htm. Accessed May 16, 2014.
47. Seedhouse D. 'Well-being': health promotion's red herring. *Health Promotion International.* 1995;10:61-67.
48. Dinham A. Raising expectations or dashing hopes? Well-being and participation in disadvantaged areas. *Community Development Journal.* 2007;42:181-193.
49. McAllister, F. Wellbeing Concepts and Challenges. Discussion Paper Prepared by Fiona McAllister for the Sustainable Development Research Network (SDRN), 2005. http://www.sd-research.org.uk/ sites/default/files/publications/Wellbeing%20Concepts%20and%20Challenges_0.pdf. Accessed May 15, 2014.
50. Ryan RM, Deci, EL. On happiness and human potentials: a review of research on Hedonic and Eudaimonic well-being. *Annu Rev Psychol.* 2001;52:141-166.
51. Ereaut G, Whiting R. What do we mean by 'wellbeing'? And why might it matter? Research Report DCSF-RW073. London, UK: Department for Children, Schools and Families; 2008.
52. Noble T, McGrath H, Wyatt T, Carbines R, Robb L. Scoping Study into Approaches to Student Wellbeing. Report to the Department of Education, Employment and Workplace Relations Australian Catholic University and Erebus International. 2008. http://www.sueroffey.com/wp-content/uploads/ import/34-scoping_study_into_approaches_to_student_wellbeing_final_report.pdf. Accessed May 16, 2014.

53. Griffiths TG, Cooper SA. Social and emotional wellbeing in schools: a review of systems' policies. Education Connect: Occasional Papers about Social and Emotional Wellbeing in Schools. 2005;1:5-11.

54. Hamilton M, Redmond G. Conceptualisation of and emotional wellbeing for children and young people, and policy implications. Sydney, Australia: Social Policy Research Centre; 2010.

55. McAuley C, Rose W. Eds. *Child Well-Being: Understanding Children's Lives*. London, UK: Jessica Kingsley Publishers; 2010.

56. Hird S. What is well-being? A brief review of current literature and concepts. Scotland: National Health Service-Scotland; 2003. http://www.mentalhealthpromotion.net/?i=training.en.bibliography.1784. Accessed April 17, 2012.

57a. Canada Well-being Measurement Act. Government of Canada Publications. 2001. http://www.publications.gc.ca/pub?id=99343&sl=0. Accessed March 30, 2012.

57b. ESRC Research Group on Wellbeing in Developing Countries (WeD). *Wellbeing and International Development: Research Statement*. Available at: www.welldev.org.uk/research/wed-res-statement.doc. Accessed May 21, 2012.

58. Child wellbeing in Africa: the true wealth of nations. *The Lancet*. 2010; 376(9757):1960. doi:10.1016/S0140-6736(10)62245-3.

59a. Federal Interagency Forum on Aging-Related Statistics. Older Americans 2004: key indicators of well-being. http://www.agingstats.gov/Main_Site/Data/2004_Documents/entire_report.pdf. Accessed October 15, 2005.

59b. Sen A. *Development as Freedom*. Oxford: Oxford University Press; 1999.

59c. World Health Organization. *International Classification of Functioning, Disability and Health*. Geneva, Switzerland: Classification, Assessment, Surveys and Terminology Team, WHO; 2001.

59d. Gough, I, McGregor, JA, editors. *Wellbeing in Developing Countries: From Theory to Research*. Cambridge: Cambridge University Press; 2007.

59e. Bradshaw J, Hoelscher P, Richardson D. An index of child well-being in the European Union. *Social Indicators Research*. 2007; 80: 133-77.

59f. Angner E. The philosophical foundations of subjective measures of well-being. In Bruni L, Comim F, Pugno M, editors. *Capabilities and Happiness*. Oxford: Oxford University Press; 2008: 286-298.

59g. Diener E. Subjective well-being. In Diener E, editor. *The Science of Well-Being*. New York: Springer; 2009; 11-58.

59h. Camfield L, Streuli N, Woodhead M. What's the use of 'well-being' in contexts of child poverty? Approaches to research, monitoring and children's participation. *The International Journal of Children's Rights*. 2009: 17(1), 65-109.

59i. Barwais F. *Definitions of Wellbeing, Quality of Life and Wellness*. 2011. http://nwia.idwellness.org/2011/02/28/definitions-of-wellbeing-quality-of-life-and-wellness/.

59j. *Gallup Healthways Well-Being Index (WBI)*. Available at: www.well-beingindex.com.

60. Cohen P, Struening EL, Muhlin GL, Genevie LE, Kaplan SR, Peck HB. Community stressors, mediating conditions and wellbeing in urban neighborhoods. *J Community Psychol*. 1982;10:377-391.

61. Argyle M. *The Psychology of Happiness*. New York, NY: Methuen and Co; 1987.

62. Koenig H, Kvale J, Ferrel C. Religion and well-being in later life. *Gerontologist*. 1988;28:18-28.

63. Burckardt CS, Woods SL, Schultz AA, Ziebarth DM. Quality of life of adults with chronic illness: a psychometric study. *Res Nurs Health*. 1989;12:347-354.

64. McConatha JT, McConatha D. An instrument to measure self-responsibility for wellness in older adults. *Educational Gerontology*. 1985;11:295-308.

65. Homel R, Burns A. Environmental quality and the well-being of children. *Social Indicators Research*. 1989;21:133-158.

66. Land K. 2011 Child and Youth Well-being Index(CWI). Durham, NC: Department of Sociology, Duke University. http://www.soc.duke.edu/~cwi/2011_FINAL_CWI_Report.pdf (accessed May 20, 2014).

67. Pybus M, Thomson M. Health awareness and health actions of parents. In: Boddy J, ed. *Health: Perspectives and Practices*. Palmerston North, New Zealand: The Dunmore Press; 1985.

68. Wilcock A. Unpublished research carried out as part of student learning about the relationship between occupation and health. University of South Australia, 1991-1995.

69. Washington State University Wellbeing Online. *Occupational Wellbeing*. https://wellbeingonline.wsu.edu. Accessed September 1, 2014.

70. Csikszentmihalyi M. *Flow: The Psychology of Optimal Experience*. New York, NY: Harper & Row; 1990.

71. Csikszentmihalyi M. Activity and happiness: towards a science of occupation. *Journal of Occupational Science: Australia*. 1993;1:38-42.

72. Csikszentmihalyi M, LeFevre J. Optimal experience in work and leisure. *J Pers Soc Psychol.* 1989;56:815-822.

73. Collins A, Sarkisian N, Winner E. Flow and happiness in later life: an investigation into the role of daily and weekly flow experiences. *J Happiness Stud.* 2009;10:703-719.

74. Ullah P. The association between income, financial strain and psychological well-being among unemployed youths. *The British Psychological Society.* 1990;63:319-330.

75. Isaksson K. A longitudinal study of the relationship between frequent job change and psychological well-being. *Journal of Occupational Psychology.* 1990;63:297-308.

76. Warr P. The measurement of well-being and other aspects of mental health. *J Occup Organ Psychol.* 1990;63(3):193-210.

77. Healthways. State of American Well-being: 2013 State, Community and Congressional District Analysis. Available from: http://info.healthways.com/wbi2014. Accessed August 31, 2014.

78. McClelland A, Pirkis J, Willcox S. *Enough to Make You Sick: How Income and Environment Affect Health.* Melbourne, AU: National Health Strategy Research 1992.

79. Watson D. The dramatic effect of poverty on death rates in the US. World Socialist Website: International Committee of the Fourth International (ICFI). Available at: http://www.wsws.org/en/articles/2011/07/pove-j13.html. Accessed May 20, 2014.

80. Whitehead M. *The Health Divide.* New York, NY: Penguin; 1988.

81. Browne K. *Introducing Sociology for AS Level.* Cambridge UK: Polity Press; 2006.

82. Csikszentmihalyi M. If we are so rich, why aren't we happy? *American Psychologist.* 1999;54:821-827.

83. Shellenbarger S. Plumbing for joy? Be your own boss. *The Wall Street Journal: Work and Family.* September 15, 2009. http://online.wsj.com/news/articles/SB20001424052970203917304574414853397450872 Accessed May 20, 2014.

84. Nordqvist C. What Is Health? What Does Good Health Mean? *Medical News Today.* May 21 2009. http://www.medicalnewstoday.com/articles/150999.php. Accessed May 20, 2014.

85. Normalbreathing.com. Normal Breathing Defeats Chronic Diseases. Available at: http://www.normalbreathing.com/e/physical-health.php. Accessed May 20, 2014.

86. Seeking and Finding Wholeness. The Definition of Physical Wellness. Available at: www.seekingwholeness.com/terms-definitions/the-definition-of-physical-wellness. Accessed April 9, 2012.

87. Doyal L, Gough I. *A Theory of Human Need.* London, UK: Macmillan; 1991.

88. Carnall D. Cycling and health promotion: a safer, slower urban road environment is the key. *BMJ.* 2000;320:888.

89. Sydney KH, Shephard RJ. Activity patterns of elderly men and women. *J Gerontol.* 1977;32:25-32.

90. Kirchman MM. The preventive role of activity: myth or reality: a review of the literature. *Physical and Occupational Therapy in Geriatrics.* 1983;2:39-47.

91. Folkins CH, Sime WE. Physical fitness training and mental health. *Am Psychol.* 1981;36:373-389.

92. Chamove A. Exercise improves behaviour: a rationale for occupational therapy. *Brit J Occup Ther.* 1986;49:83-86.

93. Morgan WP. Psychological effects of exercise. *Behavioral Medicine Update.* 1982;4:25-30.

94. Oliver J. Physical activity and the psychological development of the handicapped. In: Kane J, ed. *Psychological Aspects of Physical Education and Sport.* London, England: Routledge; 1972:187-204.

95. World Health Organization. Mental health: new understanding, new hope. *The World Health Report.* Geneva, Switzerland: World Health Organization; 2001.

96. Vaillant GE. Mental health. *Am J Psychiatry.* 2003;160:1373-1384.

97. Bech P, Gudex C, Johansen KS. The WHO (Ten) Well-Being Index: validation in diabetes. *Psychother Psychosom.* 1996;65:183-190.

98. Bech P. *Quality of Life in the Psychiatric Patient.* London, UK: Mosby-Wolfe; 1998.

99. Bech P. Male depression: stress and aggression as pathways to major depression. In: Dawson A, Tylee A, eds. *Depression: an Economic Timebomb.* London, UK: BMJ Books; 2001:63-66.

100. World Health Organization. Wellbeing Measures in Primary Health Care/ The Depcare Project. Regional Office for Europe; 1998. http://www.euro.who.int/__data/assets/pdf_file/0016/130750/E60246.pdf. Accessed May 21, 2014.

101. Myers JE, Sweeny TJ, Witmer JM. The wheel of wellness counseling for wellness: a holistic model for treatment planning. *Journal of Counseling and Development.* 2000;78:251-266.

102. ESRC Research Group on Wellbeing in Developing Countries (WeD). *Wellbeing in Developing Countries.* http://www.welldev.org.uk/research/aims.htm. Acccessed May 21, 2014.

103. Payne W, Hahn D, Lucas E. Understanding Your Health (Loose Leaf Edition). New York, NY: McGraw-Hill Humanities; 2012.

104. Kanner AD, Coyne JC, Schaefer C, Lazarus RS. Comparison of two modes of stress management: daily hassles and uplifts versus life events. *J Behav Med.* 1981;4:1-39.

105. Antonovsky A. The sense of coherence as a determinant of health. In: Matarazzo JD, Weiss SM, Herd JA, Miller N, Weiss S, eds. *Behavioral Health. A Handbook of Health Enhancement and Disease Prevention.* New York, NY: John Wiley & Sons; 1990:114-129.

106. Witmer JM, Sweeny TJ. A holistic model for wellness and prevention over the lifespan. *Journal of Counseling and Development.* 1992;71:140-148.

107. Hattie JA, Myers JE, Sweeney TJ. A factor structure of wellness: theory, assessment, analysis and practice. *Journal of Counseling and Development.* 2004;82:354-364.

108. Bradburn NM. *The Structure of Psychological Well-Being.* Chicago, IL: Aldine; 1969.

109. Andrews FM, Withey SB. *Social Indicators of Well-being: Americans' Perceptions of Life Quality.* New York, NY: Plenum Press; 1976.

110. Diener E. Subjective well-being. In Diener E, editor. The Science of Well-Being. New York: Springer; 2009; 11-58.

111. Strack F, Argyle M, Schartz N, eds. *Subjective Well-Being: An Interdisciplinary Perspective.* Oxford, UK: Pergamon Press; 1991.

112. Maslow AH. *The Farther Reaches of Human Nature.* New York, NY: Viking Press; 1971.

113. Bullock A. *The Humanist Tradition in the West.* London, UK: Norton; 1985.

114. Burnham W. *The Wholesome Personality: A Contribution to Mental Hygiene.* New York, NY: Appleton-Century; 1932.

115. Fromm E. *Man for Himself: An Inquiry into the Psychology of Ethics.* New York, NY: Holt, Rinehart and Winston; 1947.

116. Rogers C. *On Becoming a Person: A Therapist's View of Psychotherapy.* Boston, MA: Houghton Mifflin; 1961.

117. Ingleby D. Mental health. In: Kuper A, Kuper J, eds. *The Science Encyclopedia.* London, UK: Routledge; 1985:517-519.

118. Boddy J, ed. *Health: Perspectives and Practices.* New Zealand: The Dunmore Press; 1985.

119. do Rozario L. Ritual, meaning and transcendence: the role of occupation in modern life. *Journal of Occupational Science: Australia.* 1994;1:46-53.

120. Rappaport RA. *Ecology, Meaning, and Religion.* Richmond, VA: North Atlantic Books; 1979.

121. Dunbar R. Why gossip is good for you. *New Scientist.* 1992;136:28-31.

122. Well-being. *Oxford Dictionary of Geography.* Copyright © Susan Mayhew 2004. Available at: http://www.answers.com/topic/social-well-being. Accessed May 21, 2014.

123. World Health Organization. *Determinants of Health.* Copenhagen: WHO Europe; 2003.

124. World Health Organization. *Achieving Health Equity: From Root Causes to Fair Outcomes. Interim Statement.* Geneva: Commission on Determinant of Health; 2007.

125. World Health Organization. *Rio Political Declaration on Social Determinants of Health.* Rio de Janeiro, Brazil: 2011. Available at: http://www.who.int/sdhconference/declaration/Rio_political_declaration.pdf

126. Bradshaw J, Hoelscher P, Richardson D. Comparing child well-being in OECD countries: concepts and methods. Innocenti working paper. Florence: UNICEF: 2007; 135. In: Graham A. *Strengthening Young People's Social and Emotional Wellbeing.* Lismore, NSW: Australia: Southern Cross University; 2011.

127. Nutbeam D. Health promotion glossary. Health Promotion International. 1998;13:349-364.

128. Richards T. Social policy more important for health than medicines, conference told. *BMJ.* 1999;319:1592.6.

129. Hensgen S. *Planning for Health: A Study on the Integration of Health and Planning in South Australia.* Adelaide, South Australia: Planning Futures Pty Ltd.; 2009.

130. Hetzel B, McMichael T. *The L S Factor: Lifesyle and Health.* Ringwood, Victoria, Australia: Penguin; 1987.

131. Iwama M. Occupation as a cross-cultural construct. In: Whiteford GE, Wright-St Clair V, eds. *Occupation and Practice in Context.* Sydney, Australia: Elsevier/Churchill Livingstone; 2005:242-253.

132. Kronenberg F, Simo Algado S, Pollard N. *Occupational Therapy Without Borders: Learning from the Spirit of Survivors.* London, UK: Elsevier; 2005.

133. Maguire GH. An exploratory study of the relationship of valued activities to the life satisfaction of elderly persons. *Occupational Therapy Journal of Research.* 1983;3:164-172.

134. World Health Organization. *Primary Health Care. Report of the International Conference on Primary Health Care.* Alma Ata, USSR: World Health Organization; 1978.

135. Kreuter M, Lezin N. *Improving Everyone's Quality of Life: A Primer on Population Health.* Atlanta, GA: Group Health Community Foundation; 2001:7. http://www.cche.org/pubs/ghcf-publication-improving-quality-life.pdf.

136. Hamilton N, Bhatti T. *Population Health Promotion: An Integrated Model of Population Health and Health Promotion.* Ottawa, Ontario, Canada: Health Promotion Development Division; 1996.

137. Epp J. *Achieving Health for All: A Framework for Health Promotion.* Ottawa, Ontario, Canada: Health and Welfare Canada; 1986.

138. Winslow, CEA. The untilled field of public health. *Modern Medicine.* 1920;2:183-191.

139. Frank JW. Why "population health"? *Can J Public Health.* 1995;86:162-164.

140. Evans RG, Barer ML, Marmor TR. *Why Are Some People Healthy and Others Not? The Determinants of Health of Populations.* New York, NY: Aldine de Gruyter; 1994.

141a. Kindig D, Stoddart G. What is population health? *Am J Public Health.* 2003;93:380-383.

141b. Wanless D. *Securing Good Health for the Whole Population: Final Report.* London: Department of Health; 2004.

142. Health Canada. *Taking Action on Population Health.* Ottawa, Ontario, Canada: Health Canada; 1998.

143. Dunn JR, Hayes MV. Toward a lexicon of population health. *Can J Public Health.* 1999; 90(suppl 1):S7-S10.

144. Young TK. *Population Health: Concepts and Methods.* New York, NY: Oxford University Press; 1998.

145. Brown TM, Cueto M, Fee E. The World Health Organization and the transition from "international" to "global" public health. *Am J Public Health.* 2006;96:62-72.

146. Skolnik R. *Essentials of Global Health.* 2010. Sudbury, MA: Jones and Bartlett Publishers, 2008.

147. Macfarlane SB, Jacobs M, Kaaya EE. In the name of global health: trends in academic institutions. *J Public Health Policy.* 2008;29:383-401.

148. Kickbusch I. From charity to rights: proposal for five action areas of global health. *J Epidemiol Community Health.* 2004;58:630-631.

149. Kickbusch I. Working definition of global health for the Fulbright New Century Scholars Program. 2001/2002. http://old.ilonakickbusch.com/global-health/index.shtml. Accessed May 21, 2014.

150. Global Health Intiative. *Why Global Health Matters.* Washington, DC: Families USA; 2008.

151. Koplan J, Bond TC, Merson MH, et al. Towards a common definition of global health. *Lancet.* 2009;373:1993-1995.

152. Fried LP, Bentley ME, Buekens P, et al. Global health is public health. *Lancet.* 2010;375:535-537.

153. Beaglehole B, Bonita R. What is global health. *Global Health Action.* 2010;3:5142. doi:10.3402/gha.v3i0.5142.

Theme 2

"Understanding the history of health … helps the global public health community to respond to the challenges of today and helps shape a healthier future for everyone, especially those most in need."

WHO: Global Health Histories Project[1]

Chapter 2

EVOLUTION OF HEALTH BELIEFS

The chapter addresses:
- Biological Needs and Natural Health
  - Biological Needs as a Mechanism for Health
  - Natural Health
- Evolving Patterns of Life and Health
- Rules of Health
  - Ancient: Humoral Physiology and the Regimen Sanitatis
  - Modern: Public Health—Sanitation, Prevention, and Empowerment
  - Global Population Health: World Health Organization and International Initiatives
- Conclusion

To understand health in the current day, it is not only necessary to know how it is defined, but it is also useful to briefly review aspects of its origins and its rich history. Health is a complex subject, as the previous chapter demonstrates. It is important to begin to explore the labyrinth of ideas that is its foundation and makeup, so that a beginning appreciation of occupation's role is possible. The discussion here will only scratch the surface of the complexity. What makes for the complexity? At the very least, it results from the myriad opinions about the possible causes of illness, as well as ideas about health itself differing according to types of economic, cultural, and spiritual philosophies; ecology; socially dominant and individual views; and health technology available.

The discussion in this chapter focuses on the ideas, actions, and explorations about what helps to make and keep people well and what appears to cause morbidity (or makes resistance to it difficult). Health is so multifaceted that not all health-enhancing or health-risk factors have been established. There are as yet many unknown determinants of illness and perhaps even fewer of well-being. Contemporary studies performed at population level can only establish probable links. Another way to understand health better is to uncover and review the history of basic biological needs that relate to it. This is an approach taken by several notable scholars of public health such as René Dubos in the mid-20th century and Thomas McKeown, a pioneer Chair of Social Health

Wilcock AA, Hocking C.
An Occupational Perspective of Health, Third Edition (pp 32-57).
© 2015 Taylor & Francis Group.

at Birmingham University, because "clinical definitions of health cannot provide a comprehensive framework for describing the condition"[2] discussed in the last chapter.

This chapter examines the ideas about natural or inbuilt health processes, as well as approaches to individual and population health in earlier times. The basic biological health mechanisms and needs of primitive humans would initially have been largely unaffected by culturally acquired knowledge, values, and behavior. As populations increased and environments changed, experiences of health and illness also changed. Therefore, the discussion will progress to contemporary concepts of global population health to provide a foundation for development in subsequent chapters. It will also continue to uncover aspects of health that, if named and framed differently, would increase awareness of occupation's positive and negative influence. Ironically, occupational medicine is, perhaps, the oldest branch of public health, with texts on "mining" diseases being published as early as the 16th century,[3,4] and classical texts on occupational diseases in 1705[5] and 1831.[6]

Biological Needs and Natural Health

Studying the biological health mechanisms and needs of the earliest humans should assist in the understanding of the basic nature of health without excessive interference of perhaps erroneous contemporary viewpoints. To accomplish this, the health and illness experiences of the earliest peoples need to be considered. McKeown highlighted 4 key discoveries in *The Origins of Human Disease* that have contributed to the large and complex jigsaw of health:

1. "Human genetic constitution is much the same today as it was 100,000 years ago." People now "face vastly changed conditions of life with the genetic equipment of hunter gatherers."

2. "In technically advanced countries, the modern transformation of health, and the associated increase of population, began more than a century before effective medical intervention was possible, and must be attributed largely to advances in the standard of living."

3. Because of "the nature of infectious diseases," prevention is possible "by increasing resistance and reducing exposure."

4. Most classes of noncommunicable diseases "have environmental origins and are potentially preventable by changes in living conditions and behavior."[7]

BIOLOGICAL NEEDS AS A MECHANISM FOR HEALTH

Closely connected to the idea of health is that of biological needs. To survive, there is a basic requirement for all animals, including humans, to meet biological needs and to avoid serious hazards.[7] This depends on a close working link between the unconscious and the conscious: between anatomy, physiology, and action. Indeed, as Lorenz[8] suggested, the principal purpose of anatomical characteristics and behavioral patterns is survival. It is the major stimulus to engage in healthy behavior, albeit largely unconsciously.

Humans have four basic needs that are imperative to meet:

1. Oxygen: within minutes.
2. Warmth (or no excessive heat loss): within hours.
3. Water: within days.
4. Food: within weeks.

"Unlike the other essentials, food is not a given; it has to be gathered, hunted, cultivated, preserved, and at times, competed for. It is the crucial determinant of health and population growth."[7] The occupations that people followed for millennia were more often than not concentrated around the acquisition or cultivation of food. However, exploration of the environment in the search for food-rich habitats had to take into account the availability of water and shelter and that the adequate supply of oxygenated air is scarce at high altitudes. Apart from those essential requirements, humans were able to adapt to life in many different environments. Such adaptations did not necessarily meet other biological needs of almost equal importance in the most health-giving way. Indeed, because some of the needs are now obscured by millions of years of acquired values and behaviors, present-day health awareness may not reflect needs that were, and probably still are, fundamental to healthy survival.

At this point, it is useful to consider homeostasis, which is described as "a tendency to stability in the normal body states [internal environment] of the organism."[9] It "is an evolutionary strategy for preserving internal sameness by resisting and smoothing out the changes" and variations from the external environment and is especially necessary:

> *for the proper functioning of the central nervous system of animals on the higher rungs of the evolutionary ladder. Before intelligent life could appear, and well before the culminating event of consciousness, the mechanism to ensure the sameness of the internal milieu had to be in place.*[10]

Claude Bernard, a 19th century French physiologist, developed the concept that the milieu intérieur of a living organism must maintain reasonable constancy despite external circumstances. He recognized that humans, despite their apparent indifference to the environment, are "in a close and wise relationship with it, so that its equilibrium results from a continuous and delicate compensation established as if by the most sensitive balances."[11] Animals able to maintain inner sameness have greater freedom to live in many different environments and are less vulnerable to ecological change.[11] This perhaps results in their apparent indifference to the environment.

American physiologist Walter Cannon, who suggested the term *homeostasis*, recognized it as a system working cooperatively with brain and body.[12] He found that at "critical times" of environmental stress "economy is secondary to stability;" and that important substances, such as water, sugar, or salt, are eliminated to maintain constancy.[13] Cannon researched and described the way a fluid matrix provides a stable context for highly specialized cells, which, by themselves, can only survive in specific conditions to enact their part in complex, flexible, and versatile activities. He postulated that homeostasis leaves humans free to do new occupations, to be adventurous, and to seek beyond survival to the unessentials that are part and parcel of civilization (Figure 2-1).[13]

Although addressed occasionally, the study of biological needs is not currently a fashionable concept within the scientific community and has been neglected. As Allport[14] remarked about the ever-changing focus of scientific inquiry, "we never seem to solve our problems or exhaust our concepts; we only grow tired of them." The neglect may be a result of the more recent emphasis on nurture in the long-running nature versus nurture debate. Numerous need theories were hypothesized when the emphasis tended to be on nature, as it was in the 1930s[15-19] and again in the 1960s and 1970s,[20-22] in attempts to identify what motivates human behavior from a "natural" perspective.

It is necessary to discuss the concept of need to understand its role in health. Meaning a "central motivating variable," the word need made its debut into academic psychology in the early 1930s, eventually replacing the notion of instinct.[23] By the 1970s, need was described in the *Dictionary of Behavioral Science* as "the condition of lacking, wanting, or requiring something which if present would benefit the organism by facilitating behavior or satisfying a tension" and as "a construct representing a force in the brain which directs and organizes the individual's perception, thinking, and action, so as to change an existing, unsatisfying situation."[24] Unlike instinct, which is innate and undeniably goal oriented, need does not have a "repertoire of inherited, unlearned action patterns."[23] However, as Lorenz observed, although humans lack "long, self-contained chains of innate behavior patterns," they have more "genuinely instinctive impulses than any other animal."[25] In that vein, Snell bemoaned the fact that "the term instinct has gone out of fashion," but thought it was "tempting to revive the term and to say we can now relate instinct to detailed brain structure."[26]

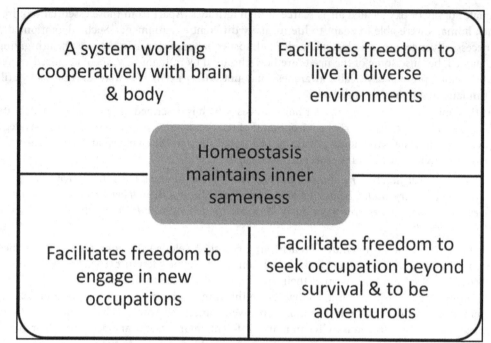

Figure 2-1. Homeostasis a health mechanism that facilitates wide ranging occupations.

Maslow's needs theory is probably the best known and most widely used, particularly in health texts. It is founded on the premise that individuals have innate needs that act as motivating forces. He identified five basic need levels related to one another in a prepotent hierarchy. At the first level are needs, such as for food, which relate to the physiological function of the human organism, followed progressively by needs for safety and security at the second level; then belonging, love, and social activity at the third level; then the need for esteem and respect at the fourth level; and, at the top of the hierarchy, self-actualization at the fifth level. His theory is that the more basic needs must be largely, but not necessarily completely, satisfied before higher level needs are activated and motivating.[22] A similar 3-level hierarchy proposed by Alderfer[21] identified existence, relatedness, and growth as the need levels. These theories articulate well with the 4-fold notion of doing, being, belonging, and becoming used in coming chapters to encapsulate the notion of occupation.

Both Maslow's[22] and Alderfer's[21] theories are compatible with notions about innate drives common in psychology for the greater part of the twentieth century but in disuse at present. Based on physiological discoveries, such as those pertaining to homeostasis, drives were seen as persistent motivations, organic in origin, which "arouse, sustain, and regulate human and animal behavior" and are distinct from external determinants of behavior, such as "social goals, interests, values, attitudes, and personality traits."[27] Dashiell illustrated this view:

> The primary drives to persistent forms of animal and human conduct are tissue conditions within the organism giving rise to stimulations exciting the organism to overt activity. A man's interest and desires may become ever so elaborate, refined, socialized, sublimated, idealistic, but the raw basis from which they are developed is found in the phenomena of living matter.[28]

More contemporary theories of human need have pointed to the importance of self-determination theory through autonomy, relatedness, and competence[29] and argued for psychological well-being through self-acceptance, autonomy, personal growth, purpose in life, positive relations with others, and environmental mastery.[30] Doyal and Gough called into question fashionable subjective and relativist approaches, arguing that health and autonomy are basic needs, the meeting of which are essential preconditions for participation in social life.[31] They recognize biological motivations or drives, but they separate them from universal needs founded on human reason. Part of their stated rationale for this separation is that physiological drives and needs can result from external sources, as in the case of someone who takes drugs needing a fix. In such cases, this is obviously not a universal need, but an acquired one.[31]

The word *need*, despite diverse common, conceptual usage, is used here to describe the mechanism by which unconscious biological requirements are communicated to neuronal systems and, specifically, to neuronal systems engaging with the external world or that alert the conscious state to the existence of some kind of disequilibrium. This usage conforms to the suggestion made by Anscombe that needs, which are a matter of objective fact, are related to what is required for living organisms—plants, animals, or humans—to fulfill potential and flourish.[32] In defining human needs, Watts agreed that "some human needs would seem to be very closely comparable with the needs of animals and plants" and are present to facilitate fulfillment of potential—to facilitate a good (physical) specimen.[33]

Such ideas infuse the needs debate with life, as does Ornstein and Sobel's account of how the brain makes countless adjustments to maintain stability between "social worlds, our mental and emotional lives, and our internal physiology."[34] To do this, each neuron produces hundreds of chemicals that, for the most part, are responsible for "keeping the body out of trouble, from commonplace problems like not falling over or walking into a wall to the myriad of tasks involved in maintaining the stability and health of the organism."[34] From the viewpoint taken in this text, this process activates biological needs that in turn promote health as people meet those needs. Therefore, biological needs are homeostatically valuable. They can be seen as inborn health agents that enable the organism as a whole to interact with the environment. They do not differentiate between physical, mental, or social issues in the way in which modern society and medical or psychological practice do, but rather work as part of a flow of processes within biological systems relating structures and function. They are integral to the collaboration between biological rhythms and homeostasis.

Because needs are subject to the scrutiny of, and adaptation by, the highly developed cognitive and intellectual capacities of humans "primitive instinctive energy can be directed from its natural goal toward alternative ends that are a greater value."[35] The cortex can override even ultradian rhythms of sleepability or wakeability. It is this process of redirection that enables the "highest achievements of humanity,"[35] and the meeting of these needs provides the essence of well-being. However, meeting such needs may not advance the experience of health at all times.

Survival of the species depends on individuals and populations being healthy, which in turn depends on built-in flexibility that allows for adaptation as contexts change. The latter is necessary to enable populations, communities, and individuals to flourish in different times, places, and environments. These ideas about biological needs suggest a simple linkage with natural health that is represented in Figure 2-2.

A brief exploration of how the natural health experience evolved to the present time discloses a broad contextual picture of positive health, morbidity, and mortality, including indication of its interaction with occupation. Ideas gained from that will be expanded in subsequent chapters.

NATURAL HEALTH

Early Oriental theories maintain that people experienced better health when they lived naturally and harmoniously with their environment. In *The Yellow Emperor's Classic of Internal Medicine*, published in China in the 4th century BC, it was supposed that in the remote past "people lived to 100 years, and yet remained active and did not become decrepit in their activities."[36] Most Taoists of Ancient China were radical believers in the possibility of "virtual immortality and eternal youth."[37] Indeed, this notion was central within the country, attracting study and writings by influential scholars, such as Lao-tzu and Chuang-tzu, who eulogized about a golden age, with

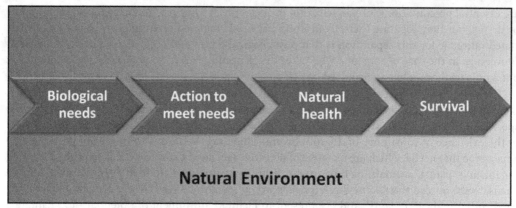

Figure 2-2. Links between biological needs, natural health, and survival.

the latter suggesting that when "the ancient men lived in a world of primitive simplicity … was a time when the yin and the yang worked harmoniously … all creation was unharmed, and the people did not die young."[37] Central notions of Taoism included temperance and quietism. The latter was exemplified by the effortless action exhibited by skilled craftsmen who achieved success with minimal effort and extended the life of their tools by clever usage.[38] In the mid-20th century, radical thinkers in the East picked up those ideas and again observed that when people had been free and uninhibited, working and resting according to need, there was little spread of contagious disease and life was usually long and death was natural.[39]

Similar beliefs were popular in Europe, particularly during the 18th century. Influenced by Rousseau's depiction of man as a noble savage corrupted by civilization, it became fashionable to suppose that a state of nature was essential to the creation of health and happiness—that civilization had spoiled people physically and corrupted them mentally.[40] Such opinions were so popular that they fostered an intellectual climate that influenced both philosophers of the Age of Reason and practical sanitarians who can be regarded as early workers in the field of public health.[41] Examples include de Cordorcet,[42] who wrote about how life could be prolonged by reducing social inequities between rich and poor, improving environments, diet, housing, and access to appropriate physical exercise, and by reducing overwork; Beddoes,[43] a British poet-physician who hypothesized that the blessed original state of health could only be recaptured by abiding by the simple order and purity of nature; Virey,[44] the 19th century French physician-philosopher who asserted that humans in a state of nature are endowed with an instinct for health that permits biological adaptation and that civilized humans have lost; and Jenner,[45] who observed that people's deviation from the natural state appears to have been a prolific source of disease. Gruman named the significant extension of life by human action prolongevity. He suggested that there is continuity from those earlier cross-cultural beliefs to the present:

> From the empirical search for herbs and drugs, and from the magical quest for potent analogies in nature, there arose pharmacy and alchemy, and from those early studies, there developed ultimately the modern sciences of pharmacology and biochemistry with their promise of truly effective methods in the effort to overcome senescence.[46]

It is tempting to accept such romantic ideas, but before doing so it is imperative to determine whether such claims have credence, at least in terms of whether early lifestyles were healthier than those of current times. Powell provided an example of one way to consider the issues in her exploration of the prehistoric society at Moundville in the United States. Interactions could have positive or negative effects; for example, diverse ecosystems include food resources as well as pathogens; hunting and fishing could enhance the quality of the diet but increase exposure to trauma; sedentism promotes population growth, as well as the accumulation of wastes and vermin;

Table 2-1

EPIDEMIOLOGICAL PERSPECTIVE OF HEALTH IN EARLY HUMAN SOCIETIES[47]

Host		Environment	Potential Stressors
Culture	**Biology**	• Quality of air	Pathologic
Subsistence technology	Age, sex, and genotype	• Water	• Parasites
Settlement pattern	Reproductive status	• Climate	• Infectious organisms
Clothing and shelter	Maintenance requirements	• Physical geography	• Metabolic disorders
Medical theory/ technology	Energy expenditure	• Flora and fauna	• Genetic disorders
Size of community	General health	• Soils	Nutritional
Other population contact	Nutritional status		• Inadequate diet
Division of labor	Immune-resistance		• Insufficient utilization of nutrients
Social organization	Adaptation to parasites		Mechanical
			• Traumatic injury
			• Degenerative disorder

Adapted from Powell ML. *Status and Health in Prehistory: a Case Study of the Mountville Chiefdom*. Washington, DC: Smithsonian Institution Press; 1988.

and division of labor encourages use of particular capacities but unequal exposure to mechanical and pathological stress.[47] The host (person) can be described in cultural and biological terms, as shown in Table 2-1, which was adapted from Powell and depicts potential stressors.

Like McKeown,[7] McMichael, a leader in the population health field, takes a historic approach to consider the nature of environmental aspects of disease. He suggested that there are "no guarantees of good health in the natural world":

> The ceaseless interplay between competing species, groups and individuals: the ubiquity of infection; the vagaries of climate, environment and food supplies; and the presence of physical hazards—these all contribute to the relentless toll of disease, dysfunction and death throughout the plant and animal kingdom.[48]

He described three interrelated and distinctive features in the "long history of human ecology and disease:"

1. The encounters of human societies with new environmental hazards
2. The recurring tension between biological needs and capacities and changes in living conditions
3. The impact of urban living and population aging on patterns of health and illness.[48]

Although dangers to health are apparent in early human cultures, there were also some advantages. Participation in the majority of occupations was directly related to maintenance of the organism and survival of individuals, their communities, and the species, and challenges were in tune with the natural world. Provision to meet the needs of survival and health through sustenance, self-care, shelter, safety, self-esteem, and life satisfaction was similar for the total population. All able-bodied people were involved first hand in the getting and preparing of food and water, with finding or devising adequate environments and shelter for safety and temperature control, and with the care and education of offspring. Few would have suffered the fate, or enjoyed the privilege, of not being able or eligible (for whatever reason) to participate in providing for themselves and others. Occupations were communal, with on-the-job training and only limited division of labor. Such simple occupational structures did not obscure innate physiological needs, but rather catered to them. The small number of people on earth did not pose a threat to ecosystems despite, even then, the obvious characteristic of seeking to control or change an environment to exploit and deplete a locality before moving on.

Unlike most other animals, humans "exploit almost every link in the food chain."[49] This characteristic supported flexibility of habitat and provided motivation for hunter-gatherers to move from "one resource to another."[49] In turn, this provided a health advantage by reducing the probability of illness due to unhygienic waste disposal and assisted physical fitness, providing communities with the type of physical activity now being rediscovered as advantageous by world health authorities. One example is provided by first nation Australians. The "practice of moving camp as they journeyed throughout the tribal land ensured that many of the health problems associated with permanent settlement sites could not develop."[50] Such hunter-gatherer nomads were constrained to balance physical exertion with sedentary and rest occupations because, at least until they learned to create and control fire to their advantage, they would have been diurnal, so following basic circadian patterns of sleeping and waking. In addition, contrary to popular belief, the obligatory occupations of providing for immediate needs was not as time-consuming as the modern 8-hour day.[51-54]

The nomadic lifestyle contributed to mental and social health benefits by providing adventure, preventing boredom, and facilitating bonding with fellow nomads. Communities were small enough not to require restrictive rules and regulations and, more so, the groups who lived together on a regular basis were probably more stable and supportive than those in later occupational eras. Survival would often have depended on the strength created by a cohesive group in combined activity. In fact, because of the constraints imposed by a nomadic way of life, the people comprising each social band constituted the movable assets of the group; that is, the people rather than material assets were valued as central to survival. Because of this advantage, any early human or community whose cooperation gene was prevalent would have both an individual and a group selection advantage: "those individuals less able to participate in group activity would have been marginalized in the survival stakes."[48] This would have influenced the development of a communal rather than an individual view of the world and of health and would have been integral to social well-being. We can look again to first-nation Australians to see this community/individual dual value reflected in the way in which their current Health Organization defined health as:

> The social, emotional, spiritual, and cultural well-being of the whole community. Health services should strive to achieve that state where every individual can achieve their full potential as human beings (Aboriginals) and thus bring about total well-being of their community as a whole.[55]

The type of lifestyle followed by all early homo species and humans for several million years provided a real test of whether engagement in occupations can sustain the health of ecosystems, as well as the well-being of people. Many consider that the occupational pursuits of the hunter-gatherer era generally would not have disturbed the environmental balance,[25,49,50] and there have been numerous positive speculations and comments about the health status of early humans from a variety of sources, most of which are supported by archaeological, anthropological, and other explorations. For example, Stephenson observed "that people living a culturally primitive life (with less medical care) are generally more physically perfect than those from affluent societies,"[49] and McNeill considered that "ancient hunters of the temperate zone were most probably healthy folk."[56] Such views are supported by reports from explorers in their initial contacts with people of primitive cultures, which suggest that they appeared happy, healthy, and vigorous.[57-59] More recent medical and anthropological surveys of "several South American tribes and undisplaced Pygmies of the Congo Basin"[60] also give credence to these views. Meindl, in considering the demography of human populations before agriculture, cited evidence that these people remain healthy and resilient, unlike many whose demographic patterns have been altered by contact with modern cultures.[60]

Despite some idealized advantages of the lifestyle, the risk of illness and early mortality for a large number of a population is believed to have been the common experience. Changes of climate, as McMichael[48] and Dobson[61] suggested, would have been more of a hazard then, especially as "older people suffer gradual loss of the ability to buffer temperature extremes."[61] So too would availability of food and water, and "parasites with high transmission rates and little or no induced immunity," such as worms, lice, ticks, and pathogens such as salmonella and trypanosoma (sleeping sickness).[60] Occupational accidents, aggression, and infanticide are also suggested causes.[60] When resources could support only a limited numbers of hunter-gatherers, it appears that social strategies, such as prolonged lactation, were used to control population numbers.[62] In addition, the abandonment of unwanted infants was probable.[63] The modern assumption that life must be preserved at all costs can sit uncomfortably with a natural ecological point of view. Those who survived and procreated were those most able to live and adapt effectively to life's demands and, in fact, could be designated healthy. In this way, "natural selection is not thwarted, and in their breeding populations they do not build up increasing loads of disabling genes."[64]

McNeill explained how early humans and their hominid predecessors, as other animals, fit into a self-balancing, self-regulating ecological system, preying on other forms of life, as they were preyed on by large-bodied organisms, parasites, and microorganisms. They were, in fact, "caught in a precarious equilibrium between the microparasitism of disease organisms and the macroparasitism of large-bodied predators."[56] In a natural state, some microparasites provoke acute disease and kill the host; some provoke immunity reactions; others achieve a stable relationship with the host, who perhaps experiences continuous, low-level malady; and others are carried by the host and are the cause of disease in others. However, it was the occasional natural disturbances, such as drought, fire, and floods, that set limits to population imbalance. Within this natural scenario, any change to one living creature is compensated for by genetic or behavioral change in co-organisms. Undisturbed biological evolution is a slow process, but when humans began to evolve culturally and to adapt to different habitats by changes in their occupation, they transformed the balance of nature and patterns of disease altered along with this occupational transformation.[56]

Such demographic and epidemiologic deductions do not contradict the claims that hunter-gatherers experienced general well-being. Rather, as with modern humans, they experienced ill health and accidents, of which their different nature coupled with lack of specialist knowledge led to early death for many. McKeown argued that "in the limited sense that they were essentially free from many diseases that are now common, our hunter gatherer ancestors may be said to have been healthy."[7] Indeed, studies of recent hunter-gatherers have shown a virtual absence of the noncommunicable diseases prevalent today, such as heart disease, dementia, osteoarthritis, cancer, diabetes, increased blood pressure, and obesity. McMichael concluded that "many of those diseases are an expression of a mismatch between human biological inheritance and current way of life" because "urban sedentariness, dietary excesses and various socialised addictive behaviors (alcohol consumption and tobacco smoking) have become prominent features of modern human ecology."[48] On that note, he referred to several other anomalies that are factors in modern-day disease and disorder resulting from a human biology attuned to the Pleistocene age (2 to 1 million years ago) when, for example, diets included only moderate amounts of plant oils and predominantly unsaturated fats or to the Pliocene age (6 to 2 million years ago), when bipedal gait was superimposed on skeletal structures attuned to quadrupedal gait.[48]

These deductions support the notion that occupation, survival, health, and illness are inextricably linked. As Gandevia claimed, "in the social environment of a man or a community occupation looms large."[65] In addition, because of their occupational nature and potential, humans were able to strive to improve survival odds and decrease the experience of ill health. Their technology, addressed the potential risk factors of a world in which people are not the fastest, strongest, largest, or best camouflaged of animals. Much has been written about fight-or-flight behavior and its appropriateness for the natural dangers facing early humans since Cannon's[66] description in the 1920s of the single automatic pattern of response of the organism to any challenge to equilibrium.

Figure 2-3. Collecting plant products with medicinal values. (© Carol Spencer 2012, otspencer@adam.com.au. Used with permission.)

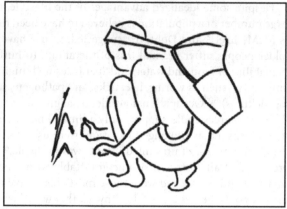

However appropriate, the response would have been unpleasant to experience and provided strong motivation to develop artifacts and social structures to overcome fear-producing situations. Social cohesion and education were used by hunter-gatherers, along with tool technology, as vehicles to improve superiority over prey and predators in the long-term.

Survival pressures provided meaning, motivation, and opportunity for engagement in a variety of individual and community occupations that addressed the obvious health risks of the day. All of this may have been largely unconscious, and it is not known whether early humans made any cognitive efforts to maintain health and prevent illness apart from shelter, sustenance, and the seeking out of substances they instinctively craved when sick, in a way similar to other animals (Figure 2-3).[67] It did lead to an eventual appreciation of "the curative values of a wide range of plant products, many of which are still in medicinal use."[49] This resulted in the acceptance of the people who were most skilled in this as medicine experts. Many records exist that point to a remarkable understanding of homeopathic medicine, notwithstanding a striking healing capacity subsequent to injury.[50]

Following this story, it is possible to see how subsequent changes in need, culture, and environment have influenced patterns of health and illness throughout time. As human hunter-gatherers began to dominate the food chain, populations increased; as they became able to overcome cold through making clothing, shelter, and fire, they were able to expand into colder environs, leaving behind many of the parasites and disease organisms. In new environments, populations escalated.[56] This was aided by the circumstance that, in nomadic life, "the small collections of human beings were too scattered to sustain micro-organisms which do not readily achieve a carrier state."[63,68]

For the greater part of human existence, people have followed a hunter-gatherer and forager lifestyle. In contrast to the earlier and perhaps romantic idea that this more natural and less complex way of life provided for healthy longevity, in recent times it has been commonly held that hunter-gatherer lifespans would have been short. This has been supported by archaeological evidence that is limited and has been attributed to a variety of reasons, such as the dangers inherent in the environment and lifestyle, as well as early human's lack of medical understanding.

However, Gurven and Kaplan suggested a characteristic lifespan of between 68 and 75 years would be more accurate.[69] This follows their cross-cultural examination of the mortality of people living premodern hunter-gatherer, forager-horticulturalist, and acculturated hunter-gatherer lifestyles. Their extensive study investigated multiple groups from various parts of the world, with a sample larger than any previous inquiry. It found that although infant and child death is much higher than in modern postindustrial societies, as previously understood, the rate of mortality remains constant until approximately age 40 years, after which mortality increases steadily. In the populations they sampled, between 57% to 67% of children born reached age 15 years. Of those, more than 60% reached age 45 years in traditional hunter-gatherer and forager-horticulturalist societies, whereas 79% did so in the acculturated hunter-gatherer sample. However, life expectancy at birth, as opposed to possible life span, was short and varied markedly between the groups sampled; the differences in early juvenile mortality largely explaining the differences in overall mortality. However, their findings suggest that at least one quarter of such populations who live away from modern health practices, and without adequate and predictable food supply are likely to live for 15 to 20 years as grandparents. They concluded that:

> human bodies are designed to function well for about seven decades in the environment in which our species evolved. Mortality rates differ among populations and among periods, especially in risks of violent death. However, those differences are small in a comparative cross-species perspective, and the similarity in mortality profiles of traditional peoples living in varying environments is impressive.[69]

Although it can be surmised from that research that the human lifespan has changed little over the millions of years humans have existed, the same is not true of life expectancy. That depends significantly on environmental factors, which differs between countries. Since the mid-19th century, improvements in population health, sanitation, and nutrition have led to an increase in average life expectancy from birth. According to data from the World Health Organization, in 2012 extremes between expected years of life ranged from 84 years in Japan to 41 years in Angola, Central African Republic and Chad,[70] whereas a 2014 estimate given in the Central Intelligence Agency (CIA) World Factbook ranged from 89.57 years in Monaco to 49.44 years in Chad.[71]

Extrapolating from that brief overview of the probable health experiences of human populations, particularly before major changes occurred to natural ways of living, it could be suggested that, apart from genetics, natural health is dependent on the environment, social structure and support, and occupation:

- The environment can provide a supply of food and water and a safe place to rest and refresh and to simply "be" between the physical and mental demands of obtaining other requirements of life.
- Natural health is also dependent on social structures and supports, for continuance of the species according to sexual needs, for assistance in providing for the other requirements of life, and for safety and support.
- Both environmental and social structure and support are dependent on occupation (i.e., on all of the things that people do to meet their needs). It is an integral part of natural health for all animals.

Evolving Patterns of Life and Health

As populations grew and occupational skills developed, fixed settlement and agriculture began to occur in some parts of the world with mixed consequences in terms of health and illness. This change is thought to have started approximately 12,000 years ago, in what is known as the Fertile Crescent, when the local people were becoming increasingly dependent on harvesting wild crops and settling where that was possible. Diamond explained that the ancestors of a large variety of what are now the world's most valuable domestic plants grew in that area.[72] For example, increasing occupational know-how with the development of stone sickles and methods for grain storage is thought to have provided a more constant access to food, reducing, comparatively, morbidity and mortality due to starvation. In addition, improved shelters provided better facilities to nurture and care for infants, the sick, and the elderly. However, the advent of farming initially led to a decline in life expectancy: people got less exercise and their diet was not as diverse. They became physically smaller and more diseased with nutritional deficiencies, dental decay, arthritis, and an increased incidence of infectious diseases.[48,72,73]

The continual development of agriculture, along with the rise of villages, towns, and cities, provided ideal conditions for hyperinfestations of various disease organisms. Diseases such as diphtheria, scarlet fever, malaria, typhus, smallpox, syphilis, leprosy, and tuberculosis caused ongoing morbidity. Plagues caused periodic but devastating tolls. Indeed, the bubonic plague, at its peak, killed 10,000 people daily in Constantinople during the 6th and 7th centuries.[74] In the 14th century, between one-third and one-half of the population of mainland Europe and the British Isles died within a few years.[75] Such epidemics and infectious diseases occurred, in part, because more distance was traveled and contact outside of a community was needed for trading. As occupations such as trading grew, along with oceanic exploration and conquest, so did the spread of disease, sometimes with disastrous consequences. For example, in 1520 smallpox arrived in Mexico along with the relief expedition for Hernán Cortés and played a major role in the outcome of the Spanish conquest.[56] A few centuries later, first-nation Australians, having "no racial experience with diseases such as measles, mumps, smallpox, chickenpox, and influenza," were devastated when exposed to these disorders during white settlement of the area.[76] Infectious diseases did not cease to be the major threat to health until the twentieth century, long after agriculture had been overtaken by industrial economies in the western world.

Increased population density, which came about with the growth of industry, led to another increase of infectious diseases and epidemics: those that had been checked by generations of adaptation gained new leases on life. The industrial revolution initially provided few health benefits for the majority of people who moved to towns and cities to find paid employment. In 1780, only 15% of the population in the United Kingdom and 5% in the United States lived in towns or cities. This had increased to 50% in the United Kingdom by 1851 and in the United States by approximately 1910.[77] Perhaps the most obvious result of this urban population explosion was overcrowding in environments not constructed for comfortable and sanitary living, which, aggravated by industrially polluted working conditions, led to a widespread increase in illness. Eversley suggested that people living in the 20th century could:

> hardly imagine the significance of pain, disfigurement, and the loss of near relations as a constant factor in every day life. Slight wounds became infected and suppurated for weeks. Fractures healed badly. Minor irritations like toothache and headache became major preoccupations, paralyzing ordinary activity ... Even where no acute injury or identifiable major disease was involved, common colds, gastric upsets from the consumption of rotten foodstuffs, and permanent septic foci such as those provided by bad teeth were common, if not universal.[78]

Many factors have brought about an improvement in this state of affairs, including public health initiatives from the mid-19th century, particularly the improvement of sanitary conditions, water supply, and housing. Other social and economic changes, such as improved nutrition, smaller families, less overcrowding, and improved education, along with major advances in medical and pharmaceutical science have also contributed to a decrease in disease and to longer life expectancy.[79] Indeed, it is possible to appreciate Gordon's suggestion that medicine's role in making life more bearable "is probably its major achievement and for this it receives little credit."[76] Making life more bearable depends, in large part, on understanding basic human needs and helping people meet these through sociopolitical and individual occupational intervention. This has been the particular focus of population health in more recent years. An anticipated focus in coming years is the health and economic concerns of an aging population.

It is possible to conclude from this overview that hazards leading to many of the current-day illnesses and the morbidity rate occur as a result of how people live and what they do. For hunter-gatherers, it was parasites, poor nutrition, and the physical dangers of occupational elements, such as the chase, exploration, and environmental dangers, that posed the greatest threats; for farmers and for early industrial workers, there was an increase of infectious diseases most likely due to fixed habitation, a greater interaction between people as travel escalated and personal and community environments became crowded, coupled with a poor understanding of sanitation and hygiene; and for people living and working in postindustrial societies, there is a predominance of noncommunicable diseases that are probably a result of changed conditions of life coupled with a genetic predisposition. As McKeown reminded us:

> We are genetically ill-equipped for the ways of life that we have made for ourselves. A school child eating potato chips while watching television, a driver steering a bus or taxi through a congested city, an adolescent smoking in front of a computer, are far removed from the conditions for which their genes had prepared them.[7]

Rules of Health

Theories about health and the working of the human body and spirit, and rules based on those theories, began to be formulated as medicine developed. It is difficult to know details about any theories held before the advent of written language. However, by the time of classical medicine, more than 2000 years ago, a physiological theory emerged that became the rationale behind much of the medical and health intervention in the western world until less than 200 years ago—humoral physiology. It has a basis in observation of mind–body occurrences, the developmental stages of people, and the natural world.

ANCIENT: HUMORAL PHYSIOLOGY AND THE REGIMEN SANITATIS

The humoral theory of physiology is said to have evolved in Ancient Greece and is a part of Aristotelian doctrine of four primal qualities, or stocheia: cold, warm, dry and wet.[80] Best known as a mathematician of Ancient Greece, Pythagoras, in the 6th century BC, is believed to be one of the originators of this long-accepted theory of health, or at least to have contributed a background of mathematical science that assisted its development. The body was said to be composed of four elements—air, fire, water, and earth—indicative of astute observation when it is recalled that the four basic needs of life identified earlier are oxygen, heat, water, and food.[7] In the theory, health was contingent on a balance between four humors: blood, phlegm, and black and yellow bile. These were believed to be the substratum of life and disease.[81] Perfect harmony, equilibrium, and balance were the guiding principles of Pythagorean theories, and numbers were thought to be the key (ie, the number four was deemed central to balance and equilibrium). In addition to the four humors, there were four temperaments: the sanguine, the phlegmatic, the bilious, and the melancholy. The humors and temperaments were known as the naturals. All were interconnected and subject to the four seasons and the four stages of human life. Disturbance of any could be a cause of disease.[81] Underlying each person's constitution and predisposition was a predominant humor and temperament that determined the probabilities and types of physical and mental illness. Factors harmful to life and health were known as contranaturals, and factors necessary for life and health were known as the nonnaturals. The nonnaturals were characterized by a high degree of individual choice and circumstance and could be subject to either balanced use or abuse. They included the following:

- Air and environment
- Activity and rest
- Food and drink
- Sleep and waking
- Evacuation and repletion, including sex
- Emotions known as "affections of the soul," such as joy, anger, fear, or distress.

Boxed Dialogue 2-1:
Introduction to the First English Translation of the *Regimen Sanitatis Salernitanum*

Redynge of olde authors and stories my most honorable lorde, I fynde, that men in tyme past were of loger lyfe, and of more propsperous helthe, than they are nowe adayes...

There are 4 necessarie thynges to conserue and prolonge mans prosperite and helthe: that is abstinence from meate, abstinence from wyne, rubbyng of the body, exercise and digestion...

Yea howe greatly are we English men bounde to the maisters of the universite of Salerne (Salerne is in the realme of Naples) which vouchesafed in our behalfe to compile thus necessari, and thus holsome a boke...

So what profiteth us a boke, be hit neuer so expedient and frutefull, if we understande hit nat...

Wherefore I consydryng the frute which myght come of this boke if hit were translated in to the englishe tongue (for why euery man understandeth nat the latine). I thought hit very expedient at some tymes, for the welthe of unlerned psones to busy my selfe there in...

Paynell T. Introduction to Regimen Sanitatis Salerni. England: 1528.

A somewhat similar humoral doctrine based on three primal essences was prevalent in Tibet until the 20th century.[80]

Hippocrates,[82] sometimes known as the Father of Medicine, is attributed with putting the humoral theory together from older sources as well as his own work. His texts *On Regimen* and *Aphorisms* provide the core for *Rules of Health,* which are based on the four humors, as well as on observations of personal, lifestyle, and environmental factors. This humoral theory was adopted within the Arabic medical tradition from the Greek and progressed through Galen to European medical authorities, including monastic-based physicians of the early medieval period.[82] During the late Middle Ages, the ideas became embedded in European Classical Medicine and in Islamic, Jewish, and Christian practices until well into the 19th century.[83]

The six rules provided for population health aimed at prevention and informed the pathology, diagnosis, and therapeutics of medical services. The difference between what was considered healthy or unhealthy depended on the quantity and quality of the six nonnatural activities. Advice was provided by authentic or self-styled physicians about the management of each, according to an individual's constitution and temperament and in conjunction with other aspects of the humoral theory. "With or without medical guidance, patients practiced self-help" and people in all walks of life acted as their own physicians until recently.[84]

The rules were disseminated in table form through what is known as the *Tacuinum Sanitatis*[85] and usually in verse as the *Regimen Sanitatis*.[86] The latter often centered on diet, with little reference to remedies for specific disorders. Personal regimes were individually tailored for those who could afford to pay a physician to create an individualized program. The creation of these flourished across Europe for royalty, the nobility, the rich of civil life, and secular and ecclesiastical gentry, in some ways similar to modern personal trainer programs. The most famous version of the *Regimen Sanitatis* is the *Regimen Sanitatis Salernitanum*, originating at the ancient University of Salerno in Southern Italy, thought to be the earliest medical school in Christian Europe. At least 160 editions of this were printed prior to 1830, each containing different versions, additions, and alterations.[84] Boxed Dialogue 2-1 provides an excerpt from the introduction to the first English translation by Thomas Paynell in 1528.[87]

The rules that provided the basis for the *Tacuinum Sanitatis* and *Regimen Sanitatis* were identifiable components in major medical texts that were also read by nonmedical individuals. In that form (ie, the printed word, which was the state of the art technology of the time), they reached the influential middle classes—the movers and shakers of their day. The six nonnaturals provided the framework for teaching about health and the prevention of illness as medical schools became established and for centuries beyond. Trainee physicians had to learn to unite knowledge of the humoral qualities that defined the somatic constitution with the temperament of individuals. They had to link the art of medicine with the fields of science and natural philosophy and with environmental and social issues. An Essay of Health and Long Life by George Cheyne provides an example of a respected medical textbook based on the nonnaturals.[88] A favorite throughout the 18th century, the text made recommendations similar to what the WHO does today—that overeating, excessive drinking, late nights, restrictive clothing, and sedentary occupations should be avoided or reduced.

Boxed Dialogue 2-2, from *Medicina Statica (IV)* by Italian physician Sanctorius Sanctorius,[89] provides a taste of how the rules relating to action and rest were based on empirical research, although we might argue with the interpretation and the lack of objective criteria.

Verse and song were the popular media of the day that could best disseminate messages to communities, and this was used to make it easier for the greater preliterate population to know and to remember the rules for health. Figure 2-4 depicts Arnaldus de Villa Nova, a celebrated 13th century physician, chemist, astrologer, and divine, presenting the rules of the *Regimen Sanitatis Salernitanum* to a broad population group. This is from an etching taken from old woodcuts in a 16th century German edition by physicians John Curio and James Crellius.[90]

Personal training manuals, professional literature, and popular media proved to be progressive methods used to promote health for more than 2000 years. Before the advent of germ theory and technologically sophisticated medicine, the content of the *Regimen* and the *Tacuinum* remained remarkably constant for many centuries, providing a consistent reminder of the way to promote health and prevent illness. The long accepted messages became disregarded and largely forgotten, and currently rules about health are more varied than those from ancient times and, perhaps, appear to be less dogmatic. There are also many sources of modern rules. These are developing and changing with the discoveries of medicine, the directives of the WHO referred to throughout this book, and the growth, research, and insights of population health.

MODERN: PUBLIC HEALTH—SANITATION, PREVENTION, AND EMPOWERMENT

The health of populations is the primary concern of public health practitioners. Although its genesis can be traced to the species' beginnings, the discipline of public health did not formally come into being until the mid-19th century. It has grown since then, addressing the causes of illness that impact the positive or negative quality of life experienced by individuals around the world and proclaiming the importance of population well-being. It is the lynchpin of WHO approaches and has become a focus in economics and political science.

Public health has roots in antiquity when, for example, the rules of health were developed and religious directives and taboos regulated behaviors relating to food, alcohol, and sex. The early recognition that safe drinking water is essential to life makes it truly appalling that in the 21st century approximately 783 million people lack access to safe water and currently more than 2.5 billion people lack access to adequate sanitation,[91] despite the Romans some 2000 years ago dealing with human waste disposal as a health issue. In Europe, the use of quarantine during the Middle Ages helped control the spread of many infectious diseases, and methods of immunity and inoculation from smallpox were pioneered in China in approximately 1000 BC. This was well ahead of early-18th century Western recognition. Vaccination did not become prevalent until the 1820s.

The industrial revolution fostered the spread of disease through large urban areas around factories. Poor lifestyles of the working poor and cramped primitive settlements that were without

---

Boxed Dialogue 2-2:
Excerpts: Medicina Statica (IV) by Sanctorius Sanctorius (1561-1636)[89]

IV. The body perspires much more lying quietly in bed than turning from one side to another by frequent agitation.

V. Cheerful and angry persons are less wearied by long travelling than the fearful and pensive: for the former perspire more healthfully, but the other less.

VI. Those bodies which are admitted to refection, (refreshment with food and drink) after immoderate exercise, receive much prejudice; because, as they are wearied and burthened with meat, they perspire less.

VII. Exercise from the seventh hour to the twelfth after refection, does insensibly dissolve more in the space of one hour than it does in three hours at any other time.

XIII. If a person who has kept his bed long be troubled with pain in the feet, the remedy is walking; if one that is upon a journey be so troubled, the remedy is rest.

XIV. There are two kinds of exercises, one of the body, the other of the mind: that of the body evacuates the sensible excrements: that of the mind the insensible rather, and especially those of the heart and brain, where the mind is seated.

XV. An excessive rest of the mind does more obstruct perspiration than that of the body.

XVI. The exercises of the mind which most conduce to the cheering up of the spirits, are anger, sudden joy, fear, and sorrow.

XVII. Men's bodies resting in bed, and agitated with a vehement motion of the mind, for the most part become more faint, and less ponderous, than if there be a tranquility of mind, with a violent motion of the body, as it happens at tennis, or any game at ball.

XIX. Violent exercise of mind and body renders bodies of lighter, hastens old age, and threatens untimely death: for, according to the philosopher, those persons that are exercised die sooner than such as are not.

XXI. By exercise the body perspires less, by sleep, more, and the belly is more loosened.

XXIV. Swimming immediately after violent exercise, is hurtful; for it very much obstructs perspiration.

XXV. Violent exercise in a place where the wind blows is hurtful.

XXVI. From the wind proceeds a difficulty of respiration, from the motion, acrimony.

XXVII. Riding relates more the perspirable matter of the parts of the body from the waist upwards, than downwards, but in riding, the amble is the most wholesome, the trot the most unwholesome, pace.

XXXII. The exercise of the top, consisting of moderate and violent motion, to-wit, walking and the agitation of the arms, promotes perspiration.

XXXIII. Moderate dancing, without any capering or jumping, comes near the commendation of moderate walking; for it moderately expels the concocted perspirable matter.

Sanctorius Sanctorius

---

organized sanitation were predisposing factors to disease. The first Public Health Act in Britain was passed in 1842 following Edwin Chadwick's enquiry into the sanitary conditions of the laboring population.[92] Chadwick, along with Thomas Southwood-Smith, was a prime mover in the

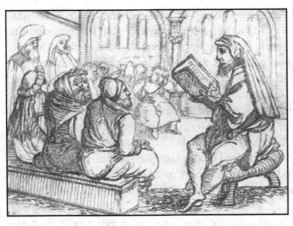

Figure 2-4. Arnaldus de Villa Nova presents the *Regimen* (from an etching taken from old woodcuts in a 16th century German edition).

reform of industrial work and mining practices, as well as other conditions of living.[93] Linking all such factors is the science of epidemiology, which is central to public health. John Snow is recognized as its founder, following his identification of a polluted well in London as the source of an outbreak of cholera in 1854. By the mid-19th century, public health programs had also begun to appear in parts of Europe and the United States:

> *Farr, Chadwick, Virchow, Koch, Pasteur, and Shattuck helped to establish the discipline on the basis of 4 factors: (1) decision making based on data and evidence (vital statistics, surveillance and outbreak investigations, laboratory science); (2) a focus on populations rather than individuals; (3) a goal of social justice and equity; and (4) an emphasis on prevention rather than curative care.[94]*

In 1892, international population health initiatives began to emerge, with an international sanitary conference held in Venice, Italy. This was followed by the founding of the Office International d'Hygiene Publique in Paris, France, in 1909. However, the Health Organisation of the League of Nations, which was established in 1920, was the first one to be truly international, with the public health role of preventing illness in all countries, all continents, and all part of the world.[95] Also anticipating the public health programs of the WHO was an international relief agency representing 44 nations known as the United Nations Relief and Rehabilitation Administration. Formed in 1943, this agency continued until 1947. It provided medical and other essential services and basic necessities for the relief of victims of war in areas hit hard by starvation, dislocation, and political chaos. It assisted displaced individuals in returning home. In addition, it offered an extensive social welfare program supplying food, fuel, clothing, shelter, tools, and farm implements to aid agricultural and economic rehabilitation. Founded prior to the current United Nations Organization, the 1943 version of the Relief and Rehabilitation Administration referred to only the united allies of World War II and initially only rendered aid to nationals of member countries. This was extended in late 1944 to include displaced Jews who had been born in Germany, and it also provided assistance further afield in China and Taiwan.[96,97] Many of its programs, and those of the Office International d'Hygiene Publique, were absorbed into the WHO, which is the United Nation's specialized agency of international public health.

In developed nations, the early 20th century saw a decrease in death rates caused by diseases such as typhoid and cholera. This was attributed, in large part, to ongoing improvements in sanitation, such as the treatment of sewage and the chlorination of drinking water.[98] However, in the majority of developing countries, these and other largely preventable infectious diseases and deaths continued, exacerbated by poverty, malnutrition, and, for babies, lack of exclusive breastfeeding in the first 6 months of life.[99,100]

In more recent times, the prevalence of infectious diseases has continued to decrease in advanced economies. Public health efforts have increasingly focused on chronic diseases, such as heart disease and cancer, road traffic accidents, work safety, and tobacco use. Since Alma Ata, interest in improving the health of populations by reducing health inequalities has led to new public health programs that address issues related to a wide range of social determinants of global health, such as where and how people live, their income, education, and social relationships. One example is provided by "healthy cities" initiatives that aim toward the creation of healthy living spaces. That focus suggests that modern population health practice has to include multidisciplinary teams of community development practitioners, architects, sociologists, engineers, lawyers, and political analysts, as well as health professionals. In this text, the term population health practitioners is used to indicate any of a range of multidisciplinary personnel. The interdisciplinary nature of global public health encourages solutions to transnational health issues and determinants, as well as those embracing curative, rehabilitative, and other aspects of clinical medicine while giving the greatest emphasis to population-based prevention, improving and achieving equity in health for all people worldwide.[94]

Most countries around the world have departments or ministries of public health that are associated with or a part of governments. They supply the rules to attain or maintain health that were provided in earlier times by texts such as the *Regimen Sanitatis*. The rules imposed by public health differ from the ancient ones, which left it to individuals or their health advisors to utilize. Increasingly since the mid-19th century, the rules of public health have been legislated as a requirement by law, government, local authority, work, or health practice and differ from place to place. These rules have reduced the incidence of illness and accidents, stopped the spread of disease or injury, and improved the environment in many cases but have also reduced, in some measure, individual freedoms. Some occupations for health benefits have been lost by restrictions of what people are able to do for themselves to meet personal, family, or community needs and wants. A selection of these will be highlighted in the subsequent chapters.

GLOBAL POPULATION HEALTH: WORLD HEALTH ORGANIZATION AND INTERNATIONAL INITIATIVES

Awareness of the interconnectedness of people across the world grew rapidly in the late 20th century. Alongside this was increased global awareness of the differences in people's health and a growing interest in the health of the Earth, which supports life:

> In a very fundamental sense, ecosystems are the planet's life-support systems—for the human species and for all other forms of life. The needs of human biology for food, water, clean air, shelter, and relative climatic constancy are basic and unalterable. Ecosystem services are indispensable to the well-being of all people, everywhere in the world. The causal links between environmental change and human health are complex because they are often indirect, displaced in space and time, and dependent on a number of modifying forces. Measures to ensure ecological sustainability would safeguard ecosystem services and therefore benefit health in the long-term.[101]

The United Nation's specialized agency for health, the WHO, is governed through the World Health Assembly, which is composed of representatives of 194 Member States. It has the objective of attaining the highest possible level of health for all people of the world.[102] This includes the right to adequate food, water, clothing, housing, health care, education, and security in the event of sickness, disability, old age, unemployment, or a lack of livelihood beyond an individual's control. In 1977, at the 30th World Health Assembly, the importance of promoting health was recognized. The year 2000 was proposed as the target for when all people would have achieved an economically productive level of health. In its definition of health discussed in the previous chapter, the WHO recognizes the close connection of social or economic issues, so the responsibility for its attainment is shared between medical and health professionals, governments and intergovernmental agencies, judiciaries, business, communities, families, and individuals. This is reflected throughout this text, with emphasis on the health outcomes of communal, corporate, and political occupations. The basic concept of the definition and the ideas embodied in the call for health of all people are addressed at Global Health Promotion Conferences, the first of which was held in Ottawa, Ontario, Canada, in 1986.

The WHO, in the spirit of Alma Ata and through the Ottawa Charter for Health Promotion, called for action in five major directions.[103] These strategies can be considered the contemporary rules for health for populations around the world:

1. Build healthy public policy.
2. Create supportive environments.
3. Strengthen community action.
4. Develop personal skills.
5. Reorient health services beyond the provision of clinical and curative services toward the pursuit of health.

The rules are holistic in their intent because they recognize "the inextricable links between people and their environment [that] constitute the basis for a socio-ecological approach to health."[103] They support and encourage "the conservation of natural resources throughout the world"; "reciprocal maintenance" through taking care of "each other, our communities, and our natural environment"; and creating conditions within "the society one lives in" toward the "attainment of health by all its members." The Charter calls for a commitment to understanding the ecological impact of ways of life so that it becomes more possible to "counteract the pressures toward harmful products, resource depletion, unhealthy living conditions, and environments." Such acknowledgement, by default, recognizes the adverse results of many current occupational structures and technology. It also recognizes the benefits of occupation. Although not using occupation-specific nomenclature, the Charter's occupation emphasis identifies that what people do affects their health. Health, it is stated, "cannot be separated from other goals" because it "is created and lived by people within the settings of their everyday life; where they learn, work, play, and love." Communities, individuals, and groups "must be able to identify and to realize aspirations, to satisfy needs, and to change or cope with the environment ... to reach a state of complete physical, mental, and social well-being."[103]

To progress those directives, subsequent World Health Promotion Conferences have reaffirmed the decisions taken at Ottawa and added the following new thoughts and details:

- The 1988 International Conference in Adelaide was based around issues of the first of the Charter's recommended strategies: healthy public policy.[104] It called for a commitment to global public health and the achievement of the "fundamental conditions for healthy living." The prerequisites of those are: "peace and social justice; nutritious food and clean water; education and decent housing; a useful role in society and adequate income; conservation of resources and the protection of the ecosystem." It described future challenges as follows:
  - "The equitable distribution of resources."
  - "The creation and preservation of healthy living and working conditions" becoming part of "all public policy decisions."
  - Recognition that "work in all its dimensions—caring work, opportunities for employment, quality of working life—dramatically affects people's health and happiness."
  - Collaboration between Nations to achieve healthy public policy toward "peace, human rights and social justice, ecology and sustainable development around the globe."[104]
- The 1991 International Conference in Sundsvall, Sweden, addressed the second of the Charter's recommended strategies—active engagement to make physical, social, economic, and political "environments more supportive of health." It identified four key public health action strategies to overcome "political decision making and industrial development" often

being based on "short-term planning and economic gains which do not take into account the true costs" to human and environmental health. These were:

- ○ Strengthen "advocacy though community action, particularly through groups organized by women."
- ○ Enable "communities and individuals to take control over their health and environment through education and empowerment."
- ○ Build alliances "to strengthen the cooperation between health and environmental campaigns."
- ○ Mediate "between conflicting interests" to ensure "equitable access" to supportive health environments.[105]

- The 4th International Conference held in Jakarta in 1997 was the first in a developing country. The Jakarta Declaration on Leading Health Promotion into the 21st Century identified five priorities:
  - ○ The promotion of social responsibility for health.
  - ○ An increase in investments for health development.
  - ○ Consolidation and expansion of partnerships for health.
  - ○ An increase of community capacity and empowerment of individuals.
  - ○ Securing the building and safeguarding of health promotion infrastructures.[106]

- The 5th International Conference held in Mexico City in 2000 agreed to decisions outlined in the Mexico Ministerial Statement for the Promotion of Health including:
  - ○ Positioning health promotion as a "fundamental priority in local, regional, national and international policies and programs."
  - ○ Ensuring the "active participation of all sectors and civil society."
  - ○ Supporting national plans of action to promote health by the identification of priorities and research and the mobilization of financial and operational resources.
  - ○ Establishing and strengthening national and international networks promoting health.[107]

- The Bangkok Charter for Health Promotion in a Globalized World records the outcome of the 6th International Conference in 2005.[108] It built on the values, principles, and action strategies of the Ottawa Charter and the recommendations of subsequent conferences. Recognizing that the global context has changed markedly since 1986, it outlined the following as critical factors:
  - ○ Increasing inequalities within and between countries
  - ○ New patterns of consumption and communication
  - ○ Commercialization
  - ○ Global environmental change
  - ○ Urbanization.

It recommended making the promotion of health central to the global development agenda; a core responsibility for all of governments; a key focus of communities and civil societies; and a requirement for good corporate practice.[108]

- The 7th Global Conference was held in Nairobi in 2009. More than 600 international participants from more than 100 countries attended. Although such interest is encouraging, the numbers of participants means that working out future directions, commitments, and strategies becomes extremely complex and difficult. Although it was recognized that health promotion has "never been more timely or more needed," it was acknowledged that "the aspirations of global health are falling short of the achievable."[109]

- The 8th Global Conference in Helsinki in 2013 was centered on a "Health in All Policies ... to improve population health and health equity." The approach is founded on health-related

Table 2-2

COMPARISON OF ANCIENT, MODERN, AND GLOBAL RULES FOR HEALTH

Ancient: Regimen Sanitatus	Public Health	Global Population Health: World Health Organization
Air and environment	Sanitation, clean air, industrial pollution control, healthy cities	Clean air, relative climatic constancy, shelter, stable ecosystem, and sustainable resources
Motion (activity/occupation) and rest	Agricultural and economic supplies, rehabilitation education, occupational health and safety	Livelihood, employment, education
Food and drink	Food, malnutrition, alcohol, breast feeding, income	Food and water, income
Sleep and waking	Noise reduction to enable sleep	Studies into sleep disturbance
Evacuation and repletion (including sexuality)	Eradication of sexually transmitted diseases	Eradication of sexually transmitted diseases
Affections of the soul (including joy, anger, fear, and distress)	Empowerment, social relationships	Mental health, social justice and equity, security in the event of sickness, disablity, old age
Mainly individually focused interventions but responsive to accepted societal understanding and community disasters	Economics, politics, housing, mainly community focused within national boundaries	Economics, politics, peace, reduction of social determinants of illness, mainly globally focused

rights and obligations for public policies to systematically address "the health implications of decisions, seek synergies, and avoid harmful health impacts."[110]

It can be observed from the brief overview above that the statements from global conferences became increasingly political and less hands on. The Ottawa Charter directives were essentially practical, providing grassroots ideas for action to change negative into more positive experiences of health. Perhaps some of the failure to reach the goals can be laid at this door or maybe the practical goals failed to reach the right political ears, workers in the field, or were not resourced.

Conclusion

This chapter has introduced the rules of health across more than 2000 years. These will be alluded to or discussed further as the book progresses. Meeting the basic needs of survival is affected by human ingenuity and occupational know-how, population size, environmental degradation, and multinational greed. The changes over that long period of time may appear major, and in many ways that is true, especially when it is considered how the world's population has increased. However, there are surprising similarities, as illustrated in Table 2-2. The themes of this chapter provide both negative and positive messages. There is obvious disappointment that "multiple charters, declarations and resolutions endorse the importance of health promotion yet implementation of these resolutions falls short of the commitments."[109]

This should suggest that more people, and especially those focusing on providing for health needs, could do much more. Changing focus toward population-based primary health care and health promotion is one important way forward, and well suited to an occupation-based approach. At the grassroots level, such change requires commitment that will override the failure of managers, resource agencies, politicians, and bureaucrats to recognize and resource more than a medicalized and individualistic understanding of health as the treatment of illness that is dominant in advanced countries because "understanding the history of health ... helps the global public health community to respond to the challenges of today and helps shape a healthier future for everyone, especially those most in need."[1]

References

1. World Health Organization. The WHO Global Health Histories Project. http://www.who.int/global_health_histories/seminars/seminars 2011.pdf. Accessed May 22, 2014.
2. Bush H, Zvelebil M, eds. *Health in Past Societies: Biocultural Interpretations of Human Skeletal Remains in Archeological Contexts.* Oxford: British Archaeological Reports International Series 567, 1991; 6.
3. Bauer G. Agricola. In: Hoover HC, Hoover HL, trans. *De re Metallica 1556.* New York, NY: Dover Publications; 1950.
4. Paracelsus. *4 Treatises of Theophrastus von Hohenheim Called Paracelsus.* 1567. Sigerist HE, ed. Temkin CL, Rosen G, Zilboorg G, Sigerist HE, trans. Baltimore, MD: Johns Hopkins Press; 1941.
5. Ramazzini B. *Of The Diseases Of Tradesmen, Shewing The Various Influence Of Particular Trades Upon The State Of Health; With The Best Methods To Avoid or Correct It,...* London, UK: Printed for Andrew Bell et al; 1705.
6. Thackrah CT. *The Effects of the Principal Arts, Trades, and Professions, and of Civic States and Habits of Living, On Health and Longevity.* London, England: Longman, Rees, Orme, Browne and Green; 1831.
7. McKeown T. *The Origins of Human Disease.* Oxford, UK: Basil Blackwell; 1988.
8. Lorenz K. *The Waning of Humaneness.* Boston, MA: Little, Brown and Co; 1987:21.
9. Homeostasis. *Dorland's Illustrated Medical Dictionary.* 25th ed. Philadelphia, PA: WB Saunders; 1974:720.
10. Lieberman P. Evolution of the speech apparatus. In: Jones S, Martin R, Pilbeam D, eds. *The Cambridge Encyclopedia of Human Evolution.* New York, NY: Cambridge University Press; 1992:136-137.
11. Bernard C. Lectures on the phenomena of life common to animals and vegetables (1878-1879). In: Langley LL, ed. *Homeostasis: Origins of the Concept.* Straudsburg, PA: Hutchinson and Ross, Inc; 1982:129-147.
12. Cannon W. *Physiological Regulation of Normal States: Some Tentative Postulations Concerning Biological Homeostasis.* Paris, France: Charles Richet; 1926.
13. Cannon WB. *The Wisdom of the Body.* New York, NY: WW Norton and Co Inc; 1939.
14. Allport GW. The open system in personality theory. *J Abnorm Soc Psychol.* 1960;61.
15. McDougall W. *The Energies of Men.* London, England: Methuen; 1932.
16. McDougall W. *An Introduction to Social Psychology.* 23rd rev ed. London, England; Methuen; 1936.
17. Lewin K. *A Dynamic Theory of Personality.* New York, NY: 1935.
18. Murray HA. *Explorations in Personality.* New York, NY: 1938.
19. Hull CL. *Principles of Behavior.* New York, NY: Appleton-Century-Crofts; 1943.
20. Madsen KB. *Theories of Motivation.* 4th ed. Kent, OH: Kent State University Press; 1968.
21. Alderfer CP. *Existence, Relatedness and Growth: Human Needs in Organizational Settings.* New York, NY: Free Press; 1972.
22. Maslow AH. *Motivation and Personality.* 2nd ed. New York, NY: Harper and Row; 1970.
23. Eysenck HS, Arnold W, Meili R. *Encyclopedia of Psychology.* New York, NY: Continuum Books, The Seabury Press; 1979:705-706.
24. Wolman B, ed. *Dictionary of Behavioral Science.* New York, NY: Van Nostand, Reinold Co; 1973:250.
25. Lorenz K. *Civilized Man's Eight Deadly Sins.* Latzke M, trans. London, England: Methuen and Co Ltd; 1974 :3-5.
26. Snell GD. *Search for a Rational Ethic.* New York, NY: Springer Verlag; 1988:147.
27. Young PT. Drives. In: Sills DL, ed. *International Encyclopedia of the Social Sciences.* New York, NY: The Macmillan Co and The Free Press; 1968.
28. Dashiell JF. *Fundamentals of Objective Psychology.* Boston, MA: Houghton Mifflin; 1928;233-234.

29. Deci E, Ryan R. The "what" and "why" of goal pursuits. Human needs and the self determination of behavior. *Psychological Inquiry.* 2000;11:227-268.
30. Ryff CD. Happiness is everything or is it? Explorations on the meaning of psychological well-being. *Journal of Personality and Social Psychology.* 1989,57:1069-1081.
31. Doyal L, Gough I. *A Theory of Human Need.* Houndmills, Hampshire: Macmillan; 1991.
32. Anscombe GEM. Modern moral philosophy. *Philosophy.* 1958;33:1-19.
33. Watts ED. Human needs. In: Kuper A, Kuper J, eds. *The Social Science Encyclopedia.* London, England: Routledge; 1985:368.
34. Ornstein RE, Sobel D. *The Healing Brain: A Radical New Approach to Health Care.* London, England: Macmillan; 1988:11-12.
35. Knight R, Knight M. *A Modern Introduction to Psychology.* London, England: University Tutorial Press Ltd; 1957.
36. Huang Ti Nei Ching Su Wen. *The Yellow Emperor's Classic of Internal Medicine.* Veith I, trans. Baltimore, MD: Williams and Wilkins; 1949:253.
37. Lao-tzu. Tao Te Ching (The Way) Circe 500 BC: Chuang-tzu. In: Dubos R, ed. *Mirage of Health: Utopias, Progress and Biological Change.* New York, NY: Harper and Row; 1959:10.
38. Gruman G. *A History of Ideas about the Prologation of Life: The Evolution of Prolongevity Hypotheses to 1800.* Philadelphia, PA: The American Philosophical Society. 1966.
39. Needham J, ed. *Science and Civilisation in China. Vol 2. History of Scientific Thought.* New York, NY: Cambridge University Press; 1956.
40. Rousseau JJ. Discourse on the origin and foundations of inequity amongst men. 1754. Johnson I, trans. Adelaide, Australia: University of Adelaide. Web edition published by eBooks@Adelaide. http://ebooks.adelaide.edu.au/r/rousseau/jean_jacques/inequality/. Last updated Thursday, March 6, 2014. Accessed May 23, 2014.
41. Dubos R, ed. *Mirage of Health: Utopias, Progress and Biological Change.* New York, NY: Harper and Row; 1959.
42. Barraclough J. (transl). *Antoine-Nicholas de Condorcet: Sketch for a Historical Picture of the Progress of the Human Mind.* New York, NY: Library of Ideas; 1955.
43. Beddoes T. *Hygeia, or Essays Moral and Medical on the Causes Affecting the Personal State of Our Middling and Affluent Classes.* 3 vols. Bristol: R Phillips; 1802-1803.
44. Virey JJ. *L'hygiene Philosophique.* Paris, France: Crochard; 1828.
45. Jenner E. *An Inquiry Into the Causes and Effects of the Variolae Vaccine or Cow Pox.* 1798. http://www.bartleby.com/38/4/1.html. Accessed May 23, 2014.
46. Gruman G. *A History of Ideas about the Prolongation of Life: The Evolution of Prolongevity Hypotheses to 1800.* Philadelphia, PA: The American Philosophical Society. 1966: 31.
47. Powell ML. *Status and Health in Prehistory: A Case Study of the Mountville Chiefdom.* Washington, DC: Smithsonian Institute Press; 1988.
48. McMichael T. *Human Frontiers, Environments and Disease: Past Patterns, Uncertain Futures.* Cambridge, MA: Cambridge University Press; 2001:xiii.
49. Stephenson W. *The Ecological Development of Man.* Sydney, Australia: Angus and Robertson; 1972.
50. King-Boyes MJE. *Patterns of Aboriginal Culture: Then and Now.* Sydney, Australia: McGraw-Hill Book Co; 1977:154-155.
51. Leakey R, Lewin R. *People of the Lake: Man: His Origins, Nature, and Future.* New York, NY: Penguin Books; 1978.
52. Leakey R. *The Making of Mankind.* London, England: Michael Joseph Ltd; 1981.
53. Falk D. As it happened: Some liked it hot. Television documentary. SBS.
54. Jones S, Martin R, Pilbeam D, eds. *The Cambridge Encyclopedia of Human Evolution.* New York, NY: Cambridge University Press; 1992.
55. Agius T. Aboriginal health in Aboriginal hands. In: Fuller J, Barclay J, Zollo J, eds. *Multicultural Health Care in South Australia.* Conference proceedings. Adelaide: Painters Prints; 1993:23.
56. McNeill WH. *Plagues and People.* London, England: Penguin Books; 1979:39.
57. Tunnes N. 1656. In: Dubos R, ed. *Mirage of Health: Utopias, Progress and Biological Change.* New York, NY: Harper and Row; 1959:11.
58. Fortuine R. The health of the Eskimos as portrayed in the earliest written accounts. *Bulletin of the History of Medicine.* 1971;45:97-114.
59. Wharton WJL, ed. *Captain Cook's Journal During His First Voyage Around the World Made in HM Bark Endeavour,* 1768-1771. London, England: Eliot Stock; 1893.

60. Meindl RS. Human populations before agriculture. In: Jones S, Martin R, Pilbeam D, eds. *The Cambridge Encyclopedia of Human Evolution*. New York, NY: Cambridge University Press; 1992.

61. Dobson A. People and disease. In: Jones S, Martin R, Pilbeam D, eds. *The Cambridge Encyclopedia of Human Evolution*. New York, NY: Cambridge University Press; 1992:411-412.

62. Landers J. Reconstructing ancient populations. In: Jones S, Martin R, Pilbeam D, eds. *The Cambridge Encyclopedia of Human Evolution*. New York, NY: Cambridge University Press; 1992:404-405.

63. Douglas M. Population control in primitive peoples. *British Journal of Sociology*. 1966;17:263-273.

64. Coon CS. *The Hunting Peoples*. London, England: Jonathan Cape Ltd; 1972:390.

65. Gandevia B. *Occupation and Disease in Australia since 1788*. Sydney: Australasian Medical publishing Co Ltd; 1971:157.

66. Cannon WB. *Bodily Changes in Pain, Hunger, Fear and Rage*. Boston, Mass: CT Branford; 1953. Original work published 1929.

67. Sigerist HE. *A History of Medicine. Vol 1. Primitive and Archaic Medicine*. New York, NY: Oxford University Press; 1955:254-255.

68. Birdsell JB. On population structure in generalized hunting and collecting populations. *Evolution*. 1958;12:189-205.

69. Gurven M, Kaplan H. Longevity among hunter-gatherers: a cross cultural examination. *Population and Development Review*. 2007;33:321-365.

70. World Health Organization. Life Expectancy: Life Expectancy Data by Country. Global Health Observatory Data Repository. http://apps.who.int/gho/data/node.main.688?lang=en. Accessed May 22, 2014.

71. Central Intelligence Agency (US). The World Factbook. Country Comparison: Life Expectancy at Birth. https://www.cia.gov/library/publications/the-world-factbook/ranko. Accessed May 22 2014.

72. Diamond J. Evolution, consequences and future of plant and animal domestication. Nature. 2002;418:700-707. http://www.nature.com/nature/journal/v418/n6898/full/nature01019.html. Accessed May 23, 2014.

73. Hetzel BS, McMichael T. *L S Factor: Lifestyle and Health*. Ringwood, Victoria: Penguin; 1987:186-187.

74. Procopius. Persian Wars 23:1. *History of the Wars*. 5 Vols. Dewing HB, trans. Cambridge, MA: Harvard University Press; 1914.

75. Mumford L. *The Condition of Man*. Secker & Warburg. London, England: Heinemann; 1963.

76. Gordon D. *Health, Sickness and Society: Theoretical Concepts in Social and Preventive Medicine*. St. Lucia, Queensland: University of Queensland Press; 1976:5,157,164,311,337,378.

77. Jones B. *Sleepers, Wake! Technology and the Future of Work*. Melbourne, Australia: Oxford University Press; 1982:16.

78. Eversley DEC. Epidemiology as social history. In: Creighton CA, ed. *History of Epidemics in Britain*. 2nd ed. London, England: Cassell; 1965:1-35.

79. Doll R. Preventive medicine: the objectives. *Ciba Found Symp*. 1985;110:3-21.

80. Biedermann H. *Medicina Magica*. Birmingham, Alabama: Classics of Medicine Library; 1986.

81. Sigerist HE. *A History of Medicine, Volume II: Early Greek, Hindu, and Persian Medicine*. New York: Oxford University Press; 1961.

82. Hippocrates. On Airs, Waters and Places (c. 400 BC). Jones WHS, trans. *On the Universe*. Cambridge, MA: Harvard University Press; 1931.

83. Berger M. *Hildegard of Bingen: On Natural Philosophy and Medicine: Selections from Cause and Cure*. Cambridge: D.S. Brewer; 1999.

84. Wilcock AA. *Occupation for Health. Volume 1. A Journey from Self Health to Prescription*. London: British College of Occupational Therapists; 2001.

85. Siraisi NG. *Medieval and Early Renaissance Medicine: An Introduction to Knowledge and Practice*. Chicago and London: University of Chicago Press; 1990:127.

86. Croke A. *Regimen Sanitatis Salernitanum: A Poem on the Preservation of Health in Rhyming Latin Verse*. Oxford: D.A. Talboys; 1830:42.

87. Paynell. T. *Introduction to Regimen Sanitatis Salerni*. England: 1528.

88. Cheyne G. *An Essay of Health and Long Life*. London and Bath: Strahan; 1724:77.

89. Sinclair J. *Code of Health and Longevity*. Edinburgh: Printed for A Constabe & Co.; 1807. https://archive.org/details/codehealthandlo00sincgoog. Accessed May 28, 2014.

90. Croke Sir A. *Regimen Sanitatis Salernitanum with the Englishman's Doctor: An Ancient Translation*. Oxford: D.A. Talboys; 1830.

91.   United Nations. Water. World Water Day 2013. http://www.unwater.org/water-cooperation-2013/water-cooperation/facts-and-figures/en/. Accessed May 22, 2014.

92.   Girling DA, ed. *Public health. New Age Encyclopaedia: Volume 23.* Sydney: Bay Books; 1983.

93.   Guy JR. *Compassion and the Art of the Possible: Dr Southwood Smith as Social Reformer and Public Health Pioneer (1993 Octavia Hill Memorial Lecture).* Cambridgeshire, England: Octavia Hill Society and Birthplace Trust; 1996.

94.   Koplan JP, Bond TC, Merson MH, et al. Towards a common definition of global health. *Lancet.* 2009;373:1993-1995.

95.   World Health Organization. Archives of the League of Nations, Health Section Files. http://www.who.int/archives/fonds_collections/bytitle/fonds_3/en/. Accessed May 23, 2014.

96.   United Nations Relief and Rehabilitation Administration (UNRRA). *Encyclopedia Britannica.* 2012. Available at: http://www.britannica.com/EBchecked/topic/616468/United-Nations-Relief-and-Rehabilitation-Adminis (accessed April 23, 2012).

97.   Hitchcock WI. *The Bitter Road to Freedom: The Human Cost of Allied Victory in World War II Europe.* New York: NYL Free Press; 2009.

98.   Cutler D, Miller G. The role of public health improvements in health advances: the twentieth-century United States. *Demography.* 2005;42:1-22.

99.   Public health. Available at: http://en.wikipedia.org/wiki/Public_health#cite_note-26. Accessed May 23, 2014.

100. World Health Organization. Fact file: 10 Facts on Breast Feeding. February 2012. Available at: http://www.who.int/features/factfiles/breastfeeding/facts/en/. Accessed May 23, 2014.

101. Ecosystems and Human Health: Some findings from the Millennium Ecosystem Assessment. Why do ecosystems matter to human health? Available at: www.millenniumassessment.org/documents/document.763.aspx.pdf. Accessed May 23, 2014.

102. World Health Organization. *Constitution of the World Health Organization.* New York, NY: World Health Organization; 1946.

103. World Health Organization, Health and Welfare Canada, Canadian Public Health Association. *Ottawa Charter for Health Promotion.* Ottawa, Canada; 1986.

104. World Health Organization. Adelaide recommendations on Healthy Public Policy. *2nd International Conference on Health Promotion.* Adelaide, Australia; 1988: 5-6.

105. World Health Organization. *International Conference on Health Promotion.* Sundsvall, Sweden: WHO; 1991.

106. World Health Organization. *Jakarta Declaration on Leading Health Promotion into the 21st Century. 4th International Conference on Health Promotion.* Jakarta, Indonesia: WHO; 1997.

107. World Health Organization. Mexico Ministerial Statement for the Promotion of Health. *5th International Conference on Health Promotion. Health Promotion: Bridging the Equity Gap.* Mexico City: WHO; 2000.

108. World Health Organization. The Bangkok Charter for Health Promotion in a Globalized World. *The Sixth International Conference on Health Promotion.* Bangkok: WHO; 2005.

109. World Health Organization. *Overview: 7th Global Conference on Health Promotion.* Nairobi, Kenya: WHO; 2009.

110. World Health Organization. 8th Global Conference on Health Promotion. Helsinki, 2013. http://www.healthpromotion2013.org/health-promotion/health-in-all-policies. Accessed March 17, 2013.

Theme 3

"A few, largely preventable, risk factors account for most of the world's disease burden ... This reflects a significant change in diet habits, physical activity levels and tobacco use worldwide as a result of industrialization, urbanization, economic development and increasing food market globalization."

WHO: Global Strategy on Diet, Physical Activity, and Health, 2003[1a]

Chapter 3

DOMINANT CONCEPTS AND CONTEMPORARY PRIORITIES

This chapter addresses:
- Illness as Disease and Infirmity
- The Origins and Purpose of Modern Medicine
  - Human Longevity
- The Prominence of the Medical Model
  - Critique of the Medical Model
  - Medical Practice Influencing Occupation
- Contemporary Priorities
  - Noncommunicable Diseases
  - Population Aging
  - Poverty
  - HIV/AIDS
- Conclusion

This chapter investigates illness as the antonym of health and introduces contemporary priorities in the pursuit of health. It explores what is meant by illness and ill-health, with a specific focus on the medical perspective that dominates channels of communication about health and its promotion. Throughout the chapter, the commentary draws attention to the need for the medical perspective to embrace occupational links. Currently, the way illness and occupation are intimately related is poorly understood; however, the relationship has been conceptualized in different ways over the centuries.

As preceding chapters make evident, the concepts of health and illness are intertwined so that prevalent understandings of health and well-being have always contained understandings about the nature and causes of ill-health. For example, in Classical Greek times, when health was conceptualized as a balance of the four bodily humors, the illness known as melancholia was attributed to an excess of black bile, one of the humors.[1b] Currently, because health is understood from a medicalized understanding of physiology, the causes of prevalent health concerns in affluent

Wilcock AA, Hocking C.
An Occupational Perspective of Health, Third Edition (pp 58-82).
© 2015 Taylor & Francis Group.

societies are often attributed to unhealthy dietary or alcohol intake, levels of exercise, or particular sex practices.

Illness, as opposed to health, has negative connotations of pain, discomfort, and curtailment of participation in occupation. Those understandings date from at least the 17th century when, consistent with current medical dictionaries, illness referred to a state of poor health or being sick.[2,3] Modern definitions often point to causative factors: a disorder of bodily or mental functions, old age, or a disease. Indeed, illness and disease are often used in combination, such as *Encyclopedia Britannica's* definition of illness, which cites the recognizable hallmarks of disease commonly exhibited by a diseased organism.[4]

Illness has meanings other than "not well; sick" or "a disease or disorder."[5] The word *ill* is a contraction of evil and, in the 18th century, illness also referred to "wickedness, depravity, immorality" and "unpleasantness, disagreeableness, hurtfulness."[6] Those ideas suggest that ill people were engaging in or conducting their occupations in ways others found offensive or damaging to their relationships. Those meanings continue into the present day. In 21st century nonmedical lexicons, ill sits with words that cross the physical, mental, and social divide, like harmful, wretched, disastrous, hostile or malevolent, unfriendly, portending danger or disaster, unfavorable, morally bad, contrary to accepted standards, improper, unsound, and disordered.[7,8] Those meanings partially explain the enduring perception held by some that tuberculosis is a divine punishment[9] and epilepsy is caused by demonic possession,[10] as well as the widespread practice of isolating people with leprosy[11] and the "contamination" of mental disorders with "images of violence, sin and laziness."[12] Acknowledging those meanings supports the concept that illness is as much a social construction about human states and undesirable or unacceptable ways of engaging in occupation as it is a biological reality.[13a]

Given that illness is as much a part of the human experience as health, it is not surprising that there are numerous words used to convey its different manifestations and the extent of its impact on people's ability to perform their everyday occupations, from slight indispositions and mild but enduring ailments through deep-seated malady to the pain and suffering of an affliction (Table 3-1). Within many of these descriptors, the consequences for occupational performance are implicit—being ill causes loss of strength, prevents people from rising from their beds, and renders them handicapped and incapable of functioning normally. In addition to the more formal terms, there are abundant colloquialisms to convey a state of ill health: feeling rotten, seedy, below par, out of sorts, off color, under the weather, or crook (used in Australia and New Zealand).[14]

Illness as Disease and Infirmity

Current understanding of illness is framed by the WHO's 1946 definition of *illness* as disease or infirmity.[15] The term *disease* derives from the Latin and means the absence of ease or "elbow room," which has connotations of impeded movement or insufficient space to perform everyday activities.[16] In the context of the modern world, diseases are understood to have a broad range of undesirable health consequences, but the connection to doing implied by restricted elbow room has all but vanished from medical knowledge. Illness is conceptualized as arising from disordered physiological functions; pathological change attributable to exposure to an infection, toxin, or prolonged stress; the presence of a developmental disorder or malfunctioning immune system or organ; genetic disorders or serious nutritional imbalances or deficiencies; or psychiatric illness. Ill-health is situated firmly in the biomedical realm by the concept of disease as a deviation from normal bodily functions that can be described and is invariant across place and time.

In the 19th century, medical discourse frequently referred to incurable diseases, including scarlet fever, typhus, cholera, consumption (tuberculosis), and lockjaw (tetanus).[17] In contrast, 20th century accounts frame diseases in terms of their prevalence, etiology and prognosis, characteristic signs (objective indicators, such as swelling) and symptoms (subjective indicators, such

Table 3-1

DICTIONARY DEFINITIONS OF ILLNESS AND ITS SYNONYMS

Illness Synonyms	Published Definitions
Ailment	A slight but often persistent illness[13b]
Affliction	A state of pain, distress, or grief; misery. Synonyms: mishap, trouble, calamity, catastrophe, disaster.[13c]
	A condition of great distress, pain, or suffering; something responsible for physical or mental suffering such as a disease, grief, etc[13d]
Debility	A weakened or enfeebled state; weakness; Debility prevented him from getting out of bed. A particular mental or physical handicap.[13e]
Disorder	A disturbance in physical or mental health or functions; malady or dysfunction.[13f]
	A disturbance or derangement that affects the function of mind or body, such as an eating disorder or abuse of a drug; to disturb the normal physical or mental health of.[13g]
Feeling poorly	In poor health. Somewhat ill or prone to illness, looking a little peaked.[13h]
Ill health	A state in which you are unable to function normally and without pain[2]
Illness	Unhealthy condition; poor health. (obsolete: wickedness).[3]
	A harmful deviation from the normal structural or functional state of an organism. A diseased organism commonly exhibits signs or symptoms indicative of its abnormal state. Thus, the normal condition of an organism must be understood in order to recognize the hallmarks of disease.[4]
Indisposition	A state of being indisposed; a slight illness.[13i]
	Sick or ill; unwilling (from Latin indispositus, disordered).[13j]
Infirmity	The condition of being feeble, frailty, lack of strength.[13k]
	A bodily ailment or weakness, especially one brought on by old age. A condition causing weakness, a failing or defect in a person's character.[13l]
	Physical weakness or debility; frailty; a moral flaw or failing.[13m]
Malady	Any disorder or disease of the body, especially one that is chronic or deep seated.[13n]
	From Latin: male habitus, doing poorly, from habēre meaning to have, hold.[13o]
Sickness	A particular disease or malady; the state or instance of being sick.[13p]

as tiredness), and preventive, curative, rehabilitative, or palliative treatment. Conceptualizing disease in this manner gives it objectivity, making it something that "doctors are able to see, touch, measure, [and] smell."[6] Occupation is recognized as a causative factor in some disease processes. However, because it exists beyond the direct influence of medicine, it is primarily addressed through narrowly focused lifestyle advice about exercise, diet, tobacco, and alcohol intake, and sexual practices that fails to account for the complex interactive determinants of people's occupational patterns. Meeting the challenge of people's immediate occupational requirements in the context of acute or chronic illness is relegated to the allied professions, with their orthotics, assistive technologies, and occupational and environmental modifications. Although those interventions could be used to enable wide-ranging health-promoting occupations, occupational therapists deployed in health and housing services are typically restricted to the safe performance of essential self-care tasks related to hygiene, nutrition, getting dressed, movement around one's home, and emergency egress. Despite the disconnection between medicine and occupation, the perception that medical interventions are available and appropriate holds true, even for conditions such as depression and schizophrenia, where the pathological origins of the disorder have not been determined.

Compared with disease, infirmity is a less prescriptive concept. Dictionary definitions again point to bodily ailments, particularly those associated with old age, but emphasis is given to the effects rather than the cause of illness. To be infirm is to be weak, frail, feeble, or debilitated and to lack strength, all of which can be interpreted as impacting life's activities. As with the concept of disease, there are connotations of being flawed by a defect in one's character or morals. That inference is reinforced by biblical references to Jesus curing "many of their infirmities and plagues, and of evil spirits" and true believers both "bearing the infirmities of the weak" and accepting their own infirmities, reproaches, distresses, and persecutions as testament to their faith.[18]

In specifying the absence of disease and infirmity, the WHO's definition of health encompasses the causes and outcomes of ill health. At the time that definition was developed, great strides were being taken toward the eradication of several deadly infectious diseases. The exigencies of World War II also hastened the implementation of several medical initiatives with dramatic effect. Following Sir Alexander Fleming's discovery of penicillin in 1929, new and more effective penicillin strains were developed and produced on an industrial scale to combat wound infections, gangrene, pneumonia, and gonorrhea. Entirely new strains of antibiotics were developed, with Selman Waksman's 1943 discovery of streptomycin providing an effective cure for tuberculosis. Although not typically described in occupational terms, those medical advances meant that many young and working-aged people were able to leave long-term and restrictive hospitalization, choose for themselves how they would spend free time, contribute to the livelihood of their family, and become productive members of society. Advances in rehabilitation meant there were also significant reductions in the number of people suffering the infirmities that had been an inevitable consequence of injuries and chronic conditions. As early as 1935, the long-standing practice of treating fractures with complete bed rest came into question. For example, this resulted in occupational therapists working to maintain and improve people's capacity to engage in occupation during recovery rather than afterward encouraging the restoration of function to atrophied muscles and stiffened joints.[19] Remarkable reductions in the length of hospitalization were achieved, with people going back home and to work in half the time.[20] Rehabilitation after stroke and for those crippled by arthritis also substantially improved people's capacity to work and perform domestic and parenting roles. During World War II, the urgent need to return injured servicemen to wartime or civilian occupations also spurred other advances, including the development of new techniques for preserving blood for use in transfusions and pioneering work in the use of skin grafts to treat burns.[21,22] Early intervention in specialist spinal injury centers and occupation-based rehabilitation improved long-term survival among returning soldiers from 10% after World War I to 90% after World War II, with many of them returning to the community to pursue educational or vocational opportunities.[23,24] In many postindustrial countries, occupation-based rehabilitation has been reduced considerably on largely economic grounds. Home-based occupations that might assist improvement of those unable to return to employment immediately is frowned on and sometimes punished, being viewed as evidence of them trying to defraud health insurance or governmental assistance.

Other breakthroughs across the spectrum of chronic and endemic illnesses that occurred in the early 1940s include the development of anti-malarial drugs and the refinement of immunizations against tetanus. Widespread use of dichlorodiphenyltrichloroethane (DDT) eradicated malaria in the United States, the Soviet Union, and Europe and markedly reduced infection rates in India, South America, and sub-Saharan Africa.[21,25] Inroads to the prevention of cancer mortality began with the introduction of routine Pap smears to diagnose cervical cancer. Perhaps most significant in this context was the identification of the correlation between diet and coronary thrombosis.[22,26] Scientific evidence was affirming what had been recognized centuries earlier: that everyday occupations such as producing, preparing, and consuming food have long-term health consequences. Against that backdrop, the possibility of delivering a future in which disease and infirmity were largely absent and the majority of people would be able to lead productive lives must have seemed

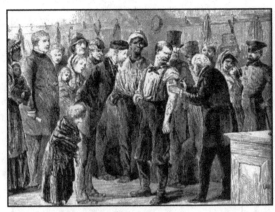

Figure 3-1. Introducing vaccinations. (From Harter J, editor. *Images of Medicine: A Definitive Volume of more than 4,800 Copyright-free Engravings Including Anatomy, General Medicine, Apothecary and Pharmaceutical, Diseases and Injuries, Therapeutics, Plus Medical Equipment, Instruments and Appliances.* New York: Bonanza Books; 1991.)

within grasp when the WHO definition of health was drafted.[15] However, the health benefits of attending to occupation as an essential component of population health was not fully realized, perhaps because it appears so commonplace. To explain further why occupation was overlooked, the history of modern medicine is traced.

The Origins and Purpose of Modern Medicine

The theoretical heart of modern Western medicine is the medical or biomedical model. This is the scientific perspective from which physicians and researchers conceptualize and study disease. The scientific process typically proceeds from observing and describing the signs and symptoms of a health condition, to being able to recognize and treat its symptoms, to identifying the specific etiology and from there to developing targeted treatments.[27] This approach is commonly described as originating with the development of germ theory in the mid to late 1800s. Louis Pasteur, a founder of microbiology, is given much of the credit for discovering microbes and viruses, as well as practical application of his discoveries. He championed health practices that are now standard procedures—pasteurization (a process to sterilize milk and wine), sanitizing hands and instruments to prevent the spread of infection, and developing vaccines for anthrax and rabies (Figure 3-1).[28] Robert Koch was also closely associated with the emergence of the medical model. In 1882, he identified the tuberculosis bacillus, thereby opening the way for the development of a vaccine. Koch also promoted the widespread adoption of Pasteur's method of sterilizing milk, which had been found to be the source of tuberculosis infection, and created health messages to curtail the spread of that disease (Figure 3-2).[29] Their work changed people's health and hygiene activities, instituted processes that food manufacturers would follow, and directly influenced the hygiene requirements and range of occupations performed by medics.

Pasteur and Koch laid a foundation of evidence to explain and treat the important health problems of the day, as well as the expectation that research into the cause and treatment of health conditions was a valuable necessity. Both men used the positivist scientific methods established by Galileo (1564-1642), Descartes (1596-1650), and Newton (1642-1727), which are characterized by empirical observation and an analytic approach to the development of knowledge. Thus reductionism became the cornerstone of the scientific method. This rigorous approach, which supports biomedicine's general view of the human body as akin to a machine, is based on: The practice of analyzing and describing a complex phenomenon in terms of its simple or fundamental constituents, especially when this is said to provide a sufficient explanation.[31]

Erving Goffman, a noted sociologist, favorably compared the medical treatment of bodily ailments with the "conduct in the tinkering trades" that repaired other finely tuned mechanisms,

Figure 3-2. Preventing the spread of tuberculosis. (Circa mid 1920s, author Rensselaer County Tuberculosis Association and the source: U.S. National Library of Medicine.)

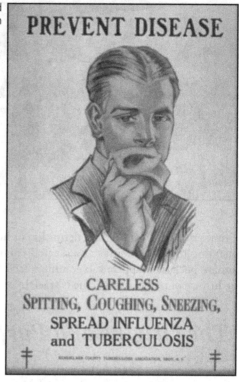

such as watches.[10] The body's complex and finely tuned mechanism is subject to physical pathologies and neurophysiologic disturbances just as machines are subject to breakdowns according to their makeup and usage.

Consistent with scientific methods, there is an assumption that biological variables fully account for disease processes because they manifest in individuals who fall ill and, in the case of infectious and contagious diseases, as they are passed from one individual to another. Recourse to social, psychological, behavioral, or occupational causes or treatment of illness is seen to "lie outside medicine's responsibility and authority."[32] It is generally assumed that remediation, or at least alleviation, of the effects of the health condition is possible using the techniques and technologies available to medicine—vaccines, medications, surgery, blood transfusions, and irradiation. With that focus, the medical model continues to drive health research into the causes and cures of physical and psychological illnesses. These sometimes touch on particular aspects of human activity. For example, by the 1980s, the link between smoking tobacco and a variety of health conditions was firmly established,[33-35] and numerous public health explorations, such as the 20-year Framingham Cohort study,[36] had produced clear evidence of the link between lifestyle and health. However, rather than the occupational perspective advanced in this book, lifestyle concerns were confined to identifying the mechanisms by which pathogenic substances enter the body (eg, cigarette smoke, salt, fat, alcohol) and the quantity of exercise rather than the physical, psychological, and social effect and combination of all activities that a person undertook.

Although medicine's grounding in positivist scientific method is relatively recent, the philosophical origins of that approach to health have a long history. The belief that the chief role of health care is to treat disease, correct imperfections, and thereby restore health is first attributed to Asclepius, the Greek god of healing. Before being elevated as a deity, Asclepius was a physician in the 12th century BC. His work had far-reaching effects as, from the 5th century BC, faith in the restorative power of health care progressively displaced the earlier health beliefs associated with the Athenian goddess Hygeia. She symbolized the belief that people would not be ill if they lived a balanced life in a pleasant environment and according to reason.[37] Hippocrates, who is widely considered to be the father of modern medicine, made some attempt to combine the approaches of Asclepius and Hygeia. He observed that a physician "was to be skilled in Nature and must strive to know what man is in relation to food, drink, occupation, and which effect each of these has on the other."[38] From an occupational perspective of health, that insight continues to hold true. However, in emphasizing the systematic gathering of information about the patient's history, conducting a physical examination to identify signs and symptoms, recording what did and did not work, and beginning to classify the conditions he treated, Hippocrates is best remembered for founding the medical procedures of today.[39] Nonetheless, his tombstone in Cos, a Greek island, is engraved:

HERE LIES HIPPOCRATES

WHO WON INNUMERABLE VICTORIES

OVER DISEASE

WITH THE WEAPONS OF HYGEIA[40]

The development of biomedicine, as it is currently practiced, is entrenched in Western rationality, a product of the Enlightenment period of the second half of the 18th century. Rational thinking favors logic over emotions and subjectivity, and is encapsulated in Rene Descartes' often quoted axiom "Cogito, ergo sum" (I think, therefore I am). Rationalism was a radical shift away from the scriptures as a primary source of knowledge. This new social order is the origin of the current belief that progress is brought about by pure reason. Increased rationality, it was believed, would "enhance social understanding, order and control, justice, moral progress, and human happiness."[41] Rationalism casts the human body as something to be controlled rather than as a part of who we are and what we do. Descartes' separation of mind and body, which partitions mental from bodily illness, is another philosophical cornerstone of biomedicine, and is equally at odds with the integrated experience of mind and body engagement in occupation that is socially constructed. According to Engel, a professor of psychiatry and medicine, medicine's mind–body dualism stems from Christianity's relegation of the body to its inferior status as the imperfect vessel for the soul. That orthodoxy opened the way for human dissections and the foundations of anatomical knowledge.[32] It also casts knowledge as something discovered within nature (rather than being a divine revelation), derived from subjective experience, or located within the practical experiences of doing, being, belonging, and becoming through occupation.

The authority that doctors of medicine enjoy derives from medical discourse, which constructs knowledge about the human body and its various disorders as objective biological realities. It is made visible when patients perceive their diagnosis as legitimizing that "something is wrong"[42] rather than them being lazy, hypochondriacal, or feigning illness to avoid work or receive some other benefit. That authority can render patients compliant, passive, or involuntary recipients of medical interventions rather than competent self-carers consulting with a health practitioner.[43] In addition, medical authority largely silences input about occupation, apart from the following:

- Gathering factual data about causation, such as drinking unsafe water or falling from scaffolding.
- Providing some diagnostic utility. For example in mental health contexts, educational and occupational problems are specified on axis IV of the *Diagnostic and Statistical Manual of Mental Disorders*.[44]

As Foucault's analysis of power in modern societies reveals, medical discourse not only legitimizes medical advice and interventions, it also influences patients' identity, and the experience of being diseased.[45] At the same time, it diverts attention from social and cultural constructs that shape the subjective experience of illness and the physical, mental, social, and occupational responses and restrictions illness generates. Medical discourse tends to overlook how public recognition of being ill endows an individual with a social role of suffering from an illness, hence deserving support to accomplish necessary occupations and meet survival and sustenance needs.[45,46]

Table 3-2

INSTANCES OF LONGEVITY RECORDED IN THE BOOK OF GENESIS[47]

Biblical Figure	Reported Lifespan (years)
Adam	930
Seth	912
Enosh	905
Kenan	910
Mahalalel	895
Jared	962
Enoch	365
Methusaleh	969
Lamech	777
Noah	950

Extracted from Gruman GJ. History of Ideas about the Prolongation of Life: the Evolution of Prolongevity Hypotheses to 1800. *Transactions of the American Philosophical Society.* 1966;56(9):5-97.

HUMAN LONGEVITY

Examination of long-held assumptions about human longevity reveals other aspects of how medicine displaced knowledge of occupation's impact on health. As noted in Chapter 2, longevity refers to the maximum lifespan humans might achieve, as opposed to life expectancy which refers to the average age at death. It is a significant concept, because it frames expectations of the ultimate purpose of medicine: prolonging human life, irrespective of capacity to engage in meaningful occupation, versus keeping people healthy until the end of their natural lifespan. The waxing and waning of those opposing outcomes is chronicled by Gerald Gruman, who was an Assistant Professor at the University of Massachusetts. His text, *History of Ideas about the Prolongation of Life: The Evolution of Prolongevity Hypotheses to 1800,* remains an authoritative source on these contradictory trains of thought.[47] Prolongevity, which refers to ideas about significantly extending human life, appears in classical and Taoist thought, as well as in Biblical references to individuals who achieved advanced long life (Table 3-2).

Longevity appears in various guises, ranging from people who are physically decrepit but enjoying great wisdom and joy to those who are eternally fit and able to engage in youthful activities. Its proponents not only draw inspiration from fables of a golden age, when people lived happy and productive lives spanning many centuries, they also debate ideas about an elixir, precious gem, ceremony, fire, or charm that confers a long life, somewhat akin to the legendary fountain of youth. The Western idea of progress restored faith in the human ability to triumph over natural forces that led to decrepitude. For example, Descartes devoted much of his time to the medical sciences and anticipated a cure for senescence:

> We could free ourselves from an infinity of maladies of body as well as mind, and perhaps also even from the debility of old age, if we had ample knowledge of their causes, and of all the remedies provided for us by nature.[48]

In a later work, Descartes made an explicit occupational link, suggesting the possibility of not only curing and preventing diseases, but also of the "retardation of aging" through modifying activity patterns.[49] Francis Bacon (1561-1626) also included an occupational focus in promoting exercise to improve the absorption of food in his specifications for achieving longevity that he held as medicine's "most noble goal."[49]

Speculation about medical prolongation of life has continued through the centuries, with Benjamin Franklin (1706-1790) recorded as one proponent of medicine's final triumph over senescence. Some have argued that rather than medical expertise, it is being busy, active, cheerful and benevolent that are the keys to resisting organic disease and prolonging life. Perhaps the clearest links between occupation and population health were offered by Condorcet (1743-1794), a French mathematician, historian, and social reformer, who identified the anxieties and overwork of the poor and the indolent lifestyle of the rich to be the primary causes of disease. He foresaw that perfection of human's physical faculties (strength, dexterity, etc) through genetic inheritance, medical advances, and social and political reform of people's occupational possibilities and demands would bring about indefinite increases in human life.[47] Of those possibilities, current attempts to increase the human lifespan have been largely confined to genetic and dietary manipulations of laboratory animals. Perhaps that is because experiments involving the manipulation of occupation are too complex, demanding observation over a long period. Alternatively, the attraction of an elixir holds sway in having no occupational or lifestyle demands. The lack of serious efforts to generate evidence of occupation's capacity to prolong health into advanced old age might also be attributable to widespread acceptance of the biblical assumption of man's allotted span of "three score years and ten." A Google search of the phrase returned approximately 25,700,000 hits. The first few pages of hits encompassed Christian and Jewish websites quoting Psalm 90, "the years of our life are seventy, or even by reason of strength eighty,"[50] as well as dictionaries and encyclopedias, blogs, talk shows, popular literature, photo sharing sites, and archival material. In the absence of hard evidence of longevity achieved through healthful occupational patterns and choices, faith in future medical breakthroughs remains strong. That belief holds despite many interventions intended to prolong life being ineffective or iatrogenic and technologies to keep people alive outstripping ethical and humanistic reasoning about whether living additional years with an increasing burden of ill health is a valued goal.

The Prominence of the Medical Model

In addition to referring to the scientific methods used to extend knowledge of disease, the term *medical model* is used to mean the problem-solving approach and set of procedures that doctors of medicine are trained to use. Those procedures are characterized by taking a medical history to elicit symptoms; performing tests and an examination to identify the biological signs of ill health; determining a diagnosis of the causative disease, condition, or syndrome; defining its treatment using pharmacotherapy and other biologically based interventions; and determining a prognosis, both with and without treatment.[51]

Medical advances are generally credited with the profound demographic shift currently occurring, when a rapidly increasing proportion of the population living in postindustrial environments survive beyond age 70 years. The considerable decline in infant mortality and childhood illnesses recorded in high-income countries over the last half century is also attributed to medicine. However, medicine's failure to arrest the marked increase in noncommunicable diseases attributable to unhealthy lifestyles, such as some cancers, diabetes mellitus, dementia, cardiovascular and respiratory disease, stress-related disorders, and mental illnesses, poses questions.[52] It is debatable as to what extent the demographic changes are due solely to medical advances, even in combination with increased health spending. Indeed, some point to the role of increased affluence delivering better sanitation and water quality, warmer houses, increased access to refrigeration, improved food processing and handling practices, safer workplaces, and fewer people engaged in back-breaking physical labor. Notwithstanding that debate, biomedicine has become institutionalized in both health systems and as the predominant folk model of health and ill health in Western societies.[32,43,53]

The pervasiveness of a medical perspective of health is apparent at the highest level and has been so for more than three-quarters of a century. The prevention of illness through medical intervention was the primary concern of the League of Nation's Health Organisation, the WHO's antecedent. Article 23 of its Covenant stipulated that state members "will endeavour to take steps in matters of international concern for the prevention and control of disease."[54] This built on the work of the International Conference of Health Experts that took place in 1920, which had determined that the science of hygiene was "making rapid strides."[54] The International Conference on Primary Health Care convened in Kazakhstan in 1978 took a broader perspective of health. It addressed the problem of meeting people's basic health needs[55] through a combined approach of "promotive, preventive, curative, and rehabilitative services."[56] The Declaration of Alma Ata, created by the representatives of 134 nations who attended that meeting, sets forth a vision for "health for all the people of the world." In defining primary health care, the Declaration of Alma Ata identified "biomedical and health services research and public health experience" as key sources of knowledge. It also specified that:

> *education concerning prevailing health problems and the methods of preventing and controlling them; ... safe water and basic sanitation; maternal and child health care ... immunization against the major infectious diseases; prevention and control of locally endemic diseases; appropriate treatment of common diseases and injuries; and provision of essential drugs.*[56]

These would be delivered and coordinated by a health team comprising physicians, nurses, and midwives, along with traditional healers, auxiliaries, and community workers as part of a comprehensive national health system.[57] For the most part, government bodies have focused on providing access to the appropriate treatment for common diseases and injuries and the availability of essential drugs to meet the absence of illness message of the Declaration, thus promoting improved access to medical services in preference to other more generic services that should be part and parcel of primary health care. This has been at the expense of political and corporate occupation-focused efforts to improve the housing, town planning, food production, transport, education, and employment sectors[58] and to coordinate endeavors to reduce occupational risk factors or, alternatively, to increase health through increased understanding that what people do in their daily lives is an important factor.

CRITIQUE OF THE MEDICAL MODEL

The medical model—as both the scientific process and the practice of medicine—has been the subject of much critique. Most vehement is that voiced in psychiatry. In 1961 Szasz, an early protagonist, asserted that "mental health is a myth" because psychiatric conditions do not align with the contemporary definition of a disease. On that basis, he urged the relegation of psychiatric practice to the new field of behavioral science, which would address the needs of people with "problems of living."[32] A decade later, that assertion was supported by psychiatrist R. D. Laing.[59] He argued that because the diagnoses of mental illness are based on a person's behavior and performance in various occupational realms rather than physical pathology, they contravene established medical procedures and fall outside the bounds of the medical model.[59] Opponents of that perspective believe that biochemical or neurophysiological causes of major mental illnesses will ultimately be discovered. This debate has continued over decades, but medical dominance has resulted in the problems of living experienced by people with mental health issues being given less consideration than biochemical anomalies.

At an individual level, medicine has been accused of failing to take account of the person with the disease.[45] That includes failing to appreciate their suffering, agency, and resistance to the illness experience and failing to understand how their activities may have contributed to ill health, acted to preserve well-being despite disease processes, or created the context in which recovery or further decline will ensue. Similarly, medicine is seen to fall short of recognizing the contribution of sociocultural, political, and historical circumstances to disease prevalence, severity, and outcomes, including those of an occupational nature. In 1970, Engel's biopsychosocial approach was an early response to such criticisms but has largely failed to gain traction in the medical sciences.[32] For example, rather than addressing the economic, social, and geographic barriers to healthy occupations that helped create addictions or obesity, medicine instead attempts to treat individuals so disadvantaged with standardized clinical interventions. Similarly, the appalling statistics about the prevalence of mental health issues among American school students reveals the problem with taking a biomedical approach, which is typified by waiting for individuals to present with a diagnosable disorder and then be brought to the attention of a highly trained professional. The delay, the expense, and the shortage of suitably qualified people ensure that only a tiny proportion of individuals receive treatment, and that service provision is largely ineffective.[60] The lack of success can be attributed to failure in initiating preventative environmental and occupational interventions that could be put in place by teachers and parents, perhaps assisted by in situ consultation or training from a suitably trained health professional.

In relation to broad understandings of health, biomedicine can also be critiqued for not providing sufficient explanation of who gets sick and who stays healthy. For example, research concentrating on why people succumb to unhealthy lifestyles and habits or continue to work in jobs that harm their health is necessary but rare, even though the final report of the WHO Commission on the Social Determinants of Health maintained that:

> Social justice is a matter of life and death. It affects the way people live, their consequent chance of illness, and their risk of premature death. We watch in wonder as life expectancy and good health continue to increase in parts of the world and in alarm as they fail to improve in others.[61]

A WHO press release at the time reported how "inequities are killing people on a grand scale":

> (The) toxic combination of bad policies, economics, and politics is, in large measure responsible for the fact that a majority of people in the world do not enjoy the good health that is biologically possible.[62]

In various part of the world, organizations not directly involved in providing health services have picked up on aspects of the report. An example from the Queensland Council of Social Service in Australia is a case in point:

> Addressing health inequalities also requires action across all areas affecting the health of the population, including investment in early childhood development, education and employment, housing and a good standard of living for all people. Action in these areas has been sporadic and lacking in cohesion.[63]

The social determinants address aspects that include occupations across many life domains. The importance of considering the latter separately as well as part of social determinants is to clarify health needs in terms of the occupational nature of all people and to obtain social conditions that support health-giving activity and development.

An occupational component hovers at the edges of many of the critiques, which amplify concerns about humans' need to engage in all of life's activities that meet their inherent needs and capacities. For example, Illich argued that "transforming pain, illness, and death from a person problem into a technical" one is a denial of humanity because it disregards the sense people make of their own experiences.[64] The humanity revealed through occupation performed despite pain or chronic ill-health that modern medicine cannot cure is an important part of understanding the human condition, yet medical perspectives focusing on isolating the cause or treating the symptoms dominate the discourse. Equally, consideration of the complex interplay of personal, environmental, psychological, physiological, and occupational factors that gives rise to ill health is all but swept away by the reductionist scientific presumption that diseases are basically mono-causal.[65] Limitations in diagnostic procedures, especially the inability to directly measure pain, are also problematic. The authenticity of health conditions for which there are no diagnostic tests (such as fibromyalgia syndrome, irritable bowel syndrome, and multiple chemical sensitivity) has been hotly contested,[66] regardless of the undeniable disruption these conditions impose on daily life. That stance impedes the development of effective medical interventions and knowledge of the ways occupation might be contributing or altered to manage troublesome symptoms. Sociologists have also observed that medical advice frequently reinforces cultural stereotypes, perhaps particularly the role and proper conduct of women.[45] In addition, medical research and technological advances, such as new drugs and high-powered medical interventions, are expensive and geared toward tertiary prevention, perhaps at the expense of primary and secondary endeavors.[43] That is, precious funds are channeled into promoting life, possibly artificially, and perhaps beyond the ability of recipients to engage in activities that made life meaningful. An alternative might be funding toward societal change that would facilitate access to occupations that promote health.

Ironically, occupational medicine is, as mentioned in the previous chapter, the oldest branch of public health.[67-70] Historically, the focus of occupational medicine has been on illness resulting from paid employment, and the prevailing public health interest reflects this limited focus, mirroring contemporary societal, political, and economic value given to that type of occupation above others.[71] It is clear from the previous chapter that occupational medicine remains biased in that direction with most other forms of human activity being considered as social determinants. Such bifurcation prevents a truly holistic perspective of the relationship between health and the combinations of all that people do.

MEDICAL PRACTICE INFLUENCING OCCUPATION

The domination of the psychological and anatomical emphasis of the medical model has several consequences in relation to the occupations of patients, people with disabilities, the population at large, and doctors themselves. Medical histories are narrowly attuned to the symptoms that might assist with diagnosis rather than the challenges ill health presents in daily living. The virtual absence of occupational perspectives persists despite patients reporting declines in performance or discomfort associated with activity, such as increased breathlessness, pain, or fatigue, that alerted them that all was not well. Equally obscured is the fact that withdrawal from occupation is a common response to ill-health, or that people have to recuperate and manage symptoms in the context of ongoing occupational demands.

The ideal of patients as blameless victims of a pathogenic process[72] can be at odds with some cultural perceptions, in that certain illnesses are stigmatized because of the nature of the symptoms or perceptions of the kind of person that typically contracts the disorder.[73,74] Any avoidance, recoiling, fear, or ostracism born of stigma has direct occupational consequences. For example, people with mental illness have high unemployment rates and people with psoriasis report being ordered out of public swimming pools on the mistaken assumption that they are infectious. Applying a diagnostic label to troublesome manifestations of ill-health can also disempower caregivers. Perceiving themselves to lack relevant medical knowledge and expertise, they are less likely to identify helpful things they might do or to persist if their efforts are not immediately successful.[60]

The authority given to medicine can have occupational consequences for other health professionals. Occupational therapists, nurses, and others working in highly medicalized spheres report that their actions are influenced and largely controlled by the dominant medical view held in their workplaces.[43] Despite the channeling of attention, a few health professionals are discovering that an occupational perspective can usefully inform prescriptions for health. For example, an investigation of the risk factors for musculoskeletal injury of mothers of young children confirmed that lifting infants in and out of baths, cots, and car seats is often a causative factor that requires attention and education.[75]

Another consequence of the importance given to the biomedical view is the way the lack of ability to successfully engage in occupations is framed as a biological dysfunction and described as a disability, which is understood to be a personal rather than a societal issue. It accrues a range of disadvantages, including decreased quality of life and increased costs of living. People with disabilities are perceived to need management by trained health professionals, including intervention and rehabilitation aimed at normalizing their functioning and participation in society through environmental modifications, skill development, and, in some cases, vocational support.[45] The medical model of disability has been critiqued as misdirecting the majority of the available funding to the medicalized healthcare system. An alternative approach would be investing in efforts or services outside medicine to promote inclusion or universal design to give people access to the occupations already available in their community.

Health is so complex that not all factors that endanger or enhance it have been established. This includes the study of the determinants or outcomes of people's wide-ranging occupations—of all that they do and strive to become. Medicine's impotence in taking an occupational perspective, particularly in some instances, is not surprising given the lack of political support in addressing the occupational risk factors and societal determinants giving rise to or compounding disorders. While the South Australian Department of Health, for example, recognizes many of the direct risk factors, the underlying occupational influences are not made clear:

> The individual behaviours and lifestyle choices that we make for ourselves are markedly influenced and impacted upon by our education, literacy levels, inclusion within society and socioeconomic position. Factors such as smoking, drinking and using illicit drugs are obvious choices that individuals make that impact greatly on their experience of health and well-being both in the short and longer term. The decision to use tobacco, alcohol and/or illicit drugs is often socially patterned by an individual's socioeconomic position. In fact, smoking behaviour is connected to the social gradient with people on the lower rungs of the gradient having the poorest smoking related health outcomes.[76]

The medical model focus on healing gives it an unambiguous perspective of health: that it equates to the absence of illness. That, along with medicine's popular acclaim and political influence, may account for the lack of emphasis generally given to physical, mental, and social well-being and the occupational determinants of health.

Contemporary Priorities

Avoiding illness shapes contemporary understandings of health risks and the health messages and actions stimulated by the WHO to address the world's most pressing health concerns. That occurs despite recognition that unplanned urbanization, globalization, and population aging are the driving force of global health.[77] In this final section of the chapter, four broad contemporary health priorities with a clear relationship to occupation are addressed: noncommunicable diseases, population aging, poverty, and HIV/AIDS.

NONCOMMUNICABLE DISEASES

One of the most important health concerns is the decrease in levels of physical activity, which is the fourth leading risk factor for global mortality and equates to 6% of deaths globally.[78] Inactivity is explicitly an occupational risk factor and, along with smoking and low fiber/high fat diets, is a

Table 3-3

ACTIVITY TYPES TO REDUCE HEALTH RISKS[81]

Age Group	Age-Specific Health Benefit	World Health Organization Activity Recommendation
Children and youth	Muscle endurance and strength, bone health, improved cardiorespiratory and metabolic biomarkers, lower body fat, reduced symptoms of anxiety and depression	Play, games, active modes of transport, recreation, sport, physical education and exercise, climbing trees, using playground equipment, running and jumping, pushing and pulling things
Adults (age 18 to 64 years)	Reduced risk of hip and vertebral fracture and osteoporosis, muscle mass, intrinsic neuromuscular activation, enhanced metabolic health	Walking and cycling integrated into daily lifestyle, sports and games, planned exercise, physically active occupations in the course of work and leisure
Older adults (age 65 years and older)	Cognitive functioning, "functional ability," decreased risk of falls, improved biomarker profile, healthier body mass and composition, enhanced bone health	Walking and cycling, leisure time physical activity, work (if still engaged in this occupation), planned exercise, games and sport, play, household chores

Adapted from World Health Organization. *Global Recommendations on Physical Activity for Health.* Geneva: WHO; 2010.

major factor in the development of the lifestyle diseases now affecting low-, medium-, and high-income countries. Regular participation in moderate- and vigorous-intensity physical occupations is advanced as reducing the risk of type-2 diabetes, hypertension, stroke and cardiovascular disease, colon and breast cancer, and depression. It also assists with weight control. Evidence of the link between inactivity and the development of noncommunicable diseases has been irrefutably established by medical science. In the 1980s, the etiology of lifestyle disorders was explained in terms of excess production of stress hormones cortisol and catecholamines, leading to cholesterol buildup, artery damage, and heart disease.[79,80] When "our responses to problems in life are excessive or deficient ... the balance is upset between us and our resident pathogens" because "the central nervous system and hormones act on our immune defences (sic) in such a way that the microbes aid and abet disease."[79]

To reduce the burden of diseases attributable to inactivity, the WHO has advised national policy makers that people require physical exertion "above and beyond the physical activity accumulated in the course of normal daily nonrecreational activities."[81] That advice applies to children, youth, adults, and older people irrespective of disability, "gender, race, ethnicity, or income level."[81] People of different ages are identified as accruing somewhat different biomedical health benefits and are expected to engage in different kinds of physically demanding occupations (Table 3-3). Aside from active modes of transport, such as walking and cycling, occupations suggested by the WHO are predominantly play or discretionary leisure activities. More productive choices, such as digging a garden, stacking firewood, or heavy household chores, are absent, although physically demanding work is listed. The WHO advises that for people of all ages, occupation needs to ensure sufficient aerobic exercise but also address strength, flexibility, and balance. It is best undertaken in the context of daily family, school, and community activities. The idea of participating in physically demanding occupations with others is apparently informed by the knowledge that "lifestyles are social practices and ways of living adopted by individuals that reflect personal, group, and socio-economic identities."[82]

In addition to concern about people's increasingly sedentary daily occupations, the WHO identified that being overweight or obese is the sixth leading risk for global mortality, killing at least 3.4 million people each year.[83] As defined medically, obesity is a body mass index of 30 kg/m^2 or

Table 3-4

GLOBAL OBESITY STATISTICS[83]

Year	Statistics (Estimates)
Since 1980	Worldwide obesity has more than doubled
2008	1.5 billtion adults (20 years and older) overweight
	200 million men and nearly 300 million women obese
	10% of the world's adult population obsese
2010	Nearly 43 million children (under 5 years) overweight

Adapted from World Health Organization. *Obesity and overweight.* Fact Sheet No311. Reviewed 2014. Available at: http://www.who.int/mediacentre/factsheets/fs311/en/ Accessed May 17, 2014.

greater, which is a level of fat accumulation that may impair health. According to the WHO, the international prevalence of individuals who are overweight is alarming, with two thirds of the world's population living in countries where more people die as a result of being overweight than underweight (Table 3-4). Causative factors are energy-dense foods, urbanization, sedentary lifestyles, and an increasing use of transport options that do not require physical exertion.[83] Although not acknowledged in biomedical contexts, obesity can impair participation in occupations that involve any form of physical exertion. Standing up, walking, bending, carrying, pulling or pushing things, and going up and down stairs can all become uncomfortable or physiologically distressing.[84] Moreover, it is known that obese children have an increased likelihood of becoming obese adults. That outcome is not surprising given the likely impact of breathlessness, increased risk of fractures, and the psychological impact of obesity on participation in physically demanding occupations. In low- and middle-income countries, obesity can coexist with infectious diseases and inadequate nutrition from high-fat, high-sugar, high-salt, and micronutrient-poor foods. Those food choices are typically cheaper[83] and, from an occupational perspective, generally require less effort and expense to acquire and prepare.

Mental health conditions often occur alongside noncommunicable diseases. They are associated with a variety of psychological, biological, and social factors and can have profound occupational outcomes, including long-term unemployment. Poverty and low levels of participation in education are the clearest associations, along with persistent socioeconomic pressures, rapid social change, gender discrimination, human rights violations, social exclusion, stressful work situations, the risk of violence, and unhealthy lifestyles.[85] The global burden of disease is defined as years lived with disability and premature death. In 2004, it was estimated that 13% of the total global burden of disease is related to mental disorders.[86] The 2012 WHO global estimate was that there were 350 million people affected by a mental disorder.[87] By 2020, it is predicted that depression across all ages will be the second largest health issue.[88] Those figures represent substantial social and economic costs and an impediment to participation in healthful occupation. The WHO has urged governments to "reach out to people with mental disorders in the design of strategies and programs that include those people in education, employment, health, social protection and poverty reduction policies."[86] The impact of attitudinal barriers, such as stigma, which prevent "full and effective participation in society," is acknowledged, and the role of sectors outside health in the promotion of mental health is recognized but remains under resourced.

Mental and physical health and functioning are mutually influential, and medical research has clarified the pathways by which that association occurs. The first pathway is direct—through neuroendocrine, immune, and other physiological systems. Occupation-specific health behaviors, such as getting adequate sleep and exertion, not smoking, and having a healthy diet, provide a second pathway. Those pathways interact with each other and the social environment, such as when anxiety adversely affects immunological functioning or healthy exercise patterns are eroded by ongoing psychological stress. Specific identified pathways include depression and low self-esteem in young people, which is linked with binge drinking, smoking, unsafe sex, and eating disorders. In adults, social isolation is more prominently associated with depression.[89] The WHO Director-General has been requested to develop a comprehensive mental health action plan to protect the rights of people with mental disorders and assess the vulnerabilities and risks of developing mental disorders. Resolution EB130.R8, which calls for a comprehensive coordinated response from health and social sectors, urges governments to address the identification, care, treatment, and recovery of people with mental illness.[86]

A biomedical perspective is highly visible in calls to respond to the needs of people with mental health disorders. However, a 2014 WHO fact sheet on mental health promotes a range of intersectoral mental health promotion strategies.[87] Those include psychosocial interventions for preschoolers, minority groups, indigenous people, migrants, and those affected by a disaster; youth development and stress prevention programs; the socioeconomic empowerment of women; social support for older people; housing improvements; and community policing initiatives.[85] These initiatives hold promise for addressing the multiple occupational impacts of mental disorders, which helps people use their abilities, engage in productive work, and contribute to family and community.

POPULATION AGING

Population demographics have changed, particularly in high-income countries, with many more people expected to live to more than age 100 years. These are "undreamed of improvements in average life expectancy that have thrust aging to the forefront of attention."[90] First predicted by Fries in 1980,[91] the compression of morbidity into later adult years is attributed to life-style improvements affecting both the length and quality of many people's lives.[92] In low-income countries, population aging is occurring alongside the insidious development of noncommunicable diseases. However, concern has been expressed that older people's health care needs will demand an ever increasing proportion of already stretched medical resources. Addressing that concern is urgent because younger cohorts are unlikely to be as healthy when they reach advanced age, given the current international trends toward decreasing levels of physical activity and rapidly increasing obesity rates. Strategies to ensure that people of all ages maintain a healthy occupational balance throughout their lives must be put in place because chronic diseases and physical decline "originate in early life, develop insidiously," and can be prevented.[93]

Recognizing population aging as a global phenomenon, the WHO has asserted that:

> Failure to deal with the demographic imperative and rapid changes in disease patterns in a rational way in any part of the world will have socioeconomic and political consequences everywhere.[94]

It rejects conventional wisdom that more people living longer means an ever feebler elderly populace and is looking beyond conventional medicine to develop strategies that bring its approach to noncommunicable diseases and health promotion together. Effective responses demand international, national, regional, and local action to create the conditions in which people can construct a health sustaining pattern of daily occupations. That agenda must become a population health priority. To that end, the WHO's policy document *Active Aging* is guided by the United Nations' principles for older people that aim at independence, participation, care, self-fulfillment, and dignity.[94] The policy was developed by the WHO's Aging and Life Course Program as a contribution to the second United Nations World Assembly on Aging, held in April 2002 in Madrid. The Active Aging policy is an ongoing theme throughout this book because it lays the basis for many health-promoting initiatives of an occupational nature.

Table 3-5	
OCCUPATION IN THE MILLENNIUM DEVELOPMENT GOALS[99]	
Millennium Goal	Occupational Aspect
Goal 1	Eradicate extreme poverty and hunger
Target 1	Halve, between 1990 and 2015, the proportion of people is income is less than one dollar a day
Goal 2	Achieve universal primary education
Target 3	Ensure that, by 2015, children everywhere, boys and girls alike, will be able to complete
Goal 3	Promote gender equality and empower women
Target 4	Eliminate gender disparity in primary and secondary education, preferably by 2005, and to all levels of education no later than 2015
Goal 7	Ensure environmental sustainability
Target 9	Integrate the principles of sustainable development into country policies and programs and reverse the loss of environmental resources
Target 10	By 2015, halve the proportion of people without sustainable access to safe drinking water

Adapted from United Nations. Resolution adopted by the General Assembly. *United Nations Millennium Declaration.* A/Res/55/2. 2000. http://www.undp.org/content/undp/en/home/mdgoverview/. Accessed May 8, 2012.

POVERTY

The WHO quotes Kofi Annan as saying that "the biggest enemy of health in the developing world is poverty."[95] Speaking bluntly, it claims that "poverty creates ill-health because it forces people to live in environments that make them sick, without decent shelter, clean water, or adequate sanitation." Poverty is essentially occupational, being the lack of a means to earn a livelihood adequate to meet basic needs for nutrition, shelter, clothing, and education. It both causes and is caused by ill-health and is aggravated when the costs of health care exceeds a family's income. For the estimated 1.2 billion people who live on less than $1 per day, there are additional environmental risks, such as pollution from solid fuels, overcrowding, and unsafe sex.[95] In some parts of the world, ill-health can be related to an increase in violence and fundamentalism, social disintegration, and instability,[96] which further reduce access to education and health care. Poor people are known to have higher rates of communicable diseases, such as tuberculosis and acute respiratory infections, malaria, diarrheal diseases, and HIV/AIDS.[97] Maternal mortality, premature preventable death, and injuries are also prevalent, along with mental, social, and spiritual illness. Poverty is associated with a lack of dignity, self-respect, freedom, and power to voice opinions and wishes. Recognizing that poor people are often best placed to generate effective solutions to poverty, the WHO is urging governments to take a rights-based approach to address the needs of the poorest poor.[98] Poverty reduction is the first of eight development goals derived from the United Nations' Millennium Declaration, which was adopted in September 2000.[99] All eight goals are directly or indirectly related to health. Those with a more occupational focus are presented in Table 3-5.

The economic impact of disease related to poverty is recognized. Countries applying for debt relief and concessional lending from the World Bank and the International Monetary Fund are required to produce Poverty Reduction Strategy Papers and outline their program of actions to meet the specific needs of the poorest poor. However, a 2004 review of 21 completed Poverty Reduction Strategy Papers revealed that there was little focus on health and that where there was, health was not always targeted in ways or to regions that would reach people living in extreme poverty.[100] Strategies that were described most often targeted access to health services rather than vocational, educational, housing, or infrastructure developments that would enhance access to occupation and reduce health risks in the short or long term. Where provision of potable water and sanitation were included as goals, those interventions were most often not identified as health-related. Both the focus on health service provision and lack of recognition of the health impact of clean water and adequate sanitation reveal a medical understanding of health, in the narrowest sense of "health sector delivery of health services."[100] Looking beyond health services and sanitation, the occupations of poor people and the environments in which they live, learn, and find employment were ignored.

Poverty is also closely related to being overweight or obese and inactivity. Strategies that deal with all three are incorporated into the WHO 2008-2013 Action Plan for the Global Strategy for the Prevention and Control of Noncommunicable Diseases.[101] In that document, Dr. Ala Alwan, an Assistant Director General of the WHO, emphasized the need for urgent action to confront the issues:

> Noncommunicable disease prevention and control programs remain dramatically under-funded at the national and global levels and have been left off the global development agenda. Despite impacting the poorest people in low-income parts of the world and imposing a heavy burden on socioeconomic development, NCD prevention is currently absent from the Millennium Development Goals. However, in all low- and middle-income countries and by any measure, NCDs account for a large enough share of the disease burden of the poor to merit a serious policy response.[102]

Aiming to "reduce premature mortality and improve quality of life," the WHO 2008-2013 Action Plan has four focuses for action by member states:

1. Monitoring the health burden of noncommunicable diseases.
2. Developing social and economic policies to reduce poverty.
3. Ensuring that policy development receives a cross-sectoral response.
4. Implementing programs that target the social determinants, particularly as they affect health in early childhood, the urban poor, and equitable access to primary health care services.[101]

The promotion of those four specific actions is aimed toward the reorientation and strengthening of national health systems. However, their capacity to respond effectively must be in doubt given the World Health Report 2006 estimate of a global deficit of health professionals, with critical shortages in sub-Saharan Africa in particular.[103] There are also specifics about tobacco control and promoting a healthy diet and physical activity. An occupational component is visible in strategies such as providing nutritional information to consumers, school-based physical activity programs, and physical environments in which it is safe to walk, cycle, play, and engage in leisure pursuits. Strengthening that focus would help avert the development of health conditions requiring medical intervention.

HIV/AIDS

Although people living in poverty are especially at risk for contracting HIV/AIDS, it affects every strata of society. Approximately 80% of young people who are HIV-positive live in sub-Saharan Africa, with women outnumbering men by a ratio of approximately 2:1. In 2000, HIV/AIDS became the leading cause of death from an infectious disease and by 2012 approximately 14.8 million children living in sub-Saharan Africa had lost one or both parents to AIDS.[104] In Africa, the occupational impacts have been profound. Of necessity, grandparents and siblings have assumed the custody and care of orphaned children. For those living in poverty, the economic and emotional burden could be overwhelming.[105] The ill-effects of HIV/AIDS include the reduced capacity or access to work due to stigma, the ongoing cost of advanced treatment regimes, and the burden of providing care over a 7- to 10-year period if treatment is not available. The socioeconomic costs include the loss of millions of adults from the workforce, as well as the diminished economic return from providing publicly funded higher education because of the proportion of graduates who are HIV-positive. Add to those the burden of grief and fear associated with the disease, criminal activity to fund healthcare,[106] and the increased incidence of rape of very young girls in the mistaken belief that it will effect a cure.

In response to the scale of the problem, the WHO's Millennium Development Goals include combating HIV/AIDS and other infectious diseases. Progress in reducing new infection rates in adults is promising, with a 19% reduction from 2000. Additionally, in the 15 to 24 age group, the reduction over the same period has been 25%.[107] Not surprisingly, a biomedical focus on prevention, intervention, and the need for efficient, effective, and comprehensive health services dominates the literature. Issues of discrimination, stigmatization, and intimate partner violence are discussed in relation to access to health services, particularly for sex workers, men who have sex with men, and transgender people. However, the occupational concerns given attention are the accidental infection of health workers and the development of housing, employment, education, immigration, and social welfare policy to avoid negative consequences for people with HIV. The sexual and reproductive rights of people with HIV are defended. However, existing difficulties with access to employment and education do not appear to rate consideration.

Conclusion

The allure of evidence generated by scientific methods and the successes achieved through identifying and defeating pathogens has led to the health discourse being dominated by medicine. Over the past century, preventative and curative technologies have come to define what health is for both the general public and the agencies charged with improving population health. It is hardly surprising that health care is aimed mainly at treating medically defined physical or mental ills. That singular focus has displaced established insights into occupation's role in maintaining health and effectively rendered us blind to the real health impacts of the noncommunicable diseases arising from modern lifestyles.

Although knowledge of the interrelationship between ill-health and occupation has been handed down since antiquity, a medicalized perspective of health has acted as a deterrent to action on the WHO's broader mandate for health as arising from the way people live. Just as in the Classical world, we are in the midst of a conflict between the opposing views of healing and health. It is confusing because both are valuable and both are on the same side. However, with the increasing costs of medical advances alongside medicine's ambiguous contribution to keeping people well, questions need to be asked about the priorities across the globe. Poverty, noncommunicable diseases, HIV/AIDS, and the aging population all point to the need for broadly focused political, social, and occupational responses to threats to population health. The WHO attempts to do so, but that raises a second question about whether the most powerful forces for health in postmodern societies listen to and follow its directives to significantly change:

> [A] few, largely preventable, risk factors [that] account for most of the world's disease burden ... reflect[ing] a significant change in diet habits, physical activity levels and tobacco use worldwide as a result of industrialization, urbanization, economic development, and increasing food market globalization.[108]

References

1a.   World Health Organization. *The Global Strategy on Diet, Physical Activity and Health.* 2003. www. who.int/dietphysicalactivity/media/en/gsfs_general.pdf. Accessed May 3, 2012.

1b.   Thase ME, Jindal R, Howland RH. Biological aspects of depression. In: Gotlib IH, Hammen CL. *Handbook of Depression.* London: Guilford Press; 2002.

2.   Ill health. (n.d.). WordNet® 3.0. Dictionary.com. http://dictionary.reference.com/browse/ill health. Accessed April 20, 2012.

3.   Illness. (n.d.). Dictionary.com Unabridged. http://dictionary.reference.com/browse/illness. Accessed April 20, 2012.

4.   Illness. (2008). Encyclopedia Britannica, Inc. http://dictionary.reference.com/browse/illness. Accessed April 19, 2012.

5.   Friel JP, ed. *Dorlands Illustrated Medical Dictionary,* 25th ed. Philadelphia: W.B.Saunders; 1974:763.

6.   Boyd KM. Disease, illness, sickness, health, healing and wholeness: exploring some elusive concepts. *Med Humanities.* 2000;26:9-17. doi:10.1136/mh.26.1.9

7.   Landau SI, chief ed. *Funk & Wagnalls Standard Desk Dictionary.* Vol 1: A-M. USA: Harper & Row, Publishers, Inc; 1984:319.

8.   Coulson J, Carr CT, Hutchinson L, Eagle D, eds. *The Standard English Desk Dictionary.* Sydney: Bay Books; 1976:419.

9.   Baral SC, Karki DK, Newell JN. Causes of stigma and discrimination associated with tuberculosis in Nepal: a qualitative study. *BMC Public Health.* 2007;7:211-219. doi:10.1186/1471-2458-7-211

10.   Shah P, Mountain D. The medical model is dead–long live the medical model. *British Journal of Psychiatry.* 2007;191:375-377. doi:10:1192/bjp.bp.107.037242

11.   World Health Organization. Leprosy: urgent need to end stigma and isolation. WHO Media Centre; 2003. http://www.who.int/mediacentre/news/releases/2003/pr7/en/index.html. Accessed April 15, 2012.

12.   World Health Organization. Mental health: advocacy. 2012. http://www.who.int/mental_health/advocacy/en/. Accessed April 15, 2012.

13a. Conrad P, Barker KK. The social construction of illness: key insights and policy implications. *Journal of Health as Social Behavior.* 2010;51(S):S67-S79.

13b. Ailment. (n.d.). *Collins English Dictionary - Complete & Unabridged.* 10th ed. Dictionary.com website: http://dictionary.reference.com/browse/ailment. Accessed April 20, 2012.

13c. Affliction. (n.d.). *Dictionary.com Unabridged.* Dictionary.com website: http://dictionary.reference.com/browse/affliction. Accessed April 20, 2012.

13d. Affliction. (n.d.). *Collins English Dictionary - Complete & Unabridged.* 10th ed. Dictionary.com website: http://dictionary.reference.com/browse/affliction. Accessed April 20, 2012.

13e. Debility. (n.d.). *Dictionary.com Unabridged.* Dictionary.com website: http://dictionary.reference.com/browse/debility. Accessed April 20, 2012.

13f. Disorder. (n.d.). *Dictionary.com Unabridged.* Dictionary.com website: http://dictionary.reference.com/browse/disorder. Accessed April 20, 2012.

13g. Disorder. (n.d.). *The American Heritage® Stedman's Medical Dictionary.* Dictionary.com website: http://dictionary.reference.com/browse/disorder. Accessed April 20, 2012.

13h. Poorly. *The Free Dictionary.* Farlax. (n.d.). http://www.thefreedictionary.com/poorly. Accessed April 20, 2012.

13i. Indisposition. (n.d.). *Dictionary.com Unabridged.* Dictionary.com website: http://dictionary.reference.com/browse/indisposition. Accessed April 20, 2012.

13j. Indisposition. (n.d.). *Collins English Dictionary - Complete & Unabridged.* 10th ed. Dictionary.com website: http://dictionary.reference.com/browse/indisposition. Accessed April 20, 2012.

13k. Infirmity. (n.d.). *Merriam-Webster Dictionary.* Retrieved April 19, 2012, from www.merriam-webster.com/dictionary/infirmity. Accessed April 20, 2012.

13l. Infirmity. (n.d.). *The American Heritage® Stedman's Medical Dictionary.* Dictionary.com website: http://dictionary.reference.com/browse/infirmity. Accessed April 20, 2012.

13m. Infirmity. (n.d.). *Collins English Dictionary - Complete & Unabridged.* 10th ed. Dictionary.com website: http://dictionary.reference.com/browse/infirmity. Accessed April 20, 2012.

13n. Malady. (n.d.). *Dictionary.com Unabridged.* Dictionary.com website: http://dictionary.reference.com/browse/malady. Accessed April 20, 2012.

13o. Malady. (n.d.). *Online Etymology Dictionary*. Dictionary.com website: http://dictionary.reference.com/ browse/malady. Accessed April 20, 2012.

13p. Sickness. (n.d.). *Dictionary.com Unabridged*. Dictionary.com website: http://dictionary.reference.com/ browse/sickness. Accessed April 20, 2012.

14. *Collins Thesaurus of the English Language*. 2nd ed. San Francisco, Calif: HarperCollins Publishers; 2002.

15. Preamble to the Constitution of the World Health Organization as adopted by the International Health Conference, New York, 19-22 June, 1946; signed on 22 July 1946 by the representatives of 61 States. Official Records of the World Health Organization. 2:100.

16. Brown L, ed. *The New Shorter English Dictionary*. Oxford: Clarendon Press; 1993.

17. Carter JB. Disease and death in the nineteenth century: a genealogical perspective. *The National Genealogical Society Quarterly*. 1988;76:289-301.

18. King James Bible. 1769. Luke 7:21, Romans 8:26, Corinthians 12:9. http://www.kingjamesbibleonline. org/. Accessed April 19, 2012.

19. McCaul G. Occupational therapy treatment for fractures. *Journal of the Association of Occupational Therapists*. 1944;7:15-18.

20. Plewes LW. Modern treatment of fractures, with particular emphasis on the rehabilitation aspect. *Occupational Therapy*. 1951;14(2):64-66.

21. Trueman C. History learning site: medicine and World War two. 2012. http://www.historylearning-site.co.uk/medicine_and_world_war_two.htm. Accessed April 29, 2012.

22. Vinas MS. Chronology of medical/technological advances. *PerfED International*.

23. Marquand H, Rt. Hon. Opening address. *Occupational Therapy*. 1951;14(4):190-196.

24. Smith MD. Occupational therapy in a spinal injury centre. *Journal of the Association of Occupational Therapists*. 1945;8(Spring):14-16.

25. Mabaso MLH, Sharp B, Lengeler C. Historical review of malarial control in southern Arfican with emphasis on the use of indoor residual house-spraying. *Tropical Medicine and International Health*, 2004;9(8):846-856.

26. Lindop E, Goldstein MJ. *America in the 1940s*. Minneapolis, MN: Twenty-First Century Books; 2010.

27. Clare AW. *Psychiatry in Dissent*. Travistock: Routledge; 1980.

28. Walsh JJ. Louis Pasteur. *Catholic Encyclopedia*. New York: Robert Appleton Company; 1913.

29. Waddington K. To stamp out "So terrible a malady": bovine tuberculosis and tuberculin testing in Britain. 1890-1939. *Med Hist*. 2004;48(1):29-48.

30. Harter J, editor. *Images of Medicine: A Definitive Volume of more than 4,800 Copyright-free Engravings Including Anatomy, General Medicine, Apothecary and Pharmaceutical, Diseases and Injuries, Therapeutics, Plus Medical Equipment, Instruments and Appliances*. New York: Bonanza Books; 1991.

31. Reductionism. Oxford dictionaries online. Oxford University Press; 2012. http://oxforddictionaries. com/definition/reductionism. Accessed April 15, 2012.

32. Engel GL. The need for a new medical model: a challenge for biomedicine. *Science*. 1977;196:129.

33. Department of Health and Human Services. *The Health Consequences of Smoking: Cancer*. Rockville, MD: 1982.

34. Department of Health and Human Services. *The Health Consequences of Smoking: Cardiovascular Disease*. Rockville, MD: 1983.

35. Department of Health and Human Services. *The Health Consequences of Smoking: Chronic Obstructive Lung Disease*. Rockville, MD: 1984.

36. Gordon T, Sorlie P, Kannel WB. Section 27, Coronary Heart Disease Atherothrombotic Brain Infarction. Intermittent Claudication. A Multivariate Analysis of Some Factors Related to Their Incidence: Framingham Study, 16 Year Follow Up. US Department of Health, Education and Welfare, Public Health Service. NIH Pub. No. 1740-0320, 1971.

37. Dubos R, ed. *Mirage of Health: Utopias, Progress and Biological Change*. New York: Harper and Row; 1959.

38. Dubos R, ed. *Mirage of Health: Utopias, Progress and Biological Change*. New York, NY: Harper and Row; 1959:138.

39. Cushing A. A piece of history: origin of the medical model. *Collegian*. 1999;6(1):4. PMID: 10401279

40. Dubos R, ed. *Mirage of Health: Utopias, Progress and Biological Change*. New York, NY: Harper and Row; 1959:139.

41. Powell JL, Owen T. The bio-medical model and aging: towards an anti-reductionist model? *The International Journal of Sociology and Social Policy*. 2005;25(9):27-40.

42. Chaufan C, Hollister B, Nazareno J, Fox P. Medical ideology as a double-edged sword: the politics of cure and care in the making of Alzheimer's disease. *Social Science and Medicine.* 2012;74:788-795. doi:10.1016/j.socscimed.2011.10.033

43. Allan JD, Hall BA. Challenging the focus on technology: a critique of the medical model in a changing health care system. *Advances in Nursing Science.* 1988;10(3):22-34.

44. American Psychiatric Association. Diagnostic and Statistical Manual of Mental Disorders, Fourth Edition - Text Revision (DSMIV-TR). Washington, DC: Author; 2000.

45. Conrad P, Barker KK. The social construction of illness: key insights and policy implications. *Journal of Health and Social Behavior.* 2010;51(S):S67-S79.

46. Marinker M. Why make people patients? *Journal of Medical Ethics.* 1975;1:84-84.

47. Gruman GJ. History of Ideas about the Prolongation of Life: the Evolution of Prolongevity Hypotheses to 1800. *Transactions of the American Philosophical Society.* 1966;56(9):5-97.

48. Gruman GJ. History of Ideas about the Prolongation of Life: the Evolution of Prolongevity Hypotheses to 1800. *Transactions of the American Philosophical Society.* 1966;56(9):78.

49. Gruman GJ. History of Ideas about the Prolongation of Life: the Evolution of Prolongevity Hypotheses to 1800. *Transactions of the American Philosophical Society.* 1966;56(9):80.

50. Bible. Psalm 90:10. English Standard Version: 2001.

51. Medical model. *Mosby's Medical Dictionary, 8th edition.* Elsevier; 2009. http://www.elsevierhealth.com.au.

52. Katz AH, Hermalin JA, Hess RE, eds. *Prevention and Health: Direction for Policy and Practice.* New York, NY: The Haworth Press; 1987.

53. Frank AW. Bringing bodies back in: a decade in review. *Theory, Culture and Society.* 1990;7(1):31-162.

54. League of Nations. Health Organization. Information Section. Geneva: 1931.

55. Black M. In Memory: EJR (Dick) Heyward 1914-2005. Quiet architect of UNICEF and international systems. *UNICEF Staff News.* 2005;3:25-32.

56. The Declaration of Alma-Ata. International Conference on Primary Health Care, Alma-Ata, USSR; 1978. www.who.int/hpr/NPH/docs/declaration_almaata.pdf. Accessed April 1, 2012.

57. Chan M. Return to Alma-Ata. *The Lancet.* 2008;372(9642):865-866.

58. World Health Organization. The Declaration of Alma-Ata. International Conference on Primary Health Care, Alma-Ata, USSR; 1998.

59. Laing RD. *The Politics of the Family and Other Essays.* London: Travistock Publications; 1971.

60. Gutkin TB. Ecological psychology: replacing the medical model paradigm for school-based psychological and psychoeducational services. *Journal of Educational and Psychological Consultation.* 2012;22:1-20.61.

61. World Health Organization. *Social Determinants of Health.* http://www.who.int/social_determinants/thecommission/finalreport/en/index.html.

62. Media Centre. World Health Organization. Inequities are Killing People on a Grand Scale, reports WHO's Commission. (Closing the Gap in a Generation: Health Equity through Action on the Social Determinants of Health.) http://www.who.int/mediacentre/news/releases/2008/pr29/en/in. Accessed April 7, 2012.

63. Queensland Council of Social Service. (QCOSS). Social Determinants of health. https://docs.google.com/viewer?a=v&q=cache:OUvTk0PLH2gJ:www.qcoss.org.au/content/april-2010 Accessed August 7, 2012.

64. Illich I. Medical nemesis. *Journal of Epidemiology & Community Health.* 1974/2003;57(12):919-923.

65. Shorter E. The history of the biopsychosocial approach in medicine: before and after Engel. In: White P, ed. *Biopsychosocial Medicine: An Integrated Approach to Understanding Illness.* Oxford: Oxford University Press; 2005:1-9.

66. Dumit J. Illness you have to fight to get: facts and forces in uncertain, emergent illnesses." *Social Science and Medicine.* 2006;62:577-590.

67. Bauer G. Agricola. In: *De re Metallica* 1556. Hoover HC, Hoover HL, trans. New York, NY: Dover Publications; 1950.

68. Paracelsus. *Four Treatises of Theophrastus von Hohenheim Called Paracelsus.* 1567. Sigerist HE, ed. Temkin CL, Rosen G, Zilboorg G, Sigerist HE, trans. Baltimore, MD: Johns Hopkins Press; 1941.

69. Ramazzini B. *Disease of Occupations.* New York, NY: Collier-MacMillan; 1980.

70. Thackrah CT. *The Effects of the Principle Arts, Trades, and Professions, and of Civic States and Habits of Living, On Health and Longevity.* London, England: Longman, Rees, Orme, Browne and Green; 1831.

71. Parmeggiani L, ed. *ILO Encyclopedia of Occupational Health and Safety.* 2 Vols. 3rd rev ed. Geneva, Switzerland: International Labour Organisation; 1983.

72. Hughes CC, Kennedy D. Beyond the germ theory: reflections on relations between medicine and the behavioral sciences. In: Ruffini J, ed. *Advances in Medical Social Science, vol. 1.* New York: Gordon and Breach; 1983:321-399.

73. Conrad P. The experience of illness: recent and new directions. *Research in the Sociology of Health Care.* 1987;6:1-31.

74. Marinker M. Why make people patients? *Journal of Medical Ethics.* 1975;1:81-84.

75. Vincent R, Hocking C. Factors that might give rise to musculoskeletal disorders when mothers lift children in the home. *Physiotherapy Research International.* 2013:18(2):81-90. doi:10.1002/pri.1530

76. Hetzel D, Page A, Glover J, Tennant S. *Inequality in South Australia: Key Determinations of Well-Being. Volume 1: The Evidence.* Adelaide: Department of Health (SA); 2004.

77. World Health Organization. *Global Recommendations on Physical Activity for Health.* Geneva: WHO; 2010.

78. Fact file: 10 facts on physical activity. World Health Organization. http://www.who.int/features/fact-files/physical_activity/facts/en/. Accessed on May 17 2014.

79. Justice B. *Who Gets Sick: Thinking and Health.* Texas: Peak Press; 1987:28-29,31-32,179.

80. Price VA. *Type A Behaviour Pattern: A Model for Research and Practice.* New York, NY: Academic Press; 1982.

81. World Health Organization. *Global Recommendations on Physical Activity for Health.* Geneva: WHO; 2010:18.

82. Al-Maskari F. Lifestyle diseases: an economic burden on health services. *UN Chronicle Online*; 2010.

83. World Health Organization. *Obesity and Overweight.* Fact Sheet No311. Reviewed 2014. Available at: http://www.who.int/mediacentre/factsheets/fs311/en/ Accessed May 17, 2014.

84. Wilson LH. Occupational consequences of weight loss surgery: a personal reflection. *Journal of Occupational Science.* 2010;17(1):47-54.

85. World Health Organization. *Fact sheet N°220: Mental Health: Strengthening our Response.* Updated April 2014. Available at: http://www.who.int/mediacentre/factsheets/fs220/en/. Accessed on May 17, 2014.

86. World Health Organization. *Global Burden of Mental Disorders and the Need for a Comprehensive, Coordinated Response from Health and Social Sectors at the Country Level* (EB 130.R8). 2012. Available at: http://www.who.int/mental_health/. Accessed on May 8, 2012.

87. *Depression. Fact sheet No369.* World Health Organization. Available at: http://www.who.int/media-centre/factsheets/fs369/en/. Accessed on May 17, 2014.

88. World Health Organization. *Mental Health: Depression.* 2012. Available at: http://www.who.int/men-tal_health/management/depression/definition/en/index.html. Accessed on May 8, 2012.

89. Herrman H, Saxena S, Moodie R. *Promoting Mental Health: Concepts, Emerging Evidence, Practice.* A report of the WHO Department of Mental Health & Substance Abuse. In collaboration with the Victorian Health Promotion Foundation & the University of Melbourne. 2005. Available at: http://www.who.int/mental_health/evidence/MH_Promotion_Book.pdf. Accessed on May 8, 2012.

90. McMurdo MET. A healthy old age: realistic or futile goal? *British Medical Journal.* 2000; 321:1149-1151.

91. Fries JF. Aging, natural death, and the compression of morbidity. *New England Journal of Medicine.* 1980;303:130-5.

92. Kalache A, Aboderin I, Hoskins I. Compression of morbidity and active aging: key priorities for public health policy in the 21st century. *Bulletin of the World Health Organization.* 2002;80(3).

93. World Health Organization. Health and aging: A discussion paper. Geneva: World Health Organization; 2001. Unpublished document WHO/NMH/HPS/01.1. In: Kalache A, Aboderin I, Hoskins I. Compression of morbidity and active aging: key priorities for public health policy in the 21st century. *Bulletin of the World Health Organization.* Geneva: World Health Organization; Accessed 2005. <Bull World Health Organvol.80no.3Genebra2002>.

94. World Health Organization's Aging and Life Course Programme. *Active Aging: A Policy Framework.* Madrid, Spain: Second United Nations World Assembly on Aging; 2002: 54.

95. World Health Organization. *Health and Development: Poverty and Health.* http://www.who.int/hdp/poverty/en/. Accessed on May 7, 2012.

96. Yach D. *Health and Illness: The Definition of the World Health Organization.* World Health Organization. http://www.who.int/. Accessed March 27, 2005.

97. World Health Organization. *Health for All in the Twenty-first Century.* Document A51/5. Geneva: World Health Organization; 1998.

98. World Health Organization. *Human Rights, Health and Poverty Reduction Strategies.* 2005. Available at: http://www.who.int/hhr/news/HRHPRS.pdf . Accessed May 3, 2012.

99. United Nations. Resolution adopted by the General Assembly. *United Nations Millennium Declaration.* A/Res/55/2. 2000. http://www.undp.org/content/undp/en/home/mdgoverview/. Accessed May 8, 2012.

100. World Health Organization. *Poverty Reduction Strategy Papers: Their Significance for Health: Second Synthesis Report.* 2004: 18. www.who.int/hdp/en/prsp.pdf. Accessed on May 3, 2012.

101. World Health Organization. *2008-2013 Action Plan for the Global Strategy for the Prevention and Control of Noncommunicable Diseases.* 2009. http://www.who.int/nmh/publications/9789241597418/en/index.html. Accessed May 8, 2012.

102. World Health Organization. *2008-2013 Action Plan for the Global Strategy for the Prevention and Control of Noncommunicable Diseases.* 2009: 5.

103. Debas HT. Global health: priority agenda for the 21st century. *UN Chronicle Online.* 2010. Available at: http://www.un.org/wcm/content/site/chronicle/home/archive/issues2010/achieving_global_health/globalhealth_priorityagendaforthe21stcentury. Accessed May 4, 2012.

104. HIV/AIDS. *One International.* 2012. http://www.one.org/c/international/issue/1118/?gclid=CPPPt6HM-bECFbBUpgodllUAVA. Accessed May 7, 2012.

105. Brodrick K. Grandmothers affected by HIV/AIDS: new roles and occupations. In: Watson R, Swartz L, eds. *Transformation Through Occupation.* London: Whurr Publishers; 233-253.

106. Coetzee Z, Swartz L. Fathers with HIV/AIDS: the struggle for occupation. In: Watson R, Swartz L. *Transformation Through Occupation.* London: Whurr Publishers; 119-128.

107. World Health Organization. *Global Health Sector strategy on HIV/AIDS 2011-2015.* 2011. Available at: www.who.int/hiv/pub/hiv_strategy/en/index.html. Accessed May 5, 2012.

108. World Health Organization. *The Global Strategy on Diet, Physical Activity and Health.* 2003. www.who.int/dietphysicalactivity/media/en/gsfs_general.pdf. Accessed May 3, 2012.

Section II

Occupation

Theme 4

"Changing patterns of life, work, and leisure have a significant impact on health. Work and leisure should be a source of health for people."

WHO: Ottawa Charter for
Health Promotion, 1986[1]

Chapter 4

AN OCCUPATIONAL THEORY OF HUMAN NATURE

This chapter addresses:
- Theories of Human Nature
- An Occupational Theory of Human Nature
  - Human Evolution and Occupation
    - Theories of Evolution
    - Occupation in Evolution
  - Important Characteristics that Help Create the Occupational Human
    - The Brain
    - Dexterity
    - Bipedal Gait and Upright Posture
    - Stereoscopic Vision
    - Complex Language
  - Changing Patterns of Occupation have a Significant Impact on Health
  - Diagnosis and Prescription
  - A Three-way Link Between Occupation, Health, and Survival
- Conclusion

The first section of the book has defined health and discussed it in relation to its historical and present priorities. This next section is about increasing understanding of occupation in relation to "all that people do" in their lives. The word *occupation* has been selected as the most appropriate to describe people's "doings." This choice is discussed at length in the following chapter because, despite its generic meaning, the word is often used to mean only paid employment, with other things that people do considered separately and often as being of less importance. A reductionist perspective of occupation as paid employment, as well as the fact that disparate professional groups study particular aspects of occupation as though they were discrete entities, prevents a holistic understanding of the relationship between doing and health. Therefore, because the vagaries of language offer alternative meanings of the word occupation, it is proposed here that the combination of all that people do throughout their lives is given inadequate attention, even though life itself is dependent on it.

Wilcock AA, Hocking C.
An Occupational Perspective of Health, Third Edition (pp 84-115).
© 2015 Taylor & Francis Group.

Figure 4-1. Obligatory and necessary, self-chosen, rest and sleep occupations for individual to global requirements.

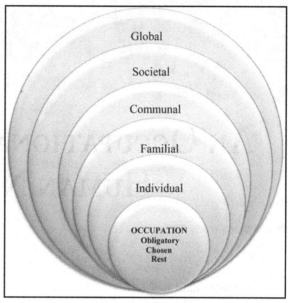

Global

Societal

Communal

Familial

Individual

OCCUPATION
Obligatory
Chosen
Rest

To draw attention to the centrality of the wide ranging occupational behavior performed by all people day by day and the fact that it is and has been a defining characteristic of humans throughout their species history, this chapter explores it in the form of a theory of human nature. This is based on the opinion that humans can be described as occupational beings, which is indisputable because all people do something all the time. To support life and maintain and enhance health, some occupations are necessary or obligatory, whereas others are chosen for particular purposes and to meet specific interests and abilities and the time spent on those is balanced with regular rest and sleep, usually occurring throughout each day. The obligatory or necessary, self-chosen, and rest and sleep occupations are performed according to individual, familial, communal, corporate, societal, and global requirements that change over time and differ from place to place (Figure 4-1). This is so because occupation provides the mechanism for people:

- To fulfill basic human needs essential for survival, including meet the active, resting, and sleep requirements for mind and body health.
- To develop and exercise genetically inherited capacities to experience physical, mental, and social well-being.
- To meet sociocultural needs and to contribute to and feel comfort and acceptance within family and community.
- To adapt to environmental conditions and environmental change.

As a counter to their active occupations, people require rest and sleep within a 24-hour continuum. Just as it is important for all of the things that people do to be considered collectively, so too is it important to recognize that active, restful, and sleep activities are integral parts of the occupation continuum. Recent research suggests that the amount of sleep necessary to function well in other aspects of occupation differs across age groups, as well as between individuals. The National Sleep Foundation of America reported that over 24 hours adults require 7 to 9 hours of sleep, teenagers require 8.5 to 9.25 hours, 5 to 10 year olds require 10 to 11 hours, and toddlers require 12 to 14 hours. Newborns to infants aged 3 months need 12 to 18 hours, and then need 14 to 15 hours for the remainder of their first year of life.[2] However, it is also recognized that individual needs will differ according to activity levels, health or disease, weight, and caffeine use and that decisions are best made according to functional requirements, productivity, health, and happiness. Short sleep durations have been linked with increased risks of motor vehicle accidents, obesity, diabetes mellitus, heart disease, depression, and substance abuse, as well as a decreased attention span and reaction times and an inability to remember new information.[3] Such medically recognized illnesses relating to sleep are addressed in Chapter 10. If for some reason people are unable to adequately meet their physical, mental, social, rest, and survival needs through what they do because of personal, social, or environmental impediments, both health and life itself are threatened. To set the scene for an occupational theory, concepts about theories of human nature will be introduced.

Theories of Human Nature

A theory, in the sense it is used here, is a system of ideas held to explain a group of facts or phenomena. It includes a "related set of principles" that "tie two or more concepts together, usually in a correlational or causal way."[4] According to Lewin's[5] three stages of theory development—the speculative, the descriptive, and the constructive—the theory that is the subject of this chapter is beyond speculation. It bridges the descriptive and the constructive stages of development: researching, testing, and trialing is progressing, as evidenced by the wide ranging material relating to occupation and health published in the *Journal of Occupational Science* since its genesis in 1993, and in the direction taken in many publications over the past decade.[6-13] Throughout this text, as in the earlier ones, the concepts, relationships, and principles of the theory are measured against a broad range of ideas and against known research.[5] For probable improvement of health across the globe in the long term, the construction of wide-ranging occupation for well-being programs are required to test the theory further. Measurement of the effectiveness of such programs can only be assessed over a long time span with large population groups.

Since this Occupational Theory of Human Nature was offered in the first edition of this book in 1998,[14] no research has become apparent that contradicts it—indeed, the opposite is the case. It has been strengthened by directives of the WHO, such as its ongoing ratification of the Ottawa Charter in subsequent Health Promotion Congresses; its policies on Active Ageing,[15] Mental Health Promotion,[16] and Physical Activity[17]; and the Rio Declaration on Social Determinants of Health.[18] The theory emphasizes the extent of the complexity and of the influence engagement in occupation has had on cultural evolution, our present circumstances, and the health of individuals and communities. People's occupational needs and behavior are such complex issues that they are worthy of a theory. That the theory is concerned with human nature may seem ambitious, but it is not unreasonable given that people are born with the physical, mental, and social equipment that facilitate and demand use through doing and the apparent importance of wide-ranging occupations to meet the prerequisites of survival, health, and comfort of all people.

Diverse theories about human nature provide the context for beliefs about the meaning and purpose of life, about visions of the future, and about what humans should or should not do.[19] Well-articulated examples of differing theories of human nature range as widely as those proposed by Plato, Marx, Freud, or Sartre, as well as those embraced in creeds as diverse as Christianity or Taoism. "The notion of human nature involves the belief that all human individuals share some common features" and characteristics that are innate.[20] This is a concept central to humanist and critical theorists in that it provides the grounds for aiming toward critical analysis of social or health environments that inhibit human potential and health.

An Occupational Theory of Human Nature

This occupational theory of human nature provides the backdrop against which the relationship between health and occupation is unraveled in the remaining chapters. The theory is based on a few arbitrary elements derived from multiple and ongoing observations. In addition, it meets the

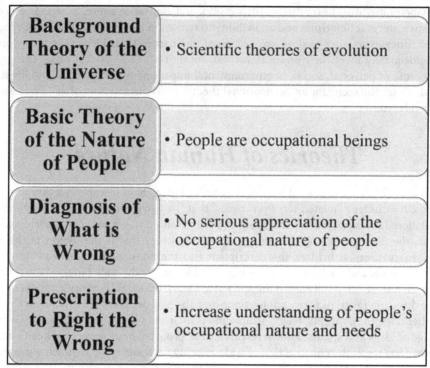

Figure 4-2. Occupational Theory of Human Nature outlined according to Stevenson and Haberman's Requirements for Theories of Human Nature.

criteria of empirical accuracy and predictive capacity required by contemporary canons of science. Stephen Hawking suggests that:

> A theory is a good theory if it satisfies two requirements; it must accurately describe a large class of observations on the basis of a model that contains only a few arbitrary elements, and it must make definite predictions about the results of future observations.[21]

The theory proposed here can definitely predict that, in the future, people will continue to engage in occupation, although the form of the occupation will change according to sociocultural and political evolution and environmental factors.

The occupational theory provided here also meets Stevenson and Haberman's[22] guidelines for such theories. In *Ten Theories of Human Nature*, they outline four constituents (Figure 4-2) that are required for a theory to be able to "offer us hope of solutions to the problems of humankind."[22] The four constituents, with a brief description of how they relate to this occupational theory, are listed below:

1. *A background theory about the world.* This theory is set within generally accepted scientific theories of the evolution of the universe and the species that inhabit it.

2. *A basic theory of the nature of human beings.* Like the majority of living creatures, people are occupational beings as a result of their biological evolution and enculturation. The degree of difference between humans and other creatures in terms of what they do depends on the particular and unique cluster of capacities that enable them to survive. The need to engage in occupation forms an integral part of innate biological systems aimed at survival; the varying potential of individuals for different occupations is mainly a result of their genetically inherited capacities; and the interest in and expression and execution of occupation is learned and modified by the ecosystem and sociocultural and personal environments in which they live. "As natural selection acts on phenotypes, not genotypes, and as phenotypes always include

an environmental component, it is of course fallacious to oppose genes and environment."[23] This concept is in accord with the views of Csikszentmihalyi and Csikszentmihalyi,[24] and Csikszentmihalyi and Massimini,[25] that human action is shaped by genetic, cultural, and self teleonomies and is supported by Snell's[26] proposal that the making of humans is about 50% genetics and 50% culture.

3. *A diagnosis of what is wrong with us.* There is inadequate understanding of occupation as all that people do. Rather, occupation as work dominates research and medico-socio-political interventions. This prevents holistic consideration of the effects of the patchwork of activities that comprise people's lives and that combine to influence health status. As a result of the restricted view, the majority of people have not seriously considered the implications or requirements of their occupational nature in relation to health and well-being from a sufficiently comprehensive perspective. This has caused deleterious effects to individual, community, population, and ecological health.

4. *A prescription for putting it right.* Addressing the lack of awareness of the requirements and outcomes of people's occupational natures could potentially result in major and beneficial changes to individual, social, corporate, political, economic, ecological, and health policies and outcomes.

HUMAN EVOLUTION AND OCCUPATION

Evolution provides the historical explanation for the diversity of life on earth. Insights from evolutionary biology are critical to ensuring the health and well-being of humans and all other forms on earth.[27]

This occupational theory of human nature is based on the fact that people have innate needs to engage in simple to complex and multiple occupations and that those needs have evolved throughout the history of the earth and its living constituents. On the whole, these needs have been overlooked in scientific inquiry and in most theories of human nature because they are so mundane. People have occupational needs that go beyond the instinctive patterned behaviors of many other animals, although for both groups these needs are related to health. In fact, they are a species' primary health mechanism. For humans they motivate the provision of other basic requirements, enabling people to use their biological capacities and potential, meet sociocultural expectations, and thereby flourish. The integrative functions of the central nervous system, which processes external and internal information which is activated by engagement in occupation, are focal to survival, the maintenance of homeostasis, and facilitating health and well-being. The adaptive capacity of the human brain allows the innate drive for purposeful occupation to respond to cultural forces and values that add a social dimension to the relationship between what people do and their health.

That engagement in occupation is innate, inborn, or natural is confirmed by the fact that all creatures in the wild have to do whatever is required for them to try to fulfill their particular survival and health requirements. Human evolution has been filled with ongoing and progressive doings that, apart from enabling the species to survive, have stimulated, entertained, and excited some people, or bored or stressed them, according to what was done; at times, they have also caused illness, death, or destruction. People spend their lives almost constantly engaged in purposeful doing, even when free of obligation or necessity. They do daily tasks, including the things they feel they must do and other things that they want to do. Occupation provides a major means of social engagement and shapes families, communities, and nations. Anthropologists describe this unique human trait as culture and suggest it is the unique blend of biology and culture that differentiates the human species from others; Leakey and Lewin[28] suggest that having a highly developed culture is not so much about what people do but more so about the fact that they can do, more or less, what they want. Indeed, doing is so much a part of everyday life that within Western cultures people frequently identify themselves and each other by what they do. For example, common forms of personal introductions name an individual's occupational pursuits, such as "Come and meet Marilyn. She is a computer 'geek' and runs marathons for fun." In some parts of the world, family surnames reflect the long-past occupations of their members, such as Smith and Barber. Frequently, children are asked, "What are you planning to do when you grow up?" or "What have you been doing?" It is as if the occupational background, present, or future of people is a major reflection of every individual, that what they do, in some ways, is who or what they are.

Theories of Evolution

The foundation of this occupational theory of human nature is based on the following brief account of biological and cultural evolutionary theory. The study of how biological life could arise from inorganic matter through natural processes is known as *abiogenesis* or *biopoiesis*.[29] Currently, it is generally accepted that abiogenesis occurred billions of years ago when living matter in the form of single-celled creatures that lacked a cell nucleus (known as prokaryotes) evolved naturally from nonliving organic molecules surrounded by a membrane-like structure (known as protobionts).[30] Over a period of perhaps 1 billion years, some electrons, protons, and neutrons combined to form atoms, which formed molecules. Some of these became "more or less well-organized aggregates," one class of which is organic matter.[30] In turn, some original microorganisms went through a "comparable hierarchical evolution" to primitive plant forms to invertebrates to vertebrates, and, in the past 60 million years, to mammals.[31]

Modern science, with cross-pollination from within the fields of chemistry, geology, paleontology, and astrophysics, plays a key role in the continuing complex discussion of life's origins. It is less concerned with why life emerged from the air, water, and rock of the barren face of the Earth than with where, when, and how. Recently, astrobiologist Robert Hazen explained many rival hypotheses of genesis, pointing to how some recent theories have suggested that microbes living in rock miles below the Earth's surface might have some answers. Hazen suggested that:

> *Crucial features of our own cells suggest an ancient cooperative merging of early, more primitive cells. If experiments establish easy synthetic pathways to both a simple metabolic cycle and to an RNA-like genetic polymer, then such a symbiosis may provide the most attractive origin scenario of all.*[32]

Other theorists have been excited by the discovery of life near hydrothermal vents deep in the ocean, leading them to propose that life may have begun there.[33] Against the background of geologist and naturalist speculation, interest and theories that were out of step with dominant Christian beliefs, Darwin's *Origin of the Species by Means of Natural Selection*[34] and *The Descent of Man and Selection in Relation to Sex*,[35] are recognized as the works that brought theories of evolution to public debate and inquiry. Darwin's evidence did not come from human beings, and only his conclusion suggested that his theory would shed light on the origin of people. Nonetheless, his hypotheses were received with moral shock, fear, and derision in the lay community, although accepted rapidly in biological science.

Dawkins suggested that although it is difficult to explain "how even a simple universe began," Darwin's theory of evolution by natural selection demonstrates a way in which "simplicity could change into complexity" and how collections of stable molecules could eventually, through "high longevity/fecundity/copying-fidelity," evolve into complex living beings.[36] Darwin's theory is based on the empirical observations that:

- There is a tendency for parental traits to be passed to their offspring.
- Despite that tendency, there are considerable and noticeable variations between individuals.
- Species are capable of a rate of generation that cannot be supported by available natural resources, requiring a struggle for existence.

	Table 4-1
	A BRIEF HISTORY OF THE DISCOVERY OF DNA

Year	Description
1869[44b]	DNA was first discovered as a microscopic substance by Miescher, a Swiss physician. He called it "nuclein."
1919[44c]	Levene suggested that DNA consisted of a short chain of nucleotide units linked together in a fixed order.
1927[44d]	Koltsov suggested that traits could be inherited via a molecule made up of two mirror strands.
1928[44e]	Frederick Griffith provided the first clear suggestion that DNA carries genetic information.
1952[44f,44g,44h]	DNA's role in heredity was confirmed by Alfred Hershey and Martha Chase.

- Because more are born than can survive, this leads to survival by natural selection of those with "certain inherited variants which increase the chances of their carriers surviving and reproducing."[37]

Spencer[38] termed the latter point as "survival of the fittest" in an often-quoted phrase that is frequently misconstrued to mean survival of those physically fit and strong rather than those with "expected reproductive success," because it is taken literally and out of context. Natural selection results in the accumulation of favored variants that will effect gradual adaptive change in every generation and, over extended periods, produce new forms of life. Diversity and individual uniqueness is the consistent message of evolutionary studies from Darwin's time to the present.[37]

Working at almost the same time as Darwin, the Austrian monk Gregor Mendel studied and experimented with plant species, which led to his formulation of biological laws of heredity. Virtually ignored at the time, his work was rediscovered in 1900 by three scientists working separately—De Vries, Correns, and Tschermak—all within a 3-month period. Mendel's work provided the answer to the "causes of the variations on which natural selection acts."[39] Shah Ebrahim, Professor of Public Health at the London School of Hygiene and Tropical Medicine, is "currently using Mendelian randomization designs to examine the unconfounded effects of environmental factors on risk of common diseases."[40]

Darwin's theory, modified in light of Mendelian genetics,[41] is known as neo-Darwinism[42] or synthetic evolution.[43] More recently, "the discovery of the structure and function of DNA (deoxyribonucleic acid) has made clear the nature of the hereditary variations upon which natural selection operates" (Table 4-1).[44a] In 1953, the elucidation of the structure of genetic DNA by Watson and Crick described how a long molecule of alternating sugar and phosphate units twisted to form a double helix that opens when chromosomes replicate.[45] Each sugar unit is attached to a base of adenine, thymine, guanine, or cytosine, which pairs with those opposite. The first two bases always pair, as do guanine and cytosine. When chromosomes replicate, new bases are added on by pairing. These form two new identical molecules. An occasional mistake during replication is known as a mutation.[46]

Occupation in Evolution

It is now acknowledged in the scientific community that humans are mammals with much in common with other animals and that, like other species, have "a certain genetic constitution that causally explains not only the anatomical features ... but also our distinctive ... behavior."[47] As Bronowski succinctly explained:

The evolution of the brain, of the hand, of the eyes, of the feet, the teeth, the whole human frame, made a special gift of man ... faster in evolution, and richer and more flexible in behavior ... he has what no other animal possesses, a jigsaw of faculties which alone ... make him creative.[48]

Bronowski's description of human difference is a useful bridge between Darwinist theories of evolution and this theory about humans as occupational beings.

The central concepts of the argument for people being described as occupational beings rely on three related sets of principles. First, all people engage in self-initiated and complex occupations, unless prevented by congenital or acquired dysfunction such as brain damage, because of their species' common combination of biological features, such as consciousness, cognitive capacity, and language. Although it is higher cortical adaptations such as these that have generated and made possible the complex occupational behavior that sets humans apart from other animals, anatomical and physiological characteristics of the body, such as bipedalism, upright posture, and hand dexterity, are vital instruments in the execution of occupation. Because of the integrated function of each, the mind and body are not seen as separate entities, but rather "simply [as] one and the same."[49] Lorenz contended that this is the only possible view "tenable for the evolutionary epistemologist" and that "the razor-edge demarcation" seen as existing between them by some disciplines is only for the purpose of understanding them.[49] Certainly, because Descartes, in the 17th century, separated the body from the mind epistemologically, generations of scientists up to the present day, have fed the assumption that the mind and body can and should be considered separately and that the treatment of people with mental disorders is separated from those with a physical disorder. This separation has hindered the growth and understanding of humans as occupational beings who, because of mind–body unity, are able to engage in occupation that integrates both.

Second, engagement in occupation is indispensable to survival, as well as being an integral part of complex health maintenance mechanisms. This hypothesis is in line with another of Lorenz's[49] suggestions—that the principal purpose of both anatomical characteristics and behavior patterns is survival—and with Ornstein and Sobel's proposition that "the major role of the brain is to mind the body and maintain health."[50] The theory held here combines these views, maintaining that a primary function of people's anatomic characteristics, particularly the brain, is to facilitate healthy survival and that occupation is a primary mechanism for this function. To this end, the whole of the brain is involved in survival and health and in engagement in occupation.

This notion does not compete with a predominant view that genomic reproduction is the principal goal of evolution, contending that because reproduction can only occur during a particular stage of the life cycle, individuals have to survive and resist disease and death to reach reproductive age and that positive health enhances survival and reproductive success. After reproduction, offspring require nurturing and education so that they can also eventually reproduce. Engagement in occupation is not only required for survival to the point of reproduction, but also for a long time after to provide support for the immature of the species, and humans have a long childhood. Views held about kin selection or gene selection, which develop the concept of Darwinian fitness to include reproductive success of individuals who share genes,[39] accounts, at least in part, for social and altruistic behaviors and occupations. It was, and in some places still is, customary or necessary for offspring support to be provided by other than biological parents. For example, programs in Australia have recently been developed to assist migrant South African fathers to develop parenting skills that were unnecessary in their homeland.

Third, the theory recognizes that, in large part, genetic traits or capacities are inherited and that there is considerable variation between individuals because of genetic recombination, which "theoretically ... can create nearly an infinite number of different organisms simply by reshuffling the immense amount of genetic differences between the DNA of any two parents."[51] The differences between people and the importance of recognizing an individual's particular range of capacities, along with sociocultural requirements, are raised in later chapters as an important issue in terms of promoting health and well-being and in preventing illness.

Integral to the three principles are ideas about the biological and sociocultural bases of behavior; the haphazard nature of evolution; the similarities and differences between species, brain size, and capacities; and the impact of occupational humans on cultural and ecological change. Those who claim that human activity depends on culture rather than genetics may criticize acceptance of a biological basis for occupational behavior. However, modern sociobiologists and ethologists contend that:

> *Within [a] gene-environmental action model, culture can be seen as the man-made part of the environment, preselected by the specifically human genome ... Culture can have no empirical referent outside of the human organisms that invent and transmit it, and, therefore, its evolution is inevitably intertwined with the biological evolution of our species.*[23]

Such contention provides "a factual background for a middle view"[26] that is in accord with the theory of human nature proposed here. It "demonstrates the importance of evolutionary origins in the behavior of the species"[52] but also maintains that, because of their biology, what people do is socioculturally determined, as sociologists claim.

Homeostasis is also fundamental to people's occupational nature because the need for sameness maintains constancy in mental processes, as well as in body physiology. To make sense of the world, psychological mechanisms seek sameness in what is received and perceived. This is facilitated by an "internal milieu, [which] seems to be more constant for the cells of the brain than for other parts of the body."[53] James claimed that the capacity to recognize sameness is a prerequisite for the existence of a sense of self and "the very keel and backbone of our thinking" because it is central to recognition, for giving meaning, and for appreciating contrast and difference.[54] Without it, every time engagement in an occupation occurred, it would appear as a new experience, take longer, and be in the nature of trial and error; no ongoing learning could occur. The evolution and health experiences of the species would indeed be different.

Because people are goal-directed and committed, by their nature, to engaging in occupation with purpose, it is difficult to appreciate that evolution may not have an ultimate purpose. The notion of predestination has led many theorists to maintain that advances in cultural evolution must progress to the enhancement of human nature. In fact, the occupational nature of humans may not be progressive in terms of ultimate "good" for the species. It may lead to less desirable outcomes for health and well-being, with occupational technology having not only the potential to destroy the earth's environment and the species, but also the means to reduce daily physical, mental, and social exercise that is, in itself, health promoting.

The remarkable advances in technology appear to increase the difficulty of accepting the undeniable similarity of humans to other species. However, the occupational nature of people is the result of evolution, as is the case for all other animals. Each species appears to have some special attributes and abilities that are paramount to its survival and influence its regular occupations; these vary between and within species. For some, it can be speed or the ability to camouflage or highly developed visual or auditory capacities, all of which are often connected with safety and procreation. Despite the complexity of human occupation, it also derives from meeting those needs. To a lesser or greater extent, all living creatures are occupational beings—all perform activities for species survival. Birds build nests, decorate bowers to attract mates, and dive from great heights for fish or prey. Some birds use stones as tools to soften or break into food. New Caledonian crows even pass on the manufacturing techniques of the insect-snagging tools they fashion from leathery pieces of torn pandanus leaf, between one another and across generations.[55] Domesticated dogs can learn that certain activities will be rewarded with food or praise or will run or play with a ball for no apparent reason except for fun, which coincidentally maintains their level of physical fitness and acuity. What animals do and how much freedom they have in the choice of occupations depends on their anatomical features; the size, structure, and capacities

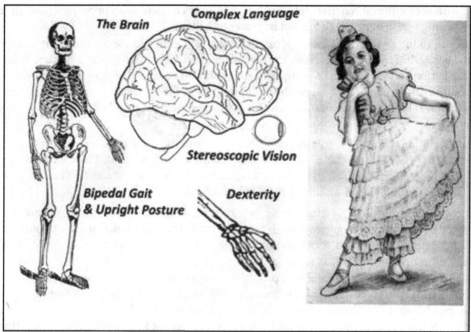

Figure 4-3. Important characteristics that help create the occupational human. Adapted from Harter J, editor. *Images of Medicine: A Definitive Volume of more than 4,800 Copyright-free Engravings Including Anatomy, General Medicine, Apothecary and Pharmaceutical, Diseases and Injuries, Therapeutics, Plus Medical Equipment, Instruments and Appliances.* New York: Bonanza Books; 1991.

of their nervous systems; and the environmental opportunities and constraints. Many animals, and particularly mammals, possess qualities and characteristics once thought unique to humans, which is not surprising because all mammalian brains have neuronal circuitry and systems that enable them to receive, attend to, interpret, communicate with, and act on information from the environment. "There is no strong evidence of unique brain-behavior relationships in any species within the class Mammalia."[56] Bronowski observed that although "every human action goes back in some part" to animal origins, an important distinction remains. He questioned: "what are the gifts that make him different?"[48]

That question suggests that to gain some appreciation of the complex nature of people as doers, it is useful to consider the most distinctive of human characteristics that create their capacity to engage in such wide ranging occupations. Evolutionary scientists, archaeologists, and anthropologists have identified, as prime examples, changes to brain structure, function, and size; the capacity to walk upright, oppose the thumb, and use hands dexterously; the ability to view their world stereoscopically; and the ability to use complex language. Campbell suggested that these particular capacities have "overwhelming significance" and when "added together separate all humans from all other animals" (Figure 4-3).[57] Each of these will now be considered.

IMPORTANT CHARACTERISTICS THAT HELP CREATE THE OCCUPATIONAL HUMAN

In beginning to explore the important and particular physical characteristics that led to people's occupational nature, it is true to say that, in isolation, no single feature is wholly responsible. Edelman explained that "the shape of an animal's body is as important to the functioning and evolution of its brain as the shape and functioning of the brain are to the behavior of that body."[58] In evolutionary terms, "the shape of cells, tissues, organs, and finally the whole animal is the largest single basis for behavior."[58] Although bearing that in mind, the functions of particular human attributes need to be considered as parts of the whole. The brain is the obvious place to start as it is this organ that coordinates and controls what people do.

The Brain

Our brain is not so much different from other brains, it is bigger. We are not a whole new experiment in the evolutionary process, but a superprimate. A quantitative change in the evolving human brain, however, has produced a qualitative change of extraordinary significance.[59]

In *The Cambridge Encyclopedia of Human Evolution*, Deacon agreed that it is "the largest primate brain that has ever existed, both in absolute terms and with respect to body size."[60]

However, its structure is typical of that of other primates, with the same cortical and subcortical structures arranged in the same configurations and composed of neurons with the same cell architecture.[60]

It is 6.3 times larger than expected for mammals of the same body size.[61] However, "comparative size of the brain may not be as important as its internal organization,"[60] nor is it indicative of its cellular composition or number of neurons. Herculano-Houzel found that although "different cellular scaling rules apply to the brains" of other creatures, the human brain contains as many neuronal and non-neuronal cells as would be expected of a primate brain of its size.[62] In addition, the "so-called overdeveloped cerebral cortex" that embodies more than 80% of the brain's mass holds only 19% of all brain neurons. Nevertheless, primate brains have evolved in a way that makes them economical and space saving, and amongst these the human brain is the largest and contains the most neurons. Therefore, it is not surprising that it is often considered outstanding among mammalian brains and the most cognitively able.[62]

Deacon concurred that the structure, configuration, and architecture is typical of other primates, despite unique anatomy and functions for special human adaptations, such as "symbolic communication, speech, tool usage, and culture."[60] Except for the neocortex, all cerebral regions have a rudimentary equivalent in reptilian brains.[63] Indeed, the brains of all animals have the same starting point. As they adapted to different habitats, climates, and subsistence demands, a "rather haphazard and seemingly disorganized set of structures" evolved in archaeological layers in the brain.[64] Each layer maintained the stability and health of the organism as conditions changed, and each layer added a new dimension to what animals were capable of doing. Herbert Spencer (1820-1903), an evolutionist social philosopher, was the first to argue that the capacity of animals to engage in a constellation of new behaviors occurred in a series of step as the brain evolved.[65] John Hughlings-Jackson (1835-1911), an English neurologist who based his work on Spencer's theory, recognized that the cortex has a special role in purposive behavior, which is supported by subcortical areas concerned with more elementary forms of the same behavior.[66]

The brainstem is the oldest part of the brain, having developed before the advent of mammals. It controls the simplest life support systems, such as breathing, heart rate, and general alerting to predators or prey. The limbic system evolved to ensure stability of the organism on land, which called for structures to maintain internal temperatures, fluid levels, and emotional reactions, such as those concerned with self-protection. The cerebellum was probably the first area to specialize in sensorimotor coordination and is integral to efficiency of skilled movement. The cerebral cortex is the most recent layer. It is here that the processes occur that make humans most different from other animals, such as their capacity to analyze, organize, understand, produce, judge, plan, activate, sense, formulate, and execute complex doing.[66] Some of the processes, such as seeing, hearing, and language comprehension are more structured than others. People can, for example think, imagine, or learn about the world, and perceive, embellish, and manipulate ideas and objects in a variety of ways.[57] Such cortical functions give humans the "capacity to adapt culturally ... to insulate themselves from the environment and to exploit the environment."[67] Unfortunately, that capacity has led to people "struggling to come to terms with humankind's place in the biosphere."[68] This is especially so in the developed world, where "culture has fostered the illusion of humans being apart from nature" in an elitist and controlling way that has been far from egalitarian or participatory.[69]

Because of their reasoning ability and social interaction skills, early hominids must have had increased chances of effectively meeting their survival needs, such as obtaining food. McMichael surmised that "selection pressure would thus have favoured more complex, hence, larger brains."[70] Because brains are metabolically expensive, their increasing size required other organs to diminish. The colon is one example of this because different food and changes to food preparation enabled it to decrease in size. The reduced need for powerful jaw muscles and strong bony anchor points also allowed for lightening of the skull, giving more space for the enlargement of the brain.[71] In addition, much of brain growth and maturation was deferred until after birth because pelvic size could not accommodate a larger, more mature organ. This led to occupational adaptations concerned with care of offspring over a comparatively longer timespan. Because of the brain's basic structure and function, there is a remarkable similarity in what all people are able to do. However, just as facial features vary between individuals, so do the brains of individuals. Even subtle variations lead to amazing differences in terms of people's interests, competence, and satisfaction.[66]

Roger Sperry, the 1981 winner of the Nobel Prize in Physiology or Medicine, explained, the growing understanding about the relationship of the brain's structure to behavior demonstrates "enormously intricate brain systems" at molecular, cellular, organismic, and transorganismic levels, all of which interconnect.[72] In the cerebral cortex alone, it has been estimated that there are between 20 and 100 billion neurons and approximately 1 million billion connections, all of which are capable of many combinations so that "the sheer number and density of neuronal networks in the brain" reaches "hyperastronomical" figures and "the brain might be said to be in touch more with itself than with anything else."[72] Indeed, "the kinds of unique individuality in our brain networks make that of fingerprints or facial features appear gross and simple by comparison."[72] Many neurons, each of which is "unusual in three respects: its shape, its electrical and chemical function, and its connectivity," have specific potential.[73] In fact, "very specific patterns of behavior are determined by very specific brain areas," with "each behavioral system probably [having] its own underlying neurophysiological mechanisms."[74]

Difference between brain structure, chemistry, and function in healthy men and women were explored by Cosgrove et al using imaging methodologies in a 25-year study undertaken between 1980 and 2006.[75] They found that male and female brains are neurochemically distinct overall according to dopaminergic, serotonergic, and gamma-aminobutyric acid markers; that brain volume and the percentage of white matter is greater in men than women; and that women have a higher percentage of global cerebral blood flow and grey matter.[75] This may have consequences not only in terms of health disorders that affect the mind, but also in terms of gender-specific occupational expectations.

Different brain areas have different cell formations that have been described in functional and cytoarchitectonic maps.[76,77] "Mapping is an important principle in complex brains," and the fibers that connect maps with each other "are the most numerous of all those in the brain."[73] Areas of the brain that have been identified with specific functions relate to the capacity to do many things, although the "complexity of the brain's structure makes it incredibly difficult to relate its components to individual capacities."[78] Even capacities themselves have incredibly complex systems. Recently, localization theories have been substantiated, with the proviso that any area with a specific function does not work in isolation. In fact, the complexities of the interactive nature of specific areas of the brain have been demonstrated by studies of brain activity from the mid-20th century onward. For example, following the inhalation of radioactive gases (zenon 133), a 2-dimensional measure of regional blood flow was taken during the doing of tasks compared with a resting state. It was found that the frontal lobes were relatively active bilaterally even at rest and that just doing simple movements of the fingers involved activity of many different areas of the brain.[79,80] Such complexity has been confirmed by 3-dimensional positron emission topography, which has been used to image the neuronal activity of both hemispheres and deeper brain structures during use.[60,81-83]

McMichael suggested that the advent of early language used to enhance social cohesion "must have accelerated the later stages of evolution of the brain."[70] As the human brain evolved, many pathways and connections remained from earlier developmental stages. Few structures have been discarded, although there may be alterations in size and function. Deacon proposed that new brain functions are the result of "systematic reorganization, elaboration, or reduction of existing structures or shifts in proportions of existing connections."[84] In answer to Bronowski's earlier question,[48] the gifts that make humans different are not only the capacities highlighted in this section of the chapter, but also the particular adaptations that evolved with increased brain size and, more specifically, the association areas of the cortex. They are responsible, in large part, for complex communication and emotional tone, language, thinking, humor, forward planning, problem-solving, analysis, judgment, and adaptation. Lorenz noted that:

> Among humans ... perceptions of depth and direction, a central nervous representation of space, Gestalt perception and the capacity for abstraction, insight and learning, voluntary movement, curiosity ... exploratory behavior [and] imitation ... are more strongly developed than any of them is among an animal species, even if they represent for those animals a fulfillment of the most vital, life-furthering functions.[85]

These highly developed capacities, along with consciousness (discussed in Chapter 7) and the particular physical characteristics discussed below, are the special survival mechanisms of humans, in that they endow unprecedented flexibility, enabling humans to adapt to and meet the challenge of many different environments and dangers. The "intelligence and skills of our forebears do not only manifest themselves in the evolutionary transformations of the brain; they can also be seen in the results of their activity."[86] It is the:

> Expansion of a standard primate brain [that has provided people with] behavioral possibilities undreamed of in other even closely related species. This brain ... gives us the human potential for making tools, talking, planning, dreaming of the future, and creating an entirely new environment for ourselves.[87]

The ongoing and progressive doings that have enabled the species to survive have stimulated and excited some people and deprived or stressed others according to what was done. That factor has health implications. Differences tend to grow or diminish according to environmental demands, enculturation, and individual opportunity: "it is the unique blend of biology and culture that makes the species Homo sapiens a truly unique kind of animal."[28] The external variables increase individual difference, in part because of structural change, which results from the neuronal demands of activity. "No two mixes of the inner and outer factors are just alike,"[26] and the inner factors alone are remarkably complex.

Dexterity

The unique capabilities of the human hand enable us to perform extremely fine movements, such as those needed to write or to thread a needle. The emergence of these capabilities was undoubtedly essential in human evolution: a combination of individually movable fingers, opposable thumbs and the ability to move the smallest finger and ring finger into the middle of the palm to meet the thumb gives us dexterity that is unparalleled in the animal kingdom.[88]

Such a hand structure, which frees the hands to do a variety of activities, is one of the special human attributes, along with the capacity to walk upright. It is fundamental to the unique ability of the species to do many things. In his 1833 Bridgewater Treatise on the hand, relating the hand's structure and function to the environment, Sir Charles Bell observed:

[the] difference in the length of the fingers (and the thumb) serves a thousand purposes, adapting the hand and fingers, as in holding a rod, a switch, a sword, a hammer, a pen or pencil, engraving tool, in all which a secure hold and freedom of motion are admirably combined.[89]

The adaptation is so important that Darwin claimed that, "man could not have attained his present dominant position in the world without the use of his hands, which are so admirably adapted to the act of obedience of his will."[90] The capacity for manipulative skill was facilitated by a refinement of specialized brain centers within the primary sensory and motor areas of the cortex. These coordinated with other brain centers, such as the basal ganglia and the cerebellum.[76,77] The part of the brain that controls voluntary movement in higher primates consists of two distinct areas. One of them is evolutionarily more recent and is essential for highly skilled movements and the emergence of manual dexterity.[88] In 2008, geneticists, Rathelot and Strick identified a short DNA sequence involved in limb development that is present in humans but not in chimpanzees or any other organisms.[88] It is thought to have been involved in the evolution of opposition of the thumb.

The anatomical advantage of hands capable of dexterity, many types of prehension, and opposition of the thumb to fingers enable them to be used as tools. However, the manufacture and use of tools is not confined to humans as was first thought. Goodall[91] and Brewer and McGrew[92] have demonstrated how chimpanzees in the wild use grasses to extract termites from their nest. In 1960 Jane Goodall discovered the primitive tool making skills of chimpanzees.[93] Chimpanzees use either a short stick to penetrate aboveground mounds or a foot forced puncturing stick to drill holes into belowground termite chambers. A separate fishing probe is used to harvest the insects. They improved the fishing probe by pulling it through their teeth to fray the end, like a paintbrush.[94]

One evolutionary explanation for the adaptation of the human hand that is necessary for complex tool use is founded on the hypothesis that "chimpanzee-like apes" threw rocks and swung clubs at adversaries. "The fossil record indicates that adaptation for throwing and clubbing began to influence hand structure at or very near the origin of the hominid lineage and continued for millions of years thereafter."[95] Over those years, this adaptation led to various anatomical changes throughout the body, including lengthening of the thumb and shortening of the fingers, which permits them to oppose in a strong and robust fashion and to engage in a wide variety of fine and gross occupations in a unique way.

Apart from rare examples, the making and using of tools intergenerationally is an essentially human characteristic. Supporting this, Benjamin Franklin is reputed to have observed that "man is a toolmaking animal."[96] Despite the truth that people are toolmakers and, without doubt, the most sophisticated of toolmakers, the phrase is less popular today, having been largely replaced with the description of humans as social animals. Humans are both, and both descriptions resonate with recognizing people as occupational beings.

Although currently the oldest stone tools are dated slightly earlier than the oldest evidence of the *Homo genus, Homo habilis* (meaning handy man) was so named in 1964 by Richard Leakey because this species was thought to represent the first manufacturers of stone tools.[97] Currently, they are the earliest known members of the Homo family, which humans belong to, and are thought to have lived 2.4 to 1.4 million years ago.[98] Although it is believed that their tools were meager, they "provide evidence about the technologies, dexterity, particular kinds of mental skills, and innovations that were within the grasp of early human toolmakers."[98] Statistical studies of the tools have shown that "their makers … had a concept of symmetry … and … planned technique."[99] Faisal et al explained "the advance from crude stone tools to elegant handheld axes was a massive technological leap for our early human ancestors,"[100] and McMichael maintained that "the early making of and use of stone and wooden tools placed a heightened premium on fine and gross motor coordination, and hence the elaboration of the motor cortex."[74] The appearance of Homo erectus, a routine toolmaker with longer legs and a larger brain, is currently dated at approximately 1.8 million years.

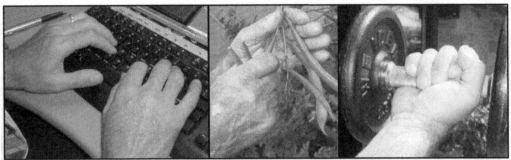

Figure 4-4. Flexible hands and tool use are central human attributes.

The use of upper limbs and hands has developed into a very specialized adaptation so that unique movements, sense of touch, reaching out, gesturing, fine manipulative capacities, and balance function can be used separately or combined in infinitely varied ways (Figure 4-4). This enables the doing of culturally derived occupations, unique to humans, to be performed. Indeed, the capacity to use hands to do a multitude of activities is integral to matters of survival and health and "one of the dominant aspects of our biological and cultural adaptation."[101] Cicero observed:

> By the manipulation of the fingers the hand is enabled to paint, to model, to carve, and to draw forth the notes of the lyre and of the flute. And besides these arts of recreation there are those of utility, I mean agriculture and building, the weaving and stitching of garments and the various modes of working bronze and iron; hence we realize that it was by applying the hand of the artificer to the discoveries of thought and observations of the senses that all our conveniences were attained. (De nat. deor. II,150)[102]

Bipedal Gait and Upright Posture

Australopithecus fossils from 4.2 to 3.9 million years ago have revealed bipedal specializations,[103] so the view that bipedalism is a relatively early hominid adaptation prior to the advent of other human traits, such as larger brains and tool use, appears to have merit.[104] It is evidence such as fragments of a 4 million-year-old thigh bone found in Ethiopia and the discovery of a trail of footprints left by three hominids in volcanic ash more than 3.5 million years ago in Laetoli that leads to the anthropological opinion that hominids stood like humans before they could think like humans. In addition to upright posture, bipedal gait appears "associated with the ecological adaptations of early hominids."[105] One explanation for the early appearance is Young's hypothesis about the physical demands of throwing and clubbing mentioned in relation to hand dexterity. Those activities called on "an innovative, instinctive, whole-body motion performed from an upright stance that begins with a thrust of the legs."[95] It is surmised that improvement in upright balance and locomotion led to its increasing use and eventual culmination in "habitual bipedalism."[95]

There are more than 200 extant primate species whose specific form of habitual posture and gait remains speculative. However, the habitual highly characteristic form of locomotion enjoyed by modern humans is now unique, although they are not alone in being bipedal. It is the combination with upright posture that provides the human difference because the greatest numbers of bipedal animals move with their backs close to horizontal and use their tails for balance. Both partial and habitual bipedalism hold several occupational advantages. There is greater efficiency for long-distance travel between clusters of food sources; the upper limbs are freed for other uses, such as carrying infants or food sharing; and there is improvement in the visual field when the head is raised. This assists animals in detecting dangers or resources farther away, reaching higher food sources, or wading in deeper water.[106]

Figure 4-5. Some occupational theories of the origin of bipedal locomotion.

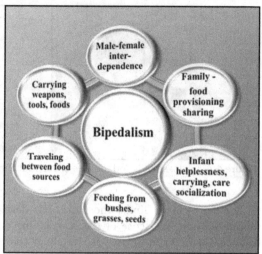

Lewin suggested one explanation of bipedalism, that upright walking was a biologically adaptive response to accessing traditional foods in a changing environment: that a more energy-efficient mode of walking was required because food sources became dispersed with climatic and subsequent environmental changes.[107] Occupation is central to that explanation, as it is to another that is favored. The second explanation is based on the fact that human young, who take a long time to mature, are dependent on their parents to carry them, unlike other primate offspring who are able to cling to their parents' long body hair. Erect standing and bipedal locomotion enabled mothers to move about while using their arms and hands to support their children.[98] However, these are only two of several plausible explanations, all of which may have influenced bipedal evolution (Figure 4-5).

Humans have developed bipedalism into an adaptation as specialized as flight in a hovering hawk, while also developing versatility.[108-110] People can run, jump, dance, climb, swim, and cope with almost any terrain. The health advantages of running, walking, dancing, and swimming, particularly with regard to the cardiovascular system, are well researched and applauded, even if not all epidemiologists agree about which form of activity is most valuable. Bipedal locomotion may be slower than quadrupedal locomotion, but people have thrived because of the occupational advantages of having the forelimbs free. "The tangled triple influence of bipedalism, brain development, and the manipulation of objects cannot be [easily] separated."[111] They work in cooperation with vision.

Stereoscopic Vision

Primates have forward-pointing eyes with an overlap between the monocular fields of both eyes. This reduces the extent of the visual field and creates a blind zone behind the head. However, the brain is provided with simultaneous information from both eyes about objects within the area of overlap. This enables stereoscopic (or depth) vision, which improves the ability to judge distances. Developments such as these in visual acuity increased the amount of processing to be performed, thus adding to the large brain size of primates.[112]

Stereoscopic vision assists people in focusing on objects that are close and to see these in 3-dimensional form, as well as enjoying the benefits of long sight. Because of the height advantage provided by an upright posture, as well as eyes positioned at the front rather than the side of the head, people are able to see for relatively long distances. This capacity has made it possible for people to manipulate and appreciate the structure of materials, to become toolmakers, and, with practice, to produce objects of great variety and complexity. In turn, that has assisted human adaptation to different environments. Coupled with visual perception, humans are able to identify objects by color, hue, brightness, and form, in different orientations, and with sufficient clarity to pick out objects from their backgrounds. They can determine whether objects are still or moving, as well as the speed, type, and direction of movement by automatically interpreting the position of shadows. This range of visual capacity has been a tool used both to assist in finding food and other necessities of life and to ensure safety from predators. It has been instrumental in the variety of occupations that people can do to give them an evolutionary advantage despite other animals having better visual faculties for their particular survival needs.

People know about their world through their senses. To many, vision is the most important sense, which is not surprising because there are estimates that between 75% and 90% of the information stored in the brain is derived from visual sources. Ornstein and Sobel explained how the brain is flooded with information because the world is in a state of constant change, yet "the eye takes in a trillionth of the energy which reaches it."[113] In addition, the visual system and the brain selects, simplifies, and organizes so that what humans see "is not so much a replication of the real world as a calculated and very selective abstraction of it."[114] This capacity prevents people from being overwhelmed by extraneous information. It helps them make sense of what they see and choose what is necessary to pay attention to. This enables more appropriate, or even fast, action to occur as necessary for survival and safety. For example, a glimpse of part of an animal or another human who may be a threat will be perceived and understood as a whole. Instead of seeing each color, shape, texture, and form of parts of a room as separate, people perceive the room as a whole coherent structure in which they can move and act.

Vision, like other capacities, is largely dependent on use and learning through experience, because "the brain constantly needs stimulation to develop, grow, and maintain its organization."[115] Sensory systems are often especially tuned in to the activities and communication systems of the same species, as a matter of survival, health, and well-being.[116,117] It is "the limitations of [human] senses [that] set the boundaries of ... conscious existence."[118]

Complex Language

There is general agreement that the origins of language are coupled with those of modern human behavior but, despite many theories, no consensus on its origin or age.[119] For example, there are continuity theories that hold that language is so complex that it must have evolved from earlier prelinguistic primate communication.[120-126] The traditional view holds that, like other characteristics, it evolved through a series of adaptive changes[127] and "may rest on neural mechanisms that are present in reduced form in other living species and that were elaborated quite early during hominid evolution."[128] In contrast, discontinuity theories maintain that human language is so unique it must have appeared fairly rapidly at some point in human evolution.[129, 130] Currently, the only prominent proponent of a discontinuity-based theory is linguist-philosopher Noam Chomsky, who suggests language is the result of "some random mutation."[131] Other theorists consider that language is largely a genetically encoded faculty, and others believe that it is learned through social interaction.[122] However, because anatomical features evolve slowly and only develop when required, the acquisition and use of complex language is mostly thought to be transitional.[132-134] Earlier language was, most probably, based on gesture, body signals, grunts, growls, cries, or even markers on trees for directional information in the hunt for food. Many hold that gesturing preceded language because:

- The cortical regions responsible for hand and mouth movement are adjacent.
- Verbal and sign language depend on similar neural structures.[135]
- The same left-hemisphere brain regions are active during sign, vocal, or written language.[136]
- People use hand and facial gesture when speaking.[137]

Speech has several occupational advantages over gesture. Communication can occur without the need to see the person speaking,[138] and as the use of tools became common, gesturing was not always possible. In addition, when a parent's hands were active with other tasks and a child was out of physical contact, they could be reassured verbally.[139] Although scholarly opinion varies about the timing of the development of primitive language, with some favoring *Homo habilis* and others favoring *Homo erectus* or *Homo heidelbergensis*, most genetic, archaeological, and paleontological evidence suggests that the development of modern language can be attributed to *Homo sapiens* less than 200,000 years ago, probably emerging in sub-Saharan Africa during the Middle Stone Age.[140]

Human language is unique among the life forms of Earth[141-143] because:

> *its complex structure affords a much wider range of possible expressions and uses than any known system of animal communication, all of which are generally closed systems, with limited functions and mostly genetically rather than socially transmitted. In contrast to non-human communication forms, human language has the properties of productivity, recursivity, and displacement. Human language is also the only system to rely mostly on social convention and learning.[144]*

Deacon reported that "language abilities may be the 'special intelligence' of humans," that the "brain has been shaped by evolutionary processes that elaborated the capacities needed for language, and not just by a general demand for greater intelligence," and that "when all such species-specific biases are taken into account, 'general intelligence' will be found to be less variable among species than once thought."[145] Regarding language, he observed that "so much of what we do, whether it's marriage, warfare, or whatever, has been transformed by this tool that has, in a sense, taken over and biased all of our interactions with the world."[146] A recent study in the United Kingdom by Faisal et al "reinforces the idea that toolmaking and language evolved together as both required more complex thought, making the end of the lower Paleolithic a pivotal time in our history. After this period, early humans left [Africa] and began to colonize other parts of the world."[100] Among the more obvious social advantages, speech would have facilitated the complex thinking abilities necessary for the production of tools. As tools became more sophisticated, sortable into different categories, and made out of more than one material, it is argued that fully developed language must have evolved to enable the transmission of manufacturing skills to the next generation.[147,148]

The brain of the toolmaker (*Homo habilis*) was larger than other hominid species of the same period. A habilis skull, estimated to be 2 million years old, was found to possess a Broca's speech area, although not as prominent a feature as that of modern humans.[149] Earlier ancestors' remains have not revealed this feature, and it is thought that their language might have depended on the limbic system. In infancy, children rely on "the workings of the limbic system to call attention to their needs ... They find temper tantrums, whimpering, or crying a much easier way ... to express [emotions] than to explain." This is despite being able to use simple speech to communicate effectively about less emotional issues. Some experts believe that human speech evolved in a similar fashion.[150]

Edelman argued that humans had the capacity to "produce and act on concepts" and to ascribe meaning prior to language acquisition.[151] Then, changes occurred in the base of the skull as a result of bipedalism at about the same time as the speech areas named after Broca and Wernicke emerged in the brain. Together these "provided a morphological basis for the evolution of...the supralaryngeal tract"[151] that was probably not completed until the emergence of modern Homo sapiens. Part of the evolutionary development was dependent on neural mechanisms involved in speech motor control and in syntax,[128] as well as adaptation of the vocal cords, tongue, palate, and teeth, that facilitated better control of air flow over the vocal cords. This "in turn allowed for the production of coarticulated sounds, the phonemes."[151] Figure 4-6 illustrates the complexities and interactions of many parts of the cortex involved in language according to electrical stimulation, cerebral blood flow, and subtractive positron emission tomography scan.

Many evolutionary scientists favor a link between doing and the evolution of language. Some emphasize the role of gesture and suggest that, as tool usage occupied hands, they became less available for communication, leading to increased use of facial gesticulation and sound.[152,153] This

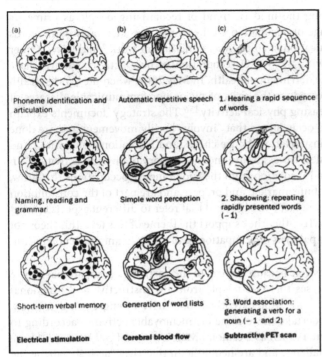

Figure 4-6. Complexities of language and the interactive nature of brain function demonstrated by various means during communication processing tasks: a) by electrical stimulation b) by zenon 133 and c) by PET scans. (Reprinted with permission from Deacon TW. The human brain. In: Jones S, Martin R, Pilbeam D, eds. *The Cambridge Encyclopedia of Human Evolution*. New York: Cambridge University Press; 1992:121.)

theory is supported by observations that hand gestures still accompany speech, and when there are difficulties in verbal communication, such as people conversing in different languages, hand and facial gestures increase. Bruner hypothesized that language is "virtually an outgrowth of the mastery of skilled action and perceptual discrimination," basing this claim on observations of ontogenetic development. From this beginning, he asserted that language is progressively freed from its original dependence on action and experience.[154] Others name hunter-gatherer activities or complex social relationships as the driving force in the evolution of language, with de Laguna suggesting that the most likely explanation lies in the need for help associated with a socio-technical way of life.[155] A combination of causes is probable—humans are both toolmakers and social animals.

Spoken language is the foundation of sociocultural occupations, because without language complex technology and social, corporate, and political structures would be impossible. Although no archaic material record or proof of this remains, reminiscence, singing, and the telling of stories, myths, and legends are central in handing down to the next generation "occupational know how," culturally sanctioned behaviors, taboos, and spiritual beliefs and doings, all of which are intimately related to survival, health, and well-being.

CHANGING PATTERNS OF OCCUPATION HAVE A SIGNIFICANT IMPACT ON HEALTH

The 2011 Rio Declaration on Social Determinants of Health draws attention to the fact that:

> Health inequities arise from the societal conditions in which people are born, grow, live, work and age ... These include early years' experiences, education, economic status, employment and decent work, housing and environment, and effective systems of preventing and treating ill health. We are convinced that action on these determinants, both for vulnerable groups and the entire population, is essential to create inclusive, equitable, economically productive and healthy societies.[18]

This Declaration, although following the modern trend of recognizing people as primarily social-beings, includes within it a range of occupational criteria that are encompassed in words such as "early years' experiences," "education," "employment and decent work," and "live." Other occupations can be added to those with the WHO recognition of how activity patterns have changed over time, in some cases to the detriment of health. In May 2004, when the World Health Assembly adopted a global strategy to reduce the risks of major noncommunicable diseases, it centered on improving diets and increasing physical activity.[156] The strategy documents explain that the term *physical activity* includes occupations that "involve bodily movement and are done as part of playing, working, active transportation, house chores and recreational activities," and that exercise specifically aimed at physical fitness is just one subcategory of physical activity.[156] In that vein, the term *diets* cannot be seen in isolation from the wide ranging occupations that grow, produce, harvest, gather, process, distribute, market, and prepare and are part of the consumption of food. Those recent WHO initiatives are just two of several that refer to different aspects of what people do as important in health terms. Together they support the theme of this text, this theory of human nature, as well as that changing patterns of occupation have a significant impact on health. This can be beneficial or detrimental.

Changing patterns of activity are possible because central to the particular occupational nature of humans are the physiological processes that free people from the instinctive and functional constraints of most animals. These activate an apparently strong drive to engage in daily, new, or adventurous occupations and to undertake unwelcome or unenjoyable activities according to sociocultural expectations. Popular writers such as Desmond Morris[157] and Lyall Watson[158] have contended that most people enjoy a challenge and are neophilic in that they "actively pursue the new and different."[158] In addition, according to Bruner[154] it is only human adults who introduce their offspring to challenging and sometimes frightening new experiences. Among both birds and other mammals, the presence of mothers is required to reduce fear of novel stimuli to enable their offspring to explore.[159] If Bruner's[154] suggestion is correct, perhaps challenging learning experiences are a necessary precursor for people to take risks to create environments in which they feel comfortable and to brave exploration of the unknown. Alternatively, this particular adult occupational behavior may be a byproduct of evolution unconnected to survival of the species.

The freedom and drive to engage in new, adventurous, or, perhaps, dangerous activities is an aspect of people's occupational nature indicative of how humans appear to go beyond survival needs.[160] The range of capacities available to humans allows them to pursue many options that may appear to have no obvious relationship to continued existence and may even result in destroying the species and the world as we know it. However, deliberation about this point has determined that some such options could be considered an integral part of healthy survival mechanisms. Engagement in wide-ranging and sometimes apparently destructive occupations enables people to hone their range of skills, their capacities, and their flexibility so that they are competent to deal with novel situations as they occur. In addition, they may provide exercise to maintain the "well working of the organism as a whole."[161]

In going beyond obvious survival needs in their pursuit of occupation, people evolve and adapt as occupational beings according to their environment, cultural values, innate capacities, and interests. The brain's capacity to adapt to social environments different from those in which humans evolved has led to culture itself creating "norms of human behavior that, in a certain sense, can step in as substitutes for innate behavior programs."[49] From birth, children, through their predominant occupation of play, seek beyond themselves for explanations of the world and their place within it. As they do this, they develop their innate capacities through learning from others, through practicing skills, and through using their minds and bodies to enable them to survive, to interact, and to choose future roles.

Humans are unable to reach a stage where they can take care of themselves from birth. However, the ability of people to adapt socioculturally enables infants at a very early age to assimilate and retain information from the environment before a conscious appreciation of meaning or significance is possible. This early absorption of observed behaviors enables ontogenetic development to be in step with sociocultural expectations. The need to connect with others, as well as the quality of relationships, motivate learning and provide infants with a sense of self and place in the world. Early learning and connecting is mainly acquired through play and having fun. Children solve problems by trial and error, discover new concepts, experiment with roles, figure out how to use language and their body, and figure out how to establish and cement effective relationships.[162] In evolutionary terms, Pellegrini et al proposed that play may have a role in human ontogeny and phylogeny. It enables the young to generate a "repertoire of innovative behaviors that may be adaptive," such as "increased exploration and cooperation, decreased aggression and stereotypic behavior, and dominance status." They suggest that "selection should favor individuals exhibiting these new phenotypes, relative to those who do not."[163]

Early dependence, coupled with the complexity of the brain, means that human babies require social support for many years to assume "full humanness." As part of this process, attitudes and occupational behaviors are absorbed and adopted. It is those formed before intellectual capacities are sufficiently advanced to allow for adequate understanding or refuting that have the strongest, albeit unconscious, hold on individuals. This mechanism would have been central to early humans' healthy survival because it allowed essential learning to occur from birth and stimulated the development of capacities.

Sociologists reason that "human beings are made, not born" because "even if someone argues that human endowments such as soul, rationality, or a tendency to aggressiveness are innate, they cannot ensure that an infant will become a truly functional human being, capable of ethical and cultural responsibility."[164] Infants have to learn as "we enact, rehearse, work, and play our way into the human condition."[164] Their view of the strength of such learned attitudes and behaviors led founding behavioral psychologists Watson[165] and Skinner[166] to argue that only physiological reflexes are inherited, with Watson going so far as to claim:

> *Give me a dozen healthy infants, well-formed, and my own specific world to bring them up in and I'll guarantee to take any one at random and train him to become any kind of specialist I might select—doctor, lawyer, artist, merchant-chief, and yes even beggar-man and thief regardless of his talents, penchants, abilities, vocations, and race of his ancestors.[165]*

Sociologists might not accept Watson's exaggerated language but a similar understanding by them has led to one of sociology's fundamental postulates: human actions are limited or determined by past and present environments and humans are the products and the victims of their society.[167]

> *Societies began historically as geographically and genetically defined groups of people who shared the occupations of survival such as hunting, gathering and defense against enemies. Today, without restrictions to geographic boundaries or genetically linked clans or tribes, there are also societies of shared interests ... Worldwide virtual groups are now connected in the shared occupations of email correspondence; synchronous or asynchronous web group discussions, online blogs and journals ... etc[168]*

Currently, sociologists generally believe that specific behaviors result from social factors that activate physiological predispositions. Although all people engage in a wide range of occupations, they develop particular occupational behavior and preferences from within their specific culture and social niche. This includes the language used, work choices, dietary choices, socialization processes and traditions, and adherence to particular rules and methods of governance. "What one culture accepts as 'normal' may vary considerably from what another culture accepts."[169] However, this rests on the fact that people have the genetic and biological capacity "to learn" and the need and will "to do," which is also part of being human. The occupational theory of human nature described in this chapter holds that, because of their particular mix of biological characteristics and capacities, humans are receptive to the process of enculturation and socialization to the extent that they can be considered products of their particular culture. As anthropologist Richard Leakey observed:

> The most pronounced differences are the way in which people do things: their dress, their architecture, their myths, their songs, their ideals and so on ... The earth is populated by one people living many different styles of life because of a unique cultural capacity. And the mind that expresses this unique capacity is the one that also universally seeks beyond itself for explanations of man himself and the nature of the world around him.[170]

It is held in this occupational theory of human nature that societies are the products of humans acting on their environment. As people engage in occupation, the physical and social environment is altered. Often, the more sophisticated the occupation, the greater the change to the environment, which in turn causes further change to and development of people. Marx suggested that "by thus acting on the external world and changing it, [man] at the same time changes his own nature,"[171] and Braverman, in the same vein, proposed that people are the special product of purposeful action.[172] He argued that occupation that "transcends mere instinctual activity is the force which created humankind and the force by which humankind created the world as we know it."[172] Neff agreed that the most revolutionary force in human history is technological change associated with the way people "wrest their living from nature."[173] He argued that social institutions are merely mirrors of technological levels. This idea, apparently well accepted in archaeological circles, supports the theory that:

- Humans are occupational beings.
- Occupation provides the nuts and bolts of technological change.
- Occupation has the potential to modify the world or the species.
- Occupation provides the mechanism to enable people to survive and adapt to biological, sociological, political, and environmental requirements.
- Occupation is central within the social determinants of health.

Consideration of humans' occupational nature from an ecological, sociological, political, or health perspective is essential. The many models of cultural evolution based on occupational technology are sometimes said not to sufficiently address the influences of other variables, such as local environments, ecology and climate, war and conquest, spiritual beliefs and social struggles, or the complexities of the interactions between them.[173] There is some truth in the criticisms because such views have been limited to economic preoccupation with work or labor perspectives. That neglects a holistic view of occupation, which, of necessity, integrates many factors. Other criticisms have been leveled at the notion of cultural evolution itself, particularly as postulated by Victorian anthropologists, such as Tylor[174] and Morgan,[175] in that it seems to imply that advanced technological societies are somehow better or "higher up the evolutionary ladder" than older cultures with less technical economies.[173] The concept of cultural superiority or the judging of other cultures by the values of one's own is known as ethnocentricity,[176] a term coined by William Sumner in 1906.[177] The notion of cultural superiority is called into question by the argument that cultures can vary independently of race and that no one culture is superior to another.[178] Similarly, the occupational nature of humans is not seen to be more evolved in technologically advanced societies in contrast to hunter-gatherer or agrarian economies, but rather expressed differently according to each culture's history and technological development.

DIAGNOSIS AND PRESCRIPTION

Stevenson and Haberman's[19] guidelines for theories of human nature call for diagnosis and prescription to be considered—any such theory has to include a diagnosis of "what is wrong with humans" and a prescription of how to "right the wrongs" from its particular perspective. As to diagnosis, although the occupational behavior of early humans and the small numbers engaged in such occupations was in tune with self-sustaining natural health and ecological balance, current directions are out of step with the natural heritage of ecology and human nature. This echoes a sentiment expressed by Alexis Carrel that modern civilization "does not suit us," being "born from the whims of scientific discoveries, from the appetites of men, their illusions, their theories, and their desires" but "without any knowledge of our real nature." He argued for a science of human individuals that views them as "an indivisible whole of extreme complexity."[179] It could be suggested that current knowledge of human nature remains rudimentary and that Carrel's science is still necessary despite an avalanche of research in various disciplines in recent decades. The occupational aspects of these need to be combined, studied, extended, and viewed from personal, familial, communal, societal, and global perspectives. In addition, the diagnosis of what is wrong has to include the health problems that have resulted as occupational behavior has changed over millennia and together with population growth threatens the world itself. Immense population growth worldwide, and changing sociocultural values and norms as occupational technology advances toward a people-driven global economy, places pressure on governments worldwide to find new and different solutions. Such changes require a fresh approach to consider how to meet people's occupational needs and wants in ways that enhance health and sustain the ecology. Current day knowledge is fragmentary and, without a real and holistic appreciation of the human need to engage in occupation, it is incomplete.

Individual and collective uniqueness, particularly in relation to how biologic characteristics and capacities, as well as social determinants, influence the biological need for engagement in occupation has not been a focal concern of political or social planners or health practitioners. However, human communities are dispersed across the globe because their individual and collective biologic capacities have developed to the extent of enabling flexible, adaptable, and wide-ranging occupations that can be modified to fit the demands of living in almost any environment. Cultural and occupational evolution, such as the use of tools and the development of agriculture, along with modern medicine, have broken through natural population restraints that maintained the population size of species at a more or less constant level over long periods of time. As a result, ecological systems have become dominated by people, many believe, to the extent of natural resources being insufficient to maintain predicted population growth.[37,39,180] Most estimates of the Earth's global population capacity are between 4 and 16 billion, and in May 2014 the population count was already in excess of 7.1 billion,[181-184] and the rapid increases of recent times are a cause for concern.[181]

As for a prescription of how to right the wrongs, addressing the lack of awareness of people's occupational natures in a way that covers all rather than part of what they do requires consideration, research, and practical trials across many domains, as well as rapid development of the multidisciplinary science of occupation. Such a science, adequately developed and resourced, has the potential to influence social, political, economic, and health policies so that they are more in tune with the holistic combination and complexities of human occupation, social determinism, self-sustaining natural health, and ecological balance. More concrete solutions do not seem advisable because prescriptive theories of human nature, even if they focus on occupational factors, do not allow sufficient flexibility for solutions to be responsive to contextual, environmental, and evolutionary change.

An occupational perspective of human nature is worthy of extensive inquiry because it appears pertinent to many of the problems the world faces, particularly how to maintain health and ensure human survival in an economic and self-sustaining way that meets the biological, sociocultural, and occupational needs of people, as well as redresses ecological degradation. Because of the nature of the approach taken, the exploration that follows can only touch on these wide-ranging issues.

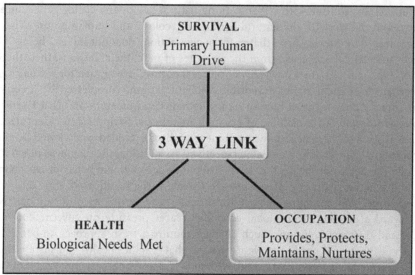

Figure 4-7. Three-way link between occupation, health, and survival.

A THREE-WAY LINK BETWEEN OCCUPATION, HEALTH, AND SURVIVAL

Unless asked to consider such factors, or some process or part of the mechanism goes amiss, people are not usually conscious of the survival and health-maintaining functions of what they do as part of their life. Like the autonomic nervous system, these factors are built into the organism to just go on working. Because of this, people are able to use their capacities for their own purposes, to explain the purpose of life in abstract rather than biological ways, and to attribute meaning to activity based on sociocultural factors. It follows that, in the current circumstances, many individuals are unable to distinguish their biological needs, which ultimately impact their health, from their wants or preferences.[185] This is believed to occur partly because the complexity of sociocultural evolution makes differentiation difficult so that "even phylogenetically evolved programs of … behavior are adjusted to the presence of a culture," which alters the significance of biological needs.[186] Fletcher goes as far as categorizing particular forms of doing to define what being human means. Along with bipedalism and toolmaking, he lists "the capacity to control fire, to interact socially with their dead, and to represent the universe in art" as marks of humanness in evolutionary terms.[187]

Our occupational nature is the result of evolution/phylogeny, genetics, ontogeny, ecological and sociocultural environments, and opportunity, all of which are centered, processed, and integrated in the brain. Forms of occupation provide the framework for daily life for all people unless prevented by disorder, external constraint, or particular forms of socialization or political expectation. This occupational theory of human nature proposes that the brain has "healthy survival" as its primary role. To facilitate healthy survival, it continually activates people's particular mix of characteristics and capacities through engagement in occupation. It is both an occupational brain and a healing brain.

Engagement in occupation forms a three-way link with health and survival (Figure 4-7). Survival is recognized as the primary drive of all animals, including humans, and is the outcome of the use of particular capacities to provide for the essential needs of the organism. This includes the occupational behavior required to develop and maintain supportive social, ecological, and material environments. The WHO recognizes those as prerequisites of health and they are the focus of the next chapter, which defines occupation in more detail. The extent and quality of survival for individuals, families, communities, and societal and global populations depends on their health and physical, mental, and social well-being; health is the outcome of each organism having all essential sustenance and safety needs met and of having physical, mental, and social capacities maintained, developed, exercised, and in balance. This is achieved through what people do. In turn, engagement in occupation depends on a level of health and its specific components, which are able to provide the energy, drive, and functional attributes necessary for engagement. In addition, survival as a healthy species depends on a humans' capacity to live in harmony with others, and within an environment that can continue to provide basic requirements, ensure the continued acquisition of these requirements, and provide safety and education for the next generation.

Conclusion

Possibly throughout human history, and certainly in current times, engagement in occupation has been dependent on and responsive to the particular adaptations that are common to the species. It is also driven by what needs to be done for individual, familial, and communal survival: to provide water, food, shelter, a place that facilitates adequate rest, and safety from predators. These were described earlier as obligatory or necessary occupations. In addition, humans have honed their skills and explored their talents and capacities through what might be described as occupations of choice, and they have offset the active periods of each day with restful activities and sleep.

Archaeologists and anthropologists recognize the strong links between what humans do, biological evolution, and survival of species. It is central to life and living and health and development and has been so throughout the evolution of the species. Human evolution through what people do has helped shape human biology, just as human biology has shaped occupations. This reciprocal and critical interaction has long-term health, illness, and survival consequences.

This occupational theory of human nature has introduced the concept that humans are occupational beings, and that "changing patterns of life, work and leisure have a significant impact on health." This is because, in common with all living creatures, healthy survival is the fundamental and evolutionary goal of humans who are adapted and socialized to engage in sophisticated and wide ranging occupations to meet the requirements of life. Because people are occupational beings, it is essential that "work and leisure should be a source of health."[1]

Further consideration of this theory will be possible as more information is uncovered about biological needs, natural health, ancient and modern rules for health, and occupational evolution. Occupation-related characteristics and capacities, occupational illness, the prevention of illness, and health and well-being will be discussed in terms of the prerequisites and social determinants of health and well-being as defined by the WHO. However, the next chapter will concentrate on clarifying and defining occupation itself, particularly in its relationship to health.

References

1. World Health Organization, Health and Welfare Canada, Canadian Public Health Association. *Ottawa Charter for Health Promotion*. Ottawa, Canada; 1986.
2. National Sleep Foundation. *Sleepmatters*. 2006;8(4). http://sleepmedicine.com/content.cfm?article=14 Accessed May 23, 2014.
3. National Sleep Foundation. *How Much Sleep Do We Really Need?* http://www.sleepfoundation.org/article/how-sleep-works/how-much-sleep-do-we-really-need. Accessed October 2, 2012.
4. Duldt BW, Giffin K. *Theoretical Perspectives for Nursing*. Boston, MA: Little, Brown and Co; 1985:47.
5. Lewin K. *Principles of Topological Psychology*. New York, NY: McGraw Hill; 1947.
6. Law M, Baum CM, Baptiste S, eds. *Occupation-based Practice: Fostering Performance and Participation*. Thorofare, NJ: Slack; 2002.

7. Letts L, Rigby P, Stewart D, eds. *Using Environments to Enable Occupational Performance.* Thorofare, NJ: Slack; 2003.
8. Molineux M, ed. *Occupation for Occupational Therapists.* Oxford, UK: Blackwell Publishing; 2004.
9. Schmid T, ed. *Promoting Health through Creativity: For Professions in Health, Art and Education.* London: Whurr Publishers; 2005.
10. Whiteford G, Wright-St Clair V, eds. *Occupation and Practice in Context.* Sydney, Australia: Elsevier/ Churchill Livingstone; 2005.
11. Christiansen CH, Townsend EA, eds. *Introduction to Occupation: The Art and Science of Living.* 2nd ed. Upper Saddle River, NJ: Prentice Hall; 2010.
12. Whiteford G, Hocking C, eds. *Occupational Science: Society, Inclusion, Participation.* Oxford, Wiley-Blackwell; 2012.
13. Matuska K, Christiansen C, eds. *Life Balance: Multidisciplinary Theories and Research.* Thorofare, NJ., Slack Inc., and AOTA Press; 2009.
14. Wilcock AA. *An Occupational Perspective of Health.* Thorofare, NJ; Slack.1998.
15. World Health Organization. *Active Ageing: A Policy Framework.* Geneva: WHO; 2002. http://www. who.int/ageing/publications/active_ageing/en/. Accessed May 28, 2014.
16. World Health Organization. *Mental Health: Strengthening our Response.* Fact sheet N°220. Updated April 2014. http://www.who.int/mediacentre/factsheets/fs220/en/. Accessed May 28, 2014.
17. World Health Organization. *Noncommunicable Diseases Fact Sheet.* Updated March 2013. http://www. who.int/mediacentre/factsheets/fs355/en/. Accessed May 28, 2014.
18. World Health Organization. *Rio Declaration on Social Determinants of Health.* Rio de Janeiro, Brazil, 21 October 2011. http://www.who.int/sdhconference/declaration/en/. Accessed May 28, 2014.
19. Stevenson L, Haberman D. *Ten Theories of Human Nature.* 3rd ed. New York & Oxford: Oxford University Press; 1998.
20. Markovic M. Human nature. In: Bottomore T, ed. *A Dictionary of Marxist Thought.* 2nd ed. Oxford, UK: Blackwell Publishers; 1991:209.
21. Hawking SW. *A Brief History of Time.* Toronto: Bantam Books; 1988:10.
22. Stevenson L, Haberman D. *Ten Theories of Human Nature.* 3rd ed. Oxford: Oxford University Press; 1998:9.
23. Van den Berghe PL. *Sociobiology.* In: Kuper A, Kuper J, eds. *The Social Science Encyclopedia.* Rev ed. London, England: Routledge; 1989:797.
24. Csikszentmihalyi M, Csikszentmihalyi IS. *Optimal Experience: Psychological Studies of Flow in Consciousness.* New York, NY: Cambridge University Press; 1988.
25. Csikszentmihalyi M, Massimini F. On the psychological selection of bicultural information. *New Ideas in Psychology.* 1985;3(2):115-138.
26. Snell GD. *Search for a Rational Ethic.* New York, NY: Springer Verlag; 1988.
27. Universitat València: Cavanilles Institute of Biodiversity and Evolutionary Biology. *Resources for Ecology, Evolutionary Biology, Systematics and Conservation Biology.* Available from: http://www. uv.es/uvweb/cavanilles-institute-biodiversity-biology/en/research/search-groups/evolutionary-genetics/technical-technological-equipment-1285894862041.html. Accessed May 28, 2014.
28. Leakey R, Lewin R. *People of the Lake: Man: His Origins, Nature and Future.* New York, NY: Penguin Books; 1978.
29. Abiogenesis. Wikipedia. Available at: http://en.wikipedia.org/wiki/Abiogenesis. Accessed May 28, 2014.
30. Zimmer C. Origins. On the origin of eukaryotes. *Science.* 2009;325(5941):666-668. doi:10.1126/science.325_666. PMID 19661396.
31. Stavrianos LS. *The World to 1500: A Global History.* 4th ed. Upper Saddle River, NJ: Prentice Hall; 1988:4.
32. Hazen RM. *Genesis: The Scientific Quest for Life's Origins.* Washington, DC: Joseph Henry Press; 2005:243.
33. Wachtershauser G. Evolution of the first metabolic cycles. *Proceedings of the National Academy of Sciences USA.* 1990;87:200-204.
34. Darwin C. *Origin of the Species by Means of Natural Selection.* Cambridge, MA: Harvard University Press; 1964. Original work published 1859.
35. Darwin C. *The Descent of Man and Selection in Relation to Sex.* New York, NY: Appleton; 1930. Original work published 1871.
36. Dawkins R. The replicators. In: Dixon B, ed. *From Creation to Chaos: Classic Writings in Science.* Oxford, UK: Basil Blackwood Ltd; 1989:39-44.

37. Jones S. The nature of evolution. In: Jones S, Martin R, Pilbeam D, eds. *The Cambridge Encyclopedia of Human Evolution.* New York, NY: Cambridge University Press; 1992:9.

38. Spencer H. *Principles of Biology. Vol 1.* New York, NY: Appleton; 1864:444.

39. Campbell BG. *Humankind Emerging.* 5th ed. New York, NY: Harper Collins Publishers; 1988:60-69,90-91,366.

40. Ebrahim S. Professor of Public Health at the London School of Hygiene and Tropical Medicine. http://www.lshtm.ac.uk/aboutus/people/ebrahim.shah. Accessed February 7, 2013.

41. Stern C, Sherwood ER, eds. *The Origin of Genetics.* San Francisco, CA: WH Freeman; 1966.

42. Medawar P. Darwinism. In: *The Fontana Dictionary of Modern Thought.* 2nd ed. London, England: Fontana Press; 1988.

43. McHenry HM. Evolution. In: Kuper A, Kuper J, eds. *The Social Science Encyclopedia.* Rev ed. London, England: Routledge; 1989.

44a. Dyson F. The argument from design. Disturbing the universe 1979. In: Dixon B, ed. *From Creation to Chaos: Classic Writings in Science.* Oxford, UK: Basil Blackwood Ltd; 1989:49.

44b. Dahm R. Discovering DNA: Friedrich Miescher and the early years of nucleic acid research. *Human Genetics.* 2008;122(6):565-81.

44c Levene P. The structure of yeast nucleic acid. *Journal of Biological Chemistry.* 1919;40(2):415-24.

44d. Soyfer V. The consequences of political dictatorship for Russian science. *Nature Reviews Genetics.* 2001;2(9):723-729.

44e. Lorenz MG, Wackernagel W. Bacterial gene transfer by natural genetic transformation in the environment. *Microbiology Review.* 1994;58(3):563-602.

44f. Hershey A, Chase M. Independent functions of viral protein and nucleic acid in growth of bacteriophage. *Journal of Genetic Physiology.* 1952;36(1):39-56.

44g. Watson J, Crick F. A structure for deoxyribose nucleic Acid. (PDF). *Nature.* 1953;171(4356):737-738.

44h. Crick F. *On Degenerate Templates and the Adaptor Hypothesis.* 1955. http://genome.wellcome.ac.uk. Accessed December 22, 2006.

45. Watson J, Crick F. Molecular structure of nucleic acids; a structure for deoxyribose nucleic acid. *Nature.* 1953;171(43560):737-738.

46. Leakey RE. Introduction. Darwin C. *The Illustrated Origin of the Species.* Abridged. London, UK: The Rainbird Publishing Co; 1979. Original work published 1859.

47. Stevenson L, Haberman D. *Ten Theories of Human Nature.* 3rd ed. New York & Oxford: Oxford University Press; 1998:137.

48. Bronowski J. *The Ascent of Man.* London, England: British Broadcasting Corp; 1973:31.

49. Lorenz K. *The Waning of Humaneness.* Boston, MA: Little, Brown and Co; 1987:5,21,57-58,93,124.

50. Ornstein R, Sobel D. *The Healing Brain: A Radical New Approach to Health Care.* London, England: MacMillan; 1988:11-12.

51. McHenry HM. Evolution. In: Kuper A, Kuper J, eds. *The Social Science Encyclopedia.* Rev ed. London, England: Routledge; 1989:280.

52. Edelman G. *Bright Air, Brilliant Fire: On the Matter of the Mind.* London, England: Penguin Books; 1992:40.

53. Campbell J. *Winston Churchill's Afternoon Nap.* London, England: Palladin Grafton Books; 1986:54.

54. James W. *The Principles of Psychology. Vol 1.* New York, NY: Dover Publications; 1890:239.

55. Pickrell J. Crows better at building than chimps, study says. *National Geographic News.* April 23, 2003. Available at: http://news.nationalgeographic.com/news/2003/04/0423_030423_crowtools.html. Aaccessed May 28, 2014.

56. Kolb B, Whishaw IQ. *Fundamentals of Human Neuropsychology.* 3rd ed. San Franscico, CA: WH Freeman; 1990:106.

57. Campbell BG. *Humankind Emerging.* 5th ed. New York, NY: Harper Collins Publishers; 1988.

58. Edelman G. *Bright Air, Brilliant Fire: On the Matter of the Mind.* London, England: Penguin Books; 1992.

59. Campbell BG. *Humankind Emerging.* 5th ed. New York, NY: Harper Collins Publishers; 1988:366.

60. Deacon TW. The human brain. In: Jones S, Martin R, Pilbeam D, eds. *The Cambridge Encyclopedia of Human Evolution.* New York, NY: Cambridge University Press; 1992:115.

61. Jerison HJ. *Evolution of the Brain and Intelligence.* New York, NY: Academic Press; 1973.

62. Herculano-Houzel S. The human brain in numbers: a linearly scaled-up primate brain. *Frontiers of Human Neuroscience.* 2009;3:31. Epub 2009 Nov. 9.

63. Rose S. *The Conscious Brain.* Rev ed. London, England: Penguin Books; 1976.

64. Ornstein R, Sobel D. *The Healing Brain: A Radical New Approach to Health Care.* London, England: Macmillan; 1988:36.

65. Spencer H. *First Principles.* 6th ed. London, Williams & Norgate; 1900.

66. Kolb B, Whishaw IQ. *Fundamentals of Human Neuropsychology.* 6th ed. New York, NY: Worth Publishers; 2008.

67. Campbell BG. *Humankind Emerging.* 5th ed. New York, NY: Harper Collins Publishers; 1988:55.

68. Campbell BG. *Humankind Emerging.* 5th ed. New York, NY: Harper Collins Publishers; 1988:374-378.

69. McMichael T. *Human Frontiers, Environments and Disease: Past Patterns, Uncertain Futures.* Cambridge, UK: Cambridge University Press; 2001;20.

70. McMichael T. *Human Frontiers, Environments and Disease: Past Patterns, Uncertain Futures.* Cambridge, UK: Cambridge University Press; 2001;49.

71. Burke J, Ornstein R. *The Axemaker's Gift: Technology's Capture and Control of our Minds and Culture.* New York, NY: Tarcher/Putnam; 1997.

72. Sperry R. *Some Effects of Disconnecting the Cerebral Hemispheres.* Les Prix Nobel; 1981:209-219.

73. Edelman G. *Bright Air, Brilliant Fire: On the Matter of the Mind.* London, England: Penguin Books; 1992:7,16-19.

74. Snell GD. *Search for a Rational Ethic.* New York, NY: Springer Verlag; 1988:140,147,165.

75. Cosgrove K, Mazure C, Staley J. Evolving knowledge of sex differences in brain structure, function, and chemistry. *Biological Psychiatry.* 2007:62(8):847-855.

76. Penfield W, Boldrey E. Somatic motor and sensory representation in the cerebral cortex as studied by electrical stimulation. *Brain.* 1958;60:389-443.

77. Brodmann K. *Vergleichended Lokalisations Lehre der Grosshirnrinde in Prinzipien Dargestellt auf Grund des Zellenbaues.* Liepzig: JA Barth; 1909.

78. Kolb B, Whishaw IQ. *Fundamentals of Human Neuropsychology.* 3rd ed. San Franscico, CA: WH Freeman and Co; 1990:4.

79. Lassen NA, Ingvar DH, Skinhoj E. Brain function and blood flow. *Scientific American.* 1978;239:62-71.

80. Roland PE. Applications of brain blood flow imaging in behavioral neurophysiology: cortical field activation hypothesis. In: Sokoloff L, ed. *Brain Imaging and Brain Function.* New York, NY: Raven Press; 1985:87-104.

81. Kety SS. Disorders of the human brain. *Scientific American.* 1979;241:202-214.

82. Mazziotta JC, Phelps ME. Human neuropsychological imaging studies of local brain metabolism: strategies and results. In: Sokoloff L, ed. *Brain Imaging and Brain Function.* New York, NY: Raven Press; 1985.

83. Restak R. *The Brain.* New York, NY: Bantam Books; 1984.

84. Deacon TW. The human brain. In: Jones S, Martin R, Pilbeam D, eds. *The Cambridge Encyclopedia of Human Evolution.* New York, NY: Cambridge University Press; 1992:123.

85. Lorenz K. *The Waning of Humaneness.* Munich, Germany: R Piper and Co Verlag; 1983:57-58.

86. Jelinek J. *Primitive Hunters.* London, England: Hamlyn; 1989.

87. Campbell BG. *Humankind Emerging.* 5th ed. New York, NY: Harper Collins Publishers; 1988:364-365.

88. Rathelot J, Strick P. Subdivisions of primary motor cortex based on cortico-motoneural cells. *Proceedings of the National Academy of Science.* 2009. doi:10.1073/pnas.0808362106

89. Bell Sir C. *The Hand: Its Mechanism and Vital Endowments as Evincing Design.* Brentwood: The Pilgrims Press; 1979:108.

90. Darwin C. *The Descent of Man and Selection in Relation to Sex.* London: Murray;. 1871:52.

91. Goodall J. *The Chimpanzees of Gombe.* Cambridge, MA: Harvard/Belknap; 1986.

92. Brewer SM, McGrew WC. Chimpanzee use of a tool-set to get honey. *Folia Primatologica.* 1990;54:100-104.

93. The Jane Goodall Institute. *Toolmaking.* http://www.janegoodall.org/chimp-central-toolmakers. Accessed May 24, 2014.

94. Trivedi B. The use of infrared, motion-triggered video cameras in the Congo. *National Geographic News.* October 6, 2004.95.

95. Young R. Evolution of the human hand: the role of throwing and clubbing. *Journal of Anatomy.* 2003;202(1):165-174. doi:10.1046/j.1469-7580.2003.00144.x.

96. Franklin B. Man is a tool-making animal. April 1778. Famous Quotations from US History - Benjamin Franklin. mr_sedivy.tripod.com/quotes13.html.

97.   Leakey L, Tobias P, Napier J. A new species of the genus homo from the Olduvai Gorge. *Nature.* 1964;4927:7-9. http://www.clas.ufl.edu/users/krigbaum/proseminar/leakey_etal_nature_1964.pdf. Accessed May 24, 2014.

98.   Smithsonian National Museum of Natural History. What does it mean to be human? *Species.* http:// humanorigins.si.edu/evidence/human-fossils/species. Accessed August 23, 2012.

99.   Jelinek J. *Primitive Hunters.* London, England: Hamlyn; 1989:24.

100. Faisal A, Stout D, Apel J, Bradley B. The manipulative complexity of lower paleolithic stone toolmaking. *PLoS ONE.* 2010;5(11):e13718. doi:10.1371/journal.pone.0013718

101. Tinkaus E. Evolution of human manipulation. In: Jones S, Martin R, Pilbeam D, eds. *The Cambridge Encyclopedia of Human Evolution.* New York, NY: Cambridge University Press; 1992:349.

102. Van Den Hoven B. *Work in Ancient and Medieval Thought: Ancient Philosophers, Medieval Monks and Theologians and their Concept of Work, Occupations and Technology.* Amsterdam: J.C. Gieben, Publisher: 1996;55.

103. McHenry H. Human evolution. In: Ruse M, Travis J. *Evolution: The First Four Billion Years.* Cambridge, MA: The Belknap Press of Harvard University Press. 2009:263.

104. Ward CV, Leakey MG, Walker A. Morphology of Australopithecus anamensis from Kanapoi and Allia Bay, Kenya. *Journal of Human Evolution.* 2001;41:255-368

105. Fleagle JG. Primate locomotion and posture. In: Jones S, Martin R, Pilbeam D, eds. *The Cambridge Encyclopedia of Human Evolution.* New York, NY: Cambridge University Press; 1992:79.

106. Harcourt-Smith W. *The Origins of Bipedal Locomotion.* Berlin, Heidelberg; Springer-Verlag: 2007. https://docs.google.com/viewer?a=v&q=cache:go00Q6qgy3IJ:evolution.binghamton.edu/evos/wp-content/uploads.

107. Lewin R. *In the Age of Mankind: A Smithsonian Book of Human Evolution.* Washington, DC: Smithsonian Books; 1988:174,179-180.

108. Watanabe H. Running, creeping and climbing: a new ecological and evolutionary perspective on human locomotion. *Mankind.* 1971;8(1):1-13.

109. Alexander RMN. Walking and running. *American Scientist.* 1984;72:348-354.

110. Alexander RMN. Characteristics and advantages of human bipedalism. In: Rayner JMV, Wootton R, eds. *Biomechanics in Evolution.* New York, NY: Cambridge University Press; 1991.

111. Campbell BG. *Humankind Emerging.* 5th ed. New York, NY: Harper Collins Publishers; 1988:230.

112. Rogers-Ramachandran D, Ramachandran VS. Seeing in stereo: illusions of depth. Scientific American. 2009; July 1. http://www.scientificamerican.com/article/seeing-in-stereo/. Accessed May 29 2014.

113. Ornstein R, Sobel D. *The Healing Brain: A Radical New Approach to Health Care.* London, England: Macmillan; 1988:105-106.

114. Watson L. *Neophilia: The Tradition of the New.* Great Britain: Hodder and Stoughton Ltd; 1989:67.

115. Ornstein R, Sobel D. *The Healing Brain: A Radical New Approach to Health Care.* London, England: Macmillan; 1988:218.

116. Hopkins CD. Sensory mechanisms in animal communication. In: Dewsbury DA, Slater PJB, eds. *Animal Behavior, Vol. 2: Communication.* New York, NY: Freeman; 1983.

117. Leger DW. *Biological Foundations for Behavior: An Integrative Approach.* New York, NY: Harper Collins Publishers; 1992.

118. Coren S, Porac C, Ward LM. *Sensation and Perception.* 2nd ed. Orlando, FL: Academic Press; 1984.

119. Origin of language. Wikipedia, the free encyclopedia. http://en.wikipedia.org/wiki/Origin_of_language. Accessed May 29, 2014.

120. Pinker S, Bloom P. Natural language and natural selection. *Behavioral and Brain Sciences.* 1990;13:707-784.

121. Pinker S. *The Language Instinct.* London: Penguin. 1994.

122. Ulbaek I. The origin of language and cognition. In: Hurford J, Studdert-Kennedy M, Knight C, eds. *Approaches to the Evolution of Language: Social and Cognitive Bases.* Cambridge: Cambridge University Press. 1998:30-43.

123. Tomasello M. The cultural roots of language. In: Velichkovsky B, Rumbaugh D. eds. *Communicating Meaning. The Evolution and Development of Language.* Mahwah, NJ: Erlbaum. 1996:275-307.

124. Pika S, Mitani J. Referential gesturing in wild chimpanzees (Pan troglodytes). *Current Biology.* 2006:16:191-192.

125. The Evolution of Language: Babel or Babble. *The Economist.* 16 April 2011:85-86. http://www.economist.com/node/18557572. Accessed May 29, 2014.

126. Cross I, Woodruff G. Music as a communication medium. In: Botha R, Knight C, eds. *The Prehistory of Language*. Oxford: Oxford University Press; 2008;77-98.

127. Lieberman P. *The Biology and Evolution of Language*. Cambridge, Mass: Harvard University Press; 1984.

128. Lieberman P. Human speech and language. In: Jones S, Martin R, Pilbeam D, eds. *The Cambridge Encyclopedia of Human Evolution*. New York, NY: Cambridge University Press; 1992:136-137.

129. Chomsky N. Language and mind: current thoughts on ancient problems. Part I & Part II. In: Jenkins L ed. *Variation and Universals in Biolinguistics*. Amsterdam: Elsevier; 2004:379-405.

130. Chomsky N. Three factors in language design. *Linguistic Inquiry*. 2005;36(1):1-22.

131. Chomsky N. *The Architecture of Language*. Oxford: Oxford University Press; 2000.

132. Ruhlen M. *Origin of Language*. New York, NY: Wiley. 1994:3.

133. Olson S. *Mapping Human History*. Boston, MA: Houghton Mifflin Books; 2002.

134. Bickerton D. *Adam's Tongue: How Humans Made Language. How Language Made Humans*. New York, NY: Farrar, Straus and Giroux; 2009.

135. Kimura D. *Neuromotor Mechanisms in Human Communication*. Oxford: Oxford University Press. 1993.

136. Newman A, et al. A critical period for right hemisphere recruitment in American sign language processing. *Nature Neuroscience*. 2002;5(1):76-80.

137. Kolb B, Whishaw I. *Fundamentals of Human Neuropsychology*. 5th ed. New York, NY: Worth Publishers; 2003.

138. Corballis M. Did language evolve from manual gestures? In: Wray A, ed. *The Transition to Language*. Oxford: Oxford University Press, 2002:161-179.

139. Falk D. Prelinguistic evolution in early Hominins: whence motherese? *Behavioral and Brain Sciences*. 2004;27:491-503.

140. Botha R, Knight C, eds. *The Cradle of Language*. Oxford: Oxford University Press; 2009.

141. Lenneberg EH. *Biological Foundations of Language*. New York, NY: Wiley; 1967.

142. John-Steiner V, Panofsky CP. Human specificity in language: socio-genetic processes in verbal communication. In: Greenberg G, ed. *Cognition, Language and Consciousness: Integrative Levels*. Hillsdale, NJ: Erlbaum; 1987:85-98.

143. Chomsky N. *The Origin of Language: Its Nature Origin and Use*. New York, NY: Praeger; 1986.

144. Language. Wikipedia. http://en.wikipedia.org/wiki/Language. Accessed May 29, 2014.

145. Deacon TW. The human brain. In: Jones S, Martin R, Pilbeam D, eds. *The Cambridge Encyclopedia of Human Evolution*. New York, NY: Cambridge University Press; 1992:115, 119, 123.

146. Deacon T. *The Co-evolution of Language and the Brain*. http://www.childrenofthecode.org/interviews/deacon.htm. Accessed September 2012.

147. Klarreich E. Biography of Richard G Klein. *Proceedings of the National Academy of Sciences of the United States of America*. 2004;101(16):5705-5707.

148. Wolpert L. *Six Impossible Things Before Breakfast. The Evolutionary Origins of Belief*. New York: Norton; 2006.

149. Leakey R. *The Making of Mankind*. London, England: Michael Joseph Ltd; 1981.

150. Campbell BG. *Humankind Emerging*. 5th ed. New York, NY: Harper Collins Publishers; 1988:360.

151. Edelman G. *Bright Air, Brilliant Fire: On the Matter of the Mind*. London, England: Penguin Books; 1992:126.

152. Hewes GW. Language origin theories. In: Rumbaugh DM, ed. *Language Learning by a Chimpanzee*. New York, NY: Academic Press; 1977.

153. Kimura D. Neuromotor mechanisms in the evolution of human communications. In: Steklis HD, Raleigh MJ, ed. *Neurobiology of Social Communication in Primates: An Evolutionary Perspective*. New York, NY: Academic Press; 1979.

154. Bruner J. Nature and uses of immaturity. *American Psychologist*. 1972;August:687-708.

155. de Laguna GA. *Speech: Its Function and Development*. Bloomington, IN: Indiana University Press; 1963. Originally published 1927.

156. World Health Organization. *Global Strategy on Diet, Physical Activity and Health*. http://www.who.int/dietphysicalactivity/pa/en/index.html. Accessed October 3, 2012.

157. Morris D. *The Human Zoo*. London, England: Jonathan Cape; 1969.

158. Watson L. *Neophilia: The Tradition of the New*. Great Britain: Hodder and Stoughton Ltd; 1989.

159. King DL. A review and interpretation of some aspects of the infant-mother relationship in mammals and birds. *Psychological Bulletin*. 1966;65:143-155.

160. Morris D. *The Human Animal*. BBC TV Production, England, 1994.

161. Kass LR. Regarding the end of medicine and the pursuit of health. In: Caplan AL, Englehardt HT, McCartney JJ, eds. *Concepts of Health and Disease: Interdisciplinary Perspectives*. Reading, MA: Addison-Wesley Publishing Co; 1981.

162. National Centre for Infants, Toddlers, and Families: Zero to Three. *Early Experiences Matter: Behavior and Development*. www.zerotothree.org/child-development/. Accessed October 12, 2012.

163. Pellegrini A, Dupuis D, Smith P. Play in evolution and development. *Developmental Review*. 2007;27:261-276.

164. Driver T. *The Magic of Ritual*. San Francisco, CA: Harper Collins Publishers; 1991:16.

165. Watson JB. *Behaviourism*. New York, NY: WW Norton; 1970:104.

166. Skinner BF. *Science and Human Behaviour*. New York, NY: Macmillan; 1953.

167. Shils E. Sociology. In: Kuper A, Kuper J, eds. *The Social Science Encyclopedia*. Rev ed. London, England: Routledge; 1989:799-810.

168. Christiansen C, Townsend E. The occupational nature of social groups. In: Christiansen C, Townsend E, eds. *Introduction to Occupation: The Art and Science of Living*. 2nd ed. Upper Saddle River, NJ; Pearson. 2010:177-178.

169. Houghton, Mifflin, Harcourt. Cliffs Notes. Sociology: Culture's Roots: Biological or Societal? http://www.cliffsnotes.com/sciences/sociology/culture-and-societies/cultures-roots-biological-or-societal. Accessed May 29, 2014.

170. Leakey R. *The Making of Mankind*. London, England: Michael Joseph Ltd; 1981:248.

171. Marx K. *Capital*. Vol 1. Hamburg, Germany: Otto Meissner; 1867:179-180.

172. Braverman H. *Labor and Monopoly Capital: The Degradation of Work in the Twentieth Century*. New York, NY: Monthly Review Press; 1974.

173. Neff WS. *Work and Human Behavior*. 3rd ed. New York, NY: Aldine Publishing Co; 1985:20.

174. Tylor EB. *Anthropology: An Introduction to the Study of Man and Civilization*. Ann Arbor, MI: University of Michigan Press; 1960.

175. Morgan LH. *Ancient Society*. Cambridge, MA: Belknap; 1964.

176. Omohundro J. *Thinking Like an Anthropologist: A Practical Introduction to Cultural Anthropology*. New York, NY: McGraw Hill; 2008.

177. Sumner W. *Folkways*. New York: Ginn; 1906.

178. Hatch E. Culture. In: Kuper A, Kuper J, eds. *The Social Science Encyclopedia*. Rev ed. London, England: Routledge; 1989:179.

179. Carrel A. *Man the Unknown*. London, England: Burns and Oates; 1935:14.

180. Suzuki D. *The Sacred Balance*. Vancouver/Toronto: Greystone Books; 2002.

181. Over Population. Wikipedia. http://en.wikipedia.org/wiki/Overpopulation. Accessed May 29, 2014.

182. U.S. Census Bureau. *World Population Clock Projection*. http://www.census.gov/popclock/. Accessed October 21, 2011.

183. British Broadcasting Corporation. *Population Seven Billion: UN set out Challenges*. http://www.bbc.co.uk/news/world-15459643. Accessed May 29, 2014.

184. The Guardian. *World's Seven Billionth Baby is Born*. http://www.theguardian.com/world/2011/oct/31/seven-billionth-baby-born-philippines. Accessed May 29, 2014.

185. Fitzgerald R, ed. *Human Needs and Politics*. Sydney, Australia: Permagon; 1977.

186. Lorenz K. *The Waning of Humaneness*. Munich, Germany: R Piper and Co Verlag; 1983:124.

187. Fletcher R. The evolution of human behaviour. In: Buranhult G, ed. *The First Humans: Human Origins and History to 10,000BC*. Australia: University of Queensland Press; 1993:17.

Theme 5

The prerequisites for health: "peace, shelter, education, food, income, a stable ecosystem, sustainable resources, social justice, and equity."

WHO: The Ottawa Charter for Health Promotion, 1986[1]

Chapter 5

DEFINING OCCUPATION IN RELATION TO HEALTH

- Defining Occupation
  - ○ Origins of Occupation and its Synonyms
  - ○ Common Definitions
- Introduction to Health-Related Definitions of Occupation
  - ○ Prerequisites of Health: A Foundational Definition
  - ○ Definitions Relating Aspects of Occupation to Health
  - ○ Definitions of Holistic Understandings of Occupation and Health
    - ➤ Time Use Researchers
    - ➤ Occupational Therapists
    - ➤ Occupational Scientists
- Defining Occupation as Doing, Being, Belonging, and Becoming
  - ○ Doing
  - ○ Being
  - ○ Belonging
  - ○ Becoming
- Conclusion

Defining Occupation

It was proposed in Chapter 4 that, as a result of their biological evolution and enculturation, people are occupational beings, and that occupation is the combination of everything that people do throughout their lives—that health and life itself is dependent upon it. To clarify the extent of what is meant by occupation in this text, this chapter starts with a review of the many different ways occupation has been discussed and defined.

Wilcock AA, Hocking C.
An Occupational Perspective of Health, Third Edition (pp 116-145).

ORIGINS OF OCCUPATION AND ITS SYNONYMS

Occupation is a word with a variety of meanings. The origin of occupation in Middle English was occupien from the 13th to 14th century when it was defined as "being employed in something," or "a particular action" and from the 15th century when it meant "trade."[2] Occupien derived from the 12th century French occupacion or occupier, which in turn derived from the Latin occupatio-nem, meaning "a taking possession, business, employment"[2] and the verb occupare, meaning "to occupy or to seize hold of." Occupare had four different applications that are still evident today. The first meaning, "a taking possession, occupying, seizure," is primarily outside the realm of this work because it mainly relates to the military occupation of a taken territory, except for in the sense of "to take or fill up space or time," as in "I was occupied this morning reading the paper."[3] The other three meanings, "a business, employment, occupation," "trivial employments," and "state affairs," are relevant.[4]

Because it has such a range of meanings, occupation has been specifically chosen as the core word in this text referring to all of the things that people do in their lives and their relationship with health. Despite the fact that it is sometimes used to mean only work, paid employment, or labor, occupation can be more inclusive of the whole range of people's doings than the other words that describe particular aspects. It has been selected instead of activity because the latter is seldom used to imply paid employment, although it is sometimes used to describe aspects of it. Occupation is seen here to embrace activity, behavior, work, labor, praxis, leisure, pastime, and rest.

Activity is derived from the Latin agere, meaning "to do."[5] This is the word most close in meaning to occupation and is often used interchangeably with it, as is sometimes the case in this text. It is defined as "the state of being active; the exertion of energy, action,"[6] and as "a condition in which things are ... being done: busy or vigorous action or movement: an action taken in pursuit of an objective: a recreational pursuit."[7] Activity is the chosen term of researchers in several health-related fields. For example, an extensive 13-year longitudinal Harvard public health study of the mortality of older Americans with regard to the participants' social and productive activities was published in the British Medical Journal in 1999.[8] The findings clearly show the long-term positive and protective impact of doing more than physical exercise. Glass et al argued:

> *While physical fitness itself is important and clearly related to health and survival, the exclusive focus on physical activity obscures the health benefits that may be associated with other, non-physical activities.*[8]

The World Health Organization (WHO) uses both activity and occupation. In the 2001 International Classification of Functioning, Disability and Health, activity in combination with participation is used to describe a "person's capacity to execute occupations (with or without assistive devices or assistance)."[9] However, in most cases, occupation is used as paid employment and the word activity is used for other occupations as in Global Recommendations on Physical Activity for Health.[10]

Behavior is another generic term that is sometimes used to describe things that people do but is less specific to people acting on their world or engaging in particular activity as responding to it in a psychological sense. It derives from the Latin habere (meaning "to have"), which led to the old French word of avoir (meaning "to have") and from the 1375 to 1425 Middle English words behaven, behavoure, or behaver. Current definitions are broad and relate to the manner in which a person behaves or conducts himself or herself, functions, or operates; anything that an organism does involving action and response to stimulation; and the response of an individual, group, or species to its environment.[11] It can be regarded as any action of an organism that changes its relationship to its environment and provides a response to the environment.[12] Behavior can be innate or learned, and current research suggests that microbes present within the body may even influence it.[13] Particular occupations may be part of behavior and, alternatively, behavior can be reflected in occupation.

Work, derived from the Old English word *weorc*, which was derived from the Old High German word *werc* and the Old Norse word *verk*, is defined in a contemporary dictionary as an "activity involving mental or physical effort done in order to achieve a result; such activity as a means of earning income; a task or tasks to be undertaken; a thing or things done or made; and the result of an action."[14] It is described by Williams as the most general word for "doing something and for something done," with its current predominant meaning of "regular paid employment being the result of the development of capitalist productive relations."[15] Currently, work is seen as the antithesis of play, leisure, rest, and recreation, implying an element of compulsion or necessary toil and earning a description as "everything we do to keep body and soul together."[16] It is "independent of any particular form of society" being "a basic condition of the existence and continuation of human life."[17]

Labor, like work, is used for activities that are, for some reason, necessary or enforced. Williams suggested that it has a "strong medieval sense of pain and toil" and that it is a harder word than work, with manual workers being described as laborers from the 13th century.[15] In the 2005 *Compact Oxford English Dictionary*, labor is defined as work, but especially as hard physical work.[14] Nineteenth century social revolutionaries deemed labor as a central issue of concern in the unhealthy and alienating conditions created by industrialization. For example, John Ruskin, a leader of the Arts and Crafts Movement, described it as a contest between material forces and a person's intellect, soul, and physical power. [18] In some ways similar, Karl Marx saw labor as:

> A process in which both man and Nature participate, and in which man of his own accord starts, regulates, and controls the material reactions between himself and Nature. He opposes himself to Nature as one of her own forces, setting in motion arms and legs, head and hands, the natural forces of his body in order to appropriate Nature's productions in a form adapted to his own wants.[19]

Likewise, a more recent socialist, Braverman, citing Aristotle's description of labor being "intelligent action," considers that it "represents the sole resource of humanity in confronting nature ... whether directly exercised or stored in such products as tools, machinery, or domesticated animals."[20] Despite those broad concepts, labor is not used for activities that are restful or playful, and, like occupation, of which it is a part, is frequently used as meaning only paid employment.

Praxis, from the Greek for "of action," "refers to almost any kind of activity that a free man is likely to perform; in particular, all kinds of business and political activity."[21] Sometimes understood as accepted practice or custom, in the *Oxford English Dictionary* praxis is defined as "doing, acting, action, practice,"[22] and in *Roget's Thesaurus* it is given as a synonym for action.[23] In a *Dictionary of Marxist Thought* Gajo Petrovic explains that Marx used praxis to describe "the free, universal, creative, and self-creative activity through which man creates (makes, produces) and changes (shapes) his historical, human world and himself."[24] This is, perhaps, the most similar usage of the word praxis to how occupation, excluding rest, is applied in this text and can be considered a valuable contributor to an occupational view of human nature. Although Marx usually opposed the use of labor to praxis, he is sometimes inconsistent, using them as one and the same. Praxis is used in various ways in scholarly or academic circumstances but is such a specialized word that it does not appear in all dictionaries and nowadays is seldom part of common communication. It is used as a descriptor for many types of action-research, such as critical praxis research or critical feminist praxis,[25,26] and praxiology—the science of efficient action—is a discipline "dealing with methods of doing anything in any way ... from the point of view of its effectiveness."[27] At the opposite end of the skill continuum, it is used in neurological terminology where apraxia (no action) refers to a lack of ability to perform purposeful activity or skilled movement when there is no apparent physical, cognitive, or emotional reason for difficulty.

Leisure stems from the Latin word *licere* meaning "permit." The word was not used in its modern sense as the opposite of work or labor until the 19th century, when the industrial revolution changed the essence of earlier occupational regimes. In medieval and early modern Europe, like the French *loisir*, the word often meant "opportunity," "an awareness of opportunity," "unstruc-tured time," or "occasion."[28] Currently, leisure time provides an opportunity to engage in occu-pations that are soothing, restorative, or invigorating as modern definitions give the meaning as "time spent in or free for relaxation or enjoyment."[14] Gerontologist Alex Comfort argued that leisure, as a time "to do trivial things," is a con for people in retirement.[29] He suggested that in affluent societies people are "shaped" to "grow old" through lack of real occupation "at an age when hairy peasants in remote areas are in midlife vigour."[30] The later years of life are a time for activism toward altering the attitudes of society, particularly about aging:

> There is an occupation ready for every retired, unemployed person. Wherever two or three
> people are gathered together to promote these changes, there should he or she be in the
> midst of them.[31]

Recreation is a word sometimes used instead of leisure. This word provides some sense of the need for occupations away from work or labor in that it is described as "a refreshment of body or mind by pleasurable exercise or amusement."[32] Another alternative is "holiday, the old word for religious festival."[15] This has implications of a contained time, such as a day or week, and for some religious affiliations it is not so much a day of leisure as a day of restraint.[33]

Pastime is a word used to describe the various and sometimes novel ways that people pass time between the serious demands of life. In both France and England, the word *passetemps*, or pastime, was coined in the 15th century[34] when it expressed a new assumption "that time was a substance which might be shaped by human will."[28] In the past, writers often associated pastimes with the affluent, Montaigne implying that time could be "annoying and contemptible,"[35] and Fielding observing "to the upper part of mankind time is an enemy, and ... their chief labour is to kill it."[36] It is true that, without pleasurable, fulfilling, or relaxing pursuits, time can appear to pass extremely slowly. People are apt to be bored, depressed, and sometimes destructive, especially if they lack both work and play.

A similar but more contemporary phrase is time-use; however, this addresses more than leisure. The earliest published use of the term was probably in 1913.[37,38] Studies in the field endeavor to quantify and qualify people's occupation across 24-hour days and across weeks, months, and even years, so they assist understanding of how to define occupation:

> Time-use studies provide crucial measures of involvement in a broad range of activities
> engaged in by individuals—such as paid work, housework and childcare, education, sleep,
> eating, socializing, games, sports, media use.[39]

Minimally they show what activities people do week to week or day to day. Maximally, they show what people are doing, where they are, who they are with, and how they feel minute to minute.[40]

Rest is a controversial addition to the doing words already described, yet the activity-rest con-tinuum is a vital aspect of occupation that is given insufficient attention. Rest and sleep provide the natural mechanism to prevent occupational overuse and a time for repair. It was one of the ancient rules of health and has been the subject of substantial exploration over recent decades. Emerging theories point to a complex relationship between sleep and what people do during waking states, suggesting that recuperation, information processing, energy conservation, and self-preservation are important aspects. Kleitman saw sleep as complementary to wakefulness as he explored and then described the day/night sequence as the "basic rest activity cycle."[41] As sleep deprivation results in symptoms, such as decreased coordination and reaction times, irritability, and blurred vision,[42] sleep appears to be necessary to effective occupation. Leger suggested that "just as musi-cians' pauses are a component of the performance, pauses from the stream of behavior are a com-ponent of the repertoire. The organism 'doing nothing' is doing something."[43] To consider sleep an occupation remains controversial, so many authorities fail to adequately consider the impact of the 24-hour activity–rest continuum. However, preparations for rest and waking up are deemed to be occupations and "disturbed sleep leads to difficulties during wakefulness."[44]

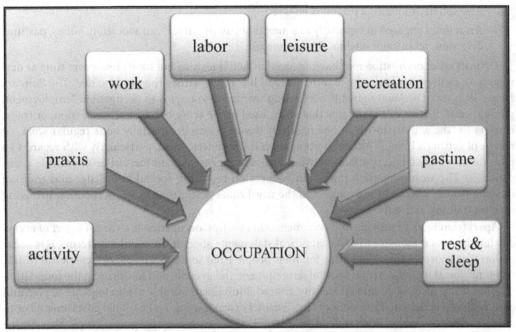

Figure 5-1. Occupation: inclusive of activity, praxis, work, labor, leisure, recreation, pastime, rest and sleep.

The range of alternatives described above gives some indication of the difficulties of defining even these aspects of occupation with any degree of accuracy. Every part appears multifaceted, as was the case when trying to define health based on apparently simple words of the WHO. Because occupation is a word that can be used instead of activity, time-use, praxis, work, labor, leisure, recreation, and pastime and can incorporate all of the things that people do, including both active and restful aspects (Figure 5-1), and because it is already in the nomenclature of health professions such as occupational therapy, occupational medicine, and occupational health and safety, it is the word of choice for this text.

Common Definitions

Occupation has several meanings that have much in common with earlier times. *The Concise Oxford Dictionary of Current English* of 1911 defined it as "occupying or being occupied, what occupies one, means of filling up one's time, temporary or regular employment, business, calling, pursuit."[45] In *Webster's Revised Unabridged Dictionary of the English Language* of 1919, the definition includes "that which occupies or engages the time and attention."[46] The printed version of the *Oxford English Dictionary* of 1989 includes "being occupied or employed with, or engaged in something."[22] In the *Compact Oxford English Dictionary* of 2005, the aspect of occupation central to this text is defined not only as a job or profession, but also as "the action, state, or period of occupying or being occupied; and a way of spending time."[14]

Of dictionary definitions, the meanings that are relevant to this work include the following:

1. To hold a position, job, rank, or office.[47]
2. An activity that serves as one's regular source of livelihood; a vocation,[48] work, calling, business, line of work, trade, post, career, situation, employment, craft, profession, pursuit, vocation, livelihood, or walk of life.
3. To engage or employ the mind or energy.[47]
4. To engage someone's attention.[49]
5. To keep someone busy or engrossed.[50]

6. Any activity in which a person is engaged.[51]

7. An activity engaged in especially as a means of passing time[48]; an avocation, hobby, pastime, diversion, relaxation, sideline, leisure pursuit.[52]

Definitions of occupation may have changed little in meaning but have grown over time as new ways have evolved to obtain the requirements of life and to satisfy the need "to do." *The Random House Webster's Dictionary* gives the following words as synonyms to occupation: "employment, pursuit, craft, métier."[3] It maintains that when used in the sense of business, profession, or trade, it refers to "the activity to which one regularly devotes oneself, especially one's regular work, or means of getting a living." Although occupation is the generic word, particularly with regard to a pleasant or congenial occupation, the word business suggests a "commercial or mercantile occupation."[53] The word *profession* infers "an occupation requiring special knowledge and training in some field of science or learning," and the word *trade* points toward an "occupation involving manual training and skill."[3]

Apart from work to provide for fundamental necessities, occupation is so much a part of everyday life that it is reasonable to make empirical statements about it. In population terms, it is occupation that provides the mechanism for what people need to do to survive or experience fulfillment, for social interaction and societal development and growth, and for forming the foundation of community, local, and national identity. Indeed, individuals are able to join together to plan and execute group activity to the extent of large business corporations and national governments or to achieve international goals for individual, mutual, and community purposes. People also engage in individual, shared, or communal occupations on a daily basis, sometimes to conform to compulsory rules and regulations or the expectations of others and sometimes with a sense of unique purpose. In all scenarios people usually think about, conceptualize, or plan (if only briefly) before commencing occupations; sometimes they act spontaneously without thinking about the effects of what they are about to do, but most have the capacity to reflect and mentally alter future activities as a result of outcomes. Not all may have the opportunity to challenge occupational restrictions or achieve health through what they do.

Occupations can demonstrate culturally sanctioned intellectual, moral, and physical attributes and those that are not culturally sanctioned. It is only by what they do that people can reveal what they are, what matters to them and to those they live among, and what they hope to be and become. Many strive toward a sense of individual achievement and for social recognition or, with others, to attain environmental, social, or political change. Accolades for achievements are often surrounded with ritualized activities, such as graduations, ticker-tape parades, and initiation ceremonies. The same need for social recognition of occupational achievements might result in some people participating in unhealthy, illegal, or dangerous activities, such as binge drinking, ram raiding commercial premises, drag racing on public roads, or criminal occupations of one sort or other. Punishment for those includes limited access to the continuation of occupations of choice. This provides another measure of occupation's significance in people's lives.

Introduction to Health-Related Definitions of Occupation

To define occupation in relation to health, it is necessary to quickly call to mind earlier discussions about the place of occupation throughout human existence, as well as the current preoccupations and bias in ideas about health. It has been noted that the occupations for early Homo species and creatures of all kinds were the lynchpin of survival and health. Murphy maintained that people achieve satisfaction by using their special human attributes: indeed they feed on them, become immersed in them, and enjoy a richer life because of them.[54] Throughout human history, experiences of morbidity, mortality, and health have been largely dependent on what and how people went about accessing the requirements of daily life to satisfy physical, mental, and social needs and to maintain and enhance their common and unique features. That remains important despite the advances of modern medicine, which have somewhat masked the relationship in affluent but not disadvantaged parts of the world.

The accepted wisdom that grew from observations about a fundamental relationship between doing and health is rarely applied currently, except with regard to the taking of medication; the appreciation that rest, exercise, and diet need to be considered; and that in advanced economies, there is regulated safety in the workplace. Rules about rest and interest in exercise as a health-giving activity have waxed and waned through the centuries, whereas fascination about the relationship between diet and health has been constant. In the present day the biochemical components of food are primary aspects of medical research. However, except in terms of hygiene and weight control, the occupations related to the getting, preparing, eating, and sharing of food have been increasingly ignored as major aspects of health. Instead, these occupations have mainly been regarded as economic or social matters, similar to some other basic health mechanisms, including the way people appear to need to find meaning, purpose, and interest in what they do and to find like-minded or agreeable people to share occupational interests.

In seeking to clarify people's beliefs, values, perceptions, and ideas about the relationship between health and occupation, it is important to remember that the medical model dominates health care, particularly in postindustrial societies. Indeed, medical science values are so integral to postindustrial cultures that it is difficult for those brought up in such a society to perceive health from a different perspective. It has already been suggested that, to some extent, this limits the study of health to ideas, beliefs, and approaches that are valued, advocated, and deemed most important by medical science. Because of this emphasis, and notwithstanding the holistic philosophy of the Ottawa Charter,[1] exploration (perhaps driven by the focus of research funding bodies) remains preoccupied with reducing the incidence of illness. This is at the expense of detailed exploration of the causes of good health and well-being, such as those of an occupational nature. Even recent interest in the social determinants of health has centered, to a large extent, on the prevention of particular illnesses, such that many people are using the terms prevention and health promotion synonymously.

Like those of any other living organism, the needs of people are related to health from the point of view of "what constitutes a good specimen" and "of how a specimen can be recognized as flourishing."[55] An understanding that humans have occupational needs that go beyond the instinctive patterned behaviors of many other animals and that these needs are related to health is outside medical science explanations. However, as Fromm maintained, needs are indispensable because they are embedded in human physiology as part of self-preservation.[56] For self-preservation, people have to meet their basic requirements through what they do. Occupation, in that sense, is physiologically conditioned and a vital aspect of human nature.[56] Occupational needs can be described as the species' primary health mechanism because they motivate the provision of other basic requirements, as well as enable individuals to use their biological capacities and potential, meet sociocultural expectations, safeguard their health and prevent illness, and, hopefully, flourish.

The integrative functions of the central nervous system, which process external and internal information, activated by engagement in occupation, are focal to survival, the maintenance of homeostasis, and facilitating health and well-being. The adaptive capacity of the human brain allows the innate drive for occupation to respond to cultural forces and values that add a social dimension to the relationship between health and occupation. Health is related to learning "how nature intended human beings to live."[57] The simplicity and complexity of health is mirrored in the simplicity and complexity of the occupational nature and needs of people.

PREREQUISITES OF HEALTH: A FOUNDATIONAL DEFINITION

The theme for this chapter provides the foundation definition of occupation in relation to health. It is an important starting point because all of the prerequisites for health identified by WHO[1]—peace, shelter, education, food, income, a stable ecosystem, sustainable resources, social justice, and equity—are intimately related to occupation in many ways. It is through engagement in occupation that people provide for their immediate and long-term needs for food, shelter, and income. It is mainly through participation in occupation with others that needs for education, peace, social justice and equity, a stable ecosystem, and sustainable resources can be pursued. Reflecting on those relationships provides a basis for appreciating the need to consider health from an occupational perspective (Table 5-1).

In terms of sustaining ecosystems, peace, equity, and social justice, it is largely interpersonal, communal, corporate, societal, and political occupations that are central. An example is provided by Rachel Thibeault's experiences in Sierra Leone as part of the United Nations' Development Program, which was supported by the World Rehabilitation Fund:

> In support of civil society, FAWE (Forum for African Women Educationalists–Sierra Leone Chapter) and CAW (Children Affected by the War) rely on occupation to promote gender equality, socio-economic development, social inclusiveness and ethical values: each step entrenched in specific occupations, brings with it a lived experience that stretches past the immediate individual and induces a new social awareness. Beyond words, occupation vividly bears witness to the largely untapped potential of severely traumatized people; it concretely demonstrates not only how they can be reintegrated within society, but also how they can contribute as active, decent citizens.[58]

DEFINITIONS RELATING ASPECTS OF OCCUPATION TO HEALTH

Defining health, specifically in relation to occupation, demands an atypical lens and an exploration of elements apart from obvious medical factors. Despite that, a first port of call has to be a medical viewpoint and the population health ideas advocated by the WHO. For both, the word occupation is used primarily in the sense of work and paid employment. Similarly the Office of the High Commission of Human Rights, with respect to discrimination relating to employment and occupation, explained that both terms "include access to vocational training, access to employment and to particular occupations, and terms and conditions of employment."[59]

Occupational medicine is especially concerned with "the prevention and treatment of diseases and injuries occurring at work or in specific occupations."[60] These are sometimes known as "occupational injuries and diseases."[61] An occupational disease is one that is "associated with a particular occupation and occurs in the workplace. Some occupations confer specific risks, such as the prevalence of black lung (byssinosis) in coal miners."[60] Such definitions illustrate that what people do or not do can have a profound negative influence on their health, as Ramazzini[62] detailed, but they do not assist in understanding the relationship between occupation and health in a positive way.

In 1950, the WHO adopted a definition of occupational health with the International Labour Organization.[63] Revised in 1995, it now reads:

> Occupational health should aim at: the promotion and maintenance of the highest degree of physical, mental and social well-being of workers in all occupations; the prevention amongst workers of departures from health caused by their working conditions; the protection of workers in their employment from risks resulting from factors adverse to health; the placing and maintenance of the worker in an occupational environment adapted to his

Table 5-1

EXAMPLES OF OCCUPATIONS TO MEET THE PREREQUISITES OF HEALTH

WHO Prerequisites of Health[1]	Examples of Occupations Meeting the Prerequisites
Peace	Seeking peaceful solutions to disputes
	Activities that build community networks: eg, cooperative ventures such as cultural festivals
	Reconciliation practices: eg, South African Truth and Reconciliation Commission following Apartheid
	Restorative justice: eg, New Zealand mediation program
	Reintegration of war victims: eg, community-based restorative occupations for peace-making in post-war Sierra Leone
	Providing practical help to and within disadvantaged countries and communities
	Participating in peace rallies
	Supporting displaced and disadvantaged people
Shelter	Self builds: simple bush dwellings, igloos, tepees, tents, mud, timber, and stone cottages
	Building industry: architecture, bricklaying, carpentering, plumbing, electrical work, engineering, laboring
	Surveying, town and council planning, local/state/national governing
Education	Family grounding in self care and life's activities
	Learning from community elders and religious practices
	Attending schools, colleges, universities, trade apprenticeship, self help and correspondence courses
	Participating in sport, recreation, and hobbies
Food	Hunting, gathering, and fishing
	Home gardening, growing, and harvesting
	Farming, animal husbandry, and crop management
	Food retailing, shopping, food storage
	Food preparation, cooking, serving, and eating
	Clearing away and hygiene practices
Income	Making a living: finding work, developing skills, apprenticeships, internships
	Work
	Social security or dole schemes
	Private income or unpaid domestic or child-rearing work supported by family
Stable ecosystem and sustainable resources	Farming, animal husbandry, mining, building, gardening, engineering practices
	Collecting and storing water
	Protecting habitats and local species of plants and wildlife
	Harnessing natural energy: sun, wind, water
	Avoiding and resisting pollutants
	Scientific experimenting to protect/save habitats, plants and animals, or to ensure future existence if geological change is unstoppable
	Urban planning, working toward healthy cities
	Use of local and renewable resources

(continued)

Table 5-1 (continued)
EXAMPLES OF OCCUPATIONS TO MEET THE PREREQUISITES OF HEALTH

WHO Prerequisites of Health	Examples of Occupations Meeting the Prerequisites
Social justice and equity	Recognizing and encouraging the occupational strengths and potential of all people
	Participation in volunteerism, civic, social, and political involvement
	Supporting individual and group rights to maintain different skills, traditions, and ways of life if they are just and equitable
	Supporting individual and group rights to change ways of doing if any are disadvantaged or if there is occupational injustice in terms of choice, opportunity, bullying, or physical, mental, or social handicap

physiological and psychological capabilities; and, to summarize, the adaptation of work to man and of each man to his job.[63]

Occupation as work is enshrined in the WHO Constitution and in the 2008-2017 Global Plan of Action on Workers Health, with the health, safety and well-being of workers being seen as dependent on the following:

- The physical work environment.
- The psychosocial work environment including organization of work and workplace culture.
- Personal health resources in the workplace.
- Ways of participating in the community to improve the health of workers, their families and other members of the community.[64]

Indeed, "the workplace, along with the school, hospital, city, island, and marketplace, has been established as one of the priority settings for health promotion into the 21st century."[64] This recognition acknowledges the direct influence of what people do, and where and how they do it, on physical, mental, economic, and social well-being. It also recognizes a follow-on effect on the health of families, communities, and society.[64]

Work has long been recognized as a likely source of physical illness and accidents, but its potential to be both a negative and a positive influence on mental and social health is also of long standing. Robert Burton (1577-1640) ended his seminal work, *The Anatomy of Melancholy*, with the conclusive phrase "Be not solitary, be not idle."[65] Those bygone ideas are supported by recent research, as well as a social-psychological analysis of 40 years of European and United States research literature on employment and unemployment undertaken by Jahoda in 1982. She found that social contact and shared purpose are vital aspects of well-being, identifying 5 important features that, in a sense, define occupation as work in relation to health:

1. Work provides meaning through shared purpose and activity within a social group.
2. Work increases the possibility of relationships beyond immediate family or neighborhood.
3. Work structures daily time. Leisure time is more valued when it is scarce.
4. Work assigns social status and clarifies personal attributes.
5. Work requires regular activity.[66]

These benefits also apply to occupations other than paid employment. Over decades, psychologists have linked mental health and well-being with employment and leisure; money, class, and education; day-to-day organization; creativity, flow, stress release, self-worth, mastery, control, confidence, happiness, and socialization; all of these are achieved through what people do and give meaning to life.[67-71]

In earlier times, the relationship between occupation other than work and positive health was also an accepted aspect of medical treatment. Doctors advised people about what they should and should not do. Thomas Southwood-Smith (1788-1861), a physician and influential sanitary reformer, wrote about health in occupational terms, as did many others.[72-74] He approached his social activist public health practice with the belief that the development of people's capacities through doing is the means to produce pleasure, which in turn positively influences health and longevity.[75] His views and activism led to major public health reforms in the 19th century that overturned child labor laws in Britain.

In the last century, Henry Sigerist, MD (1891-1957) recognized not only that "work balances our life and is therefore an essential factor of health,"[76] but also that "health is promoted by providing a decent standard of living, good labor conditions, education, physical culture, and means of rest and recreation."[77]

Sigerist, who was known as the world's leading health historian in the first half of the 20th century, called for the coordinated efforts of "the physician–expert in matters of health" with influential sectors of the population, such as "the statesman," educators, and "leaders of labor and industry," to ensure that good health through what people do (ie, through their occupations) was within reach of everyone.[77] Many of Sigerist's ideas resurfaced 30 years later in the Ottawa Charter,[1] and it is this document that clearly articulates the WHO's appreciation of the relationship between work, all the other things that people do, and health status. Key phrases that define the strong relationship between health and occupation in the generic sense include the following:

- "To reach a state of complete physical, mental and social well-being, an individual or group must be able to identify and to realize aspirations, to satisfy needs, and to change or cope with the environment."
- "Changing patterns of life, work and leisure have a significant impact on health."
- "Work and leisure should be a source of health for people."
- "Health promotion generates living and working conditions that are safe, stimulating, satisfying and enjoyable."
- "Health is created and lived by people within the settings of their everyday life; where they learn, work, play and love."[1]

Following the Rio Declaration on Social Determinants of Health,[78] in 2012 the WHO published its Health Impact Asessment, which outlined the most recent worldviews.[79] These recognize that the health of individuals and communities is a result of a combination of many factors that are often outside people's ability to control:

- "The social and economic environment."
- "The physical environment."
- "The person's individual characteristics and behaviors."[79]

This document is important in terms of understanding the links between occupation and health and in defining occupation in relation to the promotion of health. The following occupation-related factors are identified as important: income and social status; education; the physical environment, which includes employment and working conditions; social support networks, culture, customs, traditions, and beliefs; and personal behavior, activity, food, and coping skills.[79] The WHO defines health promotion as the process of enabling people to increase control over and improve their health through a "wide range of social and environmental interventions."[80]

The determinants are supported by research from a wide range of professional interests. As noted in Chapter 1, McAllister maintained there is general agreement among researchers that well-being depends on people's development and activity through meaningful work and leisure, social relationships, and material factors, such as income and wealth, as well as the more obvious impact of physical and mental health.[81] A 2005 review evaluated the relationship between physical and mental health and physical activity and exercise for men and women of different ages from diverse ethnic populations. It found that physical activity leads to "better general and health-related quality of life, better functional capacity and better mood states," as well as to better outcomes across a "variety of physical conditions."[82] Medical institutions also recognized the links, with the Mayo Clinic listing seven important health benefits from exercise or daily occupations: controlling weight; improving mood; boosting energy; promoting better sleep; improving sex-life; providing fun and enjoyment; and helping prevent or manage a wide range of health problems, including stroke, metabolic syndrome, type 2 diabetes, depression, certain types of cancer, arthritis, and falls.[83] In similar vein, the Harvard Medical School recognized that physical activity, good support systems, and relaxing with interests and hobbies reduces stress, enhances the immune system, and promotes relaxation.[84]

Several decades ago, Gandevia postulated that:

> Man's occupations are, of course, in part a function of his physical environment … are not independent of the total structure of society, its religion … its politics and legislations, its economic status, its attitudes to social problems … [and] its approach to science and research … [A]ll these factors, and others, interact to influence the concepts and practices of every occupation. Thus the relationship of every occupation to health and disease is far from fixed and immutable over any period of time: it changes.[85]

Although the focus of his work was mainly concerned with paid employment, Gandevia resisted using the term *occupational diseases* in the title because he felt it too restricting and technical, making it possible to ignore the relationship of occupation to "society's ever-changing attitudes and values." He believed that physicians are "often baffled by it" and that any definition should be dictated "by society, not by doctors: by social concepts, not by science."[85] See Table 5-2 for a summary of the definitions already discussed.

What Gandevia advanced is equally applicable to the much wider definitions of occupation discussed in the next section of this chapter, which are in tune with the WHO mandate mentioned above that "health is created and lived by people within the settings of their everyday life; where they learn, work, play and love."[1] The following are a few of the many attempts by those in some occupation-specific health professions to capture the essence of the relationship between diverse occupations and health. Definitions given by occupational health and safety practitioners have already been addressed, so they are not included in the next section and, on the whole, are confined to the health consequences of work.

DEFINITIONS OF HOLISTIC UNDERSTANDINGS OF OCCUPATION AND HEALTH

Time-use researchers, occupational therapists, and occupational scientists define and describe wide-ranging occupations in relation to health. This group of disciplines, which has a primary research or practice focus on occupation, in terms of all of the things that people do, despite many attempts has found it challenging to capture the essence of occupation in relation to health and well-being. These disciplines provide evidence of the complexity of the occupation-health nexus, but also provide an idea of the extensive range of approaches that may be valuable and need to be considered more thoroughly in the future.

Time Use Researchers

Time-use surveys offer a rich source of data on many different occupation and health-related issues. Not only do these endeavor to quantify and qualify people's occupation, they also inform health and social planners at national and international levels.[86-90] The 2006 survey conducted by the Australian Bureau of Statistics explained that:

Table 5-2

A SUMMARY OF SELECTED DESCRIPTIONS LINKING HEALTH WITH OCCUPATION

Source	Description
Robert Burton 1638[72]	Be not solitary, be not idle
Sigerist 1936, 1960[76,77]	Work balances our life and is therefore an essential factor of health
	Health is promoted by providing a decent standard of living, good labor conditions, education, physical culture, and means of rest and recreation
Gandevia 1971[85]	Occupations are a function of the physical environment ... are not independent of the total structure of society, its religion ... its politics and legislations, its economic status, its attitudes to social problems ... its approach to science and research
	The relationship of every occupation to health and disease is far from fixed and immutable over any period of time: it changes
Jahoda 1982[66]	Work: provides meaning through shared purpose and activity within a social group
	Increases the possibility of relationships beyond immediate family or neighborhood
	Structures daily time. Leisure time is more valued when it is scarce
	Assigns social status and clarifies personal attributes
	Requires regular activity
WHO 1989[1]	An individual or group must be able to identify and to realize aspirations, to satisfy needs, and to change or cope with the environment
	Work and leisure should be a source of health for people
	Living and working conditions that are safe, stimulating, satisfying, and enjoyable
	Created and lived by people within the settings of their everyday life; where they learn, work, play, and love
WHO, ILO 1995[63]	The promotion and maintenance of the highest degree of physical, mental, and social well-being of workers in all occupations
	The adaptation of work to man and of each man to his job
McAllister 2005[81]	Well-being depends on peoples' development and activity, through meaningful work and leisure, social relationships, and material factors such as income and wealth, and physical and mental health
Harvard Health Publications, 2007[84]	Mental well-being is assisted by reducing stress, enhanced immune system and promoting relaxation through physical activity, good support systems, and relaxing with interests and hobbies such as group singing
Mayo Clinic 2012[83]	Occupations control weight; help prevent or manage a wide range of health problems; improve mood; boost energy; promote a better sleep, improve sex life; and provide fun and enjoyment
	Stress control is achieved through the boosting of feel good endorphins as a result of physical activity, and distraction from everyday worries from "doing what you you love"
WHO 2012[79]	Health results from the social and economic environment, the physical environment, and the person's individual characteristics and behaviors
	Occupation-related factors related to health: income and social status; education; the physical environment that includes employment and working conditions, social support networks, culture, customs, traditions and beliefs, personal behavior, activity, food, and coping skills

Abbreviations: ILO, International Labour Organization; WHO, World Health Organization.

> *Time-use surveys collect detailed information on the daily activity patterns of people in Australia. The information is used to examine how people allocate time to activities such as paid and unpaid work and to analyze such issues as gender equality, care giving and balancing family and paid work responsibilities. The balance between paid work, unpaid work and leisure are important for a person's well-being and economic welfare.[91]*

In 1997, the Australian Bureau of Statistics provided an example of how time-use studies assist with defining health from an occupational perspective. The study on mental health and well-being, where mental health relates to emotions, thoughts, and behaviors, described:

> *A person with good mental health is generally able to handle day-to-day events and obstacles, work towards important goals, and function effectively in society. However, even minor mental health problems may affect everyday activities to the extent that individuals cannot function as they would wish, or are expected to, within their family and community.[92]*

Harvey and Pentland suggested several key terms that help in understanding what people do, including "committed time," "contracted time," "free time," and "necessary time,"[93] which was in line with Aas's sociological observations about people allocating time to committed, contracted, free, and necessary occupations on a priority basis according to personal obligation or constraints.[94] Harvey and Pentland argued that:

> *The amount of time we spend in various activities and occupations tells us very little about the quality of someone's life. It is more the attributes of engagement in the activity or occupation that have a bearing on quality of life, well-being and health.[93]*

Time-use studies not only provide help in defining occupation in relation to health,[89,90,95-98] but they also are useful resources for workers in the field, such as occupational therapists.[87,99-107] When considering the "relationships among time use, health and well-being," Pentland and McColl,[108] who are time-use researchers and occupational therapists, recognized the importance of Selye's[109] work, which defined engagement in occupation as a biological necessity for both mind and body. They also acknowledged Adolph Meyer's early contribution to the linking of health with how people use time and their day-to-day occupations.[108]

Occupational Therapists

Adolph Meyer, an American psychiatrist eminent in the first half of the 20th century and credited with providing a philosophy to occupational therapy, asserted that to maintain and balance the organism that is a person, there is a need to act in time with bodily and natural rhythms and that timely activity and rest are vital components of healthy living. In 1922, he observed that:

> *Human ideals have unfortunately and usually been steeped in dreams of timeless eternity, and they have never included an equally religious valuation of actual time and its meaning in wholesome rhythms. The awakening to a full meaning of time as the biggest wonder and asset of our lives and the valuation of opportunity and performance as the greatest measure of time; those are the beacon lights of the philosophy of the occupational worker.[110]*

Occupational therapy contends that what people do with their time, their occupation, is crucially important to their well-being. It is a person's occupation that makes life ultimately meaningful. [110]

Meyer was but one of the 19th and early 20th century medical and socialist reformers who recognized the value of human labor and who, with pragmatist philosophers such as William James, recognized the centrality of occupation to life. These principles were influential in the ideas of the modern occupational therapy profession in the United States and the United Kingdom. It was the decisive roles played by social activist Jane Addams in Chicago and medical practitioner Octavia Hill in London that led to the establishment of occupational therapy education in two different parts of the world.

The American National Society for the Promotion of Occupational Therapy was formed in 1917. Workers in the field—two architects, a social worker, a teacher, and a physician—came together at Clifton Springs, New York, to write a Certificate of Incorporation.[111] Recognizing the importance of research to back up claims about a close relationship between occupation, health, and well-being,[112] the objectives of the Society were aimed at "the advancement of occupation as a therapeutic measure; the study of the effect of occupation upon the human being; and the scientific dispensation of this knowledge."[113]

Paraphrasing George Cheyne's 18th century view that "occupation is almost as necessary to life as food and drink,"[114] Dunton, the physician in the group, proposed the creed "that occupation 'is' as necessary to life as food and drink" and added that "every human being should have both physical and mental occupations ... [and] all should have occupations which they enjoy or hobbies—at least two, one outdoor, one indoor ... [because] sick minds, sick bodies, [and] sick souls may be healed through occupation.[115] The choice of the word occupation within the profession's name perhaps reflects an earlier, more common generic use of the word when occupational therapy was developing in the first decades of the 20th century. Despite such rhetoric, the word creates some problems, even within the profession's ranks. Some Europeans neither use nor favor the word occupation because of unhappy memories of their homelands being occupied by others in times of war. In some languages, there is no identical collective word for the things that people do.[116] Even for those comfortable in the use of occupation to describe the profession's focus, there is debate about its definition (ie, what is or is not included within its boundaries) and attempts to define the difference between it and activity has been extensive.[117,118] Indeed, beginning in the 1960s and continuing for approximately 30 years, the word activity had largely, but not completely, replaced occupation in the profession's lexicon.[119] Definitions during those decades talked about how activity enables the "development and integration of the sensory, motor, cognitive, and psychological systems; serving as a socializing agent, and verifying one's efficacy as a competent, contributing member of society"[120] and how "active involvement and participation in a variety of activity and roles positively affect health and well-being.[121]

Because occupational therapists are health professionals with occupation as a primary concern, a fundamental belief to the profession's foundation philosophy was, as Meyer suggested,[110] that occupation is health giving and that it can provide treatment for people who are sick. This was extended to include the enabling of practical living skills for people with disabilities. Because of occupational therapists' fundamental belief in the close relationship between occupation, health, and well-being, it is important to consider definitions from their ranks, and there are many to choose from. These suggest a view within the profession that occupation is central to humanness. Indeed, it has been described as "a natural human phenomenon" that is taken for granted because it forms "the fabric of everyday lives,"[122] and is the means to experience social relationships and approval, as well as personal growth.[123] More specifically, it is defined as purposeful "use of time, energy, interest, and attention"[124] in work, leisure, play, self-care, rest, sleep, and social interactions.[125] It includes "activities that are playful, restful, serious, and productive" that are "carried out by individuals in their own unique ways" according to their own needs, beliefs, and preferences; "the kinds of experiences they have had; their environments; and the patterns of behavior they acquire over time."[126] It is perceived as part of personal and social identity,[127] enabling the creation of self-image and a foundation for organization of lives.[128] Occupation is subject to societal influences, and is based on an interactive process between people and their environment of "culturally valued, coherent patterns of actions" that may be either socially expected or freely chosen.[129] The current definition provided by the World Federation of Occupational Therapists[130] states that the profession is all about "promoting health and well being through occupation":

> *The primary goal of occupational therapy is to enable people to participate successfully in the activities of everyday life. Occupational therapists achieve this outcome by enabling people to do things that will enhance their ability to live meaningful lives or by modifying the environment to better support participation.*

Occupational Scientists

Occupational science was discussed briefly in the Preface. It initially sprang from a need for occupational therapists to understand better the fundamental relationship between occupation, health, and well-being that inspired the founders of the profession and to develop a recognizable scientific foundation for their work. At the University of Southern California, Mary Reilly[131] underpinned the later development of the science in the early 1960s, proposing that although the First Principle, that from which medical science draws its premise, explains that the nature of humans is to be alive, the Second Principle is for humans to grow and be productive. She maintained that the two principles "merge into a concept of function which asserts that both the existence and the unfolding of the specific powers of an organism are one and the same thing."[131] Reilly was a large influence on the work of her colleagues, one of whom (Elizabeth Yerxa) was instrumental in the development of occupational science as "a unique academic discipline sufficient in scope and importance to merit its own doctoral degree."[132] She saw the basic science of occupation as a social science akin to anthropology, sociology, and psychology and as complementary to the applied science of occupational therapy.[132] Yerxa et al defined occupational science as "the study of the human as an occupational being including the need for and the capacity to engage in and orchestrate daily occupations in the environment over the lifespan."[133]

In *An Introduction to Occupational Science*, Yerxa et al explained that occupation is culturally sanctioned, dependent on political will and environmental factors, and seen by some as "a primary organizer of time and resources," enabling humans to survive, control, and adapt to their world and to be economically self-sufficient.[134] Stimulated by the idea but prior to any published information, occupational science was also developed in Australasia.[135,136] There, in common with the region's community health focus, the science took on a broader population and social stance, different to the more individualistic application at the University of Southern California that mirrored health services in the United States. The Australasian Society of Occupational Scientists described how occupation is "a basic human need that is fundamental to health, well-being and social justice" and that it encompasses all human pursuits.[137] The International Society for Occupational Science, formed in Canberra, Australia, in 1999, described it as:

> The various everyday activities people do as individuals, in families and with communities to occupy time and bring meaning and purpose to life. Occupations include things people need to, want to and are expected to do. [138]

Other definitions explained occupation as "the ordinary and familiar things" that are done every day, with the qualification that although this reflects the "multidimensional and complex nature of daily occupation," it also "understates" it.[139] Somewhat similarly, Townsend described occupation as the active process of everyday living in the following way:

> Occupation comprises all the ways in which we occupy ourselves individually and as societies. Everyday life proceeds through a myriad of occupations, embedded in time and place, and in the cultural and other patterns that organize what we do…To live is to enfold multiple occupations which provide enjoyment, payment, personal identity and more.[140]

In line with the ideas discussed in this chapter, in 2010 Jarman hypothesized that occupational science made its debut to explore and understand occupation in terms of "nature, meaning and sociocultural structure" because it is important to understand how it is helpful in maintaining health.[141a]

The holistic view of occupation held by occupational scientists is applicable to both populations and communities at local to global levels and to individuals. The definition of occupational science in this text has been shortened to the study of people as occupational beings and is inclusive of the daily continuum of activity, rest, and sleep over the life course. A combination of definitions provided by time-use researchers, occupational therapists, and occupational scientists is displayed in Table 5-3.

Table 5-3

OCCUPATION: SELECTED DEFINITIONS RELATED TO HEALTH (HISTORICAL, TIME-USE RESEARCHERS, OCCUPATIONAL THERAPISTS, OCCUPATIONAL SCIENTISTS)

Source	Definition
Locke 1690[141b]	That which man himself ought to do, as a rational and voluntary agent, for the attainment of any ends, especially happiness
Cheyne 1724[73]	Almost as necessary to life as food and drink
Dunton 1919[115]	As necessary to life as food and drink: sick minds, sick bodies, sick souls, may be healed through occupation
Meyer 1922[110]	To maintain and balance the organism that is a person, there is a need to act in time with bodily and natural rhythms. Timely activity and rest are vital components of healthy living. What people do with their time, their occupation, is crucially important to their well-being. it is a person's occupation that makes life ultimately meaningful.
American Journal of Occupational Therapy 1972[124]	Purposeful use of time, energy, interest, and attention
Selye 1975[109]	A biological necessity for both mind and body
Fidler and Fidler 1978[120]	Enables development and integration of the sensory, motor, cognitive, and psychological systems; serving as a socializing agent, and verifying one's efficacy as a competent, contributing member of society
Yerxa et al 1989[134]	Is culturally sanctioned and a primary organizer of time and resources, enabling humans to survive, control, and adapt to their world and to be economically self-sufficient
Cynkin and Robinson 1990[122]	A natural human phenomenon that is taken for granted because it forms the fabric of everyday lives
Keilhofner 1985 1992[121,126]	Activities that are playful, restful, serious, and productive, which are carried out by individuals in their own unique ways based on societal influences; their own needs, beliefs, and preferences; the kinds of experiences they have had; their environments; and the patterns of behavior they acquire over time Active involvement and participation in a variety of activity and roles positively affect health and well-being
Turner et al 1996[127]	Is part of personal and social identity
ABS Time-use 1997[92]	Able to handle day-to-day events and obstacles, work toward important goals, and function effectively in society
Townsend 1997[140]	Comprises all the ways in which we occupy ourselves individually as societies Everyday life proceeds through a myriad of occupations, embedded in time and place, and in the cultural and other patterns that organize what we do To live is to enfold multiple occupations which provide enjoyment, payment, personal identity, and more
Cara and Macrae 1998[128]	Enables the creation of self image and is a foundation for organization of lives
International Society of Occupational Scientists 1999[138]	The various everyday activities people do as individuals, in families, and with communities to occupy time and bring meaning and purpose to life. Occupations include things people need to, want to, and are expected to do
Australasian Society of Occupational Scientists 2012[137]	It encompasses all human pursuits and it can be mental, physical, social, spiritual, restful, active, obligatory, self chosen, paid or unpaid, and is a basic human need that is fundamental to health, well-being, and social justice.

With those definitions in mind, the term occupation is being used in this text in its generic sense to refer to all of the necessary things that people are obliged to do for individual, familial, and communal survival: occupations of choice to exercise talents and interests that are offset with restful activities and sleep. In addition, it encompasses the being, belonging, and becoming components of particular occupations or the mix of them within lifestyles, namely what occupation means in a personal or communal sense; how it is integral to family, social, and economic relationships; and how people's present and future is dependent on what is done or can be done. It does not differentiate between one type of doing or another but is inclusive of all types. It encompasses the notion that everyone's uniqueness is expressed through occupations to meet different talents, interests, and capacities, as well as physical, mental, spiritual, and social needs; that occupations change with development throughout life; that throughout each day they can range through a sleep, restful, and active continuum; that they are dependent on the natural, the built, and the socio-cultural-economic-political environments; and that they differ according to life management systems, environmental capacity, socio-political regimes and requirements, and economic imperatives. It also includes group, communal, corporate, national, and global occupations where individuals come together to achieve particular occupational goals, such as work opportunities, building projects, environmental engineering, socio-political advancement, or improved health practices.

The many and varied definitions illustrate the complexity of occupation's relationship with health. In Chapter 1, the links between health, well-being, and wellness were discussed, and it became clear that they are the result of more than the absence of illness or pathology and cannot be attributed to medical expertise alone. For example, McAllister[81] lists physical health and economic growth, along with personal stability, lack of depression, relationships, development and activity, meaningful work and leisure, and material income and wealth as influencing well-being. Those ideas resonate with occupational perspectives of health, as does the claim by Greiner et al that functional health patterns that include activity-exercise, roles-relationships, and sleep-rest are integral to health.[142]

Defining Occupation as Doing, Being, Belonging, and Becoming

There are many important ideas embedded in both the discussions and definitions that have been used in this text to date, and all have value. It is apparent that occupation is an innate need of physiological and psychological significance, and that it embraces evolutionary, social, economic, and health functions. Occupations are culturally situated, so what people choose to do can be influenced by many factors other than personal need or choice from moment to moment: from skill levels to resource availability, from socioenvironmental constraints to political contexts, or from gender expectations to historical patterns.[143] The definitions that have been reviewed in this chapter illustrate that complexity.

To encapsulate some of those complexities, the terms doing, being, belonging, and becoming have been chosen as a way to discuss the meaning given to occupation in relation to health (Figure 5-2). Doing, being, belonging, and becoming will be examined separately in later chapters but are introduced at this point and encapsulated in Table 5-4 to clarify how they relate to and are inclusive of the ideas in the definitions already discussed.

Doing

The word *doing* is linked in thesauri with words such as action, getting something done, carrying out, achieving, making, executing, performing, acting, completing, fixing, preparing, organizing, and undertaking. It is also used to talk of exploits, deeds, and accomplishments, and seeing

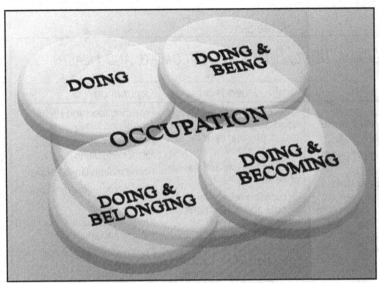

Figure 5-2. Occupation as doing, being, belonging, and becoming.

to, sorting out, or looking after. Collectively and individually, it embraces the doing of mental, physical, social, communal, spiritual, restful, active, obligatory, self-chosen, and paid or unpaid occupations. There are countless variations in what people do according to where they live; feelings about what they do; individual, family and regional interests, capacities, and talents; learned skills; education and obtainable health support; time availability or pressures; issues of personal or social control; and, during different times of life, people's social and financial status, and the norms expected by families, colleagues, or societies in particular places.[144]

BEING

The doing components of the human occupation repertoire are dependent on regular time for stillness and reflection. This quiet time is described here as being, and it is essentially a personal rather than a social aspect of occupation. Individually, it is often a period of quiet contemplation about the self and about personal past, present, and future pleasures, difficulties, and achievements. However, there are some occasions when people group together in support and reflection, such as in prayer or grief or in times of great joy and celebration that affect a community at large.

In thesauri, the word being is linked with words such as self, mind, nature, psyche, essence, true being, core, inner person, persona, soul, spirit, personality, subsistence, survival, existence, actuality, and life or living. Dictionaries define it similarly as the essential nature of someone; their substance, core or persona, and link it to occupation with examples such as "his whole being is creative."[144,145] Usually associated with mental or spiritual aspects, being embraces the thoughtful and restful facets of doing. It is the time when the meaning of what people do can be thought through and when ideas are formed, plans are formulated, and sense is made of how to go about doing what needs to be done. Being also covers the relaxation and sleep phases of the daily cycle of occupation, alternating with action and necessary toil, and can be soothing, soporific, calming, and peaceful. However, being can be disturbed by shortage of sleep, hunger, anger, conflict, guilt, boredom, over stimulation, or scarcity of active or meaningful doing. Being is the time when people reflect on their whole range of activity, including that which is communal, obligatory, self-chosen, paid or unpaid, and energetically physical, as well as the social and political.

In a different sense, it is part of common parlance to use the word being to describe a person's occupational roles or interests, such as being busy hanging out the washing or being a gardener. It is both necessary and complementary to the active phases of occupation.

Table 5-4

OCCUPATION: DOING, BEING, BELONGING, BECOMING, AND HEALTH

Word	Explained as	Health depends on	Occupation
Doing	Mental, physical, social, communal, spiritual, restful, active, obligatory Self-chosen, paid or unpaid occupations Action, participate, make, execute, prepare, organize, undertake, sort out, fix, look after Exploits, deeds, accomplishments	A decent standard of living, good labor conditions, education, physical exercise, rest and recreation[77] Work and leisure as a source of health Occupation related factors: income and social status, education, the physical environment and working conditions; social support networks, culture, customs, tradition and beliefs; personal behavior, activity, food, and coping skills[79] A biological necessity for both mind and body	Providing food and shelter for self and family Attendance at schools and further education Home maintenance/chores Food preparation/hygiene Paid work Chosen and voluntary occupations and challenges Community and political work Recreation and leisure Cultural customs and celebrations Rest and sleep Activity/affiliations and friendship through sport, arts, and service clubs
Being	Of the mind, inner person, essence, core, spirit, personality Essential nature of someone; substance Mental/spiritual self Ideas and plans formed, sense made of how to do Reflective or restful Relaxation and sleep phases of occupation Alternates with action and toil	Living and working conditions that are safe, stimulating, satisfying, and enjoyable[1] "The exclusive focus on physical activity obscures the health benefits that may be associated with other, nonphysical activities"[8]	Time out Reflecting on communal, obligatory, self chosen, paid or unpaid, energetically physical, social, and political activities Planning, deciding, organizing Making sense of doing Being an occupational being Relaxing, resting, sleeping
Belonging	Affiliation to others/places/things Being a member, a constituent, a part of something Allied, akin, attached to something Associated/connected Being in the right place, feeling right and fitting in	Created and lived by people within the settings of their everyday life; where they learn, work, play, and love[1]	Any and all occupations carried out with others, for others and as part of a family, community, national, or global group or organization Any and all occupations undertaken to become friends with someone, part of something, or attached to a place

(continued)

Table 5-4 (continued)			
OCCUPATION: DOING, BEING, BELONGING, BECOMING, AND HEALTH			
Word	Explained as	Health depends on	Occupation
Becoming	Development Transformation Become more knowledgeable or mature Realize aspirations Achieve potential Creation of communal or self image Foundation for organization of lives	To reach a state of complete physical, mental, and social well-being, an individual or group must be able to identify and realize aspirations[1] Well being: people identifying and utilizing personal capacities and strengths. Being motivated and enabled to achieve individual potential and taking part in the growth and development of beneficial social change	Any and all occupations participated in alone or with others The nature and outcome of the experience is dependent on individual, group, community, and environs

BELONGING

People are described as social beings because, throughout time, they have lived in familial, communal, and larger social groups to help meet the necessary and chosen occupations that comprise life. The term used here to describe this aspect of occupation is *belonging*. The *Oxford English Dictionary* defines belonging as the "human affiliation to other people, groups, places and things that are spiritually valuable for them."[146] In thesauri, belonging is associated with words such as being part of, a member of, an adjunct of, a constituent of, associated with, allied to, akin to, attached to, connected with, included in something, being in the right place, feeling right, and fitting in. People sometimes feel a sense of affinity for a specified place or situation to the extent that belonging extends into a sense of meaning and destiny. It can be associated with feeling acceptance of self, security, and even happiness in close relationships and nationhood, as well as within the organizations and community in which people actively participate. This is frequently experienced through shared occupations, such as family chores, work, political lobbying, attending community meetings, playing sport, painting, or making music.

BECOMING

Throughout time, humans have developed and become different through what they have done on a daily basis, occasionally, or, sometimes, only once. Groups of people have migrated from the South African "cradle of humankind" to all parts of the globe and created different cultures through what they have done; over time, they have developed the sophisticated technologies of the current day that have changed the occupational behaviors of millions of people from around the world. Day by day, individuals and communities become different through what they do, and in this text, this is explained as "becoming." In thesauri, the word *becoming* is linked with the idea of undergoing change, transformation, or development, and with words such as coming to be, changing to, emerging as, or to metamorphose (turning or growing into something or becoming somehow different, more knowledgeable, or mature). The idea of becoming resonates in the Ottawa Charter's message that "to reach a state of complete physical, mental and social well-being, an individual or group must be able to identify and to realize aspirations" and be in a position that permits people to aim toward their highest levels of personal and collective development.[1]

Boxed Dialogue 5-1:
Occupation, Health, and Well-Being

Occupation is indispensable to the well-being of all people, everywhere in the world. In a very fundamental sense, people's occupations are their personal and communal life-support systems interconnected with ecosystems. The needs of all people to engage in occupations to meet the biological requirements for food, water, clean air, shelter and relative climatic constancy are basic and unalterable. The causal links between occupation and human health are complex because they are often indirect, displaced in space and time, and dependent on many modifying forces. Measures to ensure occupational well-being would safeguard populations, communities and individuals and benefit health in the long-term.

WHO. Global Health History. www.who.int/global-health-histories/en/. Accessed 2012.

Note: In the first chapter, a quote from *WHO Global Health History* introduced some reasons for health practitioners to be responsive to ecosystem health and well-being.[1] The Boxed Dialogue 5-1 paraphrases that quote, and applies it to the occupational health and well-being needs of people.

Well-being is about people identifying and using personal and collective capacities and strengths and being motivated and enabled to achieve their potential and the good of others.

To summarize, the use of occupation to refer to all that people need, want, or are obliged to do, what it means to them, and its ever present potential as an agent of health and an agent of change (as it is used in this text) is often misunderstood. That is one reason why the next four chapters address doing, being, belonging, and becoming to assist in the understanding of the scope and depth of the concept. These will be considered alongside physical, mental, and social well-being and the absence of illness in reference to how the WHO defines health:

- Physical well-being for individuals or communities is largely, but not completely, dependent on doing and becoming and the exercise of physical capacities (Figure 5-3).
- Mental well-being for individuals or communities is largely, but not completely, dependent on being and becoming and the feelings, thoughts, and emotions that are integral to engagement in productive, creative, restful, and reflective occupations (Figure 5-4).
- Social well-being for individuals or communities is largely, but not completely, dependent on belonging and becoming and in sharing and participating in occupation with others (Figure 5-5).
- Doing, being, and belonging (alone or with others) result in some form of becoming that may occur at an individual, communal, societal, or global level.
- Absence of illness of a physical, mental, or social nature relies, to an indeterminate extent on doing, being, belonging, and becoming.

Survival, health, and well-being are affected by doing, being, belonging, and becoming (DBBB) in many ways, although the impact may never be apparent unless it is looked for and will differ as circumstances, communities, and individual physiology and genes differ. In shorthand form, db^3=shw. (Boxed Dialogue 5-1).

Chapter 1 also clearly illustrated the multidimensional nature of health. Readers may recall that the excerpt from the 2006 WHO description of "the optimal state of health of individuals and groups" includes "the realization of the fullest potential of an individual physically, psychologically, socially, spiritually and economically," as well as the "fulfillment of one's role expectations in the family, community, place of worship, workplace and other settings."[147]

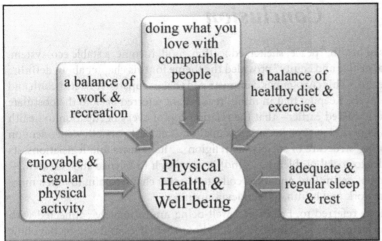

Figure 5-3. Occupation related to physical health and well-being.

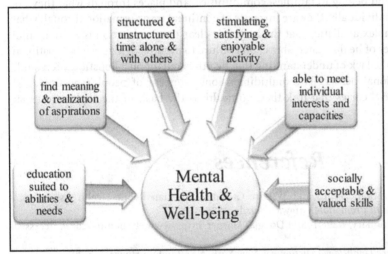

Figure 5-4. Occupation related to mental health and well-being.

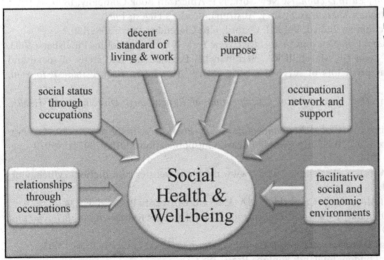

Figure 5-5. Occupation related to social health and well-being.

Conclusion

The WHO prerequisites of health: "peace, shelter, education, food, income, a stable eco-system, sustainable resources, social justice and equity" provided the theme for this chapter about defining occupation in relation to health.[1] This chapter has demonstrated that occupation affects health and well-being at fundamental levels. Keeping that in mind, readers are referred back to the postulate put forth by Gandevia and discussed earlier—that the relationship of every occupation to health and disease changes over any period of time because occupation is at least partially dependent on the physical environment, the "structure of society, its religion … its politics and legislations, its economic status, its attitudes to social problems … [and] its approach to science and research."[85] The relatively small selection of definitions and ideas collected in this chapter point to much more than a relationship between work and health, as Gandevia surmised.

Based on the several views referred to, health and well-being are intimately connected with societal and environmental factors; what people do throughout their lives and day by day; how they experience and feel about what they do and how they plan ahead, legislate, or dream; how they interact with others and belong to families, communities, and places through what they do; and how, collectively and individually, they are in a state of continual transformation through what they do. Despite such complex affiliations, at the least it is clear that occupation is fundamental to meeting the prerequisites of health noted above, and failure to even recognize the occupational nature of those continues the lack of understanding that health is reliant on a holistic understanding of people as occupational beings. The multidimensional concept of people's occupational natures and needs and the theories that link these to health is the basis of the exploration that follows.

References

1. World Health Organization, Health and Welfare Canada, Canadian Public Health Association. *Ottawa Charter for Health Promotion*. Ottawa, Canada; 1986.
2. Online Etymology Dictionary, © 2001-2014 Douglas Harper. http://www.etymonline.com/. Accessed May 29, 2014.
3. *Random House Webster's Unabridged Dictionary*. New York, NY: Random House, Inc; 2012.
4. Lewis CT. *An Elementary Latin Dictionary*. New York, NY: American Book Company; 1890.
5. *Word Finder, The Australian Thesaurus*. Sydney, Australia: Reader's Digest; 1983.
6. *The Oxford English Dictionary*. 2nd ed. Vol XII. Oxford, UK: Clarendon Press; 1989:130.
7. *Collins English Dictionary, Complete and Unabridged*. New York, NY: HarperCollins Publishers; 2003.
8. Glass TA, Mendes de Leon CF, Marotolli RA, Berkman LF. Population based study of social and productive activities as predictors of survival among elderly Americans. *British Medical Journal*. 1999;319:478-483.
9. World Health Organization. *International Classification of Functioning, Disability and Health*. Geneva: WHO; 2001.
10. World Health Organization. *Global Recommendations on Physical Activity for Health*. Geneva: World Health Organization; 2010. http://whqlibdoc.who.int/publications/2010/9789241599979_eng.pdf. Accessed May 29, 2014.
11. Behavior. *Merriam-Webster Dictionary*. http://www.merriam-webster.com/dictionary/behavior. Accessed May 29, 2014.
12. Dusenbery D. *Living at Micro Scale*. Cambridge, MA: Harvard University Press; 2009:124.
13. Forsythea P, Sudoc N, Dinand T, Taylore V, Bienenstock J. Mood and gut feelings. *Brain, Behavior and Immunity*. 2010;24(1):9-16.
14. *Compact Oxford English Dictionary of Current English*. Oxford: Oxford University Press; 2005.
15. Williams R. *Keywords*. London, England: Fontana Press; 1983.
16. Smith R. *Unemployment and Health: A Disaster and a Challenge*. Oxford, UK: Oxford University Press; 1987.

17. Parker S. *Leisure and Work*. London, England: George Allen and Unwin; 1983:13,17.
18. Ruskin J. Preface. In: Yarker PM, ed. *Ruskin: Unto This Last*. London, England: Collins Publishers; 1970.
19. Marx K. *Capital. Vol 1*. Hamburg, Germany: Otto Meissner; 1867:179-180.
20. Braverman H. *Labor and Monopoly Capital: The Degradation of Work in the Twentieth Century*. New York, NY: Monthly Review Press; 1974.
21. Lobkowicz N. *Theory and Practice: History of Concept from Aristotle to Marx*. London, England: University of Notre Dame Press; 1967:9.
22. *The Oxford English Dictionary*. 2nd ed. Vol XII. Oxford, UK: Clarendon Press; 1989:633.
23. Roget PM. *Roget's Thesaurus of Synonyms and Antonyms*. London, England: The Number Nine Publishing Company; 1972.
24. Petrovic G. Praxis. In: Bottomore T, ed. *A Dictionary of Marxist Thought*. 2nd ed. Oxford, UK: Blackwell Publishers; 1991:435.
25. Comstock D. A method of critical research. In: Bredo E, Feinberg W, eds. *Knowledge and Values in Social and Educational Research*. Philadelphia, PA: Temple University Press; 1982:370-390.
26. Lather P. Research as praxis. *Harvard Educational Review*. 1986;56(3):257-277.
27. Kotarbinski T. The goal of an act and the task of the agent. In: Gasparski W, Pszczolowski T, eds. *Praxiological Studies: Polish Contributions to the Science of Efficient Action*. Dortrecht, Holland: D. Reidel Publishing Co; 1983:22.
28. Burke P. The invention of leisure in early modern Europe. *Past & Present*. 1995;146:136-150.
29. Comfort A. *A Good Age*. London, UK; Mitchell Beazley; 1977:130.
30. Comfort A. *A Good Age*. London, UK; Mitchell Beazley; 1977:170.
31. Comfort A. *A Good Age*. London, UK; Mitchell Beazley; 1977:153.
32. Word Finder. *The Australian Thesaurus*. Sydney, Australia: Reader's Digest; 1983; 405.
33. Parker S. *Leisure and Work*. London, England: George Allen and Unwin; 1983.
34. Glasser R. *Time in French Thought*, Pearson CG trans. Manchester: Manchester University Press; 1972:150.
35. Montaigne M. *Les Essais*. C. Pinganaud, ed. Paris; Editions Arlea; 1992: bk 3, ch.13:848. Original work published 1588.
36. Fielding H. *An Enquiry into the Causes of the Late Increase of Robbers* Zirker MR, ed. Oxford, Clarendon Press; 1988:84. Original work published 1751.
37. Bevans G. *How Working Men Spend their Time*. New York: Columbia University Press; 1913.
38. Pember Reeves M. *Round about a Pound a Week*. London, England: Bell; 1913.
39. Harvey A. Guidelines for time-use data collection and analysis. In: Pentland W, Harvey A, Powell Lawton M, McColl M, eds. *Time Use Research in the Social Sciences*. New York: Kluwer Academic/ Plenum Publishers; 1999:19.
40. Harvey A, Pentland W. Time use research. In: Pentland W, Harvey A, Powell Lawton M, McColl M, eds. *Time Use Research in the Social Sciences*. Kluwer Academic/Plenum Publishers, New York: 1999:3.
41. Kleitman N. *Sleep and Wakefulness*. Chicago, IL: University of Chicago Press; 1963:188.
42. Horne JA. A review of the biological effects of total sleep deprivation in man. *Biological Psychology*. 1978;(7):55-102.
43. Leger DW. *Biological Foundations for Behavior: An Integrative Approach*. New York, NY: Harper Collins Publishers; 1992:374.
44. Christiansen C, Townsend E. *An Introduction to Occupation: The Art and Science of Living*. Upper Saddle River, NJ: Pearson Education Inc.; 2010:17.
45. *The Concise Oxford Dictionary of Current English*. Oxford, UK: Clarendon Press; 1911.
46. *Webster's Revised Unabridged Dictionary of the English Language*. London, England: G Bell and Sons Ltd; 1919.
47. Occupy. *Dictionary.com* Unabridged. http://dictionary.reference.com/browse/occupy. Accessed May 24, 2014.
48. Occupation. *The Free Dictionary*. http://www.thefreedictionary.com/occupation. Accessed May 20, 2014.
49. Engage. *The Free Dictionary*. http://www.thefreedictionary.com/engage. Accessed May 20, 2014.
50. Occupy. *Collins English Dictionary*. www.collinsdictionary.com. Accessed May 20, 2014.
51. Occupation. *Dictionary.com*. http://dictionary.reference.com/browse/occupation. Accessed May 20, 2014.
52. Occupation. Synonyms. *Collins English Dictionary*. http://www.collinsdictionary.com/dictionary/ english/occupation. Accessed May 20, 2014.

53. *Collins Thesaurus of the English Language: Complete and Unabridged.* 2nd ed. New York, NY: HarperCollins Publishers; 2002.

54. Murphy G. *Human Potentialities.* New York: Basic Books; 1958.

55. Watts ED. Human needs. In: Kuper A, Kuper J, eds. *The Social Science Encyclopedia.* Rev ed. London, England: Routledge; 1989:367-368.

56. Fromm E. *The Fear of Freedom.* London, England: Routledge and Kegan Paul Ltd.; 1960.

57. Coon CS. *The Hunting Peoples.* London, England: Jonathan Cape Ltd; 1972:393.

58. Thibeault R. Occupation and the rebuilding of civil society: Notes from the war zone. *Journal of Occupational Science.* 2002;9(1):38-47.

59. Office of the High Commission of Human Rights. *Discrimination (Employment and Occupation) Convention.* Convention (No 111) concerning Discrimination in respect of Employment and Occupation. (Adopted 25th June 1958). Geneva: United Nations; 1997-2002:2.

60. *The American Heritage Dictionary of the English Language.* 4th ed. Boston: Houghton Mifflin; 2009.

61. Occupational medicine. *The American Heritage Dictionary of the English Language.* 4th ed. Houghton Mifflin Co. http://www.answers.com/library/Dictionary. Accessed May 17, 2012.

62. Ramazzini B. *A Treatise of the Diseases of Tradesmen, and Now Done in English.* London; Andrew Bell and others; 1705.

63. Coppee GH. *Occupational Health Services and Practices.* http://www.ilo.org/safework_bookshelf/english?content&nd=857170174. Accessed May 29, 2014.

64. World Health Organization. *Workplace Health Promotion.* The workplace: A priority setting for health promotion. http://www.who.int/occupational_health/topics/workplace/en/print.html. Accessed May 29, 2014.

65. Burton R. *The Anatomy of Melancholy.* 12th ed. London; Printed for J Cuthell et al; 1821:601.

66. Jahoda M. *Employment and Unemployment: A Social-Psychological Analysis.* Cambridge: Cambridge University Press: 1982.

67. Argyle M. *The Psychology of Happiness.* London: Methuen; 1987.

68. Csikszentmihalyi M. *Beyond Boredom and Anxiety.* San Francisco: Jossey-Bass; 1975.

69. Veenhoven R. *Healthy Happiness.* Presented to European Conference on Positive Psychology. 2006. www.wellcoach.com/images/HealthyHappiness2006.pdf. Accessed October 9, 2013.

70. Peterson C, Seligman M. *Character Strengths and Virtues.* Washington, DC: American Psychological Association and Oxford University Press; 2004.

71. Seligman M. *Authentic Happiness.* New York: Free Press; 2002.

72. Burton R. *The Anatomy of Melancholy.* Oxford: Printed for Henry Cripps; 1638.

73. Cheyne G. *Essay of Health and Long Life.* London and Bath: Strahan; 1724.

74. Blundell JWF. *The Muscles and their Story from the Earliest Times (an Adaptation of the 'Ars Gymnastica') including the Whole Text of Mercurialis, and the Opinions of other Writers Ancient and Modern on Mental and Bodily Development.* London, UK: Chapman & Hall; 1864.

75. Southwood-Smith T. *The Philosophy of Health or the Exposition of the Physical and Mental Constitution of Man, with a View to the Promotion of Human Longevity and Happiness.* Vol. 1. London; Charles Knight: 1836-7.

76. Sigerist HE. The Wesley M Carpenter Lecture: Historical background of industrial and occupational diseases. October 19, 1936. In: *Henry Sigerist on the History of Medicine.* Edited and with an Introduction by Felix Marti-Ibanez. 1st ed. New York: MD Publications; 1960:46.

77. Sigerist HE. *The University at the Crossroads: Addresses and Essays.* New York, NY: Henry Schuman; 1946:127.

78. World Health Organization. *Rio Declaration on Social Determinants of Health.* Rio de Janeiro, Brazil, 21 October 2011. http://www.who.int/sdhconference/declaration/en/. Accessed May 28, 2014.

79. World Health Organization. *Health Impact Assessment: The Determinants of Health.* WHO; 2012. www.who.int/hia/evidence/doh/en. Accessed May 29, 2014.

80. World Health Organization. *Health Topics: Health Promotion.* WHO; 2012. www.who.int/topics/health_promotion/en/. Accessed May 29, 2014.

81. McAllister F. *Well-being: Concepts and Challenges.* Discussion Paper prepared for the Sustainable Development Research Network; 2005. http://www.sd-research.org.uk/well-being/documents/SDRNwell-beingpaper-Final_000.pdf. Acessed May 29, 2014.

82. Penedo F, Dahn J. Exercise and well-being: a review of mental and physical health benefits associated with physical activity. *Current Opinion in Psychiatry.* 2005:18(2);189-193.

83. Mayo Clinic. *Fitness. Exercise: 7 Benefits of Physical Activity.* Mayo Clinic; 2012. http://users.rowan. edu/~whitea13/7benefits.htm. Accessed May 29, 2014.

84. Harvard Health Publications, Harvard Medical School. *Harvard Health Letter: In Brief: Sing along for Health.* March, 2007. http://www.health.harvard.edu/newsletters/harvard_health_letter/2007/March. Accessed May 29, 2014.

85. Gandevia B. *Occupation and Disease in Australia since 1788.* Sydney: Australasian Medical Publishing Company Ltd; 1971:158.

86. Castles I. *How Australians Use Their Time.* Catalog No. 4153.0. Australian Bureau of Statistics, 1992 (embargoed to 1994).

87. Harvey AS. Quality of life and the use of time theory and measurement. *Journal of Occupational Science: Australia.* 1993;1(2):27-30.

88. Andrew C, Milroy BM, eds. *Life Spaces: Gender, Household, Employment.* Vancouver, Canada: University of Vancouver Press; 1988.

89. Robinson JP. *How Americans Use Time: A Social-Psychological Analysis of Everyday Behaviour.* New York, NY: Praeger Publishers; 1977.

90. Szalai A. *The Use of Time: Daily Activities of Urban and Suburban Populations in Twelve Countries.* The Hague: Mouton; 1972.

91. Australian Bureau of Statistics. *How Australians Use Their Time.* Canberra: Australian Bureau of Statistics; 2006. http://www.abs.gov.au/ausstats/. Accessed June 7, 2012.

92. Australian Bureau of Statistics. *Households Research Database.* Information Pack on the Mental Health and Well-being Survey 1997. Australian Bureau of Statistics. ABS Catalogue 4327AU. MH 97: Canberra, Australia: 1997.

93. Harvey A, Pentland W. What people do. In: Christiansen C, Townsend E, eds. *An Introduction to Occupation: The Art and Science of Living.* Upper Saddle River, NJ: Pearson Education; 2010:123.

94. Aas D. Designs for large scale time use studies of the 24 hour day. In: *It's About Time.* Sofia: Institute of Sociology at the Bulgarian Academy of Science; 1980.

95. Sorokin P, Berger C. *Time Budgets of Human Behaviour.* Cambridge, MA: Harvard University Press: 1939.

96. Chapin S. *Human Activity Patterns in the City.* New York: Wiley Interscience; 1974.

97. Andorka R. Time budgets and their uses. *Annals of Reviews in Sociology.* 1987;13:149-164.

98. Pentland W, Harvey A, Powell Lawton M, McColl MA, eds. *Time Use Research in the Social Sciences.* New York, NY: Kluwer Academic/Plenum Publishers; 1999.

99. Kielhofner G. The temporal dimension in the lives of retarded adults. *American Journal of Occupational Therapy.* 1979;33:161-168.

100. Neville A. Temporal adaptation: application with short-term psychiatric patients. *American Journal of Occupational Therapy.* 1980;34:328-331.

101. Rosenthal LA, Howe MC. Activity patterns and leisure concepts: a comparison of temporal adaptation among day versus night shift workers. *Occupational Therapy in Mental Health.* 1984;4:59-78.

102. Weeder TC. Comparison of temporal patterns and meaningfulness of daily activities of schizophrenics and normal adults. *Occupational Therapy in Mental Health.* 1986;6:27-45.

103. Yerxa EJ, Locker SB. Quality of time used by adults with spinal cord injuries. *American Journal of Occupational Therapy.* 1990;44:318-326.

104. Mackinnon J, Avison W, McCain G. Rheumatoid arthritis, occupational profiles and psychological adjustment. *Journal of Occupational Science: Australia.* 1994;1(4):3-10.

105. Walker C. Occupational adaptation in action: shift workers and their strategies. *Journal of Occupational Science.* 2001;12(2):69-81.

106. Gallew HA, Mu K. An occupational look at temporal adaptation: Night shift nurses. *Journal of Occupational Science.* 2004;11(1):23-30.

107. Winkler D, Unsworth C, Sloan S. Time Use following a severe traumatic brain injury. *Journal of Occupational Science.* 2005;8(1):17-24.

108. Pentland W, McColl M. Application of time-use research to the study of life with a disability. In: Pentland W, Harvey A, Powell Lawton M, McColl M, eds. *Time Use Research in the Social Sciences.* Kluwer Academic/Plenum Publishers, New York: 1999.

109. Selye H. *Stress Without Distress.* New York: New American Library: 1975.

110. Meyer A. The philosophy of occupational therapy. *Archives of Occupational Therapy.* 1922;1:1-10.

111. Woodside HH. The development of occupational therapy 1910-1929. *American Journal of Occupational Therapy.* 1971;XXV(5):226-230.

112. Schartz KB. The history of occupational therapy. In: Crepeau EB, Cohn ES, Boyt Schell BA, eds. *Willard & Spackman's Occupational Therapy.* 10th ed. Philadelphia, PA: Lipincott, Williams & Wilkins; 2003.

113. Dunton WR Jr. *Prescribing Occupational Therapy.* 2nd ed. Springfield, IL: Charles C Thomas; 1928.

114. Cheyne G. *Essay of Health and Long Life.* London and Bath: Strahan; 1724:89.

115. Dunton WR. *Reconstruction Therapy.* Philadelphia: Saunders; 1919:17.

116. Nelson DL, Jonsson H. Occupational terms across languages and cultures. *Journal of Occupational Science.* 1999;6(1):42-47.

117. Larsen E, Wood W, Clark F. Occupational science: building the science and practice of occupation through an academic discipline. Chapter 2 in: Crepeau EB, Cohn ES, Schell BAB, eds. *Willard & Spackman's Occupational Therapy.* 10th ed. Philadelphia: Lippincott Williams & Wilkins; 2003.

118. Moruno P, Iglesias E, Romero D. Activity versus occupation: two concepts for the practice of occupational therapy. In: *Action for Health in a New Millenium. Abstract Book.* Stockholm: WFOT; 2002.

119. Wilcock AA. *Occupation for Health: Volume 2 - A Journey from Prescription to Self Health.* London: COT; 2001.

120. Fidler G, Fidler H. Doing and becoming: purposeful action and self-actualization. *American Journal of Occupational Therapy.* 1978;32(5):305.

121. Kielhofner G. *The Conceptual Foundations of Occupational Therapy.* Philadelphia: F. A. Davis: 1992.

122. Cynkin S, Robinson AM. *Occupational Therapy and Activities Health: Towards Health through Activities.* Boston, MA: Little, Brown and Co; 1990.

123. Wilcock AA. *Occupational Therapy Approaches to Stroke.* Melbourne, Australia: Churchill Livingstone; 1986.

124. Occupational therapy: its definitions and functions. *American Journal of Occupational Therapy.* 1972;26:204.

125. Stein F, Roose B. *Pocket Guide to Treatment in Occupational Therapy.* San Diego, CA: Singular Publishing Co; 2000:201.

126. Kielhofner G, ed. *A Model of Human Occupation: Theory and Application.* Baltimore, MD: Williams and Wilkins; 1985.

127. Turner A, Foster M, Johnson SE, eds. *Occupational Therapy and Physical Dysfunction: Principles, Skills and Practice.* 4th ed. New York: Churchill Livingstone; 1996.

128. Cara E, Macrae A. *Psychosocial Occupational Therapy: A Clinical Practice.* New York: Delmar Publishers; 1998.

129. Humphry R. Young children's occupations: explicating the dynamics of developmental processes. *American Journal of Occupational Therapy.* 2002;56:171-179.

130. World Federation of Occupational Therapists. *Definition of Occupational Therapy.* http://www.wfot.org/AboutUs/AboutOccupationalTherapy/WhatisOccupationalTherapy.aspx). Accessed May 21, 2014.

131. Reilly M. 1961 Eleanor Clarke Slagle Lecture. Occupational therapy can be one of the great ideas of 20th-century medicine. *American Journal of Occupational Therapy.* 1962;16:1-9.

132. Larson E, Wood W, Clark F. Occupational science: building the science and practice of occupation through an academic discipline. In: Crepeau EB, Cohn ES, Boyt Schell BA, eds. *Willard & Spackman's Ocupational Therapy.* 10th ed. Philadelphia, PA: Lipincott, Williams & Wilkins; 2003.

133. Yerxa EJ, Clark F, Frank G, et al. An introduction to occupational science: a foundation for occupational therapy in the 21st century. *Occupational Therapy in Health Care.* 1989;6(4):3.

134. Yerxa EJ, Clark F, Frank G, et al. An introduction to occupational science. A foundation for occupational therapy in the 21st century. *Occupational Therapy in Health Care.* 1989;6(4):1-17.

135. Wilcock AA. *Is Occupational Science the Basis of Occupational Therapy? Presentation to the 2nd South Australian Occupational Therapy Conference.* 1989.

136. Wilcock AA. *Occupational Science.* Presentation to the World Federation of Occupational Therapists Congress, Melbourne. 1990.

137. Australasian Society of Occupational Scientists. *Key Beliefs.* http://www.anzoccsci.org. Accessed May 29, 2014.

138. International Society for Occupational Science. *Welcome to the ISOS: ISOS has a mission...;* 2009. www.isoccsci.org. Accessed May 29, 2014.

139. Christiansen C, Clark F, et al. Position paper: Occupation. *American Journal of Occupational Therapy.* 1995;49(10):1015-1018.

140. Townsend E. Occupation: potential for personal and social transformation. *Journal of Occupational Science.* 1997;46(1):18-26.

141a. Jarman J. Occupation in occupational therapy and occupational science. In: Christiansen C, Townsend E, eds. *Introduction to Occupation: The Art and Science of Living.* 2nd ed. Upper Saddle River, NJ. Pearson; 2010: 86.

141b. Locke J. *An Essay Concerning Humane Understanding.* London: Printed for Tho, Bassett, and sold by Edw. Mory at the sign of the Three Bibles in St. Paul's Church-Yard; 1690:361.

142. Greiner PA, Fain JA, Edelman CL. Health defined: objectives for promotion and prevention. In: Edelman CL, Mandle CL, eds. *Health Promotion throughout the Lifespan.* 5th ed. St Louis: Mosby; 2002:6.

143. Galvaan R. Occupational choice: the significance of socio-economic and political factors. In: Whiteford G, Hocking C, eds. *Occupational Science: Society, Inclusion, Participation.* Oxford; Wiley-Blackwell; 2012:152-162.

144. *Word Finder: Australian Thesaurus.* Sydney, Australia: Reader's Digest; 1983:56.

145. Landau SI, chief ed. *Funk & Wagnalls Standard Desk Dictionary.* Vol 1. New York: Harper & Row; 1984:58.

146. *Oxford English Dictionary.* Oxford University Press; 2013. http://public.oed.com/about/free-oed/. Accessed May 29, 2014.

147. Smith B, Tang K, Nutbeam D. WHO health promotion glossary: new terms. *Health Promotion International.* 2006 21(4):340.

Theme 6

"Health is created and lived by people within the settings of their everyday life; where they learn, work, play, and love."

WHO: The Ottawa Charter for Health Promotion, 1986[1]

Chapter 6

OCCUPATION

DOING, HEALTH, AND ILLNESS

This chapter addresses:
- Doing as a Prerequisite of Population Health
  - The Doing-Rest Continuum
  - Natural Health, Biological Needs, and Human Doing
    - Food and Income
    - Shelter
    - Education
    - Peace
    - A Stable Ecosystem and Sustainable Resources
    - Social Justice and Equity
    - Summation: Meeting the Prerequisites of Health Through Doing
- Rules for Health
  - An Ancient Doing Approach
  - A Modern Doing Approach: Ottawa Charter Directives
- Doing as a Factor in Illness, Health, and Well-being
- Conclusion

This chapter is the first of four in which occupation's basic relationship to health is examined. Despite the fact that occupation needs to be considered holistically, these chapters divide it according to the concepts of doing, being, belonging, and becoming. The division is purely arbitrary for clarity of explanation. It builds on the theory outlined in Chapter 4 and sets the scene for considering occupation that embraces a combination of the four concepts as an agent of population health.

Drawing on history to inform the present, this chapter challenges relevant policy makers and practitioners to consider the nature and place of doing within health care. Occupation-based programs in acute or residential care facilities have, more and more, been limited to the assessment and provision of aids to people with disabilities, valuable in themselves, but singular in purpose. The role of people's doings in the etiology of illness is most often overlooked, and the

Wilcock AA, Hocking C.
An Occupational Perspective of Health, Third Edition (pp 146-177).
© 2015 Taylor & Francis Group.

potential for people's doings to augment other treatments is hardly ever considered in the current, economically and time-driven, medically based health care systems. The timelines set by service providers are often too short to allow important life changes to be set in motion, yet those changes may be necessary to prevent further illness or promote well-being. However, it is probable that most opportunities to change unhealthy doing lie outside the world of medical care, where there is no funding or it is inadequate or sparse. This suggests that resources need to be developed for new areas of practice, services, or opportunities that link health with all that people do across the activity-rest continuum. The content of this chapter provides substance toward such change in direction, intervention, and research.

Doing as a Prerequisite of Population Health

People have an innate need to engage in occupations because survival and health depend on it. Although air, water, and food are essential to life, its continuance depends on people accessing and preparing those essentials, and finding shelter and safe environments in which to rest, keep their temperature at a comfortable level, and keep their bodies protected from the elements. Doing with others is important in establishing communities that can work together in supportive ways for familial and the common good, and in ways that form inclusive local and national identity and culture, providing a necessary and supportive sense of belonging.

Archaeological anthropologists suggest that having a highly developed culture really means that humans can "do more or less what they want."[2] Currently, doing is usually separated according to culturally accepted divisions, such as education, work, leisure, parenting, and rest, even within professions that espouse holism. How communities and individuals regard such segments of doing is dependent on cultural viewpoints, economic possibilities, and political imperatives. Although doing is rarely acknowledged as an entity in its own right in medical or scientific inquiry, such an oversight has not been the case in scholarly treatise or in time-use studies that supply census material and inform future governmental decisions. Although largely unacknowledged, it is the occupation of governmental, social, and corporate organizations to develop policies that will ultimately drive the occupations possible within individual lives. These also influence the doings of distant communities on the global stage. Doing provides the largely unacknowledged background of what all people can or cannot be and cannot be ignored; it is the foundation of living.

However, economics are so closely intertwined with doing that it is considered from that perspective more often than it is thought of in health terms. For example, within population health in postindustrial societies, concentration on doing has been aimed mainly at eradicating risks in paid employment—the aspect of doing that is closely tied with the economic wealth of businesses and nations. As discussed in Chapter 3, a new focus recognizes that an increase in the doing of physical activity is urgently required before obesity reaches pandemic proportions.[3] Such initiatives are vitally important, but fail to appreciate or act on occupation in the holistic way that is necessary. For example, a significant study with a sample of 2761 older Americans undertaken at Harvard over a period of 13 years found that doing social and productive occupations "that involve little or no enhancement of fitness" lowered the risk of all causes of death as much as doing exercise.[4]

Currently, despite the popularity of the idiom "doing well," too few of the world's population are doing well. For example, there is imbalance in the experience of doing between people of high- and low-income countries from various perspectives; between the rich and the poor, the employed and unemployed, the young and old, and the literate and illiterate; between genders; and between those who are free to pursue their doings unimpeded and those institutionalized or incarcerated. Opportunities or experience of doing may, of itself, lead to a lack of well-being for large numbers of people, just as the right kind of doing can be considered a prerequisite of health.

The WHO recognizes the health impact of not doing well and has addressed the issues in many of its strategy documents, which will be discussed later. It has also defined, to some extent,

Table 6-1

COMPARISON OF TERMS IN THIS TEXT AND THE INTERNATIONAL CLASSIFICATION OF FUNCTIONING, DISABILITY, AND HEALTH[5]

	ICF Explanations	Text Explanations	
Activity	A person's capacity to execute occupations (with or without assistive devices or assistance). What a person could do in an environment with no barriers to performance	Synonymous with or an aspect of occupation	Occupation Participation in any activity of a doing, being, belonging, and becoming nature to meet health, personal, societal, and survival needs and wants
Participation	A person's actual performance of occupations in his or her current environment, including problems the person experiences due to environmental barriers	Involvement in any of life's occupations that may be self as well as family or sociopolitically initiated	
Environmental factors	Physical, social, and attitudinal environment within which people live their lives, which can act as barriers to or facilitators of participation	The same: All aspects of external world including the natural human-made physical world, other people in different relationships and roles, attitudes and values, social systems and services, and policies, rules, and laws	
Personal factors	Aspects of the person not related to their health condition, including gender, race, age, lifestyle, habits, coping style, education, social background, previous experiences, psychological assets, behavior patterns, etc	The same, plus occupational history	

the notion of occupation as a combination of activity and participation. In the International Classification of Functioning, Disability and Health, there are indications of the way the WHO understands aspects of doing.[5] These are provided in Table 6-1 and are compared with how they are used in this text.

Apart from the social determinants of occupation that emanate from environmental factors, many physical factors influence doing. Several of these relating to internal mechanisms, physical attributes, and biological needs have already been noted as influential. These are known as regulatory motivators because they are physiological in nature. They prompt doing to meet some of the prerequisites of health, such as hunger and shelter. Other regulatory motivators might be fatigue, pain, or level of arousal.[6] Maslow described such needs as "Deficiency or D Needs."[7] Other forms of doing higher up his hierarchy, called "Being or B Needs," are the subject of later chapters.

One source of evidence about what people do comes from national statistics, at least in high-income countries. It is relevant for those planning to work in this area to consider these as a source of vital information because they relate not only to those populations, but also to what might occur to other populations in low- and middle-income countries in the not too distant future. More and more people cease to live traditional lifestyles and turn to industry, for good or bad. Over a lifetime, paid employment accounts for a smaller proportion of time than perhaps would be expected, given the emphasis on it within population health and the way Western countries have, until fairly recently, looked to the market economy to provide insight into people's needs. In recent years, and probably as a partial result of the women's movement, more appreciation has been given to other forms of work, such as parenting, volunteering, care-giving, and homemaking. Pentland and Harvey commented on those facts and noted "that activities and occupations vary much more among subpopulations in a given country than they do in total across countries."[8]

THE DOING-REST CONTINUUM

On average, in high-income countries, people spend more time sleeping than doing anything else. The continuum of doing and resting is an important one, both in terms of the quality and quantity of occupation and of health and well-being. It was recognized as a continuum in the ancient rules of health, yet sleep is not included in some modern theories about occupation because its apparent lack of active qualities appears to gainsay the essence of doing.[9] However, that is a simplistic perception. Preparing for sleep is an important part of daily activities, almost reaching ritualistic proportions for some people. For example, it encompasses preparations of the body, mind, and environment in undressing, relaxing, ensuring appropriate ventilation, or turning off the lights.[9] Sleep itself is a complex, active process affecting occupation components, such as memory, learning, creativity, and productivity, as well as emotional stability and physical health. From infancy to old age, inadequate sleep can have a negative effect on "the heart, lungs and kidneys; appetite, metabolism and weight control; immune function and disease resistance; sensitivity to pain; reaction time; mood; and brain function."[10] Emerging from sleep usually has a ritualistic quality that reverses relaxation and prepares the mind and body for the daily doings ahead. If sleep has been disturbed, the day ahead can also be disturbed or difficult.[11]

All sleep stages have a homeostatic function, even though the system does not operate on feedback principles but rather on intrinsic timing mechanisms.[12] These mechanisms differ slightly for each individual and change throughout the lifespan. The oldest form of sleep, known as slow-wave sleep, shows different patterns of electroencephalography for several different stages. Slow-wave sleep is responsible for replenishing the body and maintaining physiological and metabolic fitness. After a day of strenuous physical doing, slow-wave sleep increases, and it is only during slow-wave sleep that growth hormone, essential for restoring damaged tissue, is released.[13] Following sleep deprivation, slow-wave sleep takes priority in catching up. For example, studies such as those conducted by Shapiro et al on ultra-marathon runners demonstrated an increase in slow-wave sleep, as well as total sleeping time, over 4 nights following the run.[14] This effect appears most developed among people who are physically fit,[15] suggesting a close relationship between sleep patterns and other regular occupations.

Additional servicing is required for the maintenance of structures specializing in mental and social functions. This is provided by rapid eye movement (REM) sleep, when circuits are tested and neurotransmitters are replenished by being rested selectively.[12] During this stage, the brain is very active and "actually consumes more oxygen than it does during intense physical or mental activity when one is awake."[16] Speculations about other functions of REM sleep include the integration of knowledge acquired during the day, the laying down of long-term memory, assistance in dealing with emotionally charged material, and consolidation of information.[12,17,18] For example, patients in forensic care, some of whom committed crimes while mentally ill, have found that resting and sleeping allows them to dream of other life possibilities and find new meaning.[19,20] Fox speculated from animal experiments that "current information, blocked from the hippocampus and the limbic circuit during waking, is allowed in there during sleep to be 'matched' against those wired-in survival behaviors."[21] If the information is deemed relevant, it is processed "for at least 3 years in some form or other" during dreams, before being "stamped in" to long-term memory and eventually stored in the neocortex.[21] This process enables the neocortex to assess experience toward future goal-directed action. REM sleep may serve a similar purpose in humans, but Fox suggested that dreaming has been freed, to some extent, from phylogenetic and species-specific experience, allowing the matching process to relate to current prenatal and childhood experience.[21]

Duration of sleep is a need that differs from person to person. Gating mechanisms facilitate the passage between sleep and awake states.[22] REM sleep, which usually occurs 4 to 5 times per night, is seen as the easiest exit point from sleep and possibly evolved in part as a "sentinel device, a monitor in case of danger."[12] At rhythmic times during wakefulness, there are sleepability gates when it is easier to sleep. The most obvious of these is the biological slump occurring in the afternoon, which is taken as siesta time in many traditional cultures. Biphasic activity peaks are part of humans' biological heritage, are evident in the behaviors of other primates, and are probably an adaptation resulting from the need to reduce occupation during the hottest part of the day. Ultradian rhythms of arousal and nonarousal concerned with placement of sleep are easily overruled for doing obligatory or freely chosen occupations.[23] Differences in brainwaves throughout sleep and awake states appear to relate to when the organism is best fitted for different types of occupation or rest. These are flexible and can be overridden, as happens in 8-hour working days or 24-hour working shifts, which enables humans to behave as nocturnal rather than diurnal animals. Therefore, the sleep systems facilitate occupational flexibility, as well as servicing all systems so they can be used as required for whatever is being done.

NATURAL HEALTH, BIOLOGICAL NEEDS, AND HUMAN DOING

Although doing provides the means of maintaining health in a natural way, the opposite can be the case, and what people do can lead to illness and death. A greater understanding of the fine line between well-being and illness as a result of doing is imperative, particularly because doing is the inbuilt human mechanism to fulfill the requirements identified in the Ottawa Charter as a prerequisites of health: food and income, shelter, education, peace, a stable ecosystem and sustainable resources, and social justice, and equity.[1]

Food and Income

Food is a biological need that is essential to life itself. In most instances for early Homo species, it equated to income, so we find that successive economies are described according to their occupational means of procuring food: hunter-gathering, agriculture, and industry. The acquisition of daily food requirements is paramount to what has been done throughout time. Food has to be earned through what people do according to their natural abilities, degree of skill or luck, and the time and place; it is dependent on the community, an individual's beliefs about food, and the environment in which they live. Primitive hunter-gatherers usually experienced general well-being assisted by a low population density,[24] both men and women being engaged in occupations that included "intense endurance exercise."[25]

Premature death was due to a shortage of food, accidents that were possibly related to the acquisition of food, occasional natural disasters, and illnesses, many of which were similar to those of modern humans but seldom the chronic noncommunicable diseases of later life.[26-29] Hominids almost certainly subsisted principally on plant foods supplemented by animal protein of various kinds. For example, Homo habilis was probably an opportunistic omnivore, scavenging for "animal products such as birds' eggs, larvae, lizards, and small game" rather than hunting bigger prey. A systematic food-sharing economy and possibly some division of labor developed gradually, based on cooperative foraging of meat and plant foods.[30-32] Such activities provide for "an important part of the diet of present-day hunter-gatherers."[33] Even a modest intake of meat would have aided survival by provision of energy, a full range of amino acids, trace elements, and vitamin B_{12}.[26] A possible early method of attacking prey for food was stone throwing, as observed in the Hottentots in South West Africa and first-nation Australians.[34] Stone throwing may well have started for self-protection, required because of humans' physical vulnerability compared with many other animals.

Figure 6-1. Ploughing, an occupation with delayed return. (© Carol Spencer 2012, otspencer@adam.com.au. Used with permission.)

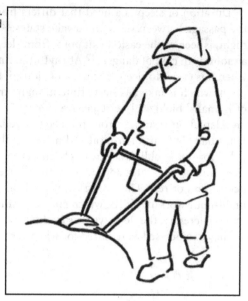

Most recent opinions seem to favor the idea that after Homo men began to take a serious interest in hunting, women, along with their child-bearing and care roles, continued to forage and gather, digging with sticks weighted with perforated round stones.[30,35] As the hunters shared their meat, the women shared their finds.[30] It has been estimated that the latter contributed more than half of the required subsistence calories and that, as a consequence, diets were very diverse, which increased the likelihood of balanced nutrition.[36,37] The use of fire, evident from at least 1.2 million years ago, increased survival and health as meats could be made more edible and the toxicity of plants reduced. Dietary modifications led to natural selection pressures regarding particular attributes, such as lighter jaws and cutting as opposed to grinding teeth, and to an increasingly complex and larger brain, smaller colon, and the modulating role of insulin in optimizing dietary glucose.[26]

"Many archaeological sequences ... show that knowledge of agriculture and domesticated plants existed long before there was a real shift from hunting and gathering."[38] Indeed, it is debatable whether there were no clear-cut distinctions between hunter-gatherers and horticulturalists, who also hunt and gather,[39] and between hunting and herding.[40] Rather, a distinction can be made between "immediate return economies," characterized as a "hand to mouth" existence such as that lived by the Hadza, who live in Tanzania,[41] and "delayed return economies" in which a time investment for the future is part of daily life.[42]

Agriculture is an example of a delayed return economy (Figure 6-1). As it became dominant and according to the societies and cultures in which they lived, men shifted the focus of their doing from hunting to farming. Although agriculture eventually provided improved continuous access to food, the diversity of food was initially reduced, leading to an initial increase in mortality and morbidity. The advent of farming heralded a change in role for many women, who increasingly became engaged in household occupations that supported the farmer and extended the nature of the food to be eaten.[43,44] In many instances, agriculture gave a different focus for combined activity too, for both individual and communal good, sometimes incorporating celebration and fun. For example, Ashton reported that, as a part of all aspects of farming activities, working parties among the Basuto "are gay, sociable affairs comprising about 10 to 50 participants of both sexes."[45] In Western agricultural societies, leisure and work were long associated with seasonal and communal food tasks.

Some hunter-gatherers did not adopt an agrarian lifestyle. This was not because they lacked the intellectual capacity to progress, as evidenced by complex social organizations and ingenious methods of obtaining foodstuffs.[46] The successful survival of the Inuit of northern Canada in an inhospitable environment is an example.[47] Their health and well-being did not deteriorate until recently when western industrial values were imposed on them and impacted their food sources. Three possible reasons for the retention of a hunter-gatherer way of life are isolation, climatic conditions not conducive to profitable agriculture, and that they did not want to change.[46] Carleton Coon, the Harvard anthropologist, suggested that societies retaining hunter-gathering economies had an eminently satisfactory way of living together in small groups, free from tedious routine, and all the food they needed. He argued that adopting agriculture would have imposed a "whole new system of human relationships that offer no easily understood advantages, and disturbs an age-old balance between man and nature and among the people who live together."[48]

Some authorities suggest that the demands of living in harsh environments with few tools other than an expanding brain made what the people of traditional societies had to do very arduous and virtually continuous; that for millions of years the struggle for existence allowed them little time for activities not immediately concerned with survival.[49,50] However, from the study of modern hunter-gatherer societies, Coon found that most individuals were "jacks of all trades," living and working mostly outdoors, their senses acute, and, like their bodies, well exercised. Their schedules and routines would seldom be monotonous and were often adventurous.[46] Others agree that this simple but effective economy provided a successful and persistent quality of life, with Marshall Sahlins of the University of Chicago naming it "the original affluent society ... in which all the people's wants are easily satisfied."[51] In the 1840s, Edward John Eyre remarked on the few hours it took for first-nation Australians, "without fatigue or labor," to procure sufficient food to last the day.[52] Studies of the !Kung San who live on the northern fringe of the Kalahari Desert also provide evidence of such observations.[53] Until recently, when this lifestyle was eroded, adults between ages 15 to 60 years only spent approximately 2.5 hours daily providing their necessities of life, even during a time of drought.[35] Now, only a few continue in traditional ways, with pressure from the government to change.

The acquisition of sufficient food and income to supply basic biological needs are now matters of huge concern for the majority of people, especially those living in low-income countries. Many still engage in subsistence occupations similar to those of early economies, but in ever degrading ecosystems changed forever by people's doings. Famine, disease, and death are constant companions that cannot be easily remediated because of the ravages of affluent nations and multicorporate greed. The call for ecologically sustainable lifestyles and a more equitable distribution of resources between the "haves and the have nots" are responses to this continuing crisis,[54] as is the increasing concern of WHO and population health in nutritional matters across the world. It has been estimated that more than 1 million children suffer from severe acute malnutrition,[55] yet worldwide obesity has more than doubled since 1980, with 65% of the world's population living in countries where being overweight and obese kills more people than does being underweight, and obesity is preventable.[56,57]

In more affluent societies, advanced social welfare systems provide income for food and other essential commodities without a doing requirement. It could be argued that this, too, may be damaging to physical, mental, or social health in the longer term. The number of young people in such societies who do not work to provide for their own needs is increasing and, alongside it, physical, mental, and social illness is manifested through increasing violence, substance abuse, and suicide.[58]

The six ancient rules for health recognized that doing (exercise, action, or motion) and food relate in terms of health outcomes. From time to time, this is remembered. For example, in 1939 Rabbinowitch proclaimed that "occupation, diet and income are intimately related."[59] He outlined that "work cannot be performed without expenditure of energy ... Man obtains his energy from his food ... When engaged in any occupation ... the primary factor which governs the need for food is the degree of muscular activity."[60] Simply providing food or income without the doing component also adds to the illness outcomes. At one extreme, it contributes to problems of obesity, such as cardiovascular disorders and diabetes mellitus, and at the other extreme it leads to decreasing opportunity and skill to provide the means of continuing to acquire provisions. In the publication *The Social Determinants of Health: The Solid Facts*, the WHO recommended "support for sustainable agriculture and food production methods that conserve natural resources and the environment" and the development of a "stronger food culture for health, especially through school education, to foster people's knowledge of food and nutrition, cooking skills, growing food and the social value of preparing food and eating together."[61] This publication reminds us that currently global markets control food supplies. This can reduce local job opportunities, which means that food being marketed does not always meet local health requirements and can lead to monopolies and the reduction of quality in the longer term. Food has become a political issue. In terms of income, and on a personal and population level, the links between food and health are clear. However, added to that are other factors, such as the links between unemployment, illness, and premature death and the links between health and well-being, job satisfaction, and security.

Shelter

There is little evidence about the earliest forms of shelter, although it is possible to speculate that the natural features of landscapes would have been used to provide protection from the elements and predators. Homo habilis is credited with building the first known stone shelters in Olduvai Gorge and carrying food to such camp sites for processing and sharing.[62] This has been queried because the gorge is an area that crocodiles might have inhabited, with Davidson and Noble claiming that there is insufficient evidence of built shelters or regular use of fire prior to 125,000 years ago. They further suggested that this may have been the time when systematic hunting also started.[63]

There is reasonable acceptance that meat eating, clothing, and a capacity to build some form of shelter and make fire enabled early expansion into colder environments. Evidence in the Central Russian Plains of semi-permanent dwellings with vaults, arches, and buttresses constructed of mammoth bones from approximately 30,000 years ago indicates that fixed habitation probably occurred in some regions thousands of years before the rapid spread of agriculture through most of the world from approximately 10,000 years ago.[62] As time progressed, shelters of many sorts were constructed according to the context, in terms of materials available and climatic conditions. These included igloos built of ice and simple bark shades; tents made of hide; structures made from conical birch bark, earth and turf, and wood or stone; and demonstrated the practical nature of hunter-gatherer health and well-being practices.

It appears to be common sense that improved shelter would enable better nurturing and care of the young and of the aged and sick when this was required. However, the nature of the shelter and surrounding circumstances could precipitate wider changes that create difficulty in terms of adjustment. For example, the !Kung San's transition from a hunter-gatherer lifestyle to agriculture led to the dispersion of shelters from villages clustered around a central, publicly shared space to more isolated shelters and individuals owning the land around them. This has changed the complex support mechanism of the older type of communities, and there has been a tendency for individuals to accumulate material goods, as well as a marked rise in birth rate. It has also resulted in an apparent decrease in social and sexual egalitarianism, a more rigid defining of male and female roles, and changed play behaviors of the children.[53] Such alterations can provide a starting point for social illness to occur. Similar changes and difficulties can be recognized in other cultures that have changed more slowly through agrarian, urban, and industrial evolution. Changes in the size, density, and type of shelter continue, with little input from research about whether such shelters meet the occupational needs and natures of people and the health consequences of not meeting those needs.

It is recognized in *The Universal Declaration of Human Rights* that housing is a fundamental aspect of an acceptable standard of living.[64] The WHO housing and health program seeks to "assess and quantify the health impact of housing conditions, identify health priorities in housing;

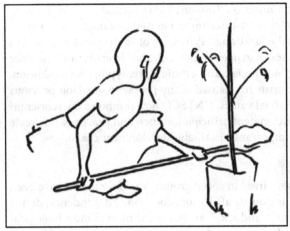

Figure 6-2. Childhood play as an integral part of day-to-day adult occupations. (© Carol Spencer 2012, otspencer@adam.com.au. Used with permission.)

develop methodologies for a cost-benefit analysis of housing rehabilitation for health gain [and] focus on specific priority technical topics."[65] Recognized as a social determinant of health, housing is acknowledged as a major environment affecting physical, mental, and social well-being in either a supportive or limiting way, even though the relationship between environmental quality, health, and well-being is not yet fully understood.[66]

Education

What is best for the safety and development of offspring is of vital importance to the species. Human young have a lot to learn and, compared with other animals, a long childhood. Learning by observing, imitating, and playing creatively provides education about doing with regard to self-care, safety, and survival. It also provides the experience of fun and the development of skills and self-worth, which are potential motivators for continued doing. Learning that occurs in the first formative years of life has significant lifelong effects; it provides children with models for their own future survival, under the protection and guidance of adults before being burdened with their responsibilities. As the species became more complex, the years of childhood, play, and education extended and changed. For example, until recent times, play and education were an integral part of the day-to-day occupations of adults and children and occurred in an environment relevant to the family's work and leisure activities (Figure 6-2).

According to *The Universal Declaration of Human Rights*, the need to promote education is fundamental.[64] As a 1996 United Nations Educational, Scientific and Cultural Organization (UNESCO) report asserts, education is the pathway to social cohesion, economic growth, and global interdependence. In promoting education as a "necessary Utopia," the document describes four pillars of education throughout the lifespan: knowing, learning to do, learning to live together, and learning to be.[67] UNESCO's Strategic Objectives for Education for 2002 to 2007 seeks to improve the quality of education through diversifying contents and methods and "the promotion of universally shared values"; to promote "experimentation, innovation and the diffusion and sharing of information"; and to promote "best practices as well as policy dialogue in education," particularly with regard to children affected by crisis.[68] Women are one target for improved education because they have the lowest levels of literacy, particularly in Asia and the Pacific and among people living in poverty. Within that, the provision of physical education for girls and women will continue to contribute to achieving the Millennium Development goals through empowering women and laying the foundation for leading physically active and healthy lives.[69]

UNESCO has acknowledged that "education has sometimes contributed to the outbreak of violent conflict" and is seeking "ways in which education can prevent such conflict or its recurrence" and to "inculcate universal values of peace and tolerance" through diverse programs.[68]

Accordingly, the 2011 United Nations' *Declaration on Human Rights Education and Training* "emphasizes that education promotes tolerance, non-discrimination and equality, "concerns all parts of society," including all levels of formal education.[70] Principles of respect and recognition are viewed as fundamental to addressing issues of gender equity, cultural diversity, and violence prevention and to eliminating gender, religious, racial, and ethnic stereotyping.[71] In addition, recognizing that the recent global economic crisis has caused many people to question previous assumptions about desirable lifestyles and personal values, UNESCO now promotes the reorientation of "education to integrate sustainable development principles, values, and practices" to create education that "empowers people to address important sustainable development challenges."[72]

Peace

Hunter-gatherers, like most modern humans, lived in social groups. Various reasons have been given for this need for social connectedness, including affiliation, coercion,[73] dependency, dominance,[74] nepotism,[75-77] reciprocity, self-esteem,[78] and sex,[35] as well as the need to meet biological needs through group activity. Social groups offer some protection against predators, and Bruner observed "there is no known human culture that is not marked by reciprocal help in times of danger and trouble, by food sharing, by communal nurturing for the young or disabled, and by the sharing of knowledge and implements for expressing skill."[79]

Within modern hunter-gatherer societies, such as those of first-nation Australians, Kalahari Bushmen, and the Birhhor of Northern India, survival needs and peaceful coexistence are major determinants of group size, with most ranging between 20 and 70 people.[80] "A group of about 25 has a good chance of surviving for perhaps 500 years" and appears to be compatible with minimal conflict. To avoid inbreeding, these groups usually form part of larger tribes of approximately 500 to 800 people.[81] Humans group together to achieve large-scale occupations and for the enjoyment that can be experienced from being with and doing things with others. People who enjoy similar occupations find pleasure and challenge in discussing and sharing their enthusiasm.

Leakey suggested that "man is not programmed to kill and make war, nor even to hunt: his ability to do so is learned from his elders and his peers when society demands it." His argument is based on the fact that no evidence of inflicted death and warfare was found before the advent of temple towns, making "this ... too recent an event to have had any influence on the evolution of human nature."[82] However Lorenz[83] asserted that in early societies not all would have been peaceful, describing "war between the generations" as part of a "species-preserving function to eliminate obsolete elements hindering new developments." In puberty, young people go through a stage of "physiological neophilia" in which everything new is attractive. When somewhat older, they experience a revival of love of tradition, or "late obedience." Lorenz's[84] explanation has some merit in that physiological neophilia at an age when physical and mental capacities are acute will facilitate experimentation and exploration across a wide spectrum of activities, which may provide survival and health advantages. In addition, later development, growth, and adaptation may be based on successful experiences and individual interest, enhancing personal capacities, health, and well-being.[84]

With greater population density came an apparent need for territorial defense, and the ever-recurring occupation of war.[85] Lorenz argued that, in common with other animals, humans are innately aggressive to maintain sufficient space for existence, to ensure the strongest males father offspring, and to establish a pecking order.[84] Others propose that an inevitable consequence of tribal bonding is hostility toward other tribes.[86] It is true that people have expended vast amounts of mental and physical effort, as well as resources, on the development and accumulation of weapons. These may be seen as an expression of a human need to feel safe, of innate aggression, or of a need to develop tool technology without being able to foresee the possible consequences of the technology produced. The weapons of war are an aspect of tool technology developing beyond and to the detriment of human well-being. This may be a reflection of the lack of planning of evolution—that adaptation to one set of environmental conditions millions of years ago may prove to be a handicap in another type of environment.[87] The expression of capacities through doing that includes ongoing experimentation and technological development is a strong force, especially when valued highly by society. The brain's ability to override biological needs with a highly developed cognitive capacity responsive to sociocultural influences has disadvantages and advantages.

Currently, conflict is a major health problem, and in Southeast Asia alone approximately 20,000 people lose their lives each year because of it. Therefore, it is apparent that "health workers in conflict areas need to learn how to function effectively without getting caught up in the disputes or being exploited by the warring parties" and to "bring parties together to solve serious health problems in conflict situations."[88] In a message to a health professionals training workshop on "Health As a Bridge for Peace" in Colombo, the WHO Director-General claimed that "health workers in conflict zones may defuse tension and build bridges for peace" because health can be "the perfect olive branch which is acceptable to almost all peoples."[88] Many have already reported that health has brought about cooperation and, sometimes, even reconciliation. The workshop was the first of its kind to be organized by the WHO and obviously met a recognized need being called for by health professionals in the field in Africa, Eastern Europe, and South America.

A Stable Ecosystem and Sustainable Resources

There is a closeness of fit between environments and the occupations of hunter-gatherers who:

> Had the energy, hardihood, and ingenuity to live and live well in every climatic region of the world not covered by icecaps. They have done so with stone tools and no firearms. In every well-documented instance, cases of hardship may be traced to the intervention of modern intruders.[89]

It is generally accepted that the advent of permanent settlements and the agrarian revolution were closely associated with environmental and climatic conditions that prevailed in different locations. Those that provided adequate food and shelter year round probably supported resident populations, greatly reducing nomadic ways of life. Major theories suggest that when the Pleistocene Ice Age ended, a major climate change occurred that produced environments conducive to agriculture. The resultant increasing social complexity resulted in a need for more formalized food production because the food procuring system of small nomadic communities became inadequate. It is also possible that the developing occupational capacity of humans was instrumental in the change. That is, as humans experimented with material resources, their skills expanded—they began to challenge the environment and adapt it to meet their own needs and comfort. This possibility is supported by the fact that as agriculture developed so did the diversity of human doings.[90]

A disadvantage of the human capacity for occupational experimentation is that agriculture changed the Earth as a result of deforestation, land clearing, ploughing, and irrigation schemes, such as blocking or moving river beds.[91] As part of the agricultural process, the domestication of animals "involved an accelerating process of elimination of the great diversity of wild animals and plants to replace them with a few species that could be easily managed and manipulated." It has also resulted in the proliferation of some to bad effect.[92] "Erosion and the alteration of the balance of species became inevitable."[93]

In Chapter 2, it was noted that agrarian development, and the permanent built environment that grew alongside it, prevented the reestablishment of natural ecosystems, providing conditions that were conducive to hyper infestations of disease organisms. For thousands of years, infectious diseases caused ongoing morbidity throughout the world, with periodic plagues resulting in catastrophic numbers of people dying. Perhaps that is indicative of the major problems still to come unless it is recognized that people's doing, ecological functioning, and health are inextricably related.

Urban environments are a powerful determinant of health because, since 2008, more than half the world's population has lived in a city.[94] Urban features, such as lack of street connectivity, decrease walking and cycling and increase car use. With every additional hour spent driving the risk of obesity increases by approximately 6%.[95] Neighborhoods with a high density of alcohol outlets and tobacco advertising work against the adoption of healthy lifestyles, as do concerns about safety and lack of ready access to places that sell fresh fruit and vegetables.[96]

The WHO claims that damage to ecosystems poses a growing threat to human health,[97] with a report from the Millennium Ecosystem Assessment (MA)[98] recognizing that the links between people's health and the environment are complex and indirect. They include constituents to well-being such as "security", "basic material for a good life", "health", and "good social relations" along with "freedom of choice and action" and "opportunities to be able to achieve what an individual values doing and being."[99] More directly, environmental change translates to illness caused by risk of water-borne infections and toxins for people in remote communities and those engaged in water-based occupations. Increasing drought brings higher rates of depression and suicide among farmers and the communities that support them. The changing environment has also been linked to altered living patterns that contribute to increasing obesity rates and to the systemic problems with work-family-life balance, consumer behavior, and loss of community, which are associated with depression.[95] As Research Australia concluded "achieving a population of healthy people requires a healthy planet to ensure the fundamentals—and healthy places in which to live, work, interact, and play."[95]

Social Justice and Equity

There has been long debate about how it was determined, in the early days of human evolution, who would do things and how. Whether any such division was equitable or just is a more modern debate. Rowley-Conway believed that although early hominids probably lived in small groups with a structure similar to that of chimpanzees, their form of scavenging required "no division of labor and does not imply sharing or any other social behavior approaching our own."[100] However, a division of what needed to be done according to gender may have been used because of differences in terms of reproductive biology, fat-to-muscle ratio, and greater variation in size than is common today; this is known as sexual dimorphism. In sexually dimorphic primate societies, monogamy is rare.

The extent of sexual dimorphism and the maturation rates of early humans set some parameters to the debate about social justice and equity.[101] Other factors reflect the concerns of the modern societies from which the ideas emanate, such as power relations, monogamy, and the nuclear family.[102] The question of why men, generally, do one thing and women another remains one of the often-addressed issues in terms of social justice and equity today, with scientists questioning the contribution of biological versus sociocultural factors. They often turn to the study of evolution in their search for answers. Lampl argued that "all human societies have defined roles for men and women that are both overt or active roles and passive roles that are learned by imitation and instruction as children."[102] Although by about 100,000 years ago dimorphism was similar to that found in modern humans,[102] evidence from primate ethology and ethnology of foragers demonstrates that male specialization in hunting and defense gives a "selective advantage to larger males" with resultant sexual dimorphism.[103]

In addition, there may be differences in the capacity to do various tasks between genders because of hormonal differences, which are under the control of genetic influences. Not only do levels of testosterone, estrogen, and progesterone account for differences in male and female activity, but also behavioral, anatomical, and neurological studies reveal that there are significant gender differences in cerebral laterality, language, and spatial skills.[104] Differences in the cerebral maturation rate appear to result in different capacities, with adolescents who mature early performing better in verbal tasks and those who mature later doing better on spatial tasks.[105] In general, men mature physically and mentally more slowly than women. The necessity for women to assume responsibility for tasks in a sequential order of those nearest to home to those farthest afield was due to child-rearing restraints.[106] There may have been a selective advantage for women who demonstrated child rearing, food gathering and preparing, and fine manipulative skills. Boserup found sexual division of labor in all the traditional societies she studied but saw no common pattern; what was considered a natural occupation for women was seemingly determined by the fact that they had "undergone little or no change for generations."[107]

In terms of inequality between social groups of quantity, quality, choice, or obligation according to what they did or did not do, it has been observed that in early hunter-gatherer lifestyles, there would be few exemptions from some kind of labor with the exception of the very young. Some believe that everyone would be primarily a hunter or gatherer and tool/household implement maker, even those with extracurricular activities, such as shamans, chiefs, or warriors.[108] Many of the complex features of our own way of life that may provide a basis for inequities to occur, such as social inequality, occupational specialization, long-distance exchange, and technological innovation, appear to have originated with hunter-gatherers.[85] These claims are supported by archeological finds that raise the possibility of "status by heredity rather than achievement"[109]; long-distance trading long before the establishment of agriculture or towns; and the early establishment of economic systems with "ritual exchange obligations."[110]

With the formation of cities, it is possible to trace occupational developments in architecture, art, writing, commerce, religion, increased technological innovation, and social administration developed to help communities cope with socioenvironmental stress, uncertainty, and unpredictability.[111] The stressors seem to have arisen from communities living in much larger, specialized populations than they had been used to and in response to possible dangers from inside and outside the community. Neff observed that during this period, what people did began to acquire distinctions and qualifications and an increasingly complicated infrastructure of evaluative meanings, including a differentiation between labor and leisure.[112]

Such complications have accelerated and increased in complexity as the years have passed, technological expertise has increased, and populations have grown out of proportion to the rest of the natural world. Social injustices and inequities have thrived and grown in those conditions, and illness and death are daily results. In terms of occupational injustice, people are prevented from gaining access to or participating in education, training, and citizen activities because of racism, discrimination, stigmatization, hostility, and unemployment. This is noted in the Social Exclusion section in the WHO's *The Social Determinants of Health: The Solid Facts*.[66] Its theme reads as follows: "Life is short where quality is poor. By causing hardship and resentment, poverty, social exclusion and discrimination cost lives. The chances of living in poverty are loaded against some social groups."[113]

Summation: Meeting the Prerequisites of Health Through Doing

Within communities throughout time, food, income, shelter, education, peace, the ecosystem, and social justice and equity can be recognized as closely related to health and illness. It is probable that community leaders addressed issues relating to health on a daily basis, although they probably thought of it in other terms. That remains the case today when political decisions are made with the well-being of a nation in mind. Erroneously, most appear to only accept decisions as health related if medical experts make them. Lack of confidence or understanding about the impact of wide ranging policies on health outcomes has grown. In part, this may result from the prescriptive nature of medicine. In the past, health experts of many persuasions, rulers, their advisors, philosophers, shaman, priests, "mouthpieces for the gods," monks, wise-women, physicians, nurses, and anyone who cared to assume the mantel of expert all prescribed, in some way, what people needed to do to be healthy or overcome illness.

Throughout their existence, it is what people have done that has provided the prerequisites for health and survival. Although less obvious in high-income industrial societies, the evidence that this remains the case is all around us. Because what people did was altered by changes within natural, sociocultural, and political environments, the experience of health was also changed. This, too, is ongoing. Both of those factors require more adequate understanding. In addition, it could be advisable to include a greater emphasis in the educational curricula of health professionals, and others, on natural mechanisms and ways of meeting the prerequisites for health.

Rules for Health

An Ancient Doing Approach

An important question to consider at this point is whether the place of doing has ever been recognized for its contribution to health or whether its economic importance has always been dominant. Consideration of Classical Greek Medicine from this point of view is a good place to start because its role has been of immense importance throughout millennia to the current day, even though much of its teachings are overlooked or considered outdated.

Authorities in Ancient Greece held a holistic view about health that included the everyday doings of its peoples and, because it made great distinction between labor associated with the requirements of living and other forms of doing, it is interesting to consider in relation to the view taken here. The Greek city-states were established by conquest during the 3rd and 2nd millennia BC, when the Greek citizen "managed to divest himself of all need to labor," leaving this to slaves, free peasants, artisans, and craftsmen who were usually the indigenous people of conquered domains.[114] Labor and work were regarded as "brutalizing the mind, making man unfit for thinking of truth or for practicing virtue; it was a necessary evil which the visionary elite should avoid."[115] In contrast, the domain of the citizen was doing intellectual, political, social, and war-like pursuits deemed worthy of free men while maintaining "a conscious abstention from all activities connected with merely being alive."[116]

Aristotle, concurring with those cultural norms, argued that without labor it is not possible to provide all the necessities of life, but that to master slaves is the human way to master necessity and thus not against nature.[117] This opinion was in line with his view of occupation as an aspect of health. In terms of doing, being, belonging, and becoming, he believed that labor, manual work, and the banausic or utilitarian arts were deleterious to the body; that because of the monetary component minds became preoccupied and degraded; and that personal development was hindered.[117] However, he approved unconditionally of money earned through medicine, architecture, teaching, and land ownership.[117,118] Hannah Arendt (1906-1975), an authority on the Greco-Roman world, recognized the lack of modern-day theory about animal laborans (ie, the labor of the body) and homo faber (ie, the work of our hands), which she found surprising because of the current attitude about work as "the source of all values."[119]

Because of the imposed boundaries to what citizens could do, the State (perhaps unconsciously) found it necessary for the health of its population to supplement the restricted occupational regimen by the establishment of gymnasia. Unlike the current day, when gymnasia have once more become popular (labor-saving devices now take the place of slaves), the Greek centers for the development of athleticism included schools for the arts and intellect as well. In these, citizens strove to attain mental and physical excellence, health, and beauty through what they did, along with superior war-making skills.

Literature, philosophy, and stories of the gods were methods of promulgating acceptable and desirable things to do as aids to health in Ancient Greece.[120] Some examples include Homer's stated belief in music, sunshine, and fresh air and his valuing of crafts, gymnastics, games, and exercises[121]; stories of Apollo, son of Zeus, the original god of healing, who used music and poetry to relieve pain and depression[122]; and the fables of Hygeia and Asclepius with subsequent oscillation between the ascendances of healing or health practices told in Chapter 3.[123,124] In medicine, Hippocrates, in *On Regimen: Book 1*, provides propositions about food, drink, environment, and labor.[125] This also includes a major digression into occupational health issues about a wide range of trades. *On Regimen: Book 2* addresses similar topics, including labor and rest, sleep and waking, inactivity and repose, fatigue from unaccustomed or excessive exercise, natural exercise, and that which is ill-timed.[120] These obviously relate to the ancient rules of health according to the nonnaturals.

The medieval version of the nonnaturals, which provided health rules for Europeans from the 11th to the 19th century, was attributed to Claudius Galen, who is particularly interesting in terms of an occupational perspective of health. Although the majority of physicians throughout the decades appear to have concentrated on the category that is concerned with food and drink, Galen paid great attention to motion and rest.[126] Indeed, in the classic 17th century *Anatomy of Melancholy*, Burton claims that "Galen prefers Exercise before all Physick, Rectification of diet, or any Regiment in what kinde soever; 'tis Natures Physician."[127] Galen based many of his prescriptions on graded physical occupations of a sporting nature and manual labor for both physical and mental disorders; for the strengthening of cognition, intellect, and body; for the maintenance of health; and for alternative ways of making a living if deemed necessary.[128]

The Classical ideal that doing what was required to stay alive was inferior to a conscious abstention from it was challenged in Medieval Christian societies. This was due, in part, to monastic rule that saw labor as one honorable way of serving God and attaining spiritual health. For example, rule XLVIII of the Benedictine order ordained that "idleness is the enemy of the soul and therefore, at fixed times, the brothers ought to be occupied in manual labor, and again at fixed times, in sacred reading."[129] Such views were based, in part, on the Hebrew notion of God as one who works and the commandment of 6 days of labor followed by a day of rest on the Sabbath.[130] Because early mortality was not uncommon and was an ever-present possibility following what would now be considered minor illnesses, faith in the afterlife tended to give an understandable primacy to spiritual rather than physical health. In addition, more credence was given at that time to doing the right thing because disease was often attributed to sin.[120] Earlier than the formal publication of the *Regimen Sanitatis Salernitanun*, the influence of Classical Medicine was still evident within the health services provided by monasteries. Benedict had founded his monastery at Monte Cassino, close by Salerno where the Regimen Sanitatis Salernitanun came into being.[131] It was there that he wrote his "Rule" organized around alternate periods of prayer, labor, and rest, which are compatible with knowledge of the six nonnaturals.

Health care in much of Europe remained centered around monasteries for centuries. In contrast to that, dissolution of monasteries in Britain led to the disappearance of health services for many people with physical, mental, or social disorders and chronic and degenerative conditions for approximately 100 years. The number of workless and homeless monastic workers and inmates increased the number of beggars so that the environment became a health hazard for beggar and citizen alike. This led to unprecedented action by concerned citizens, who apparently recognized the health benefits of productive doing. They approached a young King Edward VI, the son of Henry VIII, for the gift of Bridewell Palace as a hospital of occupations. They successfully petitioned the King, asking him to "have compassion on us, that we may lie no longer in the street for lack of harbour, and that our old sore of idleness may no longer vex us, nor grieve the commonweal."[132] Two governors oversaw the hospital occupants' work in "sciences profitable to the commonweal"[133] making gloves, coats, silk lace, shoes, nails, knives, brushes, and so forth after they had been admitted and "so be preserved from perishing."[134]

Apart from this unique establishment, which spawned replicas in some provincial British towns and throughout Europe,[134] in England it was not until the Elizabethan Poor Law Act of 1601 that it was fully recognized that the care of all the poor, infirm, and homeless rested with the government. Work was central within that Act for reasons of economy, self-respect, and health, with action and rest being deemed pivotal to health's preservation as the nonnaturals prescribed. When work was not otherwise available, local parish authorities were required to provide it and to supply the raw materials for that purpose. The original concept of local initiatives being most useful in community care was revisited in the 20th century and in the oft use phrase "think globally, act locally."[120]

Boxed Dialogue 6-1:
Cheyne's Ideas About the Nature of Occupation and its Effects Upon Productivity and Health[141]

To restore this decay and wasting of animal bodies, nature has wisely made alternate periods of labour and rest, sleeping and watching, necessary to our being; the one for the active employments of life, to provide for and take in the materials of our nourishment; the other to apply those materials to the proper wasted parts, and to supply the expenses of living.

All the nations and ages have agreed that the morning season is the proper time for speculative studies, and those employments that require the faculties of the mind.

We proceed in the next place, to the consideration of exercise and quiet, the due regulation of which is almost as necessary to health and long life, as food itself.

Of all the exercises that are or may be used for health (such as walking, riding a horseback or in a coach, fencing, dancing, playing at billiards, bowls or tennis, digging, working at a pump, ringing a dumb bell) walking is the most natural, as it would not spend too much of the spirits of the weakly.

George Cheyne, 18th Century

Although that initiative provides an example of how social health issues related to doing were tackled according to the ancient rules of health, other initiatives aimed at physical health demonstrate adherence to the same rules. Ambroise Pare (1510-1590), regarded by the French as the father of modern surgery,[135] described the health giving nature of doing in terms of motion and rest. The benefits of moderate and well-timed doing were explained in terms of strengthening respiration and body-limb function, increased tolerance, improved digestion and nourishment, expulsion of wastes, and internal cleansing.[136] He prescribed moderate doing that involved all body parts before eating, that ceased when the doer was red, perspiring, weary, or breathing heavily, and was accompanied by a cooling down activity and followed by night-time rest. Pare explained that "we see the members of a man's body by a friendly consent are always busied, and stand ready to perform those functions for which they are appointed by nature, for the preservation of the whole, of which they are parts."[137] Earlier, Hieronymous Mercurialis (1530-1606) was advocating occupation as exercise for health,[138] and a century or so later Bernadino Ramazzini (1633-1717) compiled the earliest substantial research on matters of occupational health and safety.[139] His work preempts the current preoccupation with the direct cause and effect of illness that is rare but not unknown in the case of specific occupations (Figures 6-3 and 6-4).

In England, basing his 18th century medical texts on the rules of the six nonnaturals, Cheyne also recognized the value of doing as both a reward and a cost of living in terms of population health and of wear and tear on body and mind.[140] With something of the concern of a current-day occupational scientist or, perhaps, epidemiologist, Cheyne obviously studied the nature of occupation and its effects on productivity and health. In common with many modern thinkers, he claimed that many people are able to engage better in intellectual occupations after a night's sleep. He addressed doing as part of mental health[140] and prescribed specific occupations for health in general (Boxed Dialogue 6-1).[141]

Robert Burton also addressed occupation for mental health in his famous and all-encompassing work *The Anatomy of Melancholy*. Throughout his text, and backed up by endless references, he advocates the health-giving effects of doing. For example he claims, "Nothing better than Exercise (if opportunely used) for the preservation of the Body: Nothing so bad, if it be unseasonable, violent or overmuch."[142] Maintaining that idleness (a lack of occupation) is the "sole cause of this

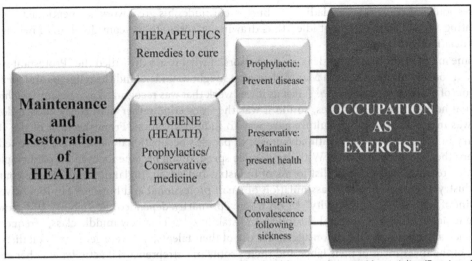

Figure 6-3. Flow chart: Occupation as exercise for health according to Mercurialis. (Reprinted with permission from Wilcock AA. *Occupation for Health. Volume 1. A Journey from Self-Health to Prescription*. London: British College of Occupational Therapists; 2001:184. Reproduced by kind permission of the British Association of Occupational Therapists.)

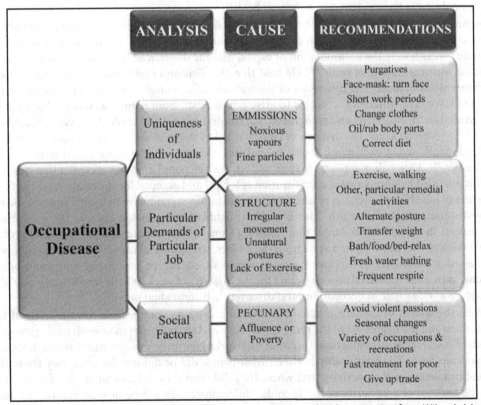

Figure 6-4. Ramazzini's occupational health approach. (Reprinted with permission from Wilcock AA. *Occupation for Health. Volume 1. A Journey from Self-Health to Prescription*. London: British College of Occupational Therapists; 2001:184. Reproduced by kind permission of the British Association of Occupational Therapists.)

[depression] and many other maladies,"[143] Burton concludes his great work, as mentioned earlier, by stating "Be not solitary, be not idle," thus drawing attention to the consideration of belonging in association with doing.[144]

Some might argue that these ideas are precursors of what is usually called the "Protestant work ethic," a concept originating with Max Weber, who sought to understand the religious and idealistic roots of modern capitalism.[145,146] Just as it was work that was recognized as a means to achieve spiritual health in medieval times, so too it was the work ethic rather than freely chosen doing that was in ascendance as agriculture gave way to industrialization. From the turn of the 18th century in the Occident, the health advantages of people's occupational nature were subjected to perhaps their greatest challenge. With remarkable speed, doing became focused on paid employment, increasingly within capitalist forms of industry. Indeed, in England, which led the change to industry, there was a "steady assimilation of small professional and business families, diverse in point of both wealth and activity" [147] on whom "primarily, depended the viability and growth of the national economy ... social flexibility and stability."[148] This new middle class, "frequently self-made and always dependent on aggressive use of their talents, ... were genuine 'capitalists' in terms of the investment of their labor and their profits in entrepreneurial activity, whether commercial or professional," who dominated what people were required to do or were not able to do.[147] Occupation, as integral to accepted rules for health, became largely disregarded and replaced with the entrepreneurial fascination with pragmatics and applied technology that lingers today. So, too, does modern economics, which also developed at this time. Indeed, it is one of the most influential forces on doing in the modern day, as it is on health.

Adam Smith (1723-1790), whose text *An Inquiry Into the Nature and Causes of the Wealth of Nations* is considered the foundation of classical economics, proposed that the keys to increasing a nation's wealth were the accumulation of capital and the division of labor, both of which would increase with the freeing of trade.[149] He held that the division of labor would enhance workers' specialist skills because "the difference of natural talents ... is not ... so much the cause, as the effect of labor. The difference ... seems to arise not so much from nature, as from habit, custom, and education." However, he also recognized that the division of labor could decrease the quality of work.[150] In a broad sense, the division of labor has led to the modern exchange economy (ie, specialization followed by exchange between specialists), which is a fundamental aspect of all modern economies.[151] Although it appears that the majority of the population has accepted that material wealth provided by occupational specialization is logical and acceptable, one could raise the basic question of whether the division of labor and specialization is conducive to health and well-being, notwithstanding material wealth. This is not a straightforward question because there are many dimensions to specialization—from that resulting from the development of personal and professional skills to that imposed by a system. In the former, strengths and capacities can be developed. In the latter, individual development may be minimalized, except for minute and meaningless actions, as in some industrial processes, and for the majority of workers little opportunity available to explore a wide range of occupations and discover their individual potential.

With the advent of modern medicine in the 20th century, coming hard on the heels of the sanitarians and the hygienists of the previous century and the ushering in of epidemiological gold standard research, earlier rules based on what had worked for millennia got, more or less, relegated to the scrap-heap. The relationship between what people did or did not do, what they ate or did not eat in relation to their activity, and where they did what they did and what they felt about it, was the concern of a minority of hardy souls. Unfortunately, in a time of reductionist, test-tube experimentation, older empirical know-how based on observation became less valued. However, the tide is slowly turning and once again we see the emergence of guidelines about living healthily. The greatest source of these on a holistic front is the WHO.

Table 6-2

OTTAWA CHARTER DIRECTIVES FOR "DOING" HEALTH[1]

Building Healthy Public Policy	Creating Supportive Communities	Strengthening Community Action	Developing Personal Skills	Reorientation of Health Services
Direct policy makers to be aware of the health conse-quences of deci-sions made	Recognize the inextricable links within societies that are complex and interrelated	Empower com-munities to own and control their endeavors and destinies	Support personal development through the provi-sion of information and education for health	Share the responsibility for health promo-tion with those in outside health services
Direct policy makers to place health promotion on all agendas	Encourage reciprocal maintenance through a socioecological approach	Empower communities to set priorities, make decisions, plan strategies to improve health	Enhance life skills to increase avail-able options for people to control their health and environs	Work with individuals, communities, and governments toward health promotion
Foster equity through coordinated health, income, and social policies	Take care of each other, our communities, and our natural environment	Promote concrete and effective community action	Enable life-long learning and preparation for life stages and cop-ing with possible illness	Move increasingly beyond clinical and curative services toward health promotion
Foster joint action, cleaner, more enjoyable environments	Advance the organization of work and leisure to help create a healthy society	Develop flexible systems to strengthen public participation on health matters	Promote action in educational, professional, com-mercial, and volun-tary bodies	Open channels between health and social, political, and economic and environs sectors
Identify and Inform of obstacles to adoption of healthy public policies and ways to overcome them	Generate safe, stimulating, satisfying, and enjoyable liv-ing and working conditions	Seek access to information, learning opportu-nities, and funding support		Engage in health research and make changes in professional education and training
	Systematically assess health impact of chang-ing work environs, technology, energy, and urbanization			Refocus on the total needs of the individual as a whole person

A MODERN DOING APPROACH: OTTAWA CHARTER DIRECTIVES

In Chapter 2, five major directives for doing well physically, mentally, and socially were identi-fied in the Ottawa Charter. These modern action rules for health require skills in advocacy, media-tion, and enablement to empower people toward understanding and acceptance of and action toward these directives, which are focused on everything that people do in their daily lives without being selective. Table 6-2 outlines the doing directives within the strategies.

Building healthy public policy is recognized as the fundamental key to improving population health across the globe. Specifically, from the perspective taken here, the general political lack of appreciation of the relationship between what people do and their health, as evidenced in recent years, requires urgent attention. To appreciate that fact, readers are asked to consider again the prerequisites of health—peace, shelter, education, food, income, a stable ecosystem and sustainable resources, social justice, and equity—and reflect on the doing/health aspects of policies that have been enacted recently about those factors. There have been policies, but each has been separate and little attention has been paid to people's occupational natures and needs and the health impacts of such lack of consideration.

What people do on a daily basis is dependent on public policy, legislation, systems of justice, fiscal measures, taxation, organizational and corporate structures, and sociocultural values that are well informed and appropriately constructed with population health and well-being in mind. The economy, in monetary terms, is important in today's world, but it can be argued that despite what politicians espouse, it is less important than individual, community, population, and environmental health and that depends, to a large extent, on what people do. It is not only the provision of sound medical care that is essential to reduce illness, it is also the provision of sound and vigilant population health and economic structures that most importantly provide for lifestyles that satisfy basic needs. That requires power brokers and policy architects to formulate and enact health and well-being policies that consider what people do, as well as balancing the "state's power to act for the community's common good and the individual rights to liberty, autonomy, and privacy."[152] Drawing the attention of policy makers to the doing components of the prerequisites of health is a job worthy of serious attention and rigorous action. When it occurs, praise should be unstinting but that should not preclude attention to the outcomes of the policy or critical analysis of the effects.

Jones suggested that "healthy public policy includes a good measure of health protection and prevention and builds on public health traditions. The main distinction is on getting the health sector to work with other sectors and agencies."[153] Economic matters often appear beyond the realm of concern for many health professionals, who become totally involved in their daily practice and tend to cope (and complain to each other) when policies of a national or local nature appear to prevent best outcomes. It needs to be remembered that it is people who enact economic policies, so there will be mistakes, as well as successes. Indeed, there has been a persistent stream of questioning of the ill effects that accompany the goods proclaimed by classical economics. For example, Lionel Robbins, a mid-20th century economist of the English neoclassical school, suggested that economists "have nothing to say on the true ends of life and that their propositions concerning what is or what can be involve, in themselves, no propositions concerning what ought to be." [154] Post-Ricardian economics have also been criticized for defending and rationalizing the interests of capitalism at the cost of impartiality, with Marxist writers describing as "vulgar economics" that which concentrates on "surface phenomena," such as "demand and supply to the neglect of structural value relationships."[155]

More than a few socio-cultural-political institutions and policy enactments fail in enabling people to experience or develop through what they do, in ways that meet different biological needs or natures as a matter of health. Rather, the majority concentrate on doing as an economic issue. Therefore, it can be queried whether socio-cultural-political systems have sufficiently recognized people's occupational differences as a means to promote health and as an important aspect of social justice.[156] Occupational justice, which can be considered a subset of social justice, is concerned with the forms of enabling, mediating, or advocating that are needed to create a doing environment that is both just and health-promoting for all, recognizing the need to empower people regardless of their differences.[157] Townsend and Wilcock suggested that occupational justice would be served only if all people have appropriate support to engage in doing in a way that provides meaning for them and is health enhancing. To attain occupational justice everywhere will require different policies and resources for different groups.[156]

Another reason that some of the strength of population/community health has dissipated in the western world is because of the philosophical acceptance of individualism[158] that emerged with the growth of capitalism. Even when no social illnesses are apparent, the type of economy, regulations, injustices, cultural or spiritual values, habits, and routines may restrict or be disadvantageous to some people's doing potential in the practical, everyday world.[159] This is true, even if individuals are viewed collectively as active agents who hold the power to ensure that resources are allocated toward visionary or ideal goals.[160] Change imposed on older economies that are more in tune with ecosystems may be counterproductive if not considered carefully with adequate and thorough consultation. If driven by more affluent nations or multi-corporate organizations, it could create more population health problems than bonuses. Structural or attitudinal change will automatically alter a population's activities and lifestyles without necessarily providing health or lifestyle benefit.

Recognition of social illness and occupational injustices requires a different mindset to recognition of individual physical or mental disorder that can be medically diagnosed. The ancient "rules of health" recognized the importance of environmental factors but did so without the current day understanding of either physiological or ecological determinants. The modern directive of the Ottawa Charter not only recognizes the inextricable links between people and their environment, but also builds on them and recommends a socioecological approach to health as the overall guiding principle for "the world, nations, regions and communities alike."[161] The protection and conservation of natural resources is central to health promotion, just as healthy public policy is. Assisting all people to understand how what they do or do not do affects the environment is important in terms of future health. Healthy environments are more than the protection of unpolluted utilities (the development of which was so important in the early days of public health). They encompass the natural, communal, personal, and built environments. Space, comfort, beauty, and facilities that encourage healthful doing have to be considered as well as clean air and water. Such ideals advocated by the new population health inspired the healthy cities movement instigated by the WHO Regional Office for Europe in 1987. The healthy cities approach is defined as:

> One that is continually creating and improving those physical and social environments and strengthening those community resources which enable people to continually support each other in performing all the functions of life and achieving their maximum potential.[162]

In recommending "systematic assessment of the health impact of a rapidly changing environment, particularly in areas of technology, work, energy production, and urbanization," the Ottawa Charter directives encourage occupation-focused initiatives tied to the everyday world of what people do. How education, media, commercial factors, gender issues, attitudinal factors, and the changing patterns of work and leisure affect health needs to be addressed in a holistic interactive way, as well as being addressed as separate issues. All people, by action or by default, influence the design, development, and effectiveness of the communities in which they live. Suitably empowered, population groups in communities can influence societal values and thereby instigate opportunities for people to engage in doing that is health-giving rather than illness producing, and that meets a community's perceived needs rather than those of bureaucracy. Wass suggested that the development of more flexible systems will assist in strengthening public participation and direction in health matters. These should provide support to community members and the concept of localism and assist communities with the provision of resources and the planning of action. "Finding the balance between working with communities through community development and working for communities is an ongoing challenge for health professional workers. Finding the appropriate balance between these requires critical reflection."[163]

An interesting example is provided by a study that analyzed beliefs about best practice in supported hostel accommodation. In-depth interviews were conducted with people from a range of disciplines who were acknowledged by their peers as experts in the field of dementia care. These revealed that best practice meets the needs of staff and management as occupational beings, as well as residents, despite the latter's progressive decline of cognitive and functional capacities. An enabling approach driven by residents' needs emerged as both a feature and a strategy of best practice. To be health promoting, the needs of all the community required attention.[164] Although it is tempting to restrict population health intervention to those who are deemed ill according to medical science criteria, this example supports the WHO's premise that all people need to be the ongoing recipients of public and private health promoting ways of life. This includes opportunity for doing well.

The early development of personal skills is largely in the hands of families and educational institutions, but, as has been observed earlier, the separation of children from families at an early age has been the norm in high-income countries since the industrial revolution. This means that skill development is largely undertaken in group situations where individual approaches are more difficult. There are political imperatives on what children should learn, at least within schools that receive public funding. That suggests there may be restrictions on the availability of some forms of occupational learning. Indeed, that factor is causing problems at present in postindustrial econo-mies where there is a shortage of skilled tradespeople and an overabundance of young people who dropped out of school early because it failed to interest them or who left past the age of wanting to take up a trade apprenticeship. Is it coincidental that some years ago technical education was downsized in schools? The greatest impact of such a move could have been on those with little interest in more intellectual activities. If that was the case, such broad-based policies failed to take into account whether the occupational needs of a large part of the population were met, in their attempts to ensure other goals, perhaps related to social equity. Another, more cynical, possibility is that it may have appeared to provide a politically expedient decrease in unemployment statis-tics. For example, some of the most interesting and successful recent social programs that have been instigated in South Australia have been those that address the problem of youthful antisocial behavior by opportunities that teach them trades or skills. An occupational justice of difference is important to bear in mind in impoverished communities as well as affluent ones. Community recognition and utilization of the strengths and capacities of individual members can be advanta-geous to everyone's well-being.

The importance of enabling "people to learn throughout life, to prepare themselves for all of its stages and to cope with chronic illness and injuries"[165] calls for culturally appropriate educa-tion that does not reinforce power differentials. Several commentators fear that approaches within a health promotional framework have the potential to be characterized by professional domi-nance.[166-168] Gorin advised that population health practitioners require belief in:

> ... *the strengths and capabilities of the client, who defines and determines health care decisions. The provider remains a resource and facilitator of this process. The client is the expert, and the provider offers useful and meaningful information and skills.*[169]

To achieve a state in which all individuals, community groups, and governments, as well as health professionals, recognize the importance of ongoing, health promoting ways of life and doing is a daunting task. It demands not only research, but also sensitivity, mutual respect, and a refocus on the total needs of people and environment.

In summary, the ancient and modern rules of health, taken together, provide the develop-ment and substance of health determinants and foundations for future action. The former relate more specifically to personal requirements (often based on individual doing), such as food, water, exercise, and rest, according to biological needs and in relationship to one another. The latter con-centrate more on the global, ecological, national, political, and population health issues in broad terms. Both are useful so that population health can be tackled and enhanced from both a minute and particular perspective to a holistic one.

Table 6-3			
THE PREREQUISITES: HEALTH AND ILLNESS CONSEQUENCES OF DOING			
Prerequisites	Examples of Doings	Examples of Health	Examples of Doings
Peace	Creating supportive envi-rons, reciprocal practical help to others, peaceful negotiation	Community development, social well-being	War, terrorism, rioting, anti-social behavior
Shelter	Building/maintaining/providing adequate safe shelter for all people to suit environs; home-making	Community development; physical, mental, and social well-being; child security	Destruction of homes for socio-political gain, not providing affordable, safe public housing
Education	Family activities, par-ticipation in community life, attending places of learning	Community development; physical, mental, and social well-being; Child and oth-ers' personal development	Not providing appropriate, engaging, or any education, dropping out of education
Food and income	Work to provide for needs of self and others, home-making, food production, eating healthily	Physical, mental, social, and occupational well-being	Not working (nonavailable or bludging), over or under-eating, substance abuse, sitting, watching electronic screens
A stable ecosystem, sustainable resources	Conserve water, grow food, native plants and trees, reuse/recycle rather than throw away, support and develop local resource-friendly economies, walk, use public transport	Community development; physical, mental, social, environmental, and occu-pational well-being	Throw away, chop down, pollute natural environs, self-drive, support multi-national firms that exploit overseas environments and cultures
Social justice and equity	Provide opportunities according to occupational interest and skill; reward people (no discrimination) for exceptional contribu-tions in any field, intellec-tual or practical	Community development; physical, mental, social, and occupational well-being	Segregate, ignore, deprive, or abuse others, reward only those with a particular type of skill, legislate to prevent some people from being able to provide for their needs

Doing as a Factor in Illness, Health, and Well-being

The theme of the previous chapter introduced the prerequisites of health as peace, shelter, education, food, income, a stable ecosystem, sustainable resources, social justice, and equity.[1] The exploration of those in terms of the things that people do and have done in their everyday lives throughout human time has indicated not only the doings but the health and illness consequences of such doing. These are summarized in Table 6-3.

To draw this chapter to a close some form of summation is required as the issues discussed are complex in the extreme. To do that, Figure 6-5 links the underlying determinants of what people are obliged, want or need to do, and the possible health or illness outcomes. The ideas about doing and health that have been explored in the chapter sustain the view that there are not only indica-tors to the positive or negative effects that result from what people do, but also underlying factors that can positively or negatively influence the doing.

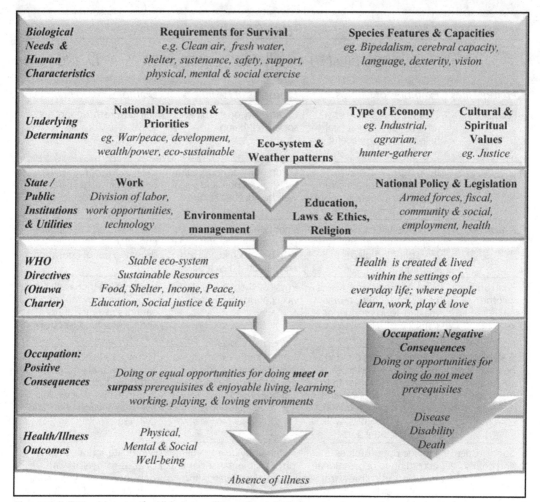

Figure 6-5. Determinants of well-being or illness through doing.

Human characteristics and biological needs are what drive people's doing. They are the force behind cultural evolution and the foundation stones of health. They have changed natural, built, and social environments, thus influencing and affecting the day-by-day experience of what people do within their ordinary lives. Over millennia, they have been instrumental in the establishment of different economies; political systems; national values, policies and priorities; institutional and cultural organizations that are themselves forms of population; and communal occupations. Combined with environmental factors, those are central to four determinants of health through doing:

1. The ecosystem and weather patterns
2. The type of economy, such as nomadic, agrarian, industrial, postindustrial, capitalist, or socialist
3. National policies and priorities, such as toward war or peace, economic growth, sustainable ecology, wealth and power of multinational organizations, or self-generated community development
4. Dominant cultural and spiritual values about what things must be done and which should not and how things must be done; about such ideas as individual freedoms, social justice, and equity as they relate to occupation, how different aspects of doing are perceived,

opportunities for leisure, the work ethic, individualistic or communal conventions, and dominant health or healing ideologies.

These underlying determinants lead to management of the environment and ecology that may be detrimental or sustaining. They also give rise to particular state and public institutions, commercial enterprises, and utilities of any given society. For example, the type of economy has direct influence on the availability and use of technology in daily life; how labor is divided between classes, genders, and age groups; the type and extent of health services; and employment and leisure opportunities. National priorities have a direct influence on legislative and fiscal institutions that provide rules by which people live, and on whether people live in fear or hope. Government agencies and policies provide the background to whether commercial enterprises flourish or have no chance, on attitudes and materialism, and on relationships and doings between communities and individuals within their geographic boundaries and with other nations. Cultural and spiritual values will affect such institutions and activities, as do the media, local regulations, social services, job creation schemes, education, worship, and health care systems.

State and public institutions and the utilities provided by them can also deliver positive or negative influence on national, community, family, or individual health. They can provide or restrict equitable opportunities for people to engage in doing that provides for the prerequisites of health. They can make opportunities available to experience learning, working, playing, and loving according to need, that exercises and nourishes the mind, body, and spirit. Being able to contribute to population health in a way that is socially valued yet maintains natural resources and recognizes the rights of all living organisms is important yet easily neglected. Underlying determinants may act as deterrents to both occupation and health, often in the name of economic advancement.

The positive or negative consequences of doing or the opportunity to do to meet the prerequisites for health are many. Positively, it can increase or improve energy and alertness; flexibility, interest, contentment, or commitment; relaxation and sleep; relationships; openness to new challenges; and a willingness to learn and grow from new challenges. Increased life expectancy and health status indicators, such as appropriate height/weight ratios and normal blood pressure, cholesterol, and lung function can result from doing wisely and well.[4] At the other end of the continuum, because the type of economy, national priorities and policies, and spiritual and cultural values create a flow-on effect, they can lead to unhealthy outcomes. Those might be a lack of health prerequisites, a lack of opportunity to exercise regularly through occupations of choice, or an inability to regularly experience well-being. There may be an imbalance between diet and activity, ongoing unresolved stress, lack of environmental resources, or the development of health risk behaviors, such as substance abuse. Such risk factors can lead to early, preclinical health disorders, such as stress; boredom; burnout; depression; decreased fitness, brain, or liver function; increased blood pressure; and changes in sleep patterns, body weight, and emotional states. All can ultimately result in disease, disability, or death.

Conclusion

Health and well-being result from what people do, being in tune with their occupational species' nature. Being responsive to biologically driven needs and doing to provide the requirements of living has, in the past, been central to maintaining homeostasis, preventing illness, and promoting health. It is relatively easy to see that there is a correlation between obvious survival occupations and health because what people do has direct bearing on their type of shelter and their access to food, clean air, and water, which are recognized as prerequisites of health. The correlation between ill-health and the natural health benefits of people's engagement in other types of occupations is more obscure and complex, and research is limited.

Doing entails more than simply acquiring requirements for survival. Because physiological and innate biological mechanisms are informed, stimulated, influenced, and adapted by conscious social processes, these too become influential determinants of human health. For positive health, people need what they do to offer meaning, choice, satisfaction, a sense of belonging, purpose, and achievement. These enable individuals, families, communities, and populations to flourish and provide the species with a survival advantage.

References

1. World Health Organization. Health and Welfare Canada. Canadian Public Health Association. *Ottawa Charter for Health Promotion.* Ottawa, Canada; 1986.
2. Leakey R, Lewin R. *People of the Lake: Man: His Origins, Nature, and Future.* New York, NY: Penguin Books; 1978:38-39.
3. World Health Organization. 2008-2013 *Action Plan for the Global Strategy for the Prevention and Control of Noncommunicable Diseases.* Geneva: WHO; 2008. http://www.who.int/nmh/publications/9789241597418/en/index.html. Accessed May 8, 2012.
4. Glass TA, Mendes de Leon CF, Marotolli RA, Berkman LF. Population based study of social and productive activities as predictors of survival among elderly Americans. *British Medical Journal.* 1999:319:478-483.
5. World Health Organization. *International Classification of Functioning, Disability and Health.* Geneva: WHO; 2001.
6. Christiansen CH. Occupation and identity: becoming who we are through what we do. In: Christiansen CH, Townsend EA, eds. *Introduction to Occupation: The Art and Science of Living.* Upper Saddle River, NJ: Prentice Hall; 2004.
7. Maslow AH. *Motivation and Personality.* New York, NY: Harper and Row; 1970.
8. Harvey AS, Pentland W. What do people do? In: Christiansen CH, Townsend EA, eds. *Introduction to Occupation: The Art and Science of Living.* Upper Saddle River, NJ: Prentice Hall; 2004:87.
9. Christiansen CH, Townsend EA, eds. *Introduction to Occupation: The Art and Science of Living.* Upper Saddle River, NJ: Prentice Hall; 2004.
10. Brody J. Personal health: Cheating ourselves of sleep. *The New York Times.* June 17; 2013.
11. Arnoff MS. *Sleep and its Secrets: The River of Crystal Light.* Los Angeles: Insight Books; 1991.
12. Lieberman P. Evolution of the speech apparatus. In: Jones S, Martin R, Pilbeam D, eds. *The Cambridge Encyclopedia of Human Evolution.* New York, NY: Cambridge University Press; 1992:136-137.
13. Sassin JF, Parker DC, Mace JW, Gotlin RW, Johnson LC, Rossman LG. Human growth hormone release: relation to slow wave sleep and sleep waking cycles. *Science.* 1969;165:513-515.
14. Shapiro CM, Bortz R, Mitchell D, Bartel P, Jooste P. Slow wave sleep: a recovery period after exercise. *Science.* 1981;214:1253-1254.
15. Foret J. To what extent can sleep be influenced by diurnal activity? *Experientia.* 1984;40:422-424.
16. Moore JC. *The Lifespan in Relation to the Nervous System.* Melbourne, Australia: Australian Association of Occupational Therapists; June 1994:188.
17. Pearlman CA. R.E.M. sleep and information processing: evidence from animal studies. *Neuroscience and Neurobehavioural Reviews.* 1979;3:57-68.
18. Smith C. Sleep states and learning: a review of the animal literature. *Neuroscience and Neurobehavioural Reviews.* 1985;9:157-168.
19. Gay J, Farnworth L, Alcorn K. *The Use of Time and its Meaning for Forensic Psychiatric Patients.* International Forensic Health Conference. Melbourne, Australia: 1999.
20. Molineux M, ed. *Occupation for Occupational Therapists.* Oxford, UK: Blackwell Publishing; 2004.
21. Fox R. *The Search for Society.* New Brunswick, NJ: Rutgers University Press; 1989:179.
22. Winson J. *Brain and Psyche: The Biology of the Unconscious.* Garden City, NY: Anchor Press/Doubleday; 1985.
23. Campbell SS. Duration and placement of sleep in a "disentrained environment." *Psychophysiology.* 1984;21(1):106-113.
24. McClellan J, Dorn H. *Science and Technology in World History.* 2nd ed. Johns Hopkins University Press, Baltimore, MD; 2006:6-12.

25. Schultz E, Lavenda R. Consequences of domestication and sedentism. In: Schultz EA, Lavenda RH, Dods RR, eds. *Cultural Anthropology: A Perspective on the Human Condition*. 2nd ed. Oxford: Oxford University Press; 2012:196-200.

26. McMichael T. *Human Frontiers, Environments and Disease: Past Patterns, Uncertain Futures*. Cambridge, UK: Cambridge University Press; 2001.

27. McNeill WH. *Plagues and People*. London, England: Penguin Books; 1979.

28. Douglas M. Population control in primitive peoples. *British Journal of Social Psychology*. 1966;17:263-273.

29. Birdsell JB. On population structure in generalized hunting and collecting populations. *Evolution*. 1958;12:189-205.

30. van der Merwe NJ. Reconstructing prehistoric diet. In: Jones S, Martin R, Pilbeam D, eds. *The Cambridge Encyclopedia of Human Evolution*. New York, NY: Cambridge University Press; 1992:369-372.

31. Wing ES, Brown AG. *Paleonutrition: Method and Theory in Prehistoric Foodways*. New York, NY: Academic Press; 1978.

32. Isaac GLI. The food sharing behaviour of protohuman hominids. *Scientific American*. 1978;238(April):90-106.

33. Buranhult G, ed. *The First Humans: Human Origins and History to 10,000BC*. Australia: University of Queensland Press; 1993:59.

34. Isaac B. Throwing. In: Jones S, Martin R, Pilbeam D, eds. *The Cambridge Encyclopedia of Human Evolution*. New York, NY: Cambridge University Press; 1992:358.

35. Leakey R, Lewin R. *People of the Lake: Man: His Origins, Nature, and Future*. New York, NY: Penguin Books; 1978.

36. Lee RB, DeVore I. *Man the Hunter*. Chicago, IL: Aldine Publishing Co; 1968.

37. Dalberg F, ed. *Woman the Gatherer*. New Haven, Conn: Yale University Press; 1981.

38. Binford LR. Subsistence—a key to the past. In: Jones S, Martin R, Pilbeam D, eds. *The Cambridge Encyclopedia of Human Evolution*. New York, NY: Cambridge University Press; 1992:365-368.

39. Ellen RF. *Environment, Subsistence and System*. New York, NY: Cambridge University Press; 1982.

40. Ingold T. *Hunters, Pasturalists and Ranchers*. New York, NY: Cambridge University Press; 1980.

41. Foley R. Studying human evolution by analogy. In: Jones S, Martin R, Pilbeam D, eds. *The Cambridge Encyclopedia of Human Evolution*. New York, NY: Cambridge University Press; 1992:336.

42. Woodburn J. Hunters and gatherers today and reconstruction of the past. In: Gellner E, ed. *Soviet and Western Anthropology*. London, England: Duckworth; 1980.

43. Ember CR. The relative decline in women's contribution to agriculture with intensification. *American Anthropologist*. 1983;85(2):285-304.

44. Burton ML, White DR. Sexual division of work in agriculture. *American Anthropologist*. 1984;86(3):568-583.

45. Ashton H. The Basuto. In: Parker S. *Leisure and Work*. London, England: George Allen and Unwin; 1983:131.

46. Coon CS. *The Hunting Peoples*. London, England: Jonathan Cape Ltd; 1972.

47. Thibeault R. Fostering healing through occupation: the case of the Canadian Inuit. *Journal of Occupational Science*. 2002;9;153-158.

48. Coon CS. *The Hunting Peoples*. London, England: Jonathan Cape Ltd; 1972:3.

49. Waechter J. *Man Before History*. Oxford, UK: Elsevier-Phaidon; 1976.

50. Neff WS. *Work and Human Behaviour*. 3rd ed. New York, NY: Aldine Publishing Co; 1985.

51. Lewin R. *In the Age of Mankind: A Smithsonian Book of Human Evolution*. Washington, DC: Smithsonian Books; 1988:190.

52. Eyre EJ. *Journals of Expeditions of Discovery into Central Australia and Overland*. London, England: T and W Boone; 1845.

53. Leakey R. *The Making of Mankind*. London, England: Michael Joseph Ltd; 1981.

54. World Health Organization. The Declaration of Alma-Ata. *International Conference on Primary Health Care*, Alma-Ata, USSR; 1998.

55. UNICEF Humanitarian Action Update: Sahel Nutrition Crisis: Burkina Faso, Cameroon, Chad, Mali, Mauritania, Niger, Nigeria & Senegal. UNICEF; 6 February 2012. http://www.unicef.org/hac2012/files/UNICEF_Humanitarian_Action_Update_-_Sahel_crisis_-_6_February_2012.pdf. Accessed May 30, 2014.

56. World Health Organization. *Obesity and Overweight. Fact sheet N°311.* WHO: May 2014. Available at: http://www.who.int/mediacentre/factsheets/fs311/en/. Accessed May 30, 2014.

57. World Health Organization. *Obesity: Preventing and Managing the Global Epidemic. A Report of a WHO Consultation* (WHO Technical Report Series 894). WHO; 2000. http://www.who.int/nutrition/publications/obesity/WHO_TRS_894/en/. Accessed May 30, 2014.

58. Queensland Health. *Social Determinants of Health: Unemployment Fact Sheet.* Available at: www.health.qld.gov.au/ph/Documents/saphs/20407.pdf. Accessed October 29, 2012.

59. Rabinowitch IM. Calories and occupation. Chapter 1. In: *Nutrition in Everyday Practice.* Toronto: Canadian Medical Association; 1939;4.

60. Rabinowitch IM. Calories and occupation. Chapter 1. In: *Nutrition in Everyday Practice.* Toronto: Canadian Medical Association; 1939;1.

61. Wilkinson R, Marmot M, eds. *Social Determinants of Health: The Solid Facts,* 2nd ed. Copenhagen, Denmark: World Health Organization Regional Office for Europe; 2003;27.

62. Jelinek J. *Primitive Hunters.* London, England: Hamlyn; 1989.

63. Davidson I, Noble W. When did language begin? In: Buranhult G, ed. *The First Humans: Human Origins and History to 10,000BC.* Australia: University of Queensland Press; 1993:46.

64. United Nations. *The Universal Declaration of Human Rights.* Adopted: Paris 1948. Available at: http://www.un.org/en/documents/udhr/. Accessed May 25, 2014.

65. World Health Organization. *Proceedings of the 2nd WHO International Housing and Health Symposium.* Vilnius, Lithuania. Geneva: WHO; 2005.

66. Wilkinson R, Marmot M, eds. *Social Determinants of Health: The Solid Facts.* 2nd ed. Copenhagen, Denmark: World Health Organization Regional Office for Europe; 2003.

67. Delors J. Learning: The Treasure Within: Report to UNESCO of the International Commission on Education for the Twenty-first Century. Paris: UNESCO; 1996. Available at: unesdoc.unesco.org/images/0010/001095/109590eo.pdf.

68. UNESCO. Medium-Term Strategy Contributing to Peace and Human Development in an Era of Globalization through Education, the Sciences, Culture and Communication 2002-2007. Fontenoy, Paris: UNESCO; 2002. http://unesdoc.unesco.org/images/0012/001254/125434e.pdf. Accessed September 3, 2014.

69. Kirk D. *Advocacy Brief: Empowering Girls and Women through Physical Education and Sport.* Bangkok: UNESCO; 2012. Available at: unesdoc.unesco.org/images/0021/002157/215707e.pdf. Accessed May 12, 2012.

70. United Nations General Assembly Resolution. *United Nations Declaration on Human Rights Education and Training.* A/RES/66/137. 2011.

71. UNESCO. *Contemporary Issues in Human Rights Education.* Paris, France: UNESCO; 2011.

72. UNESCO. *Strategy for the Second Half of the United Nations Decade of Education for Sustainable Development.* New York: UNESCO;m2010:10. www.preventionweb.net/.../15341_unescostrategy-fortheunitednations. Accessed May 13, 2012.

73. van den Berghe PL. Sociobiology. In: Kuper A, Kuper J, eds. *The Social Science Encyclopedia.* London, England: Routledge; 1985.

74. Argyle M. *The Psychology of Interpersonal Behaviour.* Harmondsworth: Penguin Books; 1967.

75. Alexander RD. *Darwinism and Human Affairs.* Seattle, Wash: University of Washington Press; 1979.

76. Chagnon N, Irons W, eds. *Evolutionary Biology and Human Social Behaviour.* North Scituate, MA: Duxbury Press; 1979.

77. Symons D. *The Evolution of Human Sexuality.* New York, NY: Oxford University Press; 1979.

78. Trivers RL. The evolution of reciprocal altruism. *Quarterly Review of Biology.* 1971;46(1):35-57.

79. Bruner JS. Nature and uses of immaturity. *American Psychologist.* 1972;August:687-708.

80. Liljegren R. Animals of ice age Europe. In: Buranhult G, ed. *The First Humans: Human Origins and History to 10,000BC.* Brisbane, Australia: University of Queensland Press; 1993.

81. Buranhult G, ed. *The First Humans: Human Origins and History to 10,000BC.* Australia: University of Queensland Press; 1993:93.

82. Leakey R. *The Making of Mankind.* London, England: Michael Joseph Ltd; 1981:242.

83. Lorenz K. *On Aggression.* London, England: Methuen; 1966:52.

84. Lorenz K. *On Aggression.* London, England: Methuen; 1966.

85. Lewin R. *In the Age of Mankind: A Smithsonian Book of Human Evolution.* Washington, DC: Smithsonian Books; 1988.

86. Morris D, Marsh P. *Tribes.* London, England: Pyramid Books; 1988:9.

87. Lorenz K. *The Waning of Humaneness*. London, England: Unwin Paperbacks; 1983.

88. Uton Muchtar Rafei, Regional Director, SEAR. World Health Organization Regional Office for South East Asia; *Health as a Bridge for Peace*. Press Release. 1999. http://www.who.int/. Accessed May 19, 2012.

89. Coon CS. *The Hunting Peoples*. London, England: Jonathan Cape Ltd; 1972:388-389.

90. Parker S. *Leisure and Work*. London, England: George Allen and Unwin; 1983.

91. Hole F. Origins of agriculture. In: Jones S, Martin R, Pilbeam D, eds. *The Cambridge Encyclopedia of Human Evolution*. New York, NY: Cambridge University Press; 1992:373-379.

92. Clutton-Brock J. Domestication of animals. In: Jones S, Martin R, Pilbeam D, eds. *The Cambridge Encyclopedia of Human Evolution*. New York, NY: Cambridge University Press; 1992:380-385.

93. Hole F. Origins of agriculture. In: Jones S, Martin R, Pilbeam D, eds. *The Cambridge Encyclopedia of Human Evolution*. New York, NY: Cambridge University Press; 1992:379.

94. United Nations Population Fund (UNFPA). *Linking Population, Poverty and Development. Urbanization: A Majority in Cities*. 2007. Available at: http://www.unfpa.org/pds/urbanization.htm. Accessed May 12, 2012.

95. Research Australia. *Healthy Planet, Places and People*. 2007; 11. http://aries.mq.edu.au/publications/other/HealthyPlanet.pdf. Accessed May 24, 2014.

96. Institute of Medicine. *Living Well with Chronic Illness: A Call for Public Health Action*. Washington, DC: Institute of Medicine; 2012. www.iom.edu/Reports/2012/Living-Well-with-Chronic-Illness.aspx. Accessed May 12, 2012.

97. World Health Organization. *Damage to Ecosystems Poses Growing Threat to Human Health*. Geneva/Brasilia; 30 March, 2005. http://www.who.int/mediacentre/news/releases/2005/pr15/en/. Accessed May 25, 2014.

98. Millennium Ecosystem Assessment. *Ecosystems and Human Well-being: Synthesis*. Washington, DC: Island Press; 2005. http://www.millenniumassessment.org/documents/document.356.aspx.pdf. Accessed May 15, 2014.

99. Millennium Ecosystem Assessment, 2005. *Ecosystems and Human Well-being: Synthesis*. Washington, DC: Island Press; 2005:11. http://www.millenniumassessment.org/documents/document.356.aspx.pdf. Accessed May 15, 2014.

100. Rowley-Conway P. Mighty hunter or marginal scavenger? In: Buranhult G, ed. *The First Humans: Human Origins and History to 10,000 BC*. Australia: University of Queensland Press; 1993:61-62.

101. Potts R. The hominid way of life. In: Jones S, Martin R, Pilbeam D, eds. *The Cambridge Encyclopedia of Human Evolution*. New York, NY: Cambridge University Press; 1992.

102. Lampl M. Sex roles in prehistory. In: Buranhult G, ed. *The First Humans: Human Origins and History to 10,000 BC*. Australia: University of Queensland Press; 1993:31.

103. Burton ML, White DR. Division of labour by sex. In: Kuper A, Kuper J, eds. *The Social Science Encyclopedia*. London, England: Routledge; 1985:206.

104. Kolb B, Whishaw IQ. *Fundamentals of Human Neuropsychology*. 3rd ed. San Francisco, CA: WH Freeman and Co; 1990:4,123.

105. Waber DP. Sex differences in cognition: a function of maturation rate? *Science*. 1976;192:572-573.

106. Brown JK. A note on the division of labor by sex. *American Anthropologist*. 1970;72(5):1073-1078.

107. Boserup E. *Women's Role in Economic Development*. New York, NY: St. Martin's Press; 1970:15.

108. Herskovits MJ. *Economic Anthropology*. New York, NY: Knopf; 1952.

109. Buranhult G, ed. *The First Humans: Human Origins and History to 10,000 BC*. Australia: University of Queensland Press; 1993:95.

110. Lewin R. *In the Age of Mankind: A Smithsonian Book of Human Evolution*. Washington, DC: Smithsonian Books; 1988:204.

111. Lewin R. *In the Age of Mankind: A Smithsonian Book of Human Evolution*. Washington, DC: Smithsonian Books; 1988:224.

112. Neff WS. *Work and Human Behaviour*. 3rd ed. New York, NY: Aldine Publishing Co; 1985.

113. Wilkinson R, Marmot M, eds. *Social Determinants of Health: The Solid Facts*. Copenhagen, Denmark: World Health Organization Regional Office for Europe; 2003;17.

114. Neff WS. *Work and Human Behaviour*. 3rd ed. New York, NY: Aldine Publishing Co; 1985:33.

115. Parker S. *Leisure and Work*. London, England: George Allen and Unwin; 1983:14.

116. Parker S. *Leisure and Work*. London, England: George Allen and Unwin; 1983:17.

117. Aristotle. Politics. In: Barnes J, ed. *The Complete Works of Aristotle*. Rev Oxford trans. UK: Princeton University Press; 1984.

118. Aristotle. *Politics*. VIII,2,1337b7-14.

119. Arendt H. *The Human Condition*. Chicago, Ill: University of Chicago Press; 1958:83-85.

120. Wilcock AA. *Occupation for Health. Volume 1. A Journey from Self Health to Prescription*. London: British College of Occupational Therapists; 2001.

121. Homer. *Iliad 800 B.C.E.* Butler S, trans. http://classics.mit.edu/Homer/iliad.html. Accessed May 24, 2014.

122. Apollo –Greek Mythology. Available at: http://www.maicar.com/GML/Apollo.html. Accessed May 24, 2014.

123. Hygeia. *Grolier Multimedia Encyclopedia*. Grolier Electronic Publishing Inc; 1995.

124. Dubos R. *The Mirage of Health: Utopias, Progress and Biological Change*. New York: Harper and Row Publishers; 1959.

125. Hippocrates. *On Regimen in Acute Diseases 400 BC*. Adams F, trans. The Internet Classics Archive. http://classics.mit.edu/Hippocrates/acutedis.html. Accessed May 24, 2014.

126. Georgii A, ed. *Ling's Educational and Curative Exercises*. London: Renshaw; 1876:11.

127. Burton R. *The Anatomy of Melancholy*. Oxford: Printed for Henry Cripps; 1651:216.

128. Macdonald EM. *World-Wide Conquest of Disabilities: The History, Development and Present Functions of the Remedial Services*. London: Bailliere Tindall; 1981:43-44.

129. Bettenson HS, ed. *Documents of the Christian Church*. New York, NY: Springer; 1963.

130. Exodus 20: verses 9-11. *The Holy Bible. Authorized King James version*. London, England: Oxford University Press; 1972.

131. Croke Sir A. *Regimen Sanitatis Salernitanum with the Englishman's Doctor: An Ancient Translation*. Oxford: D.A. Talboys; 1830.

132. *A Short History of Bridewell and Bethlem Hospitals*. London: The Bethlem Art and History Collections Trust; 1899:3-4.

133. *A Short History of Bridewell and Bethlem Hospitals*. London: The Bethlem Art and History Collections Trust; 1899:5-7.

134. Slack P. *From Reformation to Improvement: Public Welfare in Early Modern England*. The Ford Lectures Delivered in the University of Oxford 1994-1995. Oxford: Clarenden Press; 1999:20-25.

135. Isaacs A, ed. Pare, Ambroise. In: *Macmillan Encyclopedia*. London: Macmillan; 1990:926.

136. Johnson T. *The Workes of that Famous Chirurgion Ambroise Parey. Translated out of Latin and compared with the French*. Printed by Th Cotes and R Young; 1634:34-35.

137. Pare A. The Authors dedication to Henry the third, the most Christian king of France and Poland. 1579. In: Johnson T. *The Workes of that Famous Chirurgion Ambroise Parey. Translated out of Latin and compared with the French*. Printed by Th Cotes and R Young; 1634.

138. Blundell JWF. *The Muscles and their Story from the Earliest Times (an Adaptation of the 'Ars Gymnastica') including the Whole Text of Mercurialis, and the Opinions of other Writers Ancient and Modern on Mental and Bodily Development*. London, UK: Chapman & Hall; 1864.

139. Ramazzini B. *Of the Diseases of Tradesmen, Shewing the Various Influence of Particular Trades upon the State of Health; with the Best Methods to Avoid or Correct It,...*London, UK: Printed for Andrew Bell et al; 1705.

140. Cheyne G. *The English Malady*. London: Strahan and Leake; 1733.

141. Cheyne G. *Essay of Health and Long Life*. London and Bath, 1724.

142. Burton R. *The Anatomy of Melancholy*. Oxford: Printed for Henry Cripps; 1651:84-85.

143. Burton R. *The Anatomy of Melancholy*. Oxford: Printed for Henry Cripps; 1651:85-86.

144. Burton R. *The Anatomy of Melancholy*. 12th ed. London: 1821:Vol 2;601.

145. Weber M. *The Protestant Work Ethic and the Spirit of Capitalism*. Parsons T, trans. London, England: George Allen and Unwin Ltd; 1930. http://www.marxists.org/reference/archive/weber/protestant-ethic/. Accessed May 24, 2014.

146. Kalberg S. Max Weber. In: Kuper A, Kuper J, eds. *The Social Science Encyclopedia*. London, England: Routledge; 1985:892-896.

147. Langford P, Harvie C. The eighteenth century and the age of industry. In: Morgan KO, ed. *The Oxford History of Britain*. Vol IV. Oxford, UK: Oxford University Press; 1992:42,44-45.

148. Morgan KO, ed. *The Oxford History of Britain*. Vol V. Oxford, UK: Oxford University Press; 1992.

149. Smith A. In: Campbell RH, Skinner AS, Todd WB, eds. *An Inquiry into the Nature and Causes of the Wealth of Nations*. Chicago, Ill: University of Chicago Press; 1976. Original work published 1776.

150. Raphael DD. *Adam Smith*. Vol 1. Oxford, UK: Oxford University Press; 1985:17.

151. Bannock G, Baxter RE, Rees R. *The Penguin Dictionary of Economics*. 2nd ed. New York, NY: Penguin Books; 1978.

152. Gorin S. Contexts for health promotion. In: Gorin S, Arnold J, eds. *Health Promotion Handbook*. St. Louis, MO: Mosby;1998:40.

153. Jones L. The rise of health promotion. In: J. Katz J, Pederby A, eds. *Promoting Health: Knowledge and Practice*. Hampshire, UK: MacMillan; 1997:72.

154. Robbins L. *Politics and Economics, Papers in Political Economy*. London, England: Macmillan; 1963:7.

155. Desai M. Vulgar economics. In: Bottomore T, ed. *A Dictionary of Marxist Thought*. 2nd ed. Oxford, UK: Blackwell Ltd; 1991:574.

156. Townsend EA, Wilcock AA. *Occupational Justice*. In: Christiansen CH, Townsend EA, eds. *Introduction to Occupation: The Art and Science of Living*. Upper Saddle River, NJ: Prentice Hall; 2004.

157. Daniels N, Kennedy BP, Kawachi I. Why justice is good for our health: The social determinants of health inequalities. *Daedalus*. 1999;128(4):215-251.

158. Lukes S. *Individualism*. Oxford, UK: Basil Blackwell; 1973.

159. Wilcock AA, Whiteford GE. Occupation, health promotion, and the environment. In: Letts L, Rigby P, Stewart D, eds. *Using Environments to Enable Occupational Performance*. Thorofare, NJ: Slack; 2003.

160. McGary H. Distrust, social justice, and health care. *Mt Sinai Journal of Medicine*. 1999;66(4):236-240.

161. World Health Organization, Health and Welfare Canada, Canadian Public Health Association. *Ottawa Charter for Health Promotion*. Ottawa, Canada; 1986:3.

162. Frumkin H, Frank L, Jackson R. *Urban Sprawl and Public Health: Designing, Planning, and Building for Healthy Communities*. Washington, DC: Island Press; 2004;203.

163. Wass A. *Promoting Health: The Primary Care Approach*. Marrackville, NSW: Harcourt. 2000:174.

164. Pols V. *Experts' Views of What is Best Practice in Dementia Care for Hostel Residents*. Unpublished master's thesis, University of South Australia, Adelaide, South Australia.

165. World Health Organization, Health and Welfare Canada, Canadian Public Health Association. *Ottawa Charter for Health Promotion*. Ottawa, Canada; 1986:4.

166. Carey P. Community health promotion and empowerment. In: Kerr J, ed. *Community Health Promotion: Challenges for Practice*. London: Harcourt; 2000.

167. Jones L. The rise of health promotion. In: Katz J, Pederby A, eds. *Promoting Health: Knowledge and Practice*. Hampshire, UK: Macmillan; 1997.

168. Peterson A, Lupton D. *The New Public Health: Health and the Self in the Age of Risk*. London: Sage, 1996.

169. Gorin S. Contexts for health promotion. In: Gorin S, Arnold J, eds. *Health Promotion Handbook*. St Louis, MO: Mosby-Year Book; 1998:74.

Theme 7

Health depends on validation of "the uniqueness of each person and the need to respond to each individual's spiritual quest for meaning, purpose, and belonging."

WHO: Health for All in the Twenty-First Century, 1998[1]

Chapter 7

OCCUPATION

BEING ASPECTS OF DOING

This chapter addresses:
- Introduction to the Concept of Being as an Aspect of Doing
  - Consciousness
- Being and Health
  - Natural Health: Prerequisites
    - Being and Peace
    - Being and Shelter
    - Being and Education
    - Being and Food
    - Being and Income
    - Being and a Stable Ecosystem and Sustainable Resources
    - Being and Social Justice and Equity
  - Natural Health: Capacities and Creativity
    - Human Capacities
    - Creativity
- Rules for Health: Being From Ancient to Modern
  - Being and Health in Earlier Times
    - Making Use of Being: Finding Meaning and Mental Health
    - Social Change Toward Finding Meaning Through Occupation
  - Being and Health in Modern Times
    - Mental, Physical, and Social Well-Being
    - Social Change Toward Finding Meaning Through Occupation
    - Work as a Source of Well-Being
- Conclusion

Wilcock AA, Hocking C.
An Occupational Perspective of Health, Third Edition (pp 178-209).
© 2015 Taylor & Francis Group.

In this chapter, how people feel about what they do is explored. This extremely important aspect of occupation is intimately related to health. We explain it as the being component. Although being is applicable to both, it is perhaps more pertinent to individuals than communities. The WHO theme of this chapter that "health depends on the validation of the uniqueness of each person and the need to respond to each individual's spiritual quest for meaning, purpose and belonging"[1] is central to this concept of being.

Introduction to the Concept of Being as an Aspect of Doing

People are described as human beings, in this case with being referring to a state of existence. Somewhat similarly, being is frequently used alongside occupational roles to express not only a state of existence, but also the needs and interests that drive individuals. For example, people are described as being parents, being students, being a breadwinner, being creative, or being a footballer. In that way, being refers to the qualities that constitute living[2] and, as described in Chapter 5, to the essential nature of someone: their spirit, psyche, or core; their inner person or persona.[3,4] Being enables people to plan, to dream of the future, and to create entirely new environments.[5] Being also refers to the thinking that precedes or grows from occupations or, in some cases, the occupations that are associated with thought rather than action.

Aristotle was one of the early philosophers to inquire into the nature of being, and his view encompassed the idea that the true essence of any object is independent of its material form.[6] Nineteenth century existentialist philosophers also considered the concept. Hegel wrote extensively about being—describing a state in which people allow themselves to be absorbed and find repose, which he called being-within-self.[7] However, he determined that it was difficult to find the true meaning because, stripped of all its relationships with other objects and its actions, being is nothing. Saying "I am" has no meaning if it does not relate to doing something or relating to something. Heidegger continued the search to find the meaning of being and distinguished different modes for objects and people, with the latter being described as Da-sein (there-being).[8] Sartre distinguished between being-in-itself and being-for-itself to ontologically ground his concept of freedom.[9]

Psychologists have also found the concept intriguing. Abraham Maslow, a trailblazer in the field, suggested that existential notions of being address the concept and experience of identity in the science of human nature. He preferred the term identity to essence, existence, or ontology because it was easier to understand. He came to explain being as the "contemplation and enjoyment of the inner life" and noted that "being in a state of being needs no future because it is already there."[10]

Essentially, being is a concept compatible with the Romantic school of thought that emerged in the 18th century. Romantics held an organic view of nature in which people were perceived as "playful, creative, inspired, and unpredictable beings."[11] These capacities were upheld as worthy of celebration and enhancement, in contrast to rationalists who sought to control them.[11] Both romantic being and rational doing demand expression and fulfillment for people to experience physical, mental, and social well-being and to be able to resist disease as far as it is possible. The current dominance of rationalist views explains to some extent why the notion of being is difficult to appreciate, particularly in terms of health, despite the prevalent use of well-being in modern communication.

Just as active and rest occupations are part of a continuum, so to are doing and being. The different aspects of the doing to being continuum includes the need for satisfaction, meaning, fulfillment and purpose; having choice and energy; finding pleasure, balance, and opportunity; and being challenged, committed, free, creative, and able to cope. It is also a reflective aspect of occupation and a chance for time out: a time for rest, recuperation, and stillness; a time for being acutely conscious of thoughts and feelings and of "contemplation and enjoyment of the inner life," as Maslow determined.[10] Being, in this sense, is closely aligned with consciousness that refers "to the relationship between the mind and the world with which it interacts."[12]

Exploring the being aspects of doing calls for the consideration of how people as occupational beings plan, think, and feel about what they do. This aspect of occupation is integral to health despite the difficulties of coming to terms with the concept of being in the fairly concrete world of health care. Assisting people to do things alone or with others is fairly straightforward and helping them grow into what they would like to become is, at least, understandable. The idea of belonging through doing sits comfortably within the accepted challenges of the social determinants of health. In contrast, although being is a frequently used word, pondered over by great philosophers, it is seldom addressed in postmodern health care, with its emphasis on the minute and the measurable. To shed light on some of the mystique that surrounds it and to begin to appreciate its place in occupation-focused global population health, the concept requires some clarification. Therefore, in this chapter being as an aspect of doing will be studied in terms of how it can meet the biological and natural needs that are prerequisites to health. That includes consideration of higher-order capacities of consciousness and creativity because these appear to be important if people are to find meaning, as well as to meet survival needs through what they do. Such capacities are, of course, relevant to issues discussed throughout the book.

CONSCIOUSNESS

Consciousness is a state of feeling aware of both external and internal factors (Figure 7-1).[13,14] It is defined variously as "subjectivity, awareness, the ability to experience and feel, wakefulness, having a sense of selfhood"[15] or as "the state of being conscious; inward sensibility of something; knowledge of one's own existence, sensations, cognitions, etc; and the thoughts and feelings, collectively, of an individual."[15] Indeed "anything that we are aware of at a given moment forms part of our consciousness, making conscious experience at once the most familiar and most mysterious aspect of our lives."[16]

Consciousness "is a kind of continuous apprehension of an inner reality, the reality of one's mental states and activities,"[17] enabling people to experience feelings and know what they know and the outcomes of what they do. It provides a view of the world "based on sense and body information, expectations, fantasy and crazy hopes, and other cognitive processes."[18] Philosophers divide it according to experience itself or the processing of the things in experience. The first of these is known as phenomenal consciousness and the second as access consciousness.[19] However, because currently "we all use the term consciousness in many different and often ambiguous ways" and because "we have no idea how consciousness emerges from the physical activity of the brain," Robert Frackowiak, with seven other neuroscientists, claims that "to make precise definitions at this stage is premature."[20]

From an evolutionary perspective, Edelman proposed that consciousness arose through the processes of natural selection that gave rise to form and tissue patterns and facilitated behavioral foundations. From this developed a "primary repertoire of variant neuronal groups in the brain" that is involved in selection.[21] Selection "assumes that, during behavior, anatomical synaptic connections are selectively strengthened or weakened by specific biochemical processes," carving out a variety of functioning circuits.[21] "Correlation and coordination of ...selection events are achieved by 're-entrant' signalling and by strengthening of interconnections between the maps" in the brain.[21] During evolution, this selection process linked the brainstem and limbic system with the thalamocortical system, which constitutes the majority of mammalian brains. Together, these take care of bodily functions, internal states, and values, and perceive and categorize world events.[21] Through value-category memory, they enable perceptual categorization and the subsequent development of primary consciousness.[22] Higher-order consciousness evolved in conjunction with changes to the structure of the brain such as in the Broca and Wernicke areas. Edelman deduced

Figure 7-1. Utriusque cosmi maioris scilicet et minoris [···] historia, tomus II (1619), tractatus I, sectio I, liber X, De triplici animae in corpore visione. Representation of Consciousness from the 17th century. (Illustration by Robert Fludd 1619.)

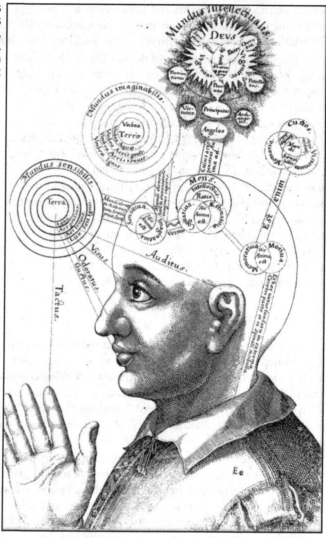

that consciousness depends on perceptual and conceptual categorization, semantics, syntax, and phonology, all of which allow learning to occur.[21]

In considering the purpose of consciousness, it seems that awareness of the possible consequences of action is necessary to ensure the survival of organisms with free will, although individuals are generally unaware of the process. This process is an essential component of being. Ornstein hypothesized that consciousness vetoes or permits every action initiated at an unconscious level. It does so despite the various and diverse types of processes within brain organization.[23] Consciousness and occupation are part of a two-way process. Complex occupational behavior would be impossible without consciousness, and the types of occupations in which individuals choose to engage can affect the states of consciousness. For example, Csikszentmihalyi has found that "when challenges are high and personal skills are used to the utmost, we experience a rare state of consciousness,"[24] which he calls flow. Flow is enjoyable, narrows attention to a clearly defined goal, and provides a sense of control over actions (although awareness of time disappears); during this time, people are absorbed and involved—they are in a state of being. "The activity can be wildly different, but when people are deeply involved [in] meeting a manageable challenge, the state of mind they report is the same the world over."[24]

From Csikszentmihalyi's point of view, consciousness depends particularly on three other capacities. He believed that "attention, awareness, and memory ... act as a buffer between genetic and cultural instructions on the one hand, and behavior on the other."[25] In addition, "consciousness frees the organism from its dependence on the forces that created it and provides a certain [if precarious] control over our behavior." It negates the need for a multitude of separate genetic programs to link stimuli and responses and "increases the possibilities" between "programmed instructions and adaptive behaviors." The self-system has a main goal to "ensure its own survival. To this effect, attention, awareness, and memory are directed to replicate those states of consciousness that are congenial to self and to eliminate those that threaten its existence."[25]

Consciousness allows humankind enormous independence and power, with the potential to destroy the environment from which they evolved and on which they depend. However, because it acts as a prompt to consider the consequences of doing, consciousness is pivotal in the balancing act between doing and being, and between occupation, health, and illness.[26-28] Similar to other capacities, its watchdog role is made complex by its susceptibility to enculturation.

Raising people's consciousness about lifestyle issues relating to ill health is integral to many agendas, such as those aimed at health education, cultural awareness, feminism, social justice, and sustainable ecology. Advocates of transpersonal psychology believe that an optimal state of consciousness is central in the achievement of positive health.[29,30] "Deep states of relaxation, increased inner awareness ... bodymind self-awareness" are enabled and effective choices are more accessible.[31] Transpersonal psychology links psychological and physiological states, incorporating notions from many Asian religions.

Similar to the pragmatic view that the brain minds the body, the psychophysiological principle claims that every conscious or unconscious change in either the physiologic or mental-emotional state is accompanied by an appropriate change in the other, and that health can be facilitated by awareness and self-regulation of normally unconscious processes.[30] Raising consciousness about the critical relationship between all-encompassing occupation and health is an important aspect of holistic health and well-being.[32-34]

Being and Health

Existential philosophy and psychology advance the notion that meaning, choice, and purpose are necessary to well-being. This suggests that a lack of meaning, choice, or purpose will result in the opposite, which is being ill. Crisp noted that although philosophers' use of well-being is usually applied to how good a person's life is for them, the "popular use of the term usually relates to health,"[35] so it is not surprising that well-being is central within the WHO definition of health. Because each person is unique within a dynamic and ever-changing social environment and the needs and feelings that drive occupational choice vary, the complexity of the relationship between occupation and health differs. The theme of this chapter highlights aspects of being in terms of meeting psychological needs that are part and parcel of what people would choose to do and of feelings of well-being. They are also integral to the prerequisites of health.

NATURAL HEALTH: PREREQUISITES

People need to meet the prerequisites of health according to their social situation, individual being, and spiritual quest for meaning and purpose in life.[1]

Being and Peace

Peace is an essential aspect of being. From the 13th century, European references can be found to peace being understood as inner tranquility, and in early English to a sense of quiet that reflects "calm, serene, and meditative approaches to family or group relationships."[36] This perception can be extended to the search for personal equanimity, inner peace, the avoidance of conflict, or tension or distress.[37] Some believe that peace is an enlightened state of consciousness and self-discovery, cultivated by prayer or meditation and coming to know one's inner nature. Experiencing such inner peace is often associated with Buddhist, Hindu, and Vedic traditions and, more recently, with some New Age movements characterized by "unbounded awareness, heightened wakefulness, and deep physical rest," such as Transcendental Consciousness.[37] For people to contemplate, review, plan, or progress toward aspirations, what has been or needs to be done requires time free from interruption, from noise that distracts, and from many of the practical demands of everyday life.

Being and Shelter

Feeling safe is an essential aspect of being. All animals need to feel safe, especially when resting according to their physiological needs, at which time they seek shelter with particular characteristics, known as a species habitat. Klinkenborg asked "when did 'home' become embedded in human consciousness?" because "for much of the earliest history of our species, home may have been nothing more than a small fire and the light it cast on a few familiar faces." Whenever that occurred, it provided "a way of organizing space in our minds. Home is home, and everything else is 'not-home.'"[38] For much of human history, homes have been constructed to meet the way people feel and think, as well as provide physical shelter. However, in many postindustrial societies, the physical construction of homes is restricted to experts who work according to rules imposed by a bureaucracy, fashioned according to available technology and trends, and increasingly expensive, and may not be suited to individual being needs. At the opposite end of the spectrum, many people throughout the world are displaced and homeless, not only without shelter but adrift and without an opportunity to fully experience the meaning, purpose, and belonging associated with home as they go about their daily lives. "Homelessness signifies much more than simply being without physical refuge" because home "constitutes, for almost all of us, simple rituals that link us with sequences of the day and patterns of time."[39]

Being and Education

UNESCO has described learning to be as one of the four pillars of education throughout the lifespan.[40] It is a lifelong process that can be either advantageous or disadvantageous in terms of health depending on how people feel, on the support and encouragement of others, on whether it meets personal interests and needs, and on whether it enables growth in terms that are individually and sociologically meaningful.[41] Creativity, which is dependent on aspects of being such as imagination and original thought, has been identified as a central aspect of education that is as important as literacy[42] because it encompasses "knowledge, ability, perception, understanding, acceptance, interaction and communication."[43,44] It can touch individuals in unique ways so that learning can be a catalyst for change and be inclusive and meaningful with the capacity to enable new beginnings for people experiencing difficulties.[43]

Being and Food

Although the International Covenant on Economic, Social and Cultural Rights (ICESCR) recognizes that people have a "fundamental right to be free from hunger,"[45] it is also important that available food is acceptable in terms of beliefs, ambiances, states of mind, and physical and mental sensitivities, as well as social, moral, and spiritual requirements and traditions. Food preparation and cooking methods are an aspect of cultural identity and local dietary habits, reflecting aesthetic and religious beliefs and feelings, as well as cultural taboos.[46] Although some people limit what they eat for more esoteric reasons, others are driven to over- or under-eat because of how they feel about themselves, their body shape, or societal norms. Others might make dietary changes to achieve a lifelong ambition or adventure. Such feelings drive what they do on a daily basis and reflect or anticipate occupational ambitions. They also influence health. This can occur in a positive way if, when feeling good about present and future occupational potential, challenge, and outcomes, they choose, prepare, and eat food wisely. However, starvation and obesity are in epidemic proportions in many different parts of the world, in many cases because of how people feel or because they have lost a meaningful sense of purpose.

Being and Income

Inequalities in the being experience also result from how people feel about the work or activity they do to achieve income. In postmodern cultures, people have shifted their ideas from expecting to work to provide for basic needs toward a right to meet interests, abilities, satisfaction, and status as well as material comforts. But, for many people, paid employment is not intrinsically satisfying.[47] The changeable fiscal climate is a compounding factor adding fear to dissatisfaction that is justified in terms of a known relationship between downward economic fluctuations and death, prison admissions, physical, and emotional illness.[48,49] In two classic texts, *Unemployment and Health: A Disaster and a Challenge* by Richard Smith[50] and *The Concept of Work: Ancient, Medieval and Modern* by Herbert Applebaum,[51] the authors claim that "most employment for most people has, since the Industrial Revolution, been hard, exhausting, boring, dirty, degrading, and, as Marx said, alienating,"[50] and that in most periods and in all urban cultures people with property and power have looked down on manual workers.[51] Such attitudes can affect the willingness to take on such work, precluding the chance that it might, unexpectedly, prove meaningful. Some people overcome constraints with or without encouragement, although others find themselves in jobs that do not fit their interests or their being. Many people who are unemployed experience a reduction in the range of occupational options outside paid work, experiencing a doubling of the effects of already limited opportunities that provide meaning and purpose.

Being and a Stable Ecosystem and Sustainable Resources

In terms of the natural environment, it is fairly recent that people's occupations have affected its systems in major ways. It has become imperative that an occupational perspective is taken in consideration of the links between the health of people, places, and the planet.[52] A stable ecosystem and sustainable resources are dependent on people giving attention to the needs of the planet rather than personal or national prosperity at whatever cost. Intellectual and emotional commitment to the development of and participation in health-giving and ecologically sustaining occupations and resource management demands new ways of thinking. This might include reflection about the maintenance or restoration of healthy relationships between what people do, human societies, other living organisms, environments, habits, and modes of life. Such thinking could be assisted by people spending more time in contemplation and the enjoyment of the natural environment than in the hectic, unnatural pursuits of city life. Being in tune with the ecosystem requires people to take opportunities for time out and stillness and for rest and recuperation—time for dreaming, reflection, contemplation, and the enjoyment of the natural world. It also calls for reflection on past doings in terms of environmental health. Contemplation of earlier health edicts that called attention to breathing fresh air, drinking clean water, and making good food choices as primary, every day, sources of health might also be helpful.[53] So too might ecologically sensitive and sensible engagement in activity, such as planning future work and leisure with environmental issues in mind, as well as slowing the pace of life by, for example, riding a bicycle, walking, or using public transportation instead of driving through traffic-congested streets.[54]

Being and Social Justice and Equity

Social justice is fundamental to health-promoting, occupation-focused being that is based on beliefs about freedoms, rights, and responsibilities that determine cultural and political foundations and governance of societies. Pelton argued for "policies that address the fundamental commonalities of all individuals: their human needs, their right to respect, and their potential to flourish when opportunity to do so is available."[55a] Occupational justice can be considered as a branch of social justice. It is about recognizing and encouraging the occupational strengths and capacities of all people, and finding ways to make possible their right to be who they want to be without discrimination, if that is just and equitable to others. It involves acknowledging and nurturing the right of individuals and groups to maintain different ideas, traditions, and ways of life, and supporting individual and group creativity. It is about supporting change if there is occupational injustice or disadvantage, such as bullying or physical, mental, or social discrimination in terms of choice or opportunity in the spiritual quest for meaning and purpose. Table 7-1 provides examples of how being aspects of occupation interact with the prerequisites for health. It presents some different examples, as well as material already discussed.

NATURAL HEALTH: CAPACITIES AND CREATIVITY

Occupation that is meaningful and purposeful is part of our biological heritage and the natural underpinning of health. As Selye observed, "our brain slips into chaos and confusion unless we constantly use it for work that seems worthwhile to us"; however, "the average person thinks he works for economic security or social status."[56] The need to nourish the mind and spirit is critical not only to meeting the prerequisites of health, but also to what people want but are not obliged to do to utilize their particular biological capacities. Frankl asserted that the quest for meaning is central to both quality of life and the human condition.[57] In meeting the spiritual quest for meaning, people engage in occupations that make use of basic biological capacities that set humans apart from other species and that provide the foundation of health.

Human Capacities

The term *human capacity* embraces an inherent aspect of individuals that lies at the heart of being. It is defined as, or used interchangeably with, other terms such as capability, faculty, characteristic, trait, talent, ability, and genetic potential. In this context, capacity is used to mean the innate and perhaps undeveloped potential with which each individual is endowed. Capacities differ between genders[58] and are the underlying building blocks that assist development of unique natures and personalities that people express through what they do. After birth, apart from obvious physical capacities such as crawling, walking,[58] and talking, "at a certain point in ontogenesis, each individual begins to realize his or her own powers to direct attention, to think, to feel, to will, and to remember. At that point a new agency develops within awareness. This is the self."[25] Being is intimately linked with self.

Capacities differ with age, "Some competencies improve with learning and practice during childhood and youth, and all do not improve at the same rate, or necessarily are perfected during a lifetime."[58]

And although individual variation is the rule, genetically endowed capacities with separate centers for specific functions are common to the species:

> *Mathematical ability is a separate talent from the ability to move gracefully; verbal agility is distinct from the previous two. There is a range of different functions, for smelling, for thinking, for moving, for calculating that the brain possesses.*[59]

Because capacities differ between people, the study of "specialized neural systems each of which possesses a rich concentration of certain abilities"[60] assists understanding of the brain's concern with health and with specific talents. One such study led Gagne to group human abilities into aptitude domains, such as intellectual, creative, socio-affective, and sensorimotor, and fields of talents, such as academic, technical, artistic, interpersonal, and athletic. He also grouped primary capacities, such as seeing, standing, perceiving color, or touching, and more complex capacities, such as problem solving, exploration, consciousness, and creativity.[61] Each capacity is "relatively independent of the others," but they may "work in concert."[62] The more complex capacities are examples of the integrative workings of many independent and interdependent systems. Capacities are capable of rapid reaction to emergency that is responsive to inner needs and external variables.

Table 7-1

EXAMPLES OF BEING TO MEET THE PREREQUISITES OF HEALTH

WHO Prerequisites of Health[55b]	"Being" to Meet the Prerequisites: Positive and Negative Examples
Being and Peace	
Peace is an essential aspect of being Inner tranquility A sense of quiet Calm, serene, meditative The search for personal equanimity, the avoidance of disputes An enlightened state of consciousness and "knowing oneself" Contemplation, planning, or review toward aspirations	Peace and war: reconciling actions with beliefs, facing the consequences, being considered a traitor, imprisonment, public condemnation or isolation Inner peace is essential to effective "doing" through "being" and is attained by reflection on the ways, means, outcomes, and effects of what has been done in the past and planned for the future. It is a necessary prerequisite to attain societal and international peace. Peace of mind is: • Dependent on people doing what they think is right and knowing that future directions will be positively influenced by present attitudes and doings. It differs from person to person. • Often dependent on means of making a living, may not necessarily appear to be "right" to others. • Familial, communal, spiritual, and national beliefs and directions, or if counter to local law/custom, with learned beliefs, respected viewpoints, and personal affiliations • Keeping true to beliefs in the face of discord • Related to healthy homeostasis; the opposite of mentally unhealthy stress or anxiety • Often overlooked as an aspect of health and well-being, although generally associated with happiness, which is, in turn, associated with health and well-being
Being and shelter	
A place giving protection from weather or danger. A refuge, asylum, haven, cover, harbor, guard or retreat All animals seek shelter in a place of safety to rest according to species needs Such shelter is known as a *species habitat* The idea of "home" has displaced species habitat, turning shelter into an intangible concept that sits comfortably with the idea of "being"	Global dispersion changed the nature and sophistication of shelters. Agrarian lifestyles led to fixed habitats, an increase in objects for comfort and decoration. Shelters became homes of increasing complexity, creating layers of cultural meaning.[39] Home has been described as a place: • "We can never see with a stranger's eyes for more than a moment"[38] • Where people feel they belong • Of refuge, relaxation, and comfort • To construct and shape memories and to remember • To share: associated with relationships, family, relatives, and friends The "doing" aspects of building a home meet individual "being" needs, but become harder to achieve as they are determined by political and legislative will outside the control of individuals. Many people are: • Displaced and homeless • Without shelter and adrift • Without opportunity to fully experience meaning, purpose and belonging associated with "home" as they go about their daily lives.

(continued)

Table 7-1 (continued)

EXAMPLES OF BEING TO MEET THE PREREQUISITES OF HEALTH

WHO Prerequisites of Health	"Being" to Meet the Prerequisites: Positive and Negative Examples
Being and Education	
"Learning to be" is one of the four pillars of education throughout the lifespan.[40] Health status often depends on how people feel about what they learn, meeting personal interests and needs, and enabling growth and success.	The need and capacity to learn about self, others, and the environment is a primary and ongoing drive. Education, like being, is dependent on contemplation, reflection, inspiration, planning, and active participation as well as support and encouragement of others. Education is a lifelong participatory process progressing through: Learning from family and friends Learning from community elders and religious practices Attending schools, higher education, courses, and trade apprenticeships Participating in sport, recreation, and hobbies Adapting and learning from mistakes and successes
Being and Food	
Apart from the "fundamental right to be free from hunger,"[45] available food has to be acceptable in terms of beliefs, states of mind, ambiances, physical and mental sensitivities, moral, and spiritual requisites and traditions.	Food preparation and cooking methods reflect cultural identity, aesthetic and religious beliefs and feelings as well as cultural taboos.[46] Food choices drive what people do on a daily basis and reflect or anticipate occupational ambitions. People may overeat, undereat, or limit what they eat for esoteric reasons, because of how they feel about themselves, their body shape, or societal norms to achieve a lifelong ambition or adventure. How people feel about food can influence health: Positively when feeling good about occupational challenges Negatively when feeling a loss of meaning or purpose
Being and income	
For most people, income and work are one and the same. Work to provide income can provide a sense of purpose and achievement, a daily time structure, social contact and status,[55b,55c] development of new directions and skills, and impetus for reflection.[178] Health can be underminded because of how people feel about work or lack of it.[203-205] Health is vulnerable to subtle economic fluctuations improving and declining with the economy.[48,49]	Paid employment is a central institution, mattering more than "government, education, religion, defense, or health."[186] Choice is frequently restricted by socioeconomic and political factors, peer pressure, and lack of time, resources, education, or training.[50] The value given to employment means people who are unemployed suffer frequent humiliations and loss of social status,[178] boredom, mental despair, apathy, deterioration,[55b,55c] with many people feeling unwanted, as if they no longer belong to society, their impoverished days having neither structure nor purpose.[50] It may be worse than "being excommunicated, disenfranchised, illiterate, conquered, or diseased."[50] Studies of unemployed report deterioration in physical and mental health;[178,189-191,198] suggest links with premature death, suicide, and deliberate self injury.[192-196] Unemployment of about 1 million people sustained for 6 years could be linked with 36,887 total deaths, 3340 prison admissions, and 4227 mental hospital admissions.[48,49]

(continued)

They are multifunctional, and the combination of specific capacities increases the potential variability of what people can do.

A single mental capacity may represent a "family of competencies."[63] A useful example is provided by the capacity for language that is central to being. Language allows individuals to explore

Table 7-1 *(continued)*

EXAMPLES OF BEING TO MEET THE PREREQUISITES OF HEALTH

WHO Prerequisites of Health	"Being" to Meet the Prerequisites: Positive and Negative Examples
Being: Stable Ecosystem and Sustainable Resources	
Enjoyment and commitment to maintenance or restoration of healthy relationships between people, human societies, other living organisms, environments, habits, and modes of life Intellectual commitment to resource management, development of, and participation in health-giving and ecologically sustaining occupations	Contemplation and enjoyment of the natural environment and its care Finding quiet, meaning, pleasure, fulfillment, and purpose in interaction with natural environments, to breathe and enjoy fresh air, "time out" and stillness, rest and recuperation, time for dreaming, reflection, and contemplation Reflecting on past doings in terms of healthy environments, protecting habitats and local species of plants and wildlife, avoiding and resisting pollutants, conserving water, harnessing natural energy: sun, wind, and water, and using local and renewable resources Slowing down and allowing time to "be" by riding a bicycle, walking, or using public transport or driving through traffic-congested streets[54]
Being: Social Justice and Equity	
Social justice based on beliefs about freedoms, rights, and responsibilities that determine cultural and political foundations and governance of societies for populations and individuals	Without discrimination, recognizing and encouraging the occupational strengths and potential of people, and their right to be who they want to be Facilitating the rights of individuals and groups to consider, develop, and maintain different ideas, skills, traditions, and ways of life if they are just and equitable to others Supporting individual and group rights to be creative or change ways of doing if any are disadvantaged or if there is occupational injustice such as bullying, or physical, mental, or social discrimination in terms of choice or opportunity

ideas, to think in abstract and concrete terms, and to incorporate new concepts into their occupational pursuits based on their unique life experience and ways of thinking. Percy Bysshe Shelley reflected that "speech created thought";[64] Lewin that "mankind's exaggerated intellectual power focuses on the need to build a better mental construct of reality …. It may have required a complex propositional language, not so much that we could converse with others, but so we could think better";[65] and Piaget that "language is not enough to explain thought, because the structures that characterize thought have their roots in action and in sensorimotor mechanisms that are deeper than linguistics."[66]

Early Greek philosophy reflects a dual interest in matters natural and spiritual, with Thales (c. 600 BC) reported as saying that "all things are full of gods."[67] It is probable that the intellectual activities now called philosophy first emerged as wonder at the natural world. The images humans left behind in cave drawings and ornamentation leads to the idea that early belief systems were based on animals and environmental forces important for survival. In addition, the earliest monumental buildings, such as those in Ur in Mesopotamia, had religious significance frequently associated with natural phenomena. Intellectual, religious, philosophical, creative, and architectural occupations that escalated as time passed all reflect a capacity for contemplation and mental creativity that are at the heart of being.

Creativity

Creativity is one of the most complex of human capacities, exciting much interest and discussion. Although the outcome of creativity is often tangible, the process itself arises from a state of being and an amalgam of other capacities and is subject to many different interpretations. Creativity may manifest as a mental phenomenon or vision, capability, innovative action or skills, tools, or as inspired, insightful, interpretive and innovative thought and action. Gordon suggested that "to create is one of man's most basic impulses."[68] Jung classified it as one of five major instinctive forces in humans;[69] Sinnott argued that it is in the inherent creativeness of people's ordinary affairs that the ultimate source of creativity is found, and that its biological basis is the "organizing, pattern forming, questing quality" of life itself.[70] Such explanations are at the heart of the relationship between being and doing for everyone. Brolin's descriptions of the particular capacities exhibited by creative people extend some of those ideas. Because creative people are attracted to complexity and obscurity and display an elevated capacity for emotional involvement during investigation, Brolin included strong motivation, endurance, intellectual curiosity, deep commitment, independence in thought and action, a strong desire for self-realization, self-confidence, openness, and sensitivity in describing their particular being characteristics.[71]

Despite various research, sources seldom agree on a definition of creativity, with one article offering more than 25 examples.[72] The word derives from the Greek *krainein*, meaning to fulfill, and the Latin *creare*, meaning to make.[73] Dictionaries describe it as the "ability to bring into existence or being ... to beget, to shape, to bring about, to invest with new character, and to be inventive."[74] A recently advanced theory of creativity integral to an occupational perspective of health that is based, to some extent, on the earlier edition of this work proposes that "humans have both the innate capacity to be creative and the biological need to express it. When creativity is adequately expressed through everyday activities, it has a major impact on health and well-being."[75]

The extent of early humans' creativity has been hard to assess. Although others disagree, Lewin, who traced examples back approximately 300,000 years, suggested that the creation of paintings, carvings, and engravings represented a true abstraction of thought and mind.[76] However, early humans appeared to possess little in the form of creative artifacts, although this may be a consequence of an unavoidable struggle between material culture and a nomadic lifestyle.[77] When the !Kung San and other first-nation peoples travel, they carry only about 12 kg each. Creativity includes being occupations such as abstract reasoning skills and the intellectual evidences of culture, as well as the manufacture of material artifacts, the stories, music and dance that are carried in the minds and recreated regularly throughout history. Whatever form creativity takes, it requires abstract conceptualization, which some describe as the ultimate human gift.

Marx argued that the collective creative activity of mankind is labor,[78] and Morris suggested that creativity is an integral part of the human contest with nature (Figure 7-2):

> A man, making something which he feels will exist because he is working at it and wills it, is exercising the energies of his mind and soul as well as of his body. Memory and imagination help him as he works. Not only his own thoughts, but the thoughts of the men of past ages guide his hands; and, as a part of the human race, he creates.[79]

In similar vein, Donald Winnicott, an early 20th century pediatrician and psychoanalyst, formulated a theory of development that places creativity as central and intrinsic to human nature, holding that cultural activity is what life is about rather than an adornment to be added to it.[80]

Despite the long history of creativity, it was not until the turn of the 20th century and the emergence of psychology that philosophical speculation and systematic study began to provide theoretical frames for investigation.[68,81-84] Theories have ranged through psychoanalytic, cognitive, behaviorist, humanist, and empirical frames of reference,[44,85-87] as well as personality,[88-90]

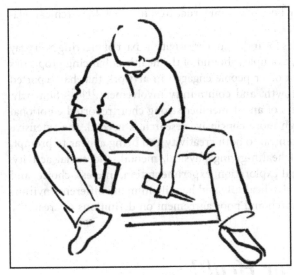

Figure 7-2. Creating in wood: an integral part of the human contest with nature. (© Carol Spencer 2012, otspencer@adam.com.au. Used with permission.)

social structure, and organizational climate models.[91-97] Early psychoanalytic theorists, Freud and Adler, reflected the early 20th century view, which limited creativity to innate talent or artistic genius stemming from neurotic tendencies.[97,98] Creativity was thought to offer the resolution or compensation for feelings of inferiority or guilt, and the creative arts were seen as socially acceptable outlets to sublimate libidinal energy and other unconscious conflicts, drives, and needs.[99-101] Despite this, Freud recognized parallels between the creative nature of children's play and the creative artist and, along with others of the psychoanalytical school, suggested that creative people were subject to both better health and, ironically, more sickness than the average person.[98,102]

Later psychologists have linked the creativity evident in all aspects of life with individual potential and the experience of health.[103] High creativity has been found to correlate with a high degree of normal, mature, and positive self-esteem,[104] and there appears to be strong links between mental well-being, creativity, and, by inference, occupation that provides meaning and purpose. Increasingly, research began to focus on the creativity of ordinary people using ethnographic, qualitative research. Eysenck claimed that studies of creative individuals have demonstrated surprising agreement over the years,[105] finding that creativity is fostered by:

- Life-long, high-level, personal self-control, sustained hard work, determination, and perseverance.[106]

- Open, supportive, and interactive environments in which people are encouraged to advance new ideas, show initiative, and take risks.[107]

Creativity is one of the inherent capacities that emerge or peak at different parts of the life cycle.[107-111] Like being itself, it can often be regarded as behavior outside conventional habits and mores, although it can be observed when people try to solve the problems of daily life. Although creative play is encouraged in young children, creative behavior is often harder to find as they grow older and reach adulthood. It is high technology with its reliance on thoughtfulness, inner contemplation, and inherent purpose that demonstrates advanced, modern, and cutting-edge creativity,[112] and, as in the industrial age, the products of the technological era have affected individual resourcefulness negatively. For example, many people buy rather than make the products that they require and, instead of thinking about and self-creating to meet their particular needs, they prefer to spend hours viewing television or manipulating images on personal computers and interactive devices that grew from someone else's mind rather than from their own. Sometimes, it appears that society suppresses creative potential that grows from being aptitudes by the encouragement of intellectual conformity.[113] Indeed, despite employers calling for graduates with thought provoking creative skills, firms may maintain traditional organization structures, in which hierarchical relationships stifle individual creativity.

The health effects of reduced opportunities for individual creativity as part of meeting everyday being needs is poorly understood. However, examples abound of the health-enhancing properties that creativity can provide, such as study of older people engaged in artwork that has reported positive effects on self-esteem, personal growth, and community involvement.[114,115] Similarly, approximately three quarters of the members of an 84-member strong choir reported emotional benefits from their involvement.[116] Although more conclusive research is needed, the extensive range of higher cortical capacities that are central to both creativity and being appear to prompt, motivate, and enable an infinite variety of health-giving physical, mental, and social activity. Purpose and meaning stimulate occupational exploration, experimentation, interest, choice, and skills that enable people to adapt to and survive healthily and happily in many different environments. However, as with being, limited research and poor agreement on definitions of creativity make it difficult to be conclusive.[117]

Rules for Health: Being From Ancient to Modern

Because health depends on more than meeting the prerequisites for survival and because, as the WHO contends, each person is unique, health is reliant on the spiritual quest for meaning and purpose that is focal to being.[1] Building on the foundation of the ancient rules for health and the modern directions of the WHO, the current discussion will focus on how meanings can change as sociocultural conditions change, despite the biological being needs remaining intact. For example, it was explained earlier how in Ancient Greece the choice of occupation (and the meaning that arose from it) was determined by citizenship status. That value changed over time, with the Stoics accepting there was no difference between Greeks and others, Seneca (c. 55 BC-AD 41) reasoning that both had the same basic human nature and need for air and water, living and dying in the same way.[118] In common with earlier ideas, Stoics explained people as only being able to experience fulfillment within the community of others. They had a natural "social responsibility" to serve others as mainly either "do-ers" or "be-ers." That could be achieved by "either by taking part in civic affairs or by leading a contemplative life, or by combining these two ways of life." Irrespective of that was the social obligation "to marry, to raise a family and to work."[118] Justice was the ultimate virtue.[119]

BEING AND HEALTH IN EARLIER TIMES

The mixed economy of hunting and gathering brought with it time for leisure,[120-122] and "a rich ceremonial life based on complex concepts and rituals."[123] As hunter-gatherer societies engaged in a variety of activities, they developed new capacities and talents, leaving behind a legacy of more than stone tools to demonstrate the range of occupations they valued. Deep in caves, they portrayed images of creatures, humans, and spirits who were part of their world and is evidence of abstract thought and a search for meaning. Wax observed that "I do not believe that any Bushman could tell us—or would be interested in telling us—which part of activity was work and which was play."[124] Meaning and satisfaction were found in doing things not just related to their continued existence, and no formal differentiation or value loading existed between labor, leisure, or self-care.

Both hunter-gatherer and early agrarian societies seem to have operated in such a way that a natural balance between activity and rest, doing, and being occurred. Their economic activities had built-in down time, such as singing and telling stories while they worked.[125] The lack of distinction was advantageous to health and well-being in that individuals were able to develop

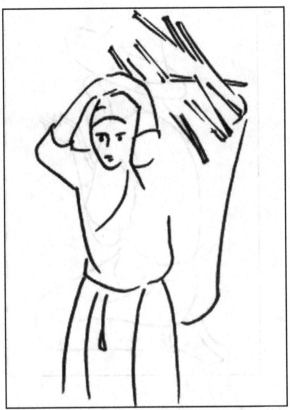

Figure 7-3. Changed methods for acquiring the necessities of life. (© Carol Spencer 2012, otspencer@adam.com.au. Used with permission.)

their own traits and capacities according to being needs or opportunity, without subjugating their choice to economic efficiencies or sociocultural rules. An example is provided by the preindustrial society of the Baluchi of Western Pakistan, who divided occupation into the sphere of obligatory duty and the sphere of one's own will, with the latter being the most valued domain.[124]

With the gradual extension of agriculture, people continued to seek satisfaction, meaning, and joy through the use of creative talents that also changed methods of acquiring the necessities of life (Figure 7-3). The use of "words, symbols and probably numbers"[126] that are essential to being as a component of doing led to the development of hammers, axes, wheels, and boats; activities such as spinning, weaving, mining, metal working, and bread and beer making; and building houses and towns. As their occupations and skills expanded, so too did mental exploration. People experimented with material resources, began to challenge the environment and adapt it to meet their perceived needs and comfort, and changed their social structures and behavior to accommodate such change. As people challenged their skills internally, the diversity of occupation flourished, along with an expansion of goods and services regarded as necessary.[125]

Occupational developments that grew from expanding being capacities became recognizable in modern terms with the advent of architecture, art, writing, commerce, religion, increased technological innovation, and social administration. That occurred with the formation of cities between 6000 and 10,000 years ago. Administrative functions, organization, and control of cities in those early days, often combined with religious activity and monumental architecture, developed to help communities cope with socioenvironmental stress, uncertainty, and unpredictability.[76] The stressors arose from living in much larger, specialized communities than people had been used to, possibly in response to dangers from outside, and that individuals had to abide by the decisions made by others more frequently, rather than depending on their own internal feelings and beliefs. That remains the case currently. Neff observed that, during that earlier time, occupation

Figure 7-4. Seeking solace in prayer. (© Carol Spencer 2012, otspencer@adam.com.au. Used with permission.)

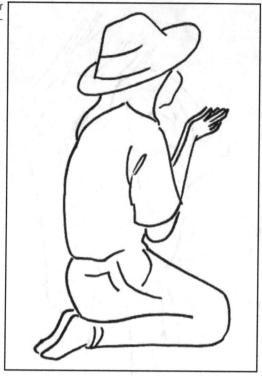

began to acquire distinctions and qualifications and an increasingly complicated infrastructure of evaluative meanings, including the distinction between the practical and reflective, between doing and being.[127]

Making Use of Being: Finding Meaning and Mental Health

Effective doing is reliant on the occupation undertaken having relevance to being needs—to expressing both meaning and purpose. In turn, meaning and purpose rely on people making use of their inherent and unique capacities and abilities to meet their needs. It is a two-way process. In this way, being is closely related to mental health.[1] Therefore, it is appropriate to briefly consider examples from history of how mental health has been pursued over time according to changing perceptions about it and about being. Examples are from the Western world, where actions to change mental illness have been perceived as humane or inhumane and as moral or immoral according to the context, the world view, and the values of those perceiving.

In Medieval times, when monasteries and nunneries provided the majority of institutional health care in the western world, a person's inner being was linked with spiritual salvation that was central to views of health. All strata of societies were advised to seek solace in reflection and prayer (Figure 7-4).[128] Physical work was deemed good for the soul rather than the body, so valuing being rather than the active doing.

John Locke equated madness with children being "unable to think straight,"[129] and Burton discussed how "minde," "passions and perturbations … work on the body." He lists a range of ideas about being causes of melancholy, such as "idleness," "loss of liberty, servitude, [and] imprisonment," and prescribes occupations that either engage the mind fully, such as shooting, swimming, mathematical studies, business, and labor, or those that permit thoughts to roam and de-stress, such as walking or enjoying pleasure gardens.[130] In line with the ancient rules for health, Santorio Sanctorius (1561-1636), a well-known Italian physician, suggested that "continual satisfaction of the mind," as well as "free perspiration" through occupation, would overcome melancholy.[131]

However, the view that "in losing his reason, the essence of his humanity, the madman had lost his claim to be treated as a human being"[132] led eminent pre-19th century doctors of the mad to use physical means and restraint to improve the being capacities that were compromised by illness.[133] Physician Francis Willis chained George III to a stake during bouts of mania. "He was frequently beaten and starved, and at best he was kept in subjection by menacing and violent language."[134]

Such atrocities began to change with the advent of the Age of Enlightenment (known sometimes as the Enlightenment), which opened a path for independent thought. The result was an intellectual and scientific revolution created with great enthusiasm and permeating nearly every facet of civilized life. The Western world was transformed, in general having a beneficial effect on opportunities for improved mental health within daily lives and, for literate citizens, the prospect of becoming increasingly self-aware and able to develop and advance their own ideas. The long-term effects of the Enlightenment improved or changed women's rights, judicial systems, educational opportunities, economic theories, literature, music, and industry. A valuing of being attributes enabled real change through the freedom of expression, which led, in turn, to new approaches to investigation, reasoning, and problem solving.[135]

A product of the Age of Enlightenment, moral treatment's genesis, success, and demise provides a fascinating but cautionary tale of improving people's mental health through them finding meaning and purpose via occupational participation. Philippe Pinel, at the Bicetre in Paris,[136-138] and William Tuke, at the Retreat in York, instituted moral treatment. This revolutionary approach was based on both being and doing factors that are part and parcel of engagement in occupation, such as self-discipline and kindness, as well as hard work.[139] Tuke valued occupation partly as a requisite of self-esteem that requires both attention and obligation.[139,140] Psychiatrist WAF Browne wrote that "[t]he whole secret of the new system and of that moral treatment by which the number of cures has been doubled may be summed up in two words, kindness and occupation."[141]

Moral treatment was also applied in other parts of Europe and the United States[142-144] until "reductionist [and] mechanical" values associated with industrialization replaced the Romantic enlightenment ideas that inspired moral treatment.[145] Medicine was reconsidering the causes of insanity in the light of new physiological knowledge, in which ideas about occupation, justice, or kindness did not seem important. Indeed, it seems almost inevitable that as positivist, medical science developed, doctors would try to make their role in the treatment of the insane fit with their view of their own skills, beliefs, meaning, and purpose. The doctor's role in moral treatment in the early days was as a wise authority figure, with Foucault stating that both Tuke and Pinel claimed "moral action was not necessarily linked to any scientific competence."[139] However, it was from their programs that madness became associated with medicine and modern notions of rehabilitation have grown. Ironically, understanding of the being aspects of activity has lessened over 2 centuries of use.

Social Change Toward Finding Meaning Through Occupation

At the time of the Industrial Revolution, the changing character of occupations and the extreme dichotomy of economic and social conditions led various intellectuals to consider the effects of the industrial era in terms of meaning. Some of their ideas were similar to those expressed by Renaissance utopians—that what people do can provide their being with a source of joy if it is creative and provides pleasure in the exercise of a range of skills.[146,147]

Because Karl Marx (1818-1883) founded much of his philosophy on the idea that "free conscious activity" (doing in accord with thoughts and beliefs) constitutes the species character of humans,[148] consideration must be given to his views. The integration of doing with finding meaning impacts on the ways people make and change themselves and their world.[147] Essentially, the combination of being and doing can be either a positive or negative experience, depending on whether it is a free, universal, creative, and self-creative activity. If prevented from mixing doing with being, individuals are unable to cultivate their unique talents; alienated from their species' need to be active, productive beings, which results in misery, exhaustion, and mental debasement.

When work is simply a process to earn a wage for the prerequisites of living and is destructive to inner being, people are alienated by it. It is a contradiction of the nature of humankind for economic conditions to become more powerful than individuals.[147]

John Ruskin and William Morris differed from Marx in that they came to social criticism from the viewpoint of creative artists. Ruskin (1819-1900) was a well-known art critic who experienced bouts of illness as a young man and found that a simple occupational regime of walking, reading, writing, and painting that met his psychological needs was remedial.[128] Starting with his publication *Unto this Last* in 1862, Ruskin turned to writing about and experimenting in the field of political economy.[149] Like Coleridge[150] and Carlyle,[151] he challenged classical political economists by accusing them of ignoring the human factor. His central theme was that the quality of life citizens enjoy is the true measure of a nation's prosperity, rather than the accumulation of wealth for its own sake. He attacked the boredom and monotony of the Victorian industrial system and the disconnection between leisure and work. He also advocated that training schools should be established at the government's expense for all children to teach the laws of health, habits of gentleness and justice, and the "calling" by which each would live.[152]

Morris (1834-1896) was also a notable social reformer.[153] As a craftsman, he deplored the machine age and the fact that commerce had become a "sacred religion," turning work from a solace into a burden and for the majority a mere drudgery.[154] He accepted that "nature does not give us our livelihood gratis; we must win it by toil of some sort or degree," but he also believed that the necessary work of society could be accomplished without overstrain or difficulty and should be enjoyed.[155] Arguing against the "stifling over-organization common to both capitalist and socialist versions of modern industrial society,"[156] Morris believed that most work could be done with actual pleasure in the doing.[157] He described a fictional utopia based on his ideas of work in which people are free and independent and where poverty, exploitation, competition, and money all disappear.[158] He recognized the importance of all people being fulfilled and satisfied and finding meaning through doing, and that this was a health issue. Morris wrote that "there are two types of work—one good, the other bad; one not far removed from a blessing, a lightening of life; the other a mere curse, a burden to life."[155] Of the first, he explained that "to all living things there is a pleasure in the exercise of their energies, and that even beasts rejoice in being lithe and swift and strong. He noted that "worthy work carries with it the hope of pleasure in rest, the hope of pleasure in using what it makes, and the hope of pleasure in our daily creative skill." He described the second type as "worthless ... mere toiling to live, that we may live to toil."[155] Morris anticipated an ecological view of health-giving being through doing that is in tune with the natural world.

Marx, Ruskin, and Morris upheld the view that doing must be inclusive of the being aspects of meaning and purpose to be true to human nature and health giving. Neither the antimodern socialist revolution focus, nor the capitalist, individualist growth focus, nor the establishment of occupational therapy was successful in creating global awareness of the need to consider people's inner being and occupational nature in future social or health planning, although all went some way in that direction. Later, the dominance of reductionist medicine led to public health practitioners being tied to a practice geared to civic sanitary conditions and control of epidemics of infectious diseases, and the diminution of broadly based, population-focused occupational approaches to health, delaying a collective consciousness of their importance.

Being and Health in Modern Times

Health and well-being are intimately related with quality of life. Quality of life is concerned with being attributes, such as ability, adaptation, control, diversity, enjoyment, flexibility, happiness, knowledge, opportunities, pleasure, satisfaction, self-esteem, socialness, and spirituality. It also addresses a range of particular being characteristics related to occupation focused life enhancement, expectations, possibilities, hopes, fulfilment, freedom, safety, and security.

Frankl asserted that the human search for meaning is fundamental to the human condition and to quality of life.[57] The concept of being relates to meaning and what some describe as the inner self, where private inner thoughts, feelings, self-awareness, and spirituality are housed. Many people use meditation, reflection, solitude, inner stillness, and silence to access their being and to awaken consciousness and find meaning. Accessing being for the purposes of doing is important in terms of occupational well-being. For example, Amabile and Kramer found that among the many emotions constituting a person's reactions during a day's work, the single most important is that the work is meaningful to those doing it. When people have positive inner work lives, they are more creative, productive, committed, and collegial in their jobs. Their studies found that when senior personnel routinely undermined meaning, creativity, productivity, and commitment, they also damaged the inner work lives of their employees.[159,160]

Another previously named aspect of finding meaning and commitment that is widely referenced in the health field and possible to relate to work and other forms of occupation is the concept of flow.[161,162] Flow is a being state characterized by complete absorption and spontaneous joy in activity—a harnessing of feelings and emotions about the doing that is beyond being pleasurably engrossed and absorbed; it is to "be in the moment," "in the zone," or "on fire" and to lose awareness of other things and even other self needs. The challenges and skills have to be high and equally matched for people to experience flow; they have to know what and how to do the activity, know they are doing it well, and be free from distractions. Flow is challenged by the being states of apathy, boredom, and anxiety.[163]

The things people do to satisfy basic being needs, experience well-being, and achieve happiness, meaning, purpose, freedom, safety, and security, underpin quality of life. Despite recognition that when absorbed in what they are doing, people appear able to resist disease and seem impervious to many problems and difficulties that beset them, there is scant acknowledgement in contemporary medical research and documentation. It is important that being aspects of occupation are not overlooked in research into minute and particular aspects of cause and effect or holistic interactions between systems, people, and social, built, and natural environments. Population health practitioners of whatever discipline have to be cognizant of, and attentive to, the possible causes of well-being, as well as disorder.

Mental, Physical, and Social Well-Being

Mental, physical, and social well-being are fostered by environments that create meaningful opportunities for people of all ages and circumstances. Whatever affects one aspect of health in turn affects other aspects, attributable to the interconnectedness of brain mechanisms. For example, unhappiness can lead to physical disorders or social problems, perhaps as often as it manifests in a depressive illness. However, because being relates more directly to people's thoughts and feelings, mental well-being is the most vulnerable.

Being characteristics relating directly to states of mental well-being are dependent on people realizing their potential, coping with normal life stresses, working productively, and contributing to their community.[164] In a negative sense, reduced opportunities to meet being needs could lead to isolation, distress, and stress, hindering the psychosocial, emotional, and cognitive development of children, adolescents, and adults. For example, the 200 million children worldwide who live on less than $2 a day are at risk of inadequate cognitive stimulation because of restricted opportunities to explore their world, play, and attend school.[165]

Acknowledging the impact of mental health on children's ability to learn and adults' ability to function at home, work, and in broader society,[166,167] the WHO has developed a framework for action toward having mental health promotion placed firmly on national agendas.[168] Mental health promotion covers a variety of strategies, such as the enhancement of socioeconomic environments and an individual's resources and capacities. Many of the macrosocial and macroeconomic factors that influence population-wide mental health lie outside the traditional health sector. Government policies and programs targeting poverty, urbanization, homelessness, unemployment, employment practices, education, and the social services and criminal justice systems are interlinked with mental health. The WHO Mental Health Policy and Service Guidance Package[169] recognizes that:

- The impact, value, and visibility of mental health promotion policies needs to be enhanced and monitored.
- "The social integration of severely marginalized groups, such as refugees, disaster victims, the socially alienated, the mentally disabled, the very old and infirm, abused children and women, and the poor" should be addressed.
- Programs are required at all stages of life to encourage creativity and promote self-esteem and self-confidence.[166]

The WHO warns of the mental health implications of recent economic reforms designed to increase flexibility of the labor force, pointing out that they decrease work time flexibility for workers and make employment more precarious,[165] which "can be particularly catastrophic for the mental health of older adults who have little prospect of re-entering the job market."[169] On the other hand, Fryer and Payne[170] found that 5% of their participants reported an improvement in their mental health—some because they escaped from jobs they disliked, whereas others had found positive aspects to unemployment.

Such requirements suggest that across high-, middle-, and low-income countries, issues about people finding meaning in their lives through what they do are neither adequately recognized nor acted upon. Occupational scientists, therapists, and population health practitioners have a mandate to bring public attention to the positive or negative health impact of occupation on being needs.

Social Change Toward Finding Meaning Through Occupation

In terms of health promotion generally, the WHO calls for action that generates living, leisure, and working conditions that are stimulating, satisfying, and enjoyable, as well as meeting health's basic prerequisites.[171,172] Currently, there are few medical or population health programs that address the potential holistic health impact of a range of occupations and the meaning they hold for people. There is ongoing research and there are programs that address illness and safety concerns in paid employment, and there are increasing programs of physical exercise to reduce the incidence of noncommunicable diseases, and more recently, to reverse the obesity epidemic in affluent countries. Programs addressing the occupational elements of work and exercise provide pointers to a significant relationship between what people do, how they feel about it, and health. However, such programs do not make all people enthusiastic and the rates of obesity and other noncommunicable diseases continue to increase. More diverse programs based on myriad factors that constitute doing and being, that have meaning for people, could be a sound alternative.

In post-modern societies, it is leisure that frequently provides opportunity for people to develop their innate capacities and creativity and fulfill "wishes at the fantasy level,"[173] as well as exercise their bodies. However, it is occupation as work that receives the most emphasis in terms of health, society appearing to value technological progress, and the material rewards of employment above all of the other forms of occupation and finding meaning.[174] Ennobling work over other aspects of activity may also have done a disservice to people's need to be true to self, diminishing opportunities for the balanced use of innate capacities to the detriment of overall well-being. As the valued domain in the post-modern world, work can take on an unhealthy, degrading, and "servile" nature when subjugation of one person to another is part of the equation, or opportunities to develop being potential is unequal; "it is not work itself that is degrading but the power relationships and social structure which surround it."[127]

Work as a Source of Well-Being

In terms of work as a source of well-being rather than simply a prerequisite of health, it is important to consider being as an important entity within occupation-focused factors. Scott, in *The Psychology of Work*, echoed Marx when he claimed that, although "at first work appears merely as a source of money—a means of earning a living ... it is the force that transforms the world and makes it either a better or a worse place in which to live ... and changes us."[175] His examination considered "what work really was, why we did it and how it affected us" and determined that, "Work is characterised by verbal communication, at a superficial level even the chatter in the canteen is important. If silence reigns, then there is something wrong with the work."[176]

Pointing to studies of tiredness to explain "the overlap between various aspects," Scott described how fatigue can be a symptom of boredom that emanates from too little to do or a lack of variety or repetition. In addition, it is often due to excessive work, with manual tasks and repetition leading to the build-up of lactic acid in muscles that lead to tenderness, swelling, pain, and physical fatigue.[177]

In modern western society, paid employment offers scope for developing new skills and decision making.[178] In addition, work "receives strongly positive valuation as a social virtue" being "dignified, natural, compatible with virtue ... a means of serving others as well as a means of exercising one's own ethical integrity."[179] Such overt valuing of work, Jenkins and Sherman claimed, has led to leisure not being considered seriously, often being confused with pleasure and being made to sound "vaguely sinful and hedonistic and frivolous enough to be frowned upon." Despite this, they observed that modern technology created a reduction in the availability of paid employment, leaving many people with up to 100% of leisure time. Eventually, Jenkins and Sherman argued, societies are going to have to come to terms with the idea that the work ethic is fast becoming redundant.[180] A need to blur work and leisure has been a constant theme of writers concerned with their study for the past 50 years.[125,181-185]

To meet the WHO directives that provide the theme for this chapter, and in terms of meaning as opposed to doing for the sake of survival, the value given to work for work's sake can be seen to be less than health enhancing. More consideration needs to be given to satisfying people's particular capacities in ways that contribute to their unique ways of thinking and being and to community. Not to develop new ways forward with such thought in mind may contribute to the increasing number of dropouts from education or regular paid work. Despite affluent societies appearing to have an abundance of occupational choices, how successfully people access opportunities may depend on their spiritual quest for meaning, as well as considerations of gender, material costs, time, resources, interest, peer pressure, place of residence, organizational structures, socio-economic, political, communal and family attitudes, and values.[186] There are inequalities of potential meaning resulting from how the nature of different work is perceived by society. This might be associated with what Radford termed *occupational culture* or *occupational fate*.[187]

People who are unemployed can experience humiliations and a loss of social status because of the value accorded to employment.[178] Therefore, it is not surprising that Smith's summary account suggests that unemployment and poor health are strongly associated—unemployment both causes and compounds health problems. People's spiritual quest for meaning and purpose are compromised by poverty, low socioeconomic status, poor education, and housing conditions that are frequently associated with both ill health and unemployment. Unemployment is also associated with emotional stressors such as high divorce rates, child and spousal abuse, unwanted pregnancies, abortions, reduced birth-weight and child growth, perinatal and infant mortality, and increased morbidity in families, although it cannot be assumed that unemployment itself is the cause for any of the associations.[188] However, Smith's findings are supported by many detailed studies. About one fifth of individuals who are unemployed report a deterioration in their mental health since being out of work,[178,189-191] and there is a link between unemployment, suicide, and deliberate self-injury.[192] Some researchers have found a link with premature death[193-196]; however, not all are convinced that this is the case.[197] There is less evidence associating unemployment with psychosis.[198] Unfortunately, unemployment is seldom an unpleasant interlude with no ongoing effect even when over, it can precipitate future self-perpetuating negative events.[199] Neither is the risk randomly distributed, but rather it is experienced by a relatively small proportion of the economically active population.[200-202]

Anxiety, apathy, and a lack of purpose often go hand in hand with the loss of socially valued and meaningful occupation leading to a decrease in well-being and increased susceptibility to illness. Studies link unemployment with physical illness,[203] and statistically significant increases in medical consultation rates and referrals to hospital outpatients for the families of people who lost jobs.[204] In Australia, unemployed men were reported as experiencing a 66% higher prevalence of disability than employed men, 21% higher prevalence of recent illnesses, 101% higher rate of days of reduced activity because of illness, and diabetes and respiratory disorders, possibly as a result of food and smoking related activities, as a more frequent cause of death. Women followed those trends but not to the same extent.[205] In recognizing that significant (and meaningful) work is conducive to well-being and preventive of illness if it complies with societal values and personal meaning, the WHO calls for strategies to improve work opportunities, such as job creation programs, the provision of vocational training, and the development of social and job seeking skills.[166]

In post-modern cultures, people have shifted their ideas from expecting to work to provide for their own needs toward an expectation that they have a right to work not only to provide themselves with material comforts, but also to meet being needs for satisfaction, meaning, and status. A prospective longitudinal study of more than 3,000 young Australians found that people dissatisfied with their employment were no better off in terms of self-esteem, levels of depression, or lack of psychological well-being than people who were unemployed.[206] The WHO provides guidelines suggesting that a "special emphasis should be given to those aspects of workplaces and the work process itself which promote mental health," which include the following:[166]

- Increasing an employer's awareness of mental health issues
- Identifying common goals and positive aspects of the work process
- Creating a balance between job demands and occupational skills
- Training in social skills
- Developing the psychosocial climate of the workplace
- Provision of counseling
- Enhancement of working capacity
- Early rehabilitation strategies.

Conclusion

Being is, arguably, the aspect of occupation that brings together, houses, coordinates, and distributes feelings of well-being. From an occupational perspective, well-being includes the spiritual quest for meaning and purpose. That sense of well-being emanates from people meeting their life needs through being creative, challenged, and finding meaning as they experience all human emotions, explore, and adapt appropriately without undue disruption. Such occupation needs to provide meaning and purpose, as well as self-esteem and motivation. Other important requirements appear to be a sufficient intellectual challenge to stimulate neuronal physiology and encourage efficient or enhanced problem solving, perception, attention, concentration, reflection, language, and memory.[207,208] Some of the practical known determinants of mental well-being are educational opportunities, appropriate economic policies, adequate housing, transport systems that promote access to employment, and assistance to move out of poverty.[209]

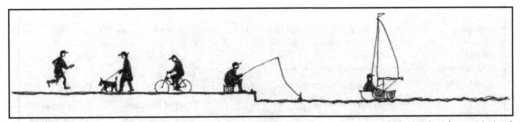

Figure 7-5. Occupations used for reflection and time to "be." (© Trevor Bywater 2013. Used with permission.)

High-powered mental doing or feeling should be interwoven with time for rest and simply being at ease with oneself.[210] A balance of occupations between mental and physical activities, intellectual challenges, spiritual experiences, emotional highs and lows, effort, relaxation, and sleep is required. Well-being will be enhanced if people, in their chosen or obligatory occupations, are able to develop spiritual, cognitive, and emotive capacities to experience timelessness and "higher-order meaning."[211] Occupation that allows people to reflect and relax may be many and various. Some of those commonly found suited to being are illustrated in Figure 7-5. Along those lines, John Hersey's admission of "feeling nourished and transformed" as a result of his literary work makes sense.[212] It appears to be important that occupational and spiritual natures and needs are intertwined and taken into consideration as a complementary whole. This calls for a balance between active doing and time for quiet and reflection. Being as an integral part of occupation will have the most obvious health promoting effects if socially sanctioned, approved, valued, and endowing social status.

Figure 7-6 provides an overview of the complex relationship between illness or physical, mental, and social well-being and being as an aspect of occupation. Human characteristics and biological needs are the foundation stones of the human need to "be," as they are of health and cultural evolution. The need to find meaning and purpose has led to the establishment of unique economies, political systems, and national values, policies, and priorities.

The utilities that emanate from those underlying institutions also provide positive or negative influence on national, community, family, or individual health by delivering or restricting occupation that provides meaning and nourishes the mind and spirit, as well as the body. The positive or negative consequences of the underlying factors or facilities that grow from them may not be the same for all communities or for all individuals. As the WHO claims, there is a "need to respond to each individual's spiritual quest for meaning, purpose and belonging" because "health depends on validation of the uniqueness of each person."[1]

This chapter on being true to the inner self, or being through occupation, has considered both the provision of the prerequisites of survival and the biological characteristics and capacities that go beyond them. Complex capacities, such as consciousness and creativity, have enabled people to not only meet their basic needs, but also to develop unique interests, seek meaning, find purpose through what they do, continually seek out the new and the different, and adapt culturally to many different natural and social environments. A brain capable of meeting a whole range of biological needs and sociocultural adaptations is common to mankind but is also unique to each individual. The next chapters will explore these ideas still further, as occupation and health are considered from the perspective of people reaching out toward belonging in their communities and becoming what they have the potential to become through what they do.

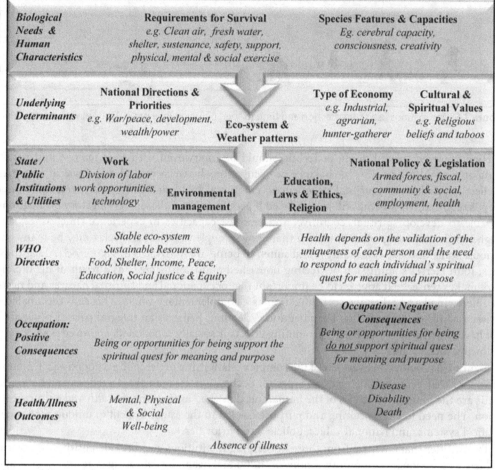

Figure 7-6. Being determinants of illness or well-being.

References

1. World Health Organization. *Health for All in the Twenty-first Century.* 1998. www.euro.who.int/__data/assets/pdf_file/0004/109759/EHFA5-E.pdf. Accessed November 2, 2005.
2. Behavior. *Merriam-Webster Dictionary.* http://www.merriam-webster.com/dictionary/behavior. Accessed May 29, 2014.
3. Landau SI, chief ed. *Funk & Wagnalls Standard Desk Dictionary.* Vol 1. Harper & Row Publishers Inc; 1984:58.
4. *Word Finder: Australian Thesaurus.* Sydney, Australia: Reader's Digest; 1983:56.
5. Campbell BG. *Humankind Emerging.* 5th ed. New York, NY: Harper Collins Publishers; 1988:364-365.
6. Cohen SM. Aristotle's metaphysics. *The Stanford Encyclopedia of Philosophy* (Spring 2009 ed). Zalta EN, ed. http://plato.stanford.edu/archives/spr2009/entries/aristotle-metaphysics/. Accessed May 14, 2012.
7. Hegel G. *The Phenomenology of Spirit.* Trans AV Miller. Oxford: Clarenden Press; 1977. Original work published 1807.
8. Heidegger M. *Sein und Zeit (Being and Time).* J Macquarie and E Robinson, trans. Oxford: Basil Blackwell; 1978. Original work published 1927.
9. Sartre J. *Stanford Encyclopedia of Philosophy.* http://plato.stanford.edu/entries/sartre/. Accessed May 13, 2014.
10. Maslow AH. *Toward a Psychology of Being.* 2nd ed. New York, NY: D Van Nostrand Co; 1968:214.

11. Hocking C. *The Relationship between Objects and Identity in Occupational Therapy: A Dynamic Balance of Rationalism and Romanticism.* Auckland University of Technology: Unpublished PhD Thesis; 2004:137.

12. Consciousness. *Internet Encyclopedia of Philosophy.* http://www.iep.utm.edu/consciou/. Accessed May 15, 2014.

13. Consciousness. *Merriam-Webster Online Dictionary.* http://www.merriam-webster.com/dictionary/consciousness. Accessed June 4, 2012.

14. van Gulick R. Consciousness. *Stanford Encyclopedia of Philosophy.* 2004. http://plato.stanford.edu/entries/consciousness/. Accessed May 28, 2014.

15. Consciousness. *The Macquarie Dictionary.* Sydney, NSW: Macquarie Dictionary Publications; 1981.

16. Velman M, Schneider S. Introduction. *The Blackwell Companion to Consciousness.* Hoboken, NJ: Wiley; 2008.

17. Churchland PM. *Matter and Consciousness.* Rev ed. Cambridge, MA: Bradford Book; 1988:73.

18. Ornstein R. *The Evolution of Consciousness: The Origins of the Way We Think.* New York, NY: Touchstone; 1991:228.

19. Block N. *Philosophical Issues about Consciousness.* http://www.nyu.edu/gsas/dept/philo/faculty/block/papers/ecs.pdf. Accessed November 5, 2005.

20. Frackowiak R. The Neural Correlates of Consciousness. In: *Human Brain Function.* Academic Press; 2004:269.

21. Edelman G. *Bright Air, Brilliant Fire: On the Matter of the Mind.* London, England: Penguin Books; 1992:83-85,117-119,134.

22. Hearn R, Granger R. Models of thalamocortical system. *Scholarpedia,* 2007; 2(11):1796.

23. Ornstein R. *The Evolution of Consciousness: The Origins of the Way We Think.* New York, NY: Touchstone; 1991.

24. Csikszentmihalyi M. Activity and happiness: toward a science of occupation. *Journal of Occupational Science: Australia.* 1993;1(1):38-42.

25. Csikszentmihalyi M, Csikszentmihalyi IS, eds. *Optimal Experience: Psychological Studies of Flow in Consciousness.* New York, NY: Cambridge University Press; 1988:20-23.

26. Dossey L. Consciousness and health: what's it all about. *Topics in Clinical Nursing.* 1982;3(Jan):1-6.

27. Newman MA. Newman's theory of health as praxis. *Nursing Science Quarterly.* 1990;3(1):37-41.

28. Burch S. Consciousness: how does it relate to health? *Journal of Holistic Nursing.* 1994;12(1):101-116.

29. Dossey BM. The transpersonal self and states of consciousness. In: Dossey BM, Keegan L, Kolkmier LG, Guzzetta CE, eds. *Holistic Health Promotion. A Guide for Practice.* Rockville, MD: Aspen Publications; 1989:32.

30. Green E, Green A. Biofeedback and transformation. In: Kunz D, ed. *Spiritual Aspects of the Healing Arts.* Wheaton, Ill: The Theosophical Publishing House; 1985:145-162.

31. Caplan M. *Eyes Wide Open: Cultivating Discernment on the Spiritual Path.* Louisville, CO: Sounds True; 2009.

32. Grimshaw A. Consciousness raising. In: Bullock A, Stalleybrass O, Trombley S, eds. *The Fontana Dictionary of Modern Thought.* 2nd ed. London, England: Fontana Press; 1988:166.

33. Koerner JG, Bunkers SS. The healing web: an expansion of consciousness. *Journal of Holistic Nursing.* 1994;12(1):51-63.

34. Smith-Campbell B. Kansans' perceptions of health care reform: a qualitative study on coming to public judgement. *Public Health Nursing.* 1995;12(2):134-139.

35. Crisp R. Well-being. *The Stanford Encyclopedia of Philosophy* (Summer 2013 Edition), Edward N. Zalta (ed.). http://plato.stanford.edu/archives/sum2013/entries/well-being/. Accessed April 9, 2005.

36. Dr Rex. *Meaning of PEACE .... starts in our brain!* http://hrexach.wordpress.com/2013/05/10/meaning-of-peace/. Posted May 10, 2013. Accessed May 27, 2014.

37. Personal Enlightenment. *Global Country of World Peace.* http://www.globalcountry.org/wp/personal-enlightenment/#. Accessed May 21, 2014.

38. Klinkenborg V. The Definition of Home. *Smithsonian Magazine,* May 2012. http://www.smithsonian-mag.com/science-nature/The-Definition-of-Home.html. Accessed May 12, 2014.

39. Cate. The Meaning of Home. *A Shelter SA Project.* July 14, 2008. http://sheltersa.wordpress.com/. Accessed November 20, 2012.

40. Delors J. Learning: The Treasure Within. *Report to UNESCO of the International Commission on Education for the Twenty-first Century.* Paris: UNESCO;1996. unesdoc.unesco.org/images/0010/001095/109590eo.pdf. Accessed February 10, 2013

41. Schofield K. 1999. In: *The Purposes of Education*. A research project commissioned by Education Queensland as a contribution to the development of Queensland State Education: 2010.

42. Robinson K. Do schools kill creativity? *Talk at the TED: Ideas worth spreading conference.* June, 2006. http://www.ted.com/index.php/talks/ken_robinson_says_schools_kill_creativity.html. Accessed August 2, 2008.

43. Kartasidou L. Creativity in its broadest sense and its role in the education of children with severe disabilities – a case study. *The Meaning of Creativity in Education – Inter-Disciplinary.Net.* http://inter-disciplinary.net/ati/education/cp/ce2/Kartasidou%20paper.pdf. Accessed November 11, 2012.

44. Craft A. *An Analysis of Research and Literature on Creativity in Education.* A Report prepared for the Qualifications and Curriculum Authority. March 2001.

45. United Nations Treaty Collection. *International Covenant on Economic, Social and Cultural Rights (ICESCR).* https://treaties.un.org/Pages/ViewDetails.aspx?src=TREATY&mtdsg_no=IV-3&chapter=4&lang=en. Accessed June 1, 2011.

46. Mead M. The changing significance of food. In: Counihan C, Van Esterik P, eds. *Food and Culture: A Reader.* UK: Routledge, 1997, 11-19.

47. Winefield AH, Tiggerman M, Goldney RD. Psychological concomitants of satisfactory employment and unemployment in young people. *Social Psychiatry and Psychiatric Epidemiology.* 1988;23:149-157.

48. Brenner MH. Health costs and benefits of economic policy. *International Journal of Health Services.* 1977;7:581-593.

49. Brenner MH. Mortality and the national economy: a review, and the experience of England and Wales. *Lancet.* 1979;ii:568-573.

50. Smith R. *Unemployment and Health: A Disaster and a Challenge.* Oxford, UK: Oxford University Press; 1987:2.

51. Applebaum H. *The Concept of Work: Ancient, Medieval and Modern.* New York: State University of New York Press; 1992.

52. Capon AG. Inaugural Ann Wilcock Lecture: Human occupations as determinants of population health: linking perspectives on people, places and planet. *Journal of Occupational Science.* 2014;21(1):8-11. doi:10.1080/14427591.2014.891430

53. Croke Sir A. *Regimen Sanitatis Salernitanum: A Poem on the Preservation of Health in Rhyming Latin Verse.* Oxford: D.A. Talboys; 1830.

54. Tranter P. The active living cure for the hurry virus: time pressure, health and the paradox of speed. *Journal of Occupational Science.* 2014;21(1):8-11. doi:10.1080/14427591.2013.865153.

55a. Pelton L. *Doing Justice: Liberalism, Group Constructs, and Individual Realities.* Albany, NY; State University of New York Press; 1999.

55b. World Health Organization, Health and Welfare Canada, Canadian Public Health Association. *Ottawa Charter for Health Promotion.* Ottawa, Canada; 1986.

55c. Jahoda M. *Employment and Unemployment.* New York, NY: Cambridge University Press; 1982.

55d. Jahoda M. Economic recession and mental health: some conceptual issues. *Journal of Social Issues.* 1988;44(4):13-23.

56. Selye H, Monat A, Lazarus RS. *Stress and Coping: An Anthology.* 2nd ed. New York, NY: Columbia University Press; 1985:28.

57. Frankl VE. *Man's Search for Meaning.* New York: Pocket Books, 1963.

58. Lieberman P. Evolution of the speech apparatus. In: Jones S, Martin R, Pilbeam D, eds. *The Cambridge Encyclopedia of Human Evolution.* New York, NY: Cambridge University Press; 1992:136-137.

59. Ornstein R, Sobel D. *The Healing Brain: A Radical New Approach to Health Care.* London, England: Macmillan; 1988:39.

60. Ornstein R, Sobel D. *The Healing Brain: A Radical New Approach to Health Care.* London, England: Macmillan; 1988:57.

61. Gagne F. Transforming gifts into talents. In: Colabango N, Davis G, eds. *Handbook of Gifted Education.* 3rd ed. Boston: Pearson Education; 1991:60-74.

62. Campbell J. *Winston Churchill's Afternoon Nap.* London, England: Palladin Grafton Books; 1986:44-54,166,194,290.

63. Gardner H. Frames of mind. *The Theory of Multiple Intelligences.* New York, NY: Basic Books; 1983:290.

64. Percy Bysshe Shelley. *Prometheus Unbound,* II, IV. London, England: C and J Ollier; 1820.

65. Lewin R. *In the Age of Mankind: A Smithsonian Book of Human Evolution.* Washington, DC: Smithsonian Books; 1988:174,179-180.

66. Piaget J. *Six Psychological Studies.* New York, NY: Random House; 1967:98.

67. Hamlyn DW. *A History of Western Philosophy*. England: Viking; 1987:15.
68. Gordon R. The creative process. In: Jennings S, ed. *Creative Therapy*. London, England: Pitman Publishing; 1975:1.
69. Jung CG. *Collected Works*. Princeton, NJ: Princeton University Press; 1959.
70. Sinnott EW. The creativeness of life. In: Vernon PE, ed. *Creativity*. London, England: Penguin Books; 1970:115.
71. Brolin C. Kreativitet och Kritiskt Tandande. Redsckap for Framtidsberedskap (Creativity and Critical Thinking. Tools for Preparedness for the Future). *Krut*. 1992: 53;64-71.
72. Morgan DN. Creativity today. *Journal of Aesthetics*. 1953;12:1-24.
73. Young JG. What is creativity? *Journal of Creative Behaviour*. 1985;19(2):77-87.
74. Creativity. *The Standard English Desk Dictionary*. 2nd ed. Oxford, UK: Oxford University Press; 1975.
75. Schmid T. *Promoting Health through Creativity: For Professionals in Health, Arts and Education*. London: Whurr Publishers; 2005: 27.
76. Lewin R. *In the Age of Mankind: A Smithsonian Book of Human Evolution*. Washington, DC: Smithsonian Books; 1988.
77. Leakey R. *The Making of Mankind*. London, England: Michael Joseph Ltd; 1981.
78. Marx K. *Karl Marx: Early Writings*. R Livingstone, G Benton, trans. London, England; Penguin Classics: 1975.
79. Morris W. 1884. In: Morton AL, ed. *Political Writings of William Morris*. London, England: Lawrence and Wishart; 1973.
80. Hand N. *D.W. Winnicott (Microform): The Creative Vision*. National Library of Australia. Distributed by ERIC Clearinghouse, 1996.
81. Skinner BF. *The Science of Behaviour*. New York, NY: Macmillan; 1953.
82. Maslow AH. *Toward a Psychology of Being*. 2nd ed. New York, NY: D Van Nostrand Co; 1968.
83. Amabile TM. *The Social Psychology of Creativity*. New York, NY: Springer Verlag; 1983.
84. Gardner H. *Creating Minds: An Anatomy of Creativity Seen through the Lives of Freud, Einstein, Picasso, Stravinsky, Eliot, Graham, and Gandhi*. New York, NY: Basic Books; 1993.
85. Freud S. Leonardo da Vinci and a memory of his childhood. In: Stachey J, ed. *The Standard Edition of the Complete Works of Sigmund Freud*. Vol 10. Hogarth Press, London; 1957:57-137. (originally published 1910)
86. Galton F, *Hereditary Genius: An Inquiry into its Laws and Consequences*. London: Macmillan; 1869.
87. Guilford J. Creativity. *American Psychologist*. 1950; 5: 444-445.
88. Getzels J, Cziksentmihalyi M. *The Creative Vision: A Longitudinal Study of Problem-Solving in Art*. Wiley; New York: 1976.
89. MacKinnon D. IPAR's contribution to the conceptualization and study of creativity. In: Taylor & Getzels, eds. *Perspectives in Creativity*. Aldine, Chicago IL; 1975:60-89.
90. Simonton D. *Genius, Creativity and Leadership: Historiometric Enquiries*. Cambridge, MA; Harvard University Press; 1984.
91. Ryhammar L, Brolin C. Creativity research: historical considerations and main lines of development. *Scandinavian Journal of Educational Research*. 1999; 43(3): 259-273.
92. Jeffrey B, Craft A. The universalization of creativity. In: Craft A, Jeffrey B, Leibling M. eds. *Creativity in Education*. London: Continuum; 2001.
93. Cziksentmihalyi M. Society, culture and person: a systems view of creativity. In: Sternberg R, ed. *The Nature of Creativity*. Cambridge: Cambridge University Press; 1998: 325-339.
94. Sternberg R. A three-facet model of creativity. In: Sternberg RJ, ed. *The Nature of Creativity*. Cambridge: Cambridge University Press; 1988.
95. Sternberg R, Lubart T. An investment theory of creativity and its development. *Human Development*. 1991;34:1-31.
96. Sternberg R, Lubart T. *Defying the Crowd. Cultivating Creativity in a Culture of Conformity*. New York: The Free Press; 1995.
97. Bruce MA, Borg B. *Frames of Reference in Psychosocial Occupational Therapy*. Thorofare, NJ: SLACK Inc; 1987.
98. Taylor IA, Getzels JW, eds. *Perspectives in Creativity*. Chicago, Ill: Aldine Publishing Co; 1975.
99. Freud S. *A General Introduction to Psychoanalysis*. Hall GS, trans. New York, NY: Boni and Liveright; 1920.
100. Freud S. *Creativity and the Unconscious*. New York, NY: Harper and Row; 1958.
101. Freud S. Creative writers and daydreaming. In: Strachey J, ed. *The Standard Edition of the Complete Psychological Works of Sigmund Freud*. Vol 9. London, England: Hogarth Press; 1959.

102. Barron F. *Creative Person and Creative Process*. New York, NY: Holt, Rinehart and Winston; 1969.

103. Maslow AH. *Motivation and Personality*. New York, NY: Harper and Row; 1954.

104. Solomon R. Creativity and normal narcissism. *Journal of Creative Behaviour*. 1985;19(1):47-55.

105. Eysenck H. Addiction, personality and motivation. *Human Psychopharmacology*. 1997;12: S79-S87.

106. Dacey J, Lennon K. *Understanding Creativity: The Interplay of Biological, Psychological and Social Factors*. Creative Education Foundation, Buffalo, NY; 2000.

107. Amabile T. Motivating creativity in organizations: On doing what you love and loving what you do. *California Management Review*. 1997:40(I);39-58.

108. Feldman D. *Beyond Universals in Cognitive Development*. Norwood, NJ: Ablex; 1980.

109. Dennis W. Creative productivity between the ages of 20 and 80 years. *Journal of Gerontology*. 1966;21:106-114.

110. Lehman H. *Age and Achievement*. Princeton, NJ: Princeton University Press; 1953.

111. Simonton DK. Sociocultural context of individual creativity: a transhistorical time-series analysis. *Journal of Personality and Social Psychology*. 1975;32:1119-1133.

112. High technology. In: Atomic Power for Europe. *The New York Times*. February 4, 1958:17. http://query.nytimes.com/gst/abstract.html?res=9803EEDA173DE53BBC4D51DFB0668383649EDE. Accessed November 5th, 2005.

113. Sternberg R. The nature of creativity. *Creativity Research Journal*. 2006;18(1):93.

114. Fisher B, Specht D. Successful aging and creativity in later life. *Journal of Aging Studies*. 1999;13:457-472.

115. Forthofer M, Hanz M, Dodge J, Clark N. Gender differences in the associations self esteem, stress and social support with functional health status among older adults with heart disease. *Journal of Women and Aging*. 2001;13:19-36.

116. Clift S, Hancox G. The perceived benefits of singing: Findings from preliminary surveys of a university college choral society. *Journal of the Royal Society for the Promotion of Health*. 2001;121:248-256.

117. Reynolds F. The effects of creativity on physical and psychological well-being: current and new directions for research. In: Schmid T. *Promoting Health through Creativity: For Professionals in Health, Arts and Education*. London: Whurr Publishers; 2005; 112-131.

118. Colish ML. *The Stoic Tradition from Antiquity to the Early Middle Ages*. (2 volumes) Leiden: E.J. Brill; 1985;40.

119. Stoics. Girling DA, ed. *New Age Encyclopaedia*. Vol. 27. Sydney, Australia: Bay Books; 1983:160-161.

120. Leakey R, Lewin R. *People of the Lake: Man: His Origins, Nature, and Future*. New York, NY: Penguin Books; 1978.

121. van der Merwe NJ. Reconstructing prehistoric diet. In: Jones S, Martin R, Pilbeam D, eds. *The Cambridge Encyclopedia of Human Evolution*. New York, NY: Cambridge University Press; 1992:369-372.

122. Leakey R. *The Making of Mankind*. London, England: Michael Joseph Ltd; 1981.

123. Buranhult G, ed. *The First Humans: Human Origins and History to 10,000BC*. Australia: University of Queensland Press; 1993:98-99.

124. Wax RH. Free time in other cultures. In: Donahue W, et al, eds. *Free Time: Challenge to Later Maturity*. Ann Arbor, MI: University of Michigan Press; 1958:3-16.

125. Parker S. *Leisure and Work*. London, England: George Allen and Unwin; 1983.

126. Jones B. *Sleepers, Wake! Technology and the Future of Work*. Melbourne, Australia: Oxford University Press; 1995:11.

127. Neff WS. *Work and Human Behaviour*. 3rd ed. New York, NY: Aldine Publishing Co; 1985:33, 35.

128. Wilcock AA. *Occupation for Health. Volume 1. A Journey from Self Health to Prescription*. London, UK: COT; 2001.

129. Locke J. *An Essay Concerning Humane Understanding*. London: Printed for Tho, Basset, and sold by Edw. Mory at the sign of the Three Bibles in St Paul's Church-Yard; MDCXC (1690).

130. Burton R. *The Anatomy of Melancholy*. Oxford: Printed for Henry Cripps; 1651: Index.

131. Sanctorius Sanctorius. Medicina Statica. In: Sinclair, Sir J. *Code of Health and Longevity*. Edinburgh: Arch Constable & Co, 1806; 184-189.

132. Scull A. Moral treatment reconsidered: some sociological comments on the episode in the history of British psychiatry. In: Scull A, ed. *Madhouses, Mad-Doctors and Madmen: The Social History of Psychiatry in the Victorian Era*. Philadelphia, PA: University of Pennsylvania Press; 1981:108,115.

133. Cullen W. First lines in the practice of physics. In: Hunter RA, MacAlpine I, eds. *Three Hundred Years of Psychiatry*. London, England: Oxford University Press; 1963.

134. Bynum W. Rationales for therapy in British psychiatry, 1780-1835. In: Scull A, ed. *Madhouses, Mad-Doctors and Madmen: The Social History of Psychiatry in the Victorian Era.* Philadelphia, PA: University of Pennsylvania Press; 1981.

135. Spark Notes: History. *The Enlightenment (1650–1800).* http://www.sparknotes.com/history/european/enlightenment/context.html. Accessed August 15, 2013.

136. Pinel P. Traite medico-philosophique sur l'alienation mentale. In: Foucault M. *Madness and Civilization: A History of Insanity in the Age of Reason.* New York, NY: Random House; 1973:258.

137. Pinel P. *A Treatise on Insanity.* Translated from the French by D. D. Davis, MD. Sheffield: Printed by W. Todd, for Messrs Cadell and Davies, Strand London: 1806. Reprinted: Birmingham, Alabama: Classics of Medicine Library, 1983:195.

138. Leuret F. 1840. On the moral treatment of insanity. In: Licht S. *Occupational Therapy Source Book.* Baltimore, MD: Williams and Wilkins; 1948.

139. Foucault M. *Madness and Civilization: A History of Insanity in the Age of Reason.* New York, NY: Random House; 1973.

140. Tuke S. *Description of the Retreat.* York: Alexander; 1813.

141. Browne WAF. *What Asylums Were, Are and Ought to Be.* Edinburgh: A. & C. Black; 1837. Reprinted: Classics in Psychiatry: Arno Press Collection. North Stratford, UK: Ayer Company Publishers; 2001:177.

142. Corsini RJ, ed. *Encylopedia of Psychology.* Vol 2. New York, NY: John Wiley and Sons; 1984:162.

143. Bockoven JS. *Moral Treatment in American Society.* New York, NY: Springer; 1963.

144. Kirkebride TS. Annual Report of the Pennsylvania Hospital for the Insane. Cited in: Tomes NJ. A generous confidence: Thomas Story Kirkebride's philosophy of asylum construction and management. In: Scull A, ed. *Madhouses, Mad-Doctors and Madmen: The Social History of Psychiatry in the Victorian Era.* Philadelphia, PA: University of Pennsylvania Press; 1981.

145. Serrett KD, ed. *Philosophical and Historical Roots of Occupational Therapy.* New York, NY: The Haworth Press; 1985.

146. Campanella T. *City of the Sun.* Donno DJ, trans. Berkeley, CA: University of California Press; 1981.

147. Marx K. *Early Writings.* New York, NY: Penguin Classics; 1992.

148. Marx K. *Early Writings.* New York, NY: Penguin Classics; 1992:328.

149. Ruskin J. *Unto This Last.* London, England: Collins Publishers; 1970. (original work published 1862.)

150. Coleridge ST. *The Friend.* New York, NY: Freeport; 1971. (original work published 1818.)

151. Carlyle T. Sartor Resartus 1833-1834. In: *Sartor Resartus, and On Heroes and Hero Worship.* London, England: Dent; 1908. Reprinted New York, NY: Dutton; 1973.

152. MacCarthy F. *William Morris: A Life for Our Time.* London, England: Faber and Faber; 1994:70-71.

153. Cole GDH. In: Selgman ERA, ed. *Encyclopaedia of Social Science.* New York, NY: Macmillan; 1933.

154. Morris W. Art and socialism. In: Morton AL, ed. *Political Writings of William Morris.* London, England: Lawrence and Wishart; 1973:110-111.

155. Morris W. Art and socialism. In: Morton AL, ed. *Political Writings of William Morris.* London, England: Lawrence and Wishart; 1973:603-604.

156. Jackson Lears TJ. *No Place of Grace: Antimodernism and the Transformation of American Culture 1880-1920.* New York, NY: Pantheon Books; 1981:63-64.

157. Morris W. Useful work versus useless toil. In: Morton AL, ed. *Political Writings of William Morris.* London, England: Lawrence and Wishart; 1973.

158. Morris W. News from nowhere. In: Morton AL, ed. *Three Works by William Morris: News from Nowhere, The Pilgrims of Hope, A Dream of John Ball.* London, England: Lawrence and Wishart; 1968.

159. Amabile T, Kramer S. *The Progress Principle.* Harvard Business Review Press; 2011.

160. Amabile T. Kramer S. How leaders kill meaning at work. *McKinsey Quarterly.* January, 2012.

161. Csikszentmihalyi M. *Good Business: Leadership, Flow, and the Making of Meaning.* New York: Penguin Books; 2003.

162. Csikszentmihalyi M. *Finding Flow: The Psychology of Engagement with Everyday Life.* New York; Basic Books. 1996.

163. Csikszentmihalyi M. *Beyond Boredom and Anxiety.* San Francisco, CA: 1975.

164. World Health Organization. *What is Mental Health? Online Q&A.* 2007. http://www.who.int/features/qa/62/en/index.html. Accessed on May 13, 2012.

165. World Health Organization Commission on Social Determinants of Health. Interim Statement. *Achieving Health Equity: From Root Causes to Fair Outcomes.* 2007. http://www.who.int/social_determinants/resources/csdh_media/cdsh_interim_statement_final_07.pdf. Accessed May 17, 2013.

166. World Health Organization. *Mental Health: Strengthening our Response.* Fact sheet N°220. Updated April 2014. http://www.who.int/mediacentre/factsheets/fs220/en/. Accessed June 24, 2014.

167. World Health Organization. *Global Burden of Mental Disorders and the Need for a Comprehensive, Coordinated Response from Health and Social Sectors at the Country Level.* EB130.R8. http://www.who.int/violence_injury_prevention/media/news/2012/20_01/en/index.html. Accessed May 10, 2012.

168. World Health Organization. Mental Health Gap Action Programme. *Scaling up Care for Mental, Neurological, and Substance Use Disorders.* 2008. http://www.who.int/mental_health/evidence/mhGAP/en/index.html. Accessed May 17, 2012.

169. World Health Organization. *Mental Health Policy and Service Guidance Package: The Mental Health Context.* Geneva: WHO; 2003. http://www.who.int/mental_health/policy/essentialpackage1/en/index.html. Accessed May 17, 2012.

170. Fryer D, Payne R. Proactive behaviour in unemployment: findings and implications. *Leisure Studies.* 1984;3:273-295.

171. World Health Organization, Health and Welfare Canada, Canadian Public Health Association. *Ottawa Charter for Health Promotion.* Ottawa, Canada, 1986.

172. World Health Organization. *Jakarta Declaration on Leading Health Promotion into the 21st Century.* 4th International Conference on Health Promotion, Jakarta, Indonesia, 21-25th July, 1997.

173. Bruner J. Nature and uses of immaturity. *Am Psychol.* 1972;August:687-708.

174. Jenkins C, Sherman B. *The Leisure Shock.* London, England: Eyre Methuen Ltd; 1981.

175. Scott D. *The Psychology of Work.* London: Duckworth; 1970;233-234.

176. Scott D. *The Psychology of Work.* London: Duckworth; 1970;228.

177. Scott D. *The Psychology of Work.* London: Duckworth; 1970;229-230.

178. Warr P. Twelve questions about unemployment and health. In: Roberts R, Finnegan R, Gallie D, eds. *New Approaches to Economic Life.* Manchester: Manchester University Press; 1985.

179. Colish ML. *The Stoic Tradition from Antiquity to the Early Middle Ages.* (2 volumes) Leiden: E.J.Brill; 1985;41.

180. Jenkins C, Sherman B. *The Leisure Shock.* London, England: Eyre Methuen Ltd; 1981:1,5.

181. Keniston K. Social change and youth in America. *Daedalus.* 1962;Winter:145-171.

182. Friedlander F. Importance of work versus non-work among socially and occupationally stratified groups. *Journal of Applied Psychology.* 1966;December:437-441.

183. Hollander P. Leisure as an American and Soviet value. *Social Problems.* 1966;3:179-188.

184. Robertson J. *Future Work.* England: Gower Publishing Co; 1985.

185. Pettifer S. Leisure as compensation for unemployment and unfulfilling work. Reality or pipe dream? *Journal of Occupational Science: Australia.* 1993;1(2):20-26.

186. Galvaan R. Occupational choice: the significance of socio-economic and political factors. In: Whiteford GE, Hocking C, eds. *Occupational Science: Society, Inclusion, Participation.* Chichester, UK; Wiley-Blackwell; 2012:152-162.

187. Radford J, ed. *Gender and Choice in Education and Occupation.* London: Routledge; 1998; iv.

188. Smith R. *Unemployment and Health: A Disaster and a Challenge.* Oxford, UK: Oxford University Press; 1987.

189. Colledge M, Bartholomew R. *A Study of the Long Term Unemployed.* London, England: Manpower Services Commission; 1980.

190. Jackson PR, Warr PB. Unemployment and psychological ill health: the moderating role of duration and age. *Psychological Medicine.* 1984;14:605-614.

191. Dowling PJ, De Cieri H, Griffin G, Brown M. Psychological aspects of redundancy: an Australian case study. *Journal of Industrial Relations.* 1987;29(4):519-531.

192. Platt S. Unemployment and suicidal behaviour: a review of the literature. *Social Science Medicine.* 1984;19:93-115.

193. Scott-Samuel A. Unemployment and health. *Lancet.* 1984;ii:1464-1465.

194. Moser KA, Fox AJ, Jones DR. Unemployment and mortality in the OPCS longitudinal study. *Lancet.* 1984;ii:1324-1329.

195. Moser KA, Goldblatt PO, Fox AJ, Jones DR. Unemployment and mortality: comparison of the 1971 and 1981 longitudinal census sample. *British Medical Journal.* 1987;294:86-90.

196. Kerr C, Taylor R. Grim prospects for the unemployed. *New Doctor.* 1993;Summer:23-24.

197. Gravelle H. *Does Unemployment Kill?* Oxford, UK: Nuffield Provincial Hospitals Trust; 1985.

198. Jaco EG. *The Social Epidemiology of Mental Disorders.* New York, NY: Russell Sage Foundation; 1960.

199. Fox A. Socio-demographic consequences of unemployment: a study of changes in individuals' characteristics between 1971 and 1981. London: City University, Social Statistics Research Unit; 1986.

200. Daniel W. How the unemployed fare after they find new jobs. *Policy Studies*. 1983; 3: 246-60.

201. Daniel W. *The Unemployed Flow*. London; Policy Studies Institute; 1990.

202. Westergaard J, Noble I, Walker A. *After Redundancy: The Experience of Economic Insecurity*. Cambridge, PolityPress; 1989.

203. Cook DG, Cummins RO, Bartley MJ, Shaper AG. Health of unemployed middle aged men in Great Britain. *Lancet*. 1982;i:1290-1294.

204. Beale N, Nethercott S. Job loss and family morbidity: a study of factory closure. *Journal of Royal College General Practitioners*. 1985;280: 510-514.

205. McClelland A, Pirkis J, Willcox S. *Enough to Make You Sick: How Income and Environment Affect Health*. National Health Strategy Research Paper No 1, National Health Strategy Unit, Commonwealth Department of Health, Housing and Community Services Canberra. 1992.

206. Aungles SB, Parker SR. *Work, Organisations and Change: Themes and Perspectives in Australia*. Sydney, Australia: George Allen and Unwin; 1988.

207. Lilley J, Jackson L. The value of activities: establishing a foundation for cost effectiveness. A review of the literature. *Activities, Adaptation and Aging*. 1990;14(4):12-13.

208. Foster P. Activities: a necessity for total health care of the long term care resident. *Activities, Adaptation and Aging*. 1983;3(3):17-23.

209. World Health Organization. *Health Impact Assessment (HIA): The Determinants of Health*. http://www.who.int/hia/evidence/doh/en/index.html. Accessed May 18, 2012.

210. do Rozario L. Ritual, meaning and transcendence: the role of occupation in modern life. *Journal of Occupational Science: Australia*. 1994;1(3):46-53.

211. Rappaport R. *Ecology, Meaning, and Religion*. Richmond, VA: North Atlantic Books; 1979.

212. Hersey J. Time's winged chariot. In: Fadiman C, ed. *Living Philosophies: The Reflections of Some Eminent Men and Women of Our Time*. New York, NY: Doubleday; 1990.

Theme 8

"Create Supportive Environments: Our societies are complex and interrelated. Health cannot be separated from other goals ... The overall guiding principle for the world, nations, regions and communities alike, is the need to encourage reciprocal maintenance—to take care of each other, our communities and our natural environment."

WHO: Ottawa Charter for
Health Promotion, 1986[1]

Chapter 8

OCCUPATION
BELONGING THROUGH DOING

This chapter addresses:
- Introduction to the Concept of Belonging as an Aspect of Doing
- Belonging and Health
  - Natural Health: Prerequisites
    - Belonging and Peace
    - Belonging and Shelter
    - Belonging and Education
    - Belonging and Food
    - Belonging and Income
    - Belonging: Stable Ecosystem and Sustainable Resources
    - Belonging: Social Justice and Equity
- Rules for Health Through Belonging: From Ancient to Modern
  - Biological Basis of Belonging and Health
    - Altruism and Belonging to Cooperative Social Groups
    - Empathy and Belonging to Cooperative Social Groups
  - Belonging and Health in Early History
  - Belonging and Health in Modern Times
    - Evaluating the Evidence for the Need to Belong
    - Belonging in Complex Social Structures
- Conclusion: Well-Being and the Quest for Belonging

The human need to belong is strongly felt. As Donne (1572-1631) asserted, "no man is an island, entire of itself; every man is a piece of the continent, a part of the main; … any man's death diminishes me, because I am involved in mankind."[2] In this chapter, the focus is on the well-being accrued from belonging. The discussion explores the sense of belonging experienced in the ease and familiarity of doing things with people you care for or have known for a long time or with others less close who share a sense of place, rather than the legal status of belonging through

Wilcock AA, Hocking C.
An Occupational Perspective of Health, Third Edition (pp 210-237).
© 2015 Taylor & Francis Group.

birthright, marriage, or citizenship. The relationships built through doing things together are pivotal because, as d'Estain asserted, "you can't build a society purely on interests, you need a sense of belonging,"[3] a sense of being interlinked with particular people and specific places. Belonging through doing, as the WHO theme for the chapter states, is about creating supportive environments in increasingly complex social and political contexts because health for all depends on taking care of each other and the natural environment.

Introduction to the Concept of Belonging as an Aspect of Doing

Doing with, alongside, and for other people fosters relationships and belonging among family, friends, organizations, and community. Even occupations performed alone are often done in relation to other people, providing feelings of connection and of being cared for and wanted.[4] Being with other people provides some of the fundamental meaning of occupation because it is through doing things with others that bonds are created and obligation, shared interests, and intimacy are experienced. Dictionaries explain that having a sense of belonging is about having the right personal and social attributes[5] to be recognized as a friend, member, supporter, or devotee of a group.[6] To a great extent, such attributes are revealed and honed through engagement in occupation, wherein important qualities such as courage, dexterity, and a sense of humor, creativity, patience, honesty, and willingness to follow directions or to take the lead are called upon.

Members of modern societies belong in multiple ways and at different times.[7] Networks of people relate to each other as family members and friends; as members of the same ethnic group, generation, or team; and as workmates, associates, volunteers, neighbors, and citizens. Figure 8-1 provides a sense of the rich array of ways in which humans come together and identify their relationship to others. Belonging is not static; rather, it is "always provisional and in process."[8] The processes by which people forge, develop, and terminate connections are rarely examined or spoken about, but require being alert to the politics of belonging and giving attention to how groups determine who can belong, who is trying to belong, how they are doing so, and for what purpose.[9]

At a personal level, belonging through doing stems from relationships that confer a sense of familiarity, affinity, kinship, commitment, affection, goodwill, and attachment.[10,11] Belonging is enacted through everyday practices, social conventions, behavioral norms, and rituals.[12] It might involve individuals doing something on behalf of others or participation in collective occupations; the domestic routines that construct a family, the productive tasks undertaken by workers and volunteers, or the shared responsibilities of office holders and organizers. Festivals, sporting events, and common concerns bring whole communities together. Subgroups get together to practice their faith, have fun, get fit, celebrate achievements and milestones, and engage in political activities. Group occupations offer opportunities for doing things together to meet a common purpose, which can enhance the pleasure and meaning derived from the doing. The sharing of values, stories, and symbols underpin the emotional response to such occupations and assists in the understanding of how to act and of their meaning.[13] There are also shared understandings of the obligations and loyalties entailed, and a sense of solidarity derived from being part of something bigger than oneself.[14]

Participating in occupations steeped in history provides a sense of belonging to something that is both shared and ongoing. For example, it has been said that crafts, such as those traditionally used by occupational therapists, "make us feel rooted, give us a sense of belonging and connect us with our history."[15] Traditional crafts bind us geographically, through their connection with the people, history, and natural resources of a particular place. The ninth generation potters of Seagrove in North Carolina are an example. Their functional, glazed earthenware preserves the style of pottery developed before the American Revolution, which uses clay and glazes sourced

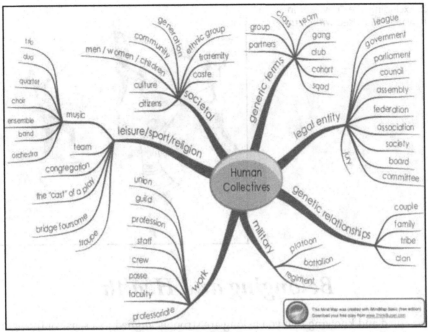

Figure 8-1. Belonging: a sample of human collectives.

from the local area, enfolding the potters in a proud family tradition. In an environmental sense, occupations embedded in a sense of place might include recycling, replanting, energy efficiency practices and research, and for some, environmental activism.

Participating in the occupations of a place gives us a sense of being in the right place[16] and of being at home; a sense that can be elicited by memories of gathering around the hearth or coming in sight of the gates of home. Being in place is to be recognized by others as an inhabitant, someone who does not need to be told when and how to do things, someone who understands the parameters and meaning of the things that are done. Belonging, in this sense, implies being able to judge what actions are appropriate to the place.[17] Occupations that belong in place encompass social, historical, and physical elements, providing the "context for who and what we are as human beings"[18] and human doers.

To the extent that they are aware of their interconnectedness at a global level, people also perceive themselves to be members of humanity—a global community. That finds occupational expression in connecting with people in other regions of the world via the Internet, phone, or as pen friends. In the global sense, belonging is also enacted through monitoring or reporting events that affect the welfare of people in distant places, giving donations to foreign aid, joining organizations that champion human rights, and working for the betterment of mankind. It is clear from those examples that belonging encompass ethical and political values,[19] which underpin and influence what people belong to and how belonging is enacted through doing.

Considering each of the ways of belonging—through occupations that provide social, historical, and geographical connections—it becomes clear that people can belong in multiple ways and at different places and times.[20] Across that shifting landscape of social locations, emotional attachments, and experiences, belonging remains central to well-being because it is intertwined with identity and being and having a place in the social world. Thus, in western societies, people typically identify themselves in relation to the groups to which they perceive themselves to belong, their locality, and their vocational, religious, national, racial, and cultural groupings.[18] All of those identifiers reveal aspects of occupation and the sense of belonging derived from doing things with, for, alongside, and because of others, in the ways they have established to belong.

Figure 8-2. Excluding the "new kid in town." (© Trevor Bywater 2013. Used with permission.)

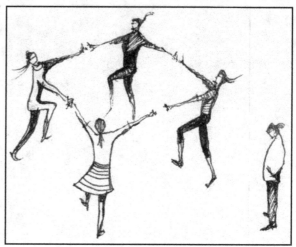

Belonging and Health

Being accepted and knowing that you belong are strongly aligned to a sense of fitting in, being suitable, or acceptable,[21] as well as being included and feeling comfortable and secure in what you are doing.[22,23] These social and mental health benefits align with the claims made about having a support network, which include experiencing mutual support and affirmation and being integrated or connected.[24,25] Belonging to a social group means that there is agreement that individuals are in their "rightful place,"[26] that they are entitled to support and their contribution to shared projects is valued by others.[27] Occupations that provide contact with others are recognized as a foundation for physical well-being and an essential element of mental well-being, as evidenced by the poor health outcomes of being isolated, shunned, or excluded—of not being able or welcome to join others in their activities (Figure 8-2). For those reasons, mental health workers consider it vital that clients participate in group and community activities in ways and to an extent that engenders a sense of belonging.

The tangible and intangible benefits of being socially connected are, at least in part, grounded in occupation. Merely sharing positive events with others can make people feel more energetic. Correlational studies show that the higher the frequency of sharing a naturally occurring pleasant occupation, the more vitality people report three weeks later.[28] Having supportive social networks also provides access to and assistance with valued occupations, giving the assurance that there is someone who can be called on for help when the challenge, cost, complexity, or emotional demand of an occupation is too great. That support is generally reciprocal. Even older people who receive formal support services simultaneously give and receive support[29] by doing things for others and having people do things for them.

The advantages derived from sharing the joy and burden of occupations helps explain population statistics that correlate a strong sense of belonging to one's local community and perceptions of good or excellent health.[30] For example, a nine-year study of 7000 Californians found that those with intimate relationships and a network of social ties extending out into the community had better health and lived longer. In contrast, participants with poorer health or who died younger tended to be socially isolated.[31] In occupational terms, those findings can be restated as the difference between people with ample opportunities to do things with people they know and people who they do not. The fact that health and belonging are interlinked has been picked up in the WHO document, *Health Impact Assessment (HIA): The Determinants of Health*, which identifies that health depends on people's circumstances and environment.[32]

Lack of belonging has long been recognized as a risk to health. Robert Burton (1577-1640) attributed melancholy to the lack or loss of belonging. Among other bodily, spiritual, and lifestyle factors, he identified the risk that voluntary solitariness might escalate to the point that company cannot be endured; that people facing adversity find themselves "left cold and comfortless" as friends and associates flee "as from a rotten wall, now ready to fall on their heads"; and that people condemned to banishment are "hated [and] rejected."[33] The injurious effect of not belonging is such that, for centuries, societies have used exile, exclusion, and imprisonment (another form of removal from society) as punishment. Next to death, solitary confinement is the most extreme punishment many societies can inflict.[34a]

Lasting damage is also inflicted at a societal level when groups are forcibly separated from their culture. For example, the faltering sense of belonging that typifies Indigenous, First Nations, or Aboriginal peoples can be attributed to their long histories of enforced abandonment of traditional occupations in favor of the imposed occupations of the colonizers. In recent times, some nonindigenous nationals of colonized countries have also questioned the legitimacy of their belonging. In response, they have sought to clarify their relationship with the indigenous people, the land, and each other,[18] which has often involved both questioning the fit of the occupational norms and practices of their forebears and greater openness to learning about and participating in the traditional occupations of other groups.

Ethnic minority and new immigrant populations can also struggle to gain a sense of belonging. One cause is the subtle or blatant behavior of members of the host community that makes newcomers feel uncomfortable, unwelcome, or excluded from occupations that confer social and material benefits, as well as responses that trivialize or denigrate the symbolism or performance of occupations from their homelands. Being known to engage in occupations in ways that are compatible with a group's values can make the difference between being welcomed, tolerated, or excluded.

NATURAL HEALTH: PREREQUISITES

Meeting the prerequisites of health identified in the Ottawa Charter for peace, shelter, education, food, income, a stable ecosystem and sustainable use of resources, social justice, and equity is both determined by the groups to which people belong and the actions of those groups. These ideas are discussed below and further elaborated in Table 8-1.

Belonging and Peace

Peace is more assured when communities have strong networks of social connectedness, include diverse people, and community members support each other to participate in occupation. In some situations, ordinary citizens take action to connect people despite political circumstances that create divisions. For example, in China, after the sense of community had been disrupted between 1949 and the 1990s, reviving Tai Chi groups and traditional dance and folk activities, such as the Lion Dance and Dragon Boat Racing, were deliberate means of enhancing community integration and endowing meaning to community life.[35] Supporting the benefits of such initiatives, there is evidence that people with a sense of belonging engage in altruistic acts to help develop their community. For example, transnational migrants who return home to Trinidad and Tobago bring technical skills, knowledge, and an entrepreneurial attitude. They also bring new ideas, such as human rights, gender equality, and community empowerment. Because of their deeply felt sense of belonging to their ancestral home, many are committed "to give something back" and persist in their efforts to establish new businesses and influence occupational norms despite frustrations and disappointments when they encounter institutional barriers and local distrust of outsiders.[36]

People are categorized as insiders or outsiders, as belonging or not, with formal and informal processes determining what people belong to and on whose terms.[37] Accepting that people need to belong explains a lot about patterns of group conformity. It also sheds light on the reasons people

Table 8-1

EXAMPLES OF BELONGING TO MEET THE PREREQUISITES OF HEALTH

WHO Prerequisites of Health	"Belonging" to Meet the Prerequisites: Positive and Negative Examples
Belonging and Peace	
Community cohesion Reciprocal support networks Diverse people are recognized as belonging (gender, race, nationality) Inclusive policies (employment, immigration, anti-discrimination legislation, poverty reduction)	Peace: inclusion is fostered, income gap between rich and poor is narrowed. Peaceful co-existence across national borders fostered by building a sense of regional belonging, with economic well-being, dependent on shared values, identity and interests. Strengthening regional trade links, educational and research exchanges, regional sports and cultural events and aid agreements, open immigration policies, and mutual recognition of qualifications. Peaceable belonging within a country fostered by: • Helping others to feel that they belong, but are not required to assimilate into the majority group • Engaging in cultural/sports events that build cross-cultural understanding and tolerance, and strengthen community networks • Valuing the economic and cultural contribution of immigrants and different regions to national interests • Positive attitudes toward intermarriage War: Enemies and minority groups portrayed as "foreign," a threat, dirty, lacking intelligence, cruel, subhuman, which justifies torture, confinement in concentration camps, rape, mass murder
Belonging and Shelter	
A place where family and friends congregate Communally owned "shelters" for culturally significant occupations; the arts, sports, civic affairs, religious services	Agrarian lifestyles and the growth of cities mean people now belong to increasingly stratified societies with increasing behavior controls[45] Home is perceived to be: • "One's rightful place," a refuge • A place to share occupations that strengthen family and other relationships • A place from which to venture to other places where one belongs (school, workplace, community) Belonging is fostered by: • Supporting homeless families to integrate into their new neighborhood (sustainable outcomes) • The Homeless World Cup soccer competition fosters belonging, achievement, and pride with a high proportion of participants moving into permanent accomodation[34b] • Taking action to provide adequate housing to people living in poverty, to address alienation arising from social disparities Alienation and disconnection fostered by: • Apartheid policies and discrimination blocking access to adequate housing • Dangerous neighborhoods

(continued)

Table 8-1 (continued)

EXAMPLES OF BELONGING TO MEET THE PREREQUISITES OF HEALTH

WHO Prerequisites of Health	"Belonging" to Meet the Prerequisites: Positive and Negative Examples
Belonging and Education	
Absence of discrimination in entry criteria Accessible schools Inclusive practices and curriculum Teaching, respect, tolerance, and recognition at all levels of education	Emphasis on belonging in Australia's national curriculum for early childhood education responds to desire for connectedness and open discussion about how belonging is fostered[12] Improve access to education for children with disabilities using universal design principles Proactive programs to increase social connections of bullies and victims of bullying contribute to well-being of all students Negatively: At-risk children less likely to experience acceptance and belonging at school[33c] Children who cannot speak the national language when they enroll in school achieve lower educational outcomes, poor quality work, with increased risk of alienation and hostility between ethnic enclaves and minority society[40] Older immigrants barred from English language classes aimed at "working age" migrants cannot integrate and experience occupational derivation and increased rates of depression[33d]
Belonging and Food	
Traditional foods of culture engender belonging Family meals Dishes associated with religious/other festivals	Inducting children into the "taste and smell" of traditional foods of their culture[33e] Modifying Christmas menu in New Zealand as forging a national identity separate from country of origin settlers[33f] People explore and encompass the shift from a monocultural national identity to embracing cultural diversity and multiculturalism, through consumption of diverse culinary styles (local, ethnic, rural)[55] Preference for "western" diet over traditional food reduces immigrant children's ties to their culture of origin Shared family routines, including family meals, strengthen family bonds and identity[33g] Negatively: Inability to provide traditional foods to their children compounds sense of alienation of women in asylum centers[33h] Eating meals alone increases risk of mental disorders amongst teenagers[33i]
Belonging and Income	
Belonging to the workforce gives identity and positive health benefits as well as income	Micro loans to women in Africa generate income spent on family nutrition and education and enhance their status within families and communities[60] Muslim Albanian immigrants in Switzerland who hold blue-collar jobs display their commitment to providing for their family through their belief that "Everything I do I do for my family"[33j] Negatively: Insufficient disposable income to access iconic occupations of the culture compound sense of alienation Decline in union membership accounts for approximately 30% of increases in income inequity[33k] Belonging to social networks with high unemployment levels reduces individuals' chances of gaining employment; in India that effect is compounded by segregation along caste lines.[33l]

(continued)

Table 8-1 (continued)

EXAMPLES OF BELONGING TO MEET THE PREREQUISITES OF HEALTH

WHO Prerequisites of Health	"Belonging" to Meet the Prerequisites: Positive and Negative Examples
Belonging and Stable Ecosystem/Sustainable Resource	
Habitat Indigenous peoples' deep sense of belonging to the environment, and everything within it	Experience belonging by consuming traditional foods of the place, while also reducing "food miles," the distance between where food is produced and where it is consumed
	UNEP Programme survey of young adults indicates different preferences for ownership versus shared/communal use of resources such as cars or community gardens[33m]
	Habitat for Humanity brings communities together to build affordable, ecofriendly housing for low-income families
	Negatively:
	Belonging needs met through participation in binge-drinking culture, with risk of acute alcohol poisoning, alcohol-related accidents, children with fetal-alcohol syndrome, long-term brain damage
Belonging and Social Justice and Equity	
Being accorded the full enjoyment of the benefits of belonging to society	Gender inequity, racism and ethnocentrism are challenged, consistent with principles of respect, tolerance, and recognition[48]
Experiencing reciprocity and the mutual benfits of belonging	Having access to the resources, relationships, places, and insider knowledge required to participate in the rituals, conventions, and practices that affirm belonging to family, school, workplace, and society
Freedom from discrimination or being categorized as belonging to less valued groups (indigenous female, illiterate, black, gay, impoverished, minority ethnic group, noncitizen, low caste)	Women's movement opened up educational and employment options and challenged gender discrimination, including gender-based pay differentials
	Legislation mandating education of children with disabilities in regular classrooms promotes inclusion
	Actions that preserve one's own language, in written and spoken forms, oratory and song, in educational, work, and cultural settings
	Engaging asylum seekers in community theater to share their stories with others is an example of community development and resisting legal and attitudinal barriers to belonging[33n]
	Negatively:
	Dowry system makes daughters a burden on family of origin, increasing risk of malnutrition and limited access to education; perpetuates social attitudes about low value of women
	Impoverished rural people move to cities seeking employment and experience loss of supportive relationships and resources, increasing risk of exploitation

form subgroups and join cults, and why they participate in occupations that undermine community cohesion, such as violence, vandalism, and graffiti, when these occupations are viewed as prerequisites to acceptance and belonging in cultural subgroups.[38,39] Therefore, although occupations that engender a sense of belonging can be described as fostering cohesion and peaceful coexistence, attention must be paid to the terms of belonging, and who is excluded. Externally imposed criteria for belonging include gender, sexuality, class, ethnicity, and nationality or citizenship. The social, political, economic, and health impact of discrimination and exclusion is evident in people's status in society, the resources and entitlements they can draw on, the type of work they can access, and their state of health relative to other groups in society. Exclusion and its accrued disadvantages are the genesis of societal division, distrust, and the radicalization of disaffected groups.[40]

Belonging and Shelter

The strength of the relationship between having a place to shelter and a sense of belonging is perhaps most evident when the conditions of acquiring it are stringent or access is insecure. Admission to Medieval Benedictine monasteries and nunneries required giving up all vestiges of one's former life (ie, name, possessions, and social status) and committing to a life of prayer, study, hard work, celibacy, and isolation from the outside world. In exchange, nuns and monks were allocated a bare cell, the simplest of food and clothing, entry to a closely bonded group, and, after death, the promise of joining the heavenly throng.[41] The provision of shelter to people recognized as belonging to a community has a long history. For example, the Alms Houses built for older residents of English villages were recognition that they were part of the place where they had spent their lives and that other members of the community bore some responsibility for their welfare.

Perhaps less austere than monasteries, but also less secure than Alms Houses, are the current day shelters established for homeless people, women escaping domestic violence, migrants, and victims of natural disasters. Although intended to provide warmth and protection from the elements, a large number of studies attest that people establish a sense of identity, belonging, and community within the shelter. Creating a home-like space is achieved by using possessions to claim shared space, filling the space with shared activities, and communally and individually decorating the space.[42] In some shelters in North America, residents develop a sense of solidarity, mutual acceptance, companionship, and commitment to the group that counters feelings of social exclusion. In creating their own place, they collaborate to survive but, incidentally, become more reluctant to move into independent living away from the shelter.[43]

Belonging and Education

The relationship between belonging and education is reciprocal, in the sense that access to education is an indicator of inclusion, whereas higher or lower literacy rates and the level of education in a population are important markers of the kind of society to which one belongs. Historically, once printing presses made books more readily available, education enabled people to read things for themselves and formulate their own views. Freed from the traditional ways of thinking promoted by the monarchy, clergy, and universities of the time, the assumption that individuals indelibly belonged to the social class into which they were born was steadily eroded.[44] Printing presses also contributed to the emergence of a new sense of belonging to a nation, as British and European kings, who controlled the presses, imposed the use of a national language rather than local dialects. That trend was reinforced as schools adopted the practice of using the local language as the vehicle of instruction, rather than using Latin textbooks.[45]

British citizens, of course, were not equal in terms of access to educational and income opportunities. For example, Andrew Bell, an ex-Colonial Office administrator in India, successfully championed the idea of establishing schools for the children of Britain's factory workers in the early 19th century. Although ostensibly improving workers' prospects, their reliance on rote learning and monitors to record the improvement, morals, cleanliness, and good order of the pupils reveal their real intent of preparing disciplined factory workers with the bare minimum level of literacy to function in that environment.[45] Belonging to society as a literate person means having a greater capability to participate in commerce and civil affairs and, for women, substantially higher survival rates for their children.[46] Access to education is most tenuous for girls living in poverty, reflecting not just the constraints of family income, but also societal understandings that women belong in the domestic sphere, and after marriage, will belong to their husband's family.

Such attitudes perpetuate female disenfranchisement and make their existence perilous if they fail to marry or are widowed.[47]

Belonging, being, and becoming are given prominence in Australia's early childhood national curriculum, which goes beyond investigating how people make a place in the world, to consider "how people make their places open to 'others.'"[12] That emphasis responds to people's desire for connectedness and opens discussion about what belonging means in educational contexts, how it can be fostered, and how it relates to inclusion. Those concerns echo the United Nations' *Declaration on Human Rights Education*, adopted in December 2011.[48] It directs all educational providers, from the preschool to tertiary level, to teach the principles of respect, tolerance, and recognition. In doing so, the United Nations intends to foster peace by creating communities in which diverse people can belong and concerned citizens challenge discrimination and injustice.

Applying those principles to schools themselves will mean opening the doors to all children, regardless of difference, and supporting them to develop to their potential. The universal right to education has only recently been secured for children with disabilities living in some western countries; in others, it remains a distant dream. Exclusion from education robs these children of opportunities to develop innate capacities and form social connections beyond their family. Teaching respect, tolerance, and recognition may also address bullying, a much discussed problem in current-day educational contexts. Bullying is an occupation with unhealthy consequences for both the perpetrator and the victim. Children who are the victims of bullying often have less cohesive friendships, lower levels of attachment to their parents, lower sense of belonging to their school, and no involvement in occupations organized by neighborhood clubs. Such a lack of engagement in occupations with others makes them an easy target. As a consequence of being bullied, they withdraw further from shared occupations and become more socially isolated.[49,50]

Belonging and Food

Participants of any social grouping actively shape occupations that engender a sense of belonging and cohesiveness. The food that parents prepare for their children inducts them into a culture of familiar tastes and smells, creating a sense of belonging at a visceral level. In early human history, the available food supply dictated practical limits on how many people could belong to a group and the density of those groups in a defined geographic area.[51] Transitioning from hunter-gatherer to agrarian lifestyles allowed communities to generate food surpluses, which meant they could support people who did not themselves produce food.[45] That technological advance radically changed the human landscape, culminating in 21st century reality of the majority of the population belonging to urban groups numbering in the hundreds of thousands or millions. Against that backdrop, parents invest considerable energy into maintaining daily routines that coordinate their family's activities, achieve necessary tasks, and strengthen family bonds and identity. The sense of belonging created by ensuring the family regularly spends time together over meals and establishing a shared identity confers behavioral and mental health benefits and fosters social well-being.[52-54]

At a societal level, people who live in increasingly multicultural countries are forging a more encompassing national identity as they taste and accept ethnic dishes into their everyday diet. For members of the European Union, and perhaps others, that shift in daily food practices can be viewed as an outcome of a political, economic, and consumerist agenda toward higher levels of regional integration.[55] A similar trend toward integration has been observed amongst first-generation immigrants, who actively create a transnational identity. They seek to find a place within the labor market of their country of residence but simultaneously recreate a sense of home in decorating their homes with things they brought with them and buying and preparing food from their country of origin. The success with which they manage to sustain this dual attachment impacts both their sense of belonging in their new country and the food served on the family's dining table.[56]

Belonging and Income

In an effort to ensure all people belong to peaceful, just, and prosperous societies, the *United Nations' Millennium Declaration* had a major focus on poverty reduction.[57] For indigenous populations, who feature prominently in international statistics for poverty and poor health, that demands more than economic advancement and modernization. Because past developmental initiatives have led to destruction of cultural, social, economic, and political structures, and the associated occupations, the United Nations' Declaration on the Rights of Indigenous People draws attention to their right to self-determination.[58] In Australia, that declaration is interpreted as empowering Aboriginal and Torres Strait Islanders to choose which economic activities are culturally appropriate, best preserve their cultural heritage, and care for their traditional lands and fisheries.[59] That is, they are being recognized as having the right and responsibility to create the kind of society to which they wish to belong, and by implication, the occupations they place value on.

Other disadvantaged groups are benefitting from ventures directed toward reducing poverty by establishing work cooperatives. A broad range of social benefits are reported. For example, the Manyakabi Area Cooperative Enterprise in southwestern Uganda was established to improve agricultural practices and productivity. In addition to the tangible outcome of increased income, female members reported improved confidence, "negotiating skills, the ability to be of service to their communities through transferring skills to non-members, and the ability to take control of certain household decisions when dealing with men."[60] Some self-help initiatives create spaces that bring people together to address their own concerns. Grandmothers Against Poverty and Aids (GAPA) is one example. Established in 2001 to address the increasing despair of grandmothers struggling to raise their grandchildren in poverty in South Africa's informal townships, it grew from humble beginnings as a patchwork group and, by 2004, there were 19 groups in Khayelitsha, teaching practical skills including growing vegetables, nursing their dying children, and running a business. Income generation projects exist alongside educational workshops about HIV/AIDS, human rights, elder abuse, and applying for grants. A sense of belonging is actively fostered by new members being introduced to the group via existing members, and support meetings still being held in the everyday environments of members' homes. In 2005, empowered by their mutual support and increasing knowledge, members of GAPA made a submission on the proposed Older Persons Bill.[61]

The sense of belonging engendered by GAPA and the Manyakabi cooperative demonstrates that belonging is enhanced when people are empowered within their intimate relationships at home and at societal levels. Belonging is both dynamic and responsive to shifts in individual and community connectedness and political agendas.[11] Accordingly, calls have been made for policies to address the social exclusion of forced migrants. Whether fleeing humanitarian and climate change crises, many experience social disadvantages and relative poverty after resettlement, with resultant poor mental health.[62] Irrespective of people's ethnic background or their pathway into poverty, the daily burden it creates is associated with higher levels of social isolation and a lower sense of belonging to their community compared with people with higher levels of income. That is, poverty in itself adds an additional layer of stigma and exclusion.[63]

Belonging: Stable Ecosystem and Sustainable Resources

Belonging includes a sense of being connected to places, traditions, and practices, as well as to people. For example, although their significance is easily overlooked, "the rituals that surround gathering food, cooking for ourselves or our families, washing, eating, sleeping and cleaning connect us to almost all of humanity ... and link us to the diverse but collective experience of 'home.'"[64] Home is not only a place of shelter, but also a place to be nurtured and protected so that it can be a place one leaves from and returns to. For indigenous peoples, home is a place one listens to; a place that calls on "visitors to identify themselves"; and a place that one responds to when it sings, cries out, or feels abandoned or violated.[65] Maintaining an environment so that it continues to flourish in its original or improved state maintains the essence of its spirit. Spiritual belonging is the connection to a birthplace, to sites of religious artifacts and spiritual guardians, to the resting places of the dead, and to the creators. Long association, childhood memories, inter-generational connections, and knowledge of how one's actions have altered a landscape or cared for the land also generate a sense of belonging to place. Belonging in this sense may be experienced as a deeply felt moral and ethical responsibility to look after the land or a sense of entitlement to be there born of a history of accomplishment, sacrifice, tragedy, or bloodshed. Felt belonging might also be embedded in the sights, sounds, smell, color, or texture of the place or the embodied knowledge of doing things there.[66] When occupations are undertaken with sustainability in mind, people express feelings of belonging and responsibility toward all life forms on the planet. Other occupations seem unsustainable at both individual and societal levels. Excessive alcohol consumption has social effects that undermine community cohesion. It decreases the safety of engaging in occupation at home and in the community by, for example, increasing the incidence of dangers in the built environments where large populations cohabit, such as traffic, workplace and home accidents, violence, unwanted pregnancies, and sexually transmitted diseases.[32]

Belonging: Social Justice and Equity

Social justice is essential if everyone is to experience a sense of belonging in the society in which they live, yet history is replete with incidental and deliberate instances of injustices and inequities. For example, as people in different regions took up agrarian lifestyles, women's role and status in society was particularly undermined. That occurred because their knowledge of food gathering was rendered obsolete, allowing power to be concentrated in the hands of the men, who controlled the food surpluses and acquired territory by force.[45] In addition to such shifts in power, in some circumstances the way things are done perpetuates divisions between people. Women's lower pay rates and representation on company boards and political office across the western world is a case in point. It is important yet challenging to consider how boundaries are articulated and arbitrated, and how flexible or permeable they are.[67] Equally challenging are questions about how people resist barriers to belonging, and how they contest imposed categories of belonging, so that new possibilities for relationships between individuals, groups, and communities are created.[68,69]

Although issues of sustainability and equity have been considered separately, there is growing acceptance of their interrelationship. Barbier was the first to propose that economic development necessarily overlaps with social and environmental conditions. Accordingly, he held that sustainability demands maximizing biological, economic, and social goals. In making that assertion, he brought together conventional development approaches, which maximize only economic goals, and Marxist economics, which maximizes only economic and social goals.[70] Later elaboration of his model identified that sustainable development requires viable, equitable, and bearable solutions (Figure 8-3). In relation to the idea that health rests, in part, on having a sense of belonging, achieving bearable social conditions seems a minimum requirement.

Rules for Health Through Belonging: From Ancient to Modern

Contemplating belonging in relation to the prerequisites for survival reveals shifting patterns, with some people enjoying the health and material benefits of social connectedness, whereas others belong to resource-poor networks or experience degrees of isolation. Although the interconnection of belonging and health seems intuitive, the following sections interrogate that relationship in more depth.

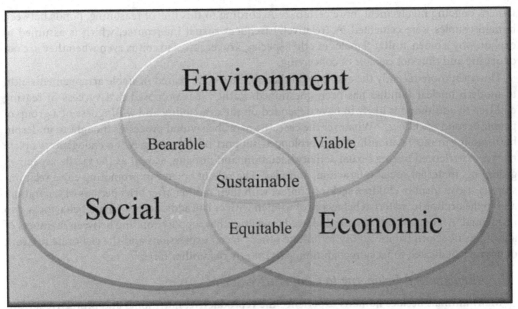

Figure 8-3. Sustainable social, environmental, and economic relationships.

BIOLOGICAL BASIS OF BELONGING AND HEALTH

From the dawn of human history until 10,000 BC, the entire human population lived as hunters, gatherers, or fishermen.[71] In those foraging societies, as now, men and women lived in close proximity. The study of current-day hunter-gatherers and the examination of archaeological remains suggest that early humans lived in bands of up to 50 members but averaged about 25, which is considered optimal for an egalitarian group. In geographic regions where the available food supply supported large numbers, more bands formed rather than larger ones. Membership was fluid, as individuals moved between established groups to find marriage partners and split off to form new bands.[51] In biological terms, early humans were compelled to live in groups to meet their nutritional needs. The wild food on which they depended might be scattered over a wide area, requiring the cooperative effort of all members of the clan to locate it in sufficient quantity.

Killing larger game animals also required the cooperation of a group of skilled hunters. Because there was little or no stored food and no crops or domesticated animals to draw from, the only people exempt from the daily toil of food gathering were infants and those who were too old or unwell to participate. Examination of skeletal remains and other indicators of health, from various parts of the world, reveal that their varied diet enabled early humans to grow to full height and enjoy remarkable health.[72] For humans, as with other species of diurnal primates, it is also thought that belonging to a band offered protection against predators (including hostile bands of people) by making it more likely that a threat would be noticed and providing increased resources to defend themselves. This proposal further supports the evolutionary advantage of belonging.[73]

Belonging to a group of people was also necessitated by the helplessness of human infants, who need to be taught even the most basic self-care, communication, and social skills. That requires input over many years, making the burden of rearing children very high. In addition, the climatic change that occurred in eastern Africa approximately 1.6 million years ago resulted in a significantly drier climate and probably decreased the available food. Those factors favor increased male involvement in families, and it appears that hominid men have a long history of supporting women and their offspring to a greater extent than other primates. One mechanism posited as promoting continued male input is the strong sexual bonding between men and women.[74] Forming monogamous couples, it is argued, gave relatively high confidence about children's paternity, making the father's ongoing involvement more certain.[72] According to this line of reasoning, bonds between human couples were cemented by (relatively) frequent sexual intercourse, which is assumed to explain why women, unlike females of other species, are receptive to coitus even when they are not ovulating and thus not capable of conceiving.

However, more recently the assumption that children were reared in stable arrangements akin to modern nuclear families has been questioned. Rather, it is proposed that success in rearing children to adulthood is likely to have depended on the availability and willingness of a group of people beyond the father.[75] Whatever the case, the neurobehavioral processes thought to underpin both monogamous relationships and prolonged support of the young is the endogenous opiate release experienced during sexual activity, lactation, and nursing, as well as the tactile aspects of grooming, maternal social interaction, and play. The role of opiates in promoting close relationships is also evident in children seeking contact with their mother after brief periods of separation, and in the decline in maternal behaviors of women with opiate addictions.[76] Infant behavior is also influential. Among the biologically endowed capacities that support bonding between members of a group is newborn babies' ability to imitate others' facial expressions and the elaborate network of neurons dedicated to facial recognition, particularly of familiar faces.[77]

Altruism and Belonging to Cooperative Social Groups

Many animals besides humans experience the reproductive, nutritional and protective advantages of belonging to a colony, herd, pride, troupe, or other collective. Belonging, in that sense, may or may not be subjectively experienced but does involve behaviors beyond simply existing in the same location. In some species, such as bees and ants, cooperative behavior seems largely instinctual. In animals higher on the evolutionary scale, observed behaviors that indicate awareness of belonging to a group are deliberate acts. Those behaviors are consistent, despite sometimes having high costs for an individual. For example, giving a distress signal when a predator is sighted protects the group but reveals the individual's position and thus increases the risk for the one that raised the alarm.[77] Raising the alarm is just one example of altruistic behavior recorded in many group-living species. Among monkeys and apes, it also includes grooming, assistance with raising young, and going to others' assistance when they are attacked.

There is some evidence that altruistic responses are more likely to occur between individuals who are closely related, but other alliances have been observed. Altruism has long been assumed to have a genetic basis. However, that assumption requires some explanation because it would seem that altruistic individuals might be less successful in reproducing given the risks to which they expose themselves. On that basis, altruism would be an evolutionary disadvantage, and even more so in species where some members of the group assist with raising others' young rather than breeding themselves. However, in 1964, WD Hamilton mathematically proved that is not the case. His concept, inclusive fitness, proposed that altruistic behaviors toward kin increase their survival rate, thus ensuring that the genes they share are handed on.[78]

Charles Darwin (1809-1882) first proposed the genetic basis of altruism in humans, arguing that tribes with "a greater number of courageous, sympathetic and faithful members, who were always ready to warn each other of danger, to aid and defend each other ... would spread and be victorious over other tribes."[79] Although cooperation features in many species, humans appear to establish "large-scale cooperation among genetically unrelated strangers" to a greater extent.[80] However, through most of the 20th century, scientists tended to deny the existence of altruism in humans. Apparent acts of altruism were generally explained as motivated by selfish intent. The expectation of return favors, a reward, praise, or earning a place in heaven were all cited as explanations. However, experimental evidence consistently failed to support such interpretation, and from the 1990s helping behavior founded on a genuine capacity for caring increasingly came to be a scientifically accepted human characteristic.[81]

A further argument for a genetic basis to altruism revisited Darwin's thesis, assembling archaeological evidence of catastrophic warfare between bands of hunter-gatherers in the late Pleistocene and early Holocene periods. Conflict is known to have intensified at that time, with rapid climatic change forcing bands to relocate into areas where they came into contact with groups with whom they did not share a language or have established patterns of interaction. It is estimated that armed conflict accounted for up to 14% of adult deaths. That scenario supports the proliferation of a genetic disposition toward altruism, at least in regions where groups lived in close proximity.[82,83]

Empathy and Belonging to Cooperative Social Groups

In addition to altruism and cooperation, prosocial behaviors associated with a sense of belonging include empathy, sympathy, and morality. To feel empathy toward another member of your species requires the capacity to identify with the other and to metaphorically "put yourself in their shoes." That capacity stems from the mirror neuron system recently discovered in monkey, ape, and human brains. Recent studies using functional magnetic resonance imaging confirm that mirror neurons not only fire when individuals perform goal-related actions, but also when watching others doing things. That neural activity simulates the observer doing the same thing and, in mirroring the other's actions, gives insight into their actions, intentions, and emotions. For example, in children who are developing in a typical way, neural activity is stimulated in areas of the brain related to emotions (anterior insula, amygdala) and imitation (pars opercularis) by observing and imitating the facial expression of others. That neural activity correlates with children's level of social development, particularly in terms of whether they empathize with others.[84] The capacity to empathize has also been proposed as an explanation of the highly cooperative behavior of children younger than age 2 years.[75] Confirming those findings, adolescents with conduct disorders exhibit both impaired capacity for empathy and significantly smaller anterior insular cortex and left amygdala neural structures.[85]

Individuals are connected by the ability to imitate the emotions of others and display protective, caring, and empathetic responses. This ability has been observed in a broad range of species, including elephants, dolphins, and lemurs. For example, monkeys can make sense of the distress others display, and even predict it—such as a mother taking action to deflect her infant away from an aggressive individual. In humans, empathic responses to the distress of others are associated with heightened metabolic activity in the medial and frontal gyrus, occipito-temporal cortices, thalamus, and the cerebellum. Involvement of the cerebellum suggests that empathy has cognitive and affective components.[86] That fits with observed empathetic responses in the animal kingdom, which are more likely if it is a relative or friend who needs assistance and become more selective as individuals age. In humans, and perhaps apes, vicarious understanding of others' situation involves recognizing their distress while maintaining the distinction between self and others. Indeed, the capacity to be empathic seems to be related to the ability to recognize such separateness. Monkeys from species without the capacity to recognize themselves in a mirror are rarely observed to console or reassure other members of their species after the initial signs of distress diminish. Human children begin to display empathy at around the same time as they recognize separateness.[81]

Because the benefits of cooperative occupations are more apparent in smaller rather than larger collectives, a link can be made between altruism and living in small groups. Accordingly, cooperative individuals are thought likely to prefer and seek out such environments.[87] The development of parochial altruism—where people inside (but not outside) the group are offered help irrespective of family ties—is supported by several social mechanisms including:

- Memories of previous help.
- A person's reputation for helping other people.
- The shunning of and refusal to help people who do not help others.
- The punishing or, more powerfully, the threat of punishment for not doing things to help others.[80]

Recent scientific evidence confirms the existence of strong empathic responses to the suffering of members of one's own group. Neuroimaging techniques show that in addition to the increased affective neural activity observed when people feel empathetic toward others, favoritism for people from one's own social group is exhibited by stronger recruitment of the cognitive neural processes seated in the medial prefrontal cortex.[88] Similar responses have been recorded when research subjects witness instances of social exclusion, with resultant prosocial responses directed toward the victim.[89] Those findings support the idea that humans evolved to live cooperatively, with the ability to share and respond to others' emotional states and provide assistance toward the completion of essential cooperative tasks.

The human capacity for empathy is surely related to morality that is concerned with whether behaviors toward others have good or bad intent, with right or wrong being judged according to values such as truth, compassion, and fairness.[90] Morality arises from being able to "anticipate the consequences of one's own actions; … make value judgments; and … choose between alternative courses of action," with moral codes being influenced by culture.[91] That morality is created by humans and entirely absent from the natural world has been a dominant view since the 19th century and typified by biologist Thomas Henry Huxley (1825-1895).[34] Huxley was one of Darwin's contemporaries and a noted critic of his theory of evolution. Darwin held the antithetical view that it was highly probable "that any animal whatever, endowed with well-marked social instincts, would inevitably acquire a moral sense or conscience as soon as its intellectual powers had become as well-developed, or anything like as well-developed as in man."[92] As for altruism, Darwin saw an evolutionary advantage for tribes that had a high standard of morality, compared with tribes that did not.[90] Current-day research supports Darwin's argument, with evidence that animals as well as humans deliberately act in ways that benefit another, even when they know that they will be worse off as a consequence. Those prosocial tendencies include consoling others, reciprocity, empathy, and fairness.[34] However, attributing morality to animals remains contentious because it seems to require the capacity for abstract thought, free will, and being able to anticipate what will happen in the future.

Bringing these arguments together, it seems apparent that belonging to a cooperative social group is supported, in an evolutionary and practical sense, by feelings of compassion, altruistic behaviors, the capacity to make moral choices, and culturally based values of right and wrong. Although these capacities are now seen to confer an evolutionary advantage, the question remains of why they arose in the first place. One proposition rests on the argument that the development of extensive social networks, marriages, and shifting alliances between group members is a uniquely complex proposition. To assess shifts in those relationships and predict how others will respond in different circumstances, sophisticated cognitive abilities are required. The need to understand kinship and social relationships and others' reactions is characteristic of human, macaque, and baboon societies.[81] In humans, some believe that complexity drove the evolution of human intelligence because "the most important—and most intellectually challenging—components in an individual's reality are other individuals."[93] The evolutionary emergence of language, which supports the development of the sophisticated social behaviors demanded by group belonging, is associated with "the unique adaptations of the [human] brain that make possible the symbolic structuring of our world."[94]

The ultimate expression of human intelligence, and essential to belonging and being, is consciousness, as described in the previous chapter. Consciousness is integral to belonging as "the tool of the social animal … We are not only self-aware, but conscious of being so."[95] It is "the key … [and] the power which motivates and drives all human affairs."[96] With it comes an increased need to conform to others of the species and to demonstrate particular skills and capacities that are socioculturally valued. Being self-conscious enables us to understand what others are thinking and feeling and, because we understand, to feel sympathy, empathy, and compassion for them. These are the foundations of social cooperation and reciprocity, which developed into rules governing how to behave and shared understandings of right and wrong.[93] Human intelligence and consciousness can be considered the structures on which belonging is enacted, giving people the capacity to fit in and be acceptable to the groups to which they belong, to gauge how well integrated and connected they are, and to support and affirm others' attachment to the group.

BELONGING AND HEALTH IN EARLY HISTORY

Philosophers have long recognized the interrelationship of people and place, with Aristotle (384-322 BC) voicing the belief that "everything [including occupation] is somewhere and in place"[97] and Archytus (circa 400 to 365 BC), who is credited as the first person to apply mathematical principles to mechanics, declaring that "to be is to be in place."[18] However, being in place is not the same as having equivalent claims of belonging. In ancient Roman society, sharp divisions were drawn between citizens, foreigners, slaves, and freedmen, or ex-slaves. In addition to legal barriers, such as those forbidding senators from marrying outside their class, differences in status separated these groups. Citizens enjoyed the dignity of having personal power and being free, whereas slaves were considered to be their master's property and were expected to be subservient. Freedmen, somewhere in between, needed to show gratitude to their ex-masters, who expected a share of their income and retained the right to berate or beat them. Having little legal standing did not prevent some freedmen from holding essential administrative positions or amassing considerable fortunes. That success did not protect them from the disdain of the elite, who resented their social mobility and considered them tasteless and unworthy. In resisting that oppression, freedmen inscribed their epitaphs and tombs with their occupational title, thus proclaiming an identity as generous, virtuous, competent, and useful citizens. In this way, they also proclaimed their cultural belongingness to the city that granted them citizenship.

In Mayan society, which flourished in Mexico between approximately 700 BC and the early 1500s, belonging was also cemented in built structures. The architectural tradition included a central platform-pyramid complex, with pillow shaped, large block masonry, rounded corners, vaults and decorative hieroglyphics. In the most politically powerful sites mapped to date, the basal platforms might measure as much as 200 by 130 feet, with the superstructure up to 125 feet tall. Although the exact purpose of these megalithic structures is unknown, their scale suggests they served important religious and political functions that expressed the religious belief system and legitimized the sovereign's power. Participating in the construction and use of these sacred spaces was a requirement of community membership: a political and a social act. The Mayan people literally built social cohesion and a sense of belonging to a specific community. That identity was cast in opposition to neighboring communities, who built and maintained their own constructions, albeit expressing the same underlying ideology.[98]

In contrast, within a traditional American Indian worldview, belonging is expressed through an ideology of interdependence and interrelatedness. Family, community, the tribe, and the universe, including the physical environment, are all connected in the Circle of Life.[99] "All belong to one another and should be treated accordingly."[100] Universal connectedness is manifest in talking circles, peacemaking circles, and healing circles, which create a nonhierarchical space within which everyone present can take their turn to speak and be listened to respectfully. Contributions are regulated by the passing around of a talking piece—a symbolic object that confers the right to speak without interruption.[101] Belonging was experienced as a deep spiritual connection to traditional ways of life, ancestors, the Creator, land, the environment, community, and family. Communal activities fostered belonging. Those included traditional storytelling, giving meaning and life to the community by reconnecting people to their tribal history and with nature.[102] As part of a prolonged process of disruption, the Indian Removal Act of 1830 fragmented their sense of belonging by forcing tribes off their land and confining them to reservations. The various stages of disruption had progressed through:

- The destruction of life-ways at the time of first contact.
- Economic competition.
- Invasion under the U.S. government extermination policies.

- The subjugation and reservation period, which introduced life on reservations.
- A boarding school period which disrupted family networks, traditions, and prospects of community survival.
- Forced relocations, characterized as cultural genocide.

These sociohistorical events continue to affect American Indians' sense of belonging.[103]

BELONGING AND HEALTH IN MODERN TIMES

Influential Austrian psychiatrist, Sigmund Freud (1856-1939), whose theories came to define psychoanalytic theory from the beginning of the 20th century, asserted the need for interpersonal contact. True to his professional leanings, Freud narrowly attributed that need to humans' sex drive and to filial bonds.[104] His ideas continue to be influential. For example, Bowlby's attachment theory, published in the late 1960s, can be read as supporting an innate need to belong. He regarded this as stemming from infants' intimate relationship with their mothers, at least in his early work.[105] More expansive views had been promoted by John Dewey (1859-1952), an American educator, philosopher, and social activist. Dewey positioned belonging in people's relationship with the world, firmly rejecting the possibility that people are separate from or merely contained within their environment. Although elements of people, their doings, and the environment might be separated out, to understand or explain their interaction, he insisted that the environment and people are continuously interactive. Each affects and is affected by the other, such that all human activity is a transaction with the environment: people and environments codefine and coconstitute each other.[106] That relationship is directly enacted through occupations such as maintaining one's environment, which constitutes a literal imprinting of oneself on the physical environment that creates a sense of home.

Similarly, Martin Heidegger's (1889-1976) concept of "being-in-the-world" posits that people are inextricably embedded in place; "The world is that to which we are already given over and in which we are taken up."[107] The Statue of Liberty and Big Ben, iconic symbols of American and British society, respectively, encapsulate this sense of a cultural place that individuals take up without thought of how it came to be (Figure 8-4). These insights point to both the ideas people adopt and their understandings of how the people who belong there go about their everyday round of activities. Such ideas maintain their currency. Belonging to place has given rise to theories explaining the environment's influence on human activity and health. For example, environmental determinism proposes that geography and climate shape human economies, culture, economics, and religion. More directly addressing health issues, Wilson's biophilia hypothesis asserts a biological basis for the influence the natural environment has on human well-being, such that doing things in, or even in sight of, natural spaces improves cognitive, physical, emotional, and spiritual well-being.[108]

Aligning with those philosophers, a sense of belonging is commonly assumed to be a basic human need, akin to the need for food and shelter.[24] However, Maslow's hierarchical ordering of human needs, placed love and belonging after more basic needs for food and shelter had been satisfied but ahead of self-esteem and self-actualization (which are addressed in the following chapter on becoming).[109] Although Maslow's theory has been highly influential, he offered no empirical data to support the existence of a need to belong.[110] Nonetheless, other psychologists continue to advance theories to explain the need and research findings support a relationship between a sense of belonging and health promoting behaviors.[111]

Evaluating the Evidence for the Need to Belong

Addressing the long-standing debate about whether the need to belong is indeed innate, Baumeister and Leary undertook a far-reaching review of the evidence generated by psychologists.[110] They hypothesized that if the need to belong were universal, it would confer survival and reproductive benefits and stimulate thought- and goal-directed activity toward forming and

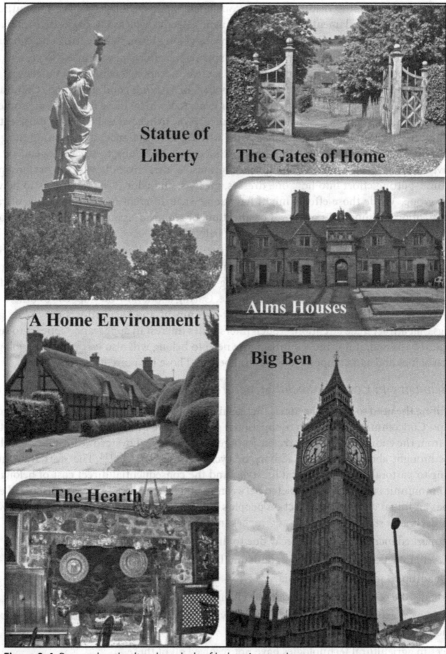

Figure 8-4. Personal and cultural symbols of belonging to place.

sustaining mutual social bonds. Furthermore, it would generate emotional responses to strengthening and weakening relationships, and being socially deprived would cause some ill effect, whether the deprivation cause was behavioral, psychological, or health related. Finally, once the need for belonging was satisfied, the motivation to form relationships would diminish. On the basis of the evidence available to them in 1995, all aspects of the hypothesis were supported, to a greater or lesser extent. They found that people in all cultures readily form bonds, resist breaking them, and spend a lot of time thinking about relationships. Deficits in belonging are associated with physical and psychological health problems, including anxiety, depression, and loneliness, plus behavioral pathologies, such as eating disorders. They concluded that psychologists have not sufficiently appreciated humans' fundamental need for "frequent, effectively pleasant, or positive interactions with the same individuals" occurring "in a framework of long-term, stable caring and concern."[112]

At a more everyday level, the need to belong explains the efforts people make to present themselves in ways others will find acceptable and attractive. Acceptable behavior, in a general sense, might be summed up in the concept of "being polite" or "having good manners." Cultural subgroups develop variations on what is acceptable or expected, which, like a high five, are sometimes accepted into mainstream society. Knowing the correct way to behave and enacting it correctly signals familiarity with group norms and a general attitude of compliance, thus earning the group's endorsement and protection.[113] Gaining entry to a group to belong to it can depend on being attractive to existing members. Although perceptions of attractiveness vary across groups and across time, putting effort into how one dresses, grooms, and adorns oneself seems to be valued in every group. While those efforts might have somewhat different intents, including attracting others' attention, earning their approval or affection, or simply dressing in a manner appropriate to one's occupation, the overall message is one of belonging.

Capitalizing on the human need to belong, the fashion and cosmetics industries thrive on people's concern with their appearance. That concern is not confined to humans: given an opportunity, apes inspect themselves in a mirror, taking the opportunity to look at their teeth and other body parts that are otherwise more difficult to see. Caring about how they appear to others is also apparent in female chimpanzees' interest in self-adornment and their efforts to see the genital swellings that attract male attention.[81] Such interspecies interest in appearance appears to support a biological basis and, if it is indeed innate, the need to belong will also be evident in biologically based capacities and as a component of natural health. Those ideas are now explored.

Belonging in Complex Social Structures

Fulfilling the need to belong becomes increasingly problematic as people live in larger and larger groups. Concommittant shifts in occupational patterns have been initiated by a combination of factors from the ending of the most recent Ice Age to serious local overcrowding and to ecological changes brought about by human activity or cyclic climate change.[114] The shift from hunter-gathering to pastoral and agricultural lifestyles and the consequential direct cost of belonging to larger communities was all but completed between 10,000 BC and 1500 AD.[71] As discussed earlier, there was an initial detrimental effect on people's physical health. These included the following:

- A decline in stature—as much as 7 inches in men and 5 inches in women.
- A marked increase in dental decay due to dietary increase of carbohydrates.
- Severe undernourishment of pregnant and lactating women.
- Quadrupled incidence of anemia.
- About 70% of the adult population developing osteoarthritis.[72]
- Increased exposure to infectious diseases, which require a sufficient number and concentration of humans to sustain them.[115]

Advances in agricultural technologies have not resolved all of these.

The socio-occupational consequences of belonging to larger, settled communities were also marked. The increased cultural stability that came with settlement is also thought to have given rise to the major language families: Afro-Asiatic, Indo-European, Elamo-Dravidian, Sino-Tibetan, and Austronesian.[45] As agricultural techniques and traditions diversified, individuals increasingly identified with their own group and recognized outsiders as being from other places. Anthropologists have noted that this tendency extends to judging people's physical attractiveness by criteria that align with one's own physical appearance (skin color, hair color and texture, facial features, stature, and patterns of fat distribution). The preference for specific, genetically determined features is one basis of mate selection and having a sense of belonging within a family and broader ethnic grouping.[72]

Agricultural breakthroughs, such as irrigating crops to increase the yield and decrease the risk of crop failure, intensified social reorganization. This geographic stability changed the nature of belonging to place in that it was now a single location that was irretrievably modified by human doing. The chiefs, scribes, doctors, and craftsmen had skills and knowledge others did not share, enabling more of the social and decision-making authority to be concentrated in their hands. Communities to which people belonged had layers of social authority that had not previously existed, with new occupational requirements. The emergence of writing, initially developed to predict the seasons and later to record the quantity of surplus food stocks and who owned them, intensified the escalation of social control. For the population at large, belonging to a community was associated not only with protection, but also with being called on to assert and enlarge the chief's position. Skeletal remains reveal that the latter enjoyed privileges that ensured them better health and longevity than others who were subjected to increasingly stringent social controls. In part, that control was asserted by religious leaders, whose authority increased as religions became institutionalized and assumed powers to judge and punish individuals for errant thoughts and deeds.

The scale of social transformation brought about by the adoption of a sedentary agricultural lifestyle has only been matched by the creation of the first states, approximately 5000 years ago, and the still unfolding process of modernization, which transformed the political, philosophical, and technological basis of life in western countries.[114] Over the centuries, the evolution of technology played an important role in shaping people's thoughts, such that belonging to western societies is now characterized by valuing rational explanation over intuition or religious doctrine, and using analytic methods to solve practical, social, and existential problems.[44] One aspect of rationalization is the trend toward the standardization of information. This is evident in almanacs, which, from the 1600s, contained information about the tides, sunrise, the lunar cycle, astrological tables, and more. As the only publications thought to rival the circulation of religious texts, almanacs were influential in bringing about uniformity in commodity prices, wage rates, weights and measures, and across any number of specialist vocations, from farmers to midwives and from merchants to seaman.[45] Thereby, the occupations contingent on belonging became increasingly conformist and homogenous, a trend that would be accelerated by the emergence of science and the scientific method.

Another rapidly changing parameter of belonging is the transition from rural to urban living. In 1990, the WHO estimated that less than 40% of the global population were city dwellers.[116] That shifted to more than half by 2010 and is expected to have increased to 70% by 2050. In developing countries, the urban population increases by an average of 1.2 million every week. Most cities house 100,000 to 500,000 people, but 10% of urban dwellers live in megacities of more than 10 million.[116] The health and belonging effects of living among such a large number of people have been viewed differently by different authorities. Some perceive overcrowding as deleterious to health, arguing that people become exhausted by interhuman relationships as the superabundance of social contact overstrains capacity, causing people to become aggressive and to shut themselves off.[117] This point of view suggests challenges for belonging. Others proclaim a love of cities—the bigger and more polluted the better.[118] From this perspective, living among an abundance of people might be seen as offering a wealth of opportunities to belong. Moderating these extremes, French sociologist Emile Durkheim (1858-1917) proposed that people need intermediate structures that bring people into society. Such structures must be relatively stable, provide a sense of connection by addressing shared issues of social life, and be small enough to provide a sense of community but large enough to be perceived as connecting people to the larger society. Finally, they must provide opportunities to interact and identify with each other.[119]

Given that more than half of humans now live in the anonymity of large cities, belonging is enacted within contexts that allow or withhold inclusion depending on prevalent ethical and political values. The fact that connections must be forged within an environment filled with strangers reminds us that not all claims of belonging are considered valid and they are not always desirable.[120] For example, the 2005 anti-Islamist riots in Australia saw people who looked Middle Eastern being attacked by mobs of young residents of Sydney.[121] Those attacks revealed that many, perhaps the majority, of Australians reject Muslim immigrants' desire to be included as citizens and welcomed in public spaces, such as beaches. Their rejection reveals cultural, racial, and religious stereotyping of Muslims as potential terrorists. Equally, youths who tag public buildings to earn gang membership generate significant costs for mainstream society, from the price of removing it to the stress generated by living in neighborhoods no longer perceived to be safe.[38]

Conclusion: Well-Being and the Quest for Belonging

Every aspect of human doing, across all countries and irrespective of age, gender, income and other parameters of difference, is in relation to other people. Doing and being enable the maintenance and development of satisfying and stimulating relationships with family members and associates and within the community in which people live. Whether our doings engender a sense of belonging is a matter of health and well-being, not just of individuals and communities, but also of the health and well-being of the whole planet, because human life is embedded within the global environment. Human evolution, which has inexorably brought people together in larger and larger groupings, brings increasing challenge to achieving a sense of belonging and increasing cost to not achieving that.

Where culturally diverse populations have come into contact, cultural and population genocide has often been the result. Colonization, dispossession of land, forced relocation, and apartheid policies leave a legacy of alienation of peoples whose own culture is profoundly disrupted and find no easy place in the culture that has overtaken them. Voluntary and forced migrants are also found to experience ongoing discrimination, with economic and health consequences that can continue over generations. Within cultures, discrimination and stigma continue to exclude some, with measurable impacts on health and well-being. Resisting domination often draws the divisions even deeper, as communities blame and punish those who resort to destruction of property or violence, or sink into substance abuse, learned helplessness, manipulativeness, compulsive gambling, and suicide.[99]

As the World Health Organization recognizes, globalization, "the increased interconnectedness and interdependence of peoples and countries ... has the potential for both positive and negative effects on development and health."[122] In 1986, when nations came together to agree on the principles of the Ottawa Charter, they recognized that creating supportive environments in which people could have a sense of belonging was fundamental to health yet inseparable from the achievement of other goals. In adopting a resolution to teach the principles of respect, tolerance, and recognition at all levels of education, the United Nations is laying a pathway to achieving nations, regions, and communities that take care of each other and the natural environment. In that supportive environment, there is hope that belonging through doing might be achieved.

References

1. World Health Organization, Health and Welfare Canada, Canadian Public Health Association. *Ottawa Charter for Health Promotion*. Ottawa, Canada; 1986.
2. Donne J. Devotions upon Emergent Occasions: Meditation 17. *The Works of John Donne* (vol III). Henry Alford, ed. London: John W. Parker, 1839;574-5.
3. Belonging. *Valery Giscard d'Estain*. Wikispaces. http://yeartwelvebelonging.wikispaces.com/ Belonging+-+Quotes. Accessed May 9, 20112.

4. Reed K, Hocking C, Smythe L. The interconnected meanings of occupation: the call, being-with, possibilities. *Journal of Occupational Science*. 2010;17(3):140-149. doi:10.1080/14427591.2010.9686688

5. Belong. *Oxford dictionaries*. http://oxforddictionaries.com/definition/belong. Accessed June 8, 2012.

6. Belonging. *Memidex dictionary/thesaurus*. http://www.memidex.com/belonging. Accessed June 8, 2012.

7. Christiansen F, Hedetoft U, eds. *The Politics of Multiple Belonging: Ethnicity and Nationalism in Europe and East Asia*. Aldershot: Ashgate; 2004.

8. Mee K. A space to care, a space of care: public housing, belonging, and care in inner Newcastle, Australia. *Environment and Planning*. 2009;41(4):844.

9. Yuval-Davis N. Belonging and the politics of belonging. *Patterns of Prejudice*. 2006;40(3):197-214.

10. Belonging. *Collins Dictionary*. www.collinsdictionary.com/dictionary/english/belonging. Accessed June 6, 2012.

11. Belonging. *Merriam-Webster*. Available at: http://www.merriam-webster.com/thesaurus/belonging. Accessed June 6, 2012.

12. Sumsion J, Wong S. Interrogating 'belonging' in belonging, being and becoming: the early years learning framework for Australia. *Contemporary Issues in Early Childhood*. 2011;12(1):28-45. doi:10.2304/ciec.2011.12.1.28

13. Read P. *Belonging: Australians, place and Aboriginal ownership*. Cambridge; Cambridge University Press, 2000.

14. Clinton B. Raising children to be citizens of the world. *Early Childhood Matters*. 2008;111:32-36.

15. George P. Quote. http://www.brainyquote.com/quotes/keywords/belonging.html#d0E1rtFTptIDpZW3.99. Accessed June 8, 2012.

16. Belong. *Macmillan British Dictionary*. www.macmillandictionary.com/dictionary/british/belong. Accessed June 8, 2012.

17. Cresswell T. *In Place Out of Place: Geography, Ideology and Transgression*. Minneapolis, MN: University of Minnesota Press, 1996.

18. Miller L. *Being and Belonging*. Doctoral thesis, University of Tasmania: 8. Available at: http://eprints.utas.edu.au/7952/. Accessed on June 9, 2012.

19. Yuval-Davis N. Belonging and the politics of belonging. *Patterns of Prejudice*. 2006;40(3):197-214.

20. Christiansen F, Hedetoft U, eds. *The Politics of Multiple Belonging: Ethnicity and Nationalism in Europe and East Asia*. Aldershot: Ashgate; 2004.

21. Belonging. *WordReference.com*. http://www.wordreference.com/definition/belonging. Accessed June 8, 2012.

22. Belong. *Cambridge Dictionary*. dictionary.cambridge.org/dictionary/british/belong. Accessed June 6, 2012.

23. Belonging. *Answers.com*. http://www.answers.com/topic/belonging. Accessed June 7, 2012.

24. Pelletier K. *Sound Mind, Sound Body: A New Model for Lifelong Health*. New York: Simon and Shuster; 1994.

25. Rebeiro KL, Day D, Semeniuk B, O'Brien M, Wilson B. Northern initiative for social action: an occupation-based mental health program. *American Journal of Occupational Therapy*. 2001;55:493-500.

26. Mee K. A space to care, a space of care: Public housing, belonging, and care in inner Newcastle, Australia. *Environment and Planning A*. 2009;41(4):843. doi:10.1068/a40197

27. Duggan CH, Dijkers M. Quality of life - peaks and valleys: a qualitative analysis of the narratives of persons with spinal cord injuries. *Canadian Journal of Rehabilitation*. 1999;12:181-191.

28. Lambert NM, Gwinn AM, Fincham FD, Stillman TF. Feeling tired? how sharing positive experiences can boost vitality. *International Journal of Wellbeing*. 2011;1(3):307-314. doi:10.5502/ijw.v1i3.1

29. Dunér A, Nordstrom M. The roles and functions of the informal support networks of older people who receive formal support: A Swedish qualitative study. *Ageing & Society*. 2007;27:67-85.

30. Statistics Canada. *Perceived Health, 2010*. http://www.statcan.gc.ca/pub/82-625-x/2011001/article/11465-eng.htm. Accessed June 9, 2012.

31. Hafren BQ, Karren KJ, Frandsen KJ, Smith NK. *Mind/body Health: The Effects of Attitudes, Emotions, and Relationships*. Boston: Allyn and Bacon; 1996.

32. World Health Organization. *Health Impact Assessment (HIA): The Determinants of Health*. 2012. Available at: http://www.who.int/hia/evidence/doh/en/index.html. Accessed May 18, 2012.

33. Burton R. *The Anatomy of Melancholy, What it is: With all the Kinds, Causes, Symptomes, Prognostickes, and Several Cures of it. In Three Maine Partitions with their several Sections, Members, and Subsections, Philosophically, Medicinally, Historically, Opened and Cut Up. 12th edition, corrected.* Vol. 1. London: Thomas Davison, Whitefriars; 1821: 236-237, 254. Original work published 1621.

34a. De Waal F. *The Age of Empathy: Nature's Lessons for a Kinder Society.* New York: Three Rivers Press; 2009.

34b. *Homeless World Cup: Beating Homelessness through Football.* 2013. Available at: http://www.homeless-worldcup.org/9. Accessed August 3, 2013.

34c. Beck M, Malley J. A pedagogy of belonging. *Reclaiming Children and Youth.* 1998;7(3):133-137.

34d. Brown CA. The implications of occupational deprivation experienced by elderly female immigrants. *Diversity in Health and Social Care.* 2008;5:65-69.

34e. Sered SS. Food and holiness: cooking as a sacred act among Middle-Eastern Jewish women. *Anthropological Quarterly.* 1988;61(3):129-139.

34f. Hocking C, Wright-St Clair, V, Bunrayong W. The meaning of cooking and recipe work for older Thai and New Zealand women. *Journal of Occupational Science.* 2002;9(3):117-127. doi:10.1080/14427591.2002.9686499

34g. Denham SA. Relationships between family rituals, family routines, and health. *Journal of Family Nursing.* 2003;9(3):305-330.

34h. Steindl C, Winding K, Runge U. Occupation and participation in everyday life: women's experiences of an Austrian refugee camp. *Journal of Occupational Science.* 2011;15(1):36-42. doi:10.1080/14427591.2008.9686605

34i. Han WJ, Miller DP. Parental work schedules and adolescent depression. *Health Sociology Review.* 2009;18(1):36-49.

34j. Heigl F, Kinebanian A, Josephsson S. I think of my family, therefore I am: perceptions of daily occupations of some Albanians in Switzerland. *Scandinavian Journal of Occupational Therapy.* 2011;18:36-48.

34k. Luhby T. Union membership down, income inequality up. CNN Money. *Economy Now.* 2012. Available at: http://economy.money.cnn.com/2012/08/30/unions-income-inequality/. Accessed August 3, 2013.

34l. Nandi TK. Social networks and employment in India. *Economics Bulletin.* 2010;30(4):2769-2778.

34m. United Nations Environment Programme. *Vision for Change: Recommendations for Effective Policies on Sustainable Lifestyles.* 2011. Sweden: Ministry for the Environment.

34n. Horghagen S, Josephsson S. Theatre as liberation, collaboration and relationship for asylum seekers. *Journal of Occupational Science.* 2010;17:168-176. doi:10.1080/14427591.2010.9686691

35. Youmin L. Making sense of good life: Local modernity from a traditional industrial-commercial region in Southern China. *International Journal of Business Anthropology.* 2012;3(1):82-101.

36. Conway D, Potter RB, St. Bernard G. Diaspora return of transnational migrants to Trinidad and Tobago: The additional contributions of social remittances. *International Development Planning Review.* 2012;34(2):189-209. doi:10.3828/idpr.2012.12

37. Schein R H. *Belonging through Land/scape. Environment and Planning A.* 2009;41(4):811-826. doi:10.1068/a41125

38. Russell E. Writing on the wall: the form, function and meaning of tagging. *Journal of Occupational Science.* 2008;15:87-97.

39. Haines C, Smith TM, Baxter MF. Participation in the risk-taking occupation of skateboarding. *Journal of Occupational Science.* 2010;17:239-245.

40. Mueller C. Integrating Turkish communities: a German dilemma. *Population Research and Policy Review.* 2006; 25:419-441.

41. Kelly N. *Heinemann History: The Medieval Realms.* Oxford: Heinemann Educational Publishers, 1991.

42. Sirah KS. *A Stone in the Brook: Aesthetics of Home in the Narratives, Memory, and Arts of Homeless Persons from a Southern Shelter Community.* Unpublished master's thesis. Chapel Hill, North Carolina: University of North Carolina at Chapel Hill. ProQuest, UMI Dissertations Publishing, 2013. 1538142.

43. Bell M. *Safe Haven: The Role of Social Support and Community Inclusion in Fostering Feelings of Belonging in a Homeless Shelter.* Unpublished master's thesis. Calgary, Canada: University of Calgary. ProQuest, UMI Dissertations Publishing: 2011.

44. Tarnas R. *The Passion of the Western Mind: Understanding the Ideas that have Shaped our Worldview.* London, UK: Pimlico; 1991.

45. Burke J, Ornstein R. *The Axemaker's Gift: Technology's Capture and Control of our Minds and Culture.* New York: Tarcher Penguin; 1997.

46. Commission on Social Determinants of Health. *Achieving Health Equity: From Root Causes to Fair Outcomes.* Geneva: World Health Organization; 2007.

47. Nussbaum MC. *Creating Capabilities: The Human Development Approach.* Cambridge, MA: The Belknap Press; 2011.

48. United Nations General Assembly. *Declaration on Human Rights Education and Training.* A/RES/66/137; 2011. Retrieved from http://www.un.org/documents/instruments/docs_en.asp?type=declarat

49. Demanet J, van Houtte M. The impact of bullying and victimization on students' relationships. *American Journal of Health Education.* 2012;43(2):104-113.

50. Morgan A, Malam S, Muir J, Barker R. *Health and Social Inequalities in English Adolescents: Exploring the Importance of School, Family and Neighbourhood. Findings from the WHO Health Behaviour in School-aged Children Study.* London: National Institute for Health and Clinical Excellence. 2006. www.hbscengland.com/pdf/HSBC_Final_10-03-06.pdf. Accessed June 9, 2012.

51. Landers J. Reconstructing ancient populations. In: Jones S, Martin R, Pilbeam D, Bunney S, editors. *The Cambridge Encyclopedia of Human Evolution.* Cambridge: Cambridge University Press; 1992:402-405.

52. Evans J, Rodger S. Mealtimes and bedtimes: windows to family routines and rituals. *Journal of Occupational Science.* 2008;15:98-104.

53. Larson EA, Zemke R. Shaping the temporal patterns of our lives: The social coordination of occupation. *Journal of Occupational Science.* 2003;10(2):80-89.

54. Segal R. Family routines and rituals: a context for occupational therapy interventions. *American Journal of Occupational Therapy.* 2004;58(5):499-508.

55. Yiakoumaki V. Local, ethnic, and rural food: on the emergence of cultural diversity in post-EU-accession Greece. *Journal of Modern Greek Studies.* 2006;24(2):415-429.

56. Philipp A, Ho E. Migration, home and belonging: South African migrant women in Hamilton, New Zealand. *New Zealand Population Review.* 2010;36:81-97.

57. UN General Assembly Resolution A/RES/55/2. *United Nations Millennium Declaration.* 2000.

58. United Nations. *UN Declaration on the Rights of Indigenous People.* 61/295. 2007. www.un.org/esa/socdev/unpfii/documents/DRIPS_en.pdf. Accessed on June 2, 2012.

59. Australian Human Rights Commission. *Community Guide to the UN Declaration on the Rights of Indigenous Peoples. Part 8: Participation, Development and Economic and Social Rights.* 2010. www.culturalsurvival.org/files/declaration_guide2010.pdf. Accessed on June 7, 2012.

60. Ferguson H, Kepe T. Agricultural cooperatives and social empowerment of women: a Ugandan case study. Development in Practice. 2011;21(3):421-429. doi:10.1080/09614524.2011.558069.

61. *GAPA: Grandmothers Against Poverty and Aids.* http://www.gapa.org.za/. Accessed December 4, 2012.

62. Davidson GR, Carr SC. Forced migration, social exclusion and poverty: introduction. *Journal of Pacific Rim Psychology.* 2010;4(1):1-6. doi:10.1375/prp.4.1.1.

63. Stewart MJ, Makwarimba E, Reutter LI, Veenstra G, Raphael D, Love R. Poverty, sense of belonging and experiences of social isolation. *Journal of Poverty.* 2009;13(2):173-195. doi:10.1080/10875540902841762.

64. Cate. *The Meaning of Home. A Shelter SA Project.* July 14, 2008. http://sheltersa.wordpress.com/ Accessed December 9, 2012.

65. Read P. *Belonging: Australians, Place and Aboriginal Ownership.* Cambridge; Cambridge University Press, 2000; 85.

66. Fenster T. Gender and the city: The different formulations of belonging. In: Seager J, Nelson L, eds. *A Companion to Feminist Geography.* Malden, MA: Blackwell. 2005:242-256.

67. Yuval-Davis N, Kannabiran K, Vieten UM. Introduction: Situating contemporary politics of belonging. In: Yuval-Davis N, Kannabiran K, Vieten UM, eds. *The Situated Politics of Belonging.* London: Sage; 2006:1-14.

68. Yuval-Davis N. Belonging and the politics of belonging. *Patterns of Prejudice.* 2006;40(3):197-214. doi:10.1080/00313220600769331.

69. Probyn E. *Outside Belongings.* New York: Routledge, 1996.

70. Barbier EB. The concept of sustainable economic development. *Environmental Conservation.* 1987;14(2):101-110. doi:10.1017/S0376892900011449.

71. Barnard A. Hunters and gatherers. In: Kuper A, Kuper J, eds. *The Social Science Encyclopedia.* New York, NY: Routledge; 1989:372-373.

72. Diamond J. *The Rise and Fall of the Third Chimpanzee: How our Animal Heritage Affects the Way We Live.* London: Vintage; 1988.

73. Jones S, Martin R, Pilbeam D, Bunney S, eds. *The Cambridge Encyclopedia of Human Evolution.* Cambridge: Cambridge University Press; 1992.

74. Potts R. The hominid way of life. In: Jones S, Martin R, Pilbeam D, Bunney S, editors. *The Cambridge Encyclopedia of Human Evolution.* Cambridge: Cambridge University Press; 1992:325-334.

75. Ehrlich PR, Ornstein RE. *Humanity on a Tightrope: Thoughts on Empathy, Family, and Big Changes for a Viable Future.* Lanham: Rowman & Littlefield Publishers; 2010.

76. Depue RA, Morrone-Strupinsky JV. A neurobehavioral model of affiliative bonding: Implications for conceptualizing a human trait of affiliation. *Behavioral and Brain Science.* 2005;28:313-395.

77. Dunbar R. Social behaviour and evolutionary theory. In: Jones S, Martin R, Pilbeam D, Bunney S, eds. *The Cambridge Encyclopedia of Human Evolution.* Cambridge: Cambridge University Press; 1992:145-147.

78. Hamilton WD. Discriminating nepotism: Expectable, common and overlooked. In: Fletcher DJC, Michener CD, eds. *Kin Recognition in Animals.* New York: Wiley; 1987:417-437.

79. Darwin C. *The Descent of Man.* Amherst, NY: Prometheus Books; 1998:156. First published 1871.

80. Pennisi E. On the origin of cooperation. *Science.* 2009;325:11196.

81. De Waal F. *Good Natured: The Origins of Right and Wrong in Humans and Other Animals.* London: Harvard University Press; 1996.

82. Bowles S. Group competition, reproductive levelling, and the evolution of human altruism. *Science.* 2006;314:1569-1572.

83. Bowles S. Did warfare among ancestral hunter-gatherers affect the evolution of human social behaviors? *Science.* 2009;324:1293-1298.

84. Pfeifer JH, Iacoboni M, Mazziotta JC, Dapretto M. Mirroring others' emotions relates to empathy and interpersonal competence in children. *NeuroImage.* 2008;39:2076-2085.

85. Sterzer P, Stadler C, Poustka F, Kleinschmidt A. A structural neural deficit in adolescents with conduct disorder and its association with lack of empathy. *NeuroImage.* 2007;37:335-342.

86. Shamay-Tsoory SG, Lester H, Chisin R, Israel O, Bar-Salom R, Peretz A, Tomer R, Tsitrinbaum Z, Aharn-Peretz J. The neural correlates of understanding other's distress: A positron emission tomography investigation of accurate empathy. *NeuroImage.* 2005;27:468-472.

87. Szathmáry E. To group or not to group? *Science.* 2011;334:1648-1649.

88. Mather VA, Harada T, Lipke T, Chiao JY. Neural basis of extraordinary empathy and altruistic motivation. *NeuroImage.* 2010;51:1468-1475.

89. Masten CL, Morelli SA, Eisenberger NI. An fMRI investigation of empathy for 'social pain' and subsequent prosocial behavior. *NeuroImage.* 2011;55(1):381-388.

90. Morality. *The Hutchinson Dictionary of Ideas.* Oxford: Helicon; 1994.

91. Ayala FJ. The difference of being human: morality. *Proceedings of the National Academy of Sciences in the United States of America.* 2010;107(Suppl. 2):9018.

92. Darwin CR. *The Descent of Man, and Selection in Relation to Sex.* New York: Appleton and Company; 1871:68-69.

93. Leakey R, Lewin R. *Origins Reconsidered: In Search of What Makes Us Human.* London: Little, Brown and Co.; 1992.

94. Pilbeam D. What makes us human? In: Jones S, Martin R, Pilbeam D, Bunney S, eds. *The Cambridge Encyclopedia of Human Evolution.* Cambridge: Cambridge University Press; 1992:4.

95. Lewin R. *In the Age of Mankind: A Smithsonian Book of Human Evolution.* Washington, DC: Smithsonian Books; 1988:179-180.

96. Watson L. *Neophilia: The Tradition of the New.* Great Britain: Hodder and Stoughton Ltd; 1989:43.

97. Grant E. Aristotle on void space. In: Grant E, editor. *Much Ado about Nothing: Theories of Space and Vacuum from the Middle Ages to the Scientific Revolution.* Cambridge: Cambridge University Press. 2001; 5-8. Chapter doi:10.1017/CBO9780511895326.003 Available at: http://ebooks.cambridge.org/chapter.jsf?bid=CBO9780511895326&cid=CBO9780511895326A008. Accessed June 9, 2012.

98. Glover JB. The Yalahau region: a study of ancient Maya sociopolitical organization. *Ancient Mesoamerica.* 2012;23:271-295.

99. Hill DL. Sense of belonging as connectedness, American Indian worldview, and mental health. *Archives of Psychiatric Nursing.* 2006;20(5):210-216.

100. Roberts R, Harper R, Tuttle-Eagle Bull D, Heideman-Provost L. The native American medicine wheel and individual psychology: common themes. *Journal of Individual Psychology.* 1998;54(1):135-145.

101. Umbreit M. *Talking Circles*. Centre for Restorative Justice and Peacemaking, School of Social Work: University of Minnesota; 2003. www.cehd.umn.edu/ssw/rjp/resources/rj...Circles/Talking_Circles. pdf. Accessed on June 23, 2012.

102. Hodge F, Pasqua A, Marquez C, Geishirt-Cantrill B. Utilizing traditional storytelling to promote wellness in American Indian communities. *Journal of Transcultural Nursing*. 2002;13(1):6-11.

103. Duran E, Duran B, Brave Heart MYH, Yellow Horse DS. Healing the American Indian soul wound. In: Danieli Y, editor. *International Handbook of Multigenerational Legacies of Trauma*. New York: Plenum Press; 1998:341-354.

104. Freud S. *Civilization and its Discontents*. J Riviere, Trans. London: Hogarth Press.

105. Bowlby J. *Attachment and Loss: Vol. 1. Attachment*. New York: Basic Books; 1969.

106. Cutchin MP, Dickie V. Transactionalism: occupational science and the pragmatic attitude. In: Whiteford GE, Hocking C, eds. *Occupational Science: Society, Inclusion, Participation*. Oxford: Wiley-Blackwell. 2012:23-37.

107. Heidegger M. *Being and Time*. (J Macquarie & E Robinson, Trans.). New York: Harper; 1962:84.

108. Maller C, Townsend M, St Leger L, Henderson-Wilson C, Pryor A, Prosser L, Moore M. *Healthy Parks, Healthy People: The Health Benefits of Contact with Nature in a Park Context*. Burwood, Melbourne: Deakin University. 2008.

109. Maslow AH. *Toward a Psychology of Being*. New York: Van Nostrand; 1968.

110. Baumeister RF, Leary MR. The need to belong: desire for interpersonal attachments as a fundamental human motivation. *Psychological Bulletin*. 1995;117(3):497-529.

111. Acton G, Malathum P. Basic need status and health-promoting self-care behavior in adults. *Western Journal of Nursing Research*. 2000;22(7):796-811.

112. Baumeister RF, Leary MR. The need to belong: desire for interpersonal attachments as a fundamental human motivation. *Psychological Bulletin*. 1995;117(3):520.

113. Galvaan R. Occupational choice: the significance of socio-economic and political factors. In: Whiteford GE, Hocking C, eds. *Occupational Science: Society, Inclusion, Participation*. Oxford, UK: Wiley-Blackwell; 2012:152-162.

114. Chirot D. Social change. In: Kuper A, Kuper J, editors. *The Social Science Encyclopedia*. New York, NY: Routledge; 1989:760-763.

115. Venkatapuram S. *Health Justice: An Argument from a Capabilities Approach*. Cambridge: Polity Press; 2011.

116. WHO. *Global Health Observatory: Urban Population Growth*. http://www.who.int/gho/urban_health/situation_trends/urban_population_growth_text/en/. Accessed August 11, 2013.

117. Lorenz K. *Civilized Man's Eight Deadly Sins*. Latzke M, trans. London, England: Methuen and Co Ltd; 1974:8-9,76.

118. Dubos R. In: Hinrichs N, ed. *Population, Environment and People*. New York, NY: McGraw-Hill; 1971:xi.

119. Christiansen CH, Townsend EA, eds. *Introduction to Occupation: The Art and Science of Living*. Upper Saddle River, NJ: Prentice Hall; 2004.

120. Giugni M. Becoming worldly: an encounter with the early years learning framework. *Contemporary Issues in Early Childhood*. 2011;12(1):11-27.

121. Kennedy L, Murphy D. Racist furore as mobs riot. *The Age*. 2005. http://www.theage.com.au/news/national/racist-furore-as-mobs-riot/2005/12/11/1134235948497.html. Accessed on July 27, 2012.

122. WHO. *Health Topics: Globalization*. WHO; 2013. http://www.who.int/topics/globalization/en/. Accessed on July 29, 2012.

Theme 9

"To reach a state of complete physical, mental and social well-being, an individual or group must be able to identify and to realize aspirations."

WHO: Ottawa Charter for Health Promotion, 1986[1]

Chapter 9

OCCUPATION

BECOMING THROUGH DOING

This chapter addresses:
- Becoming: Explaining the Concept
- Becoming: Biological Needs, Natural Health, and Reaching Potential
  - Becoming and an Aging Population
  - Lack of Understanding the Biological Need for Occupation
- Becoming: Its Place in Population Health
  - As a Prerequisite of Health
    - Becoming and Peace
    - Becoming and Shelter
    - Becoming and Education
    - Becoming and Food
    - Becoming and Income
    - Becoming: A Stable Income and Sustainable Resources
    - Becoming: Social Justice and Equity
- Negative Becoming as a Factor in Illness: Occupational Alienation
- Marx, Alienation, and Industry
- Alienation as Social, Mental, And Physical Illness
- Becoming: Early and Current Guidelines for Health
- Conclusion

This chapter begins to clarify some of the mystique that surrounds becoming, to appreciate its place in occupation-focused population health. The idea of becoming adds a sense of future to the notions of doing, being, and belonging. From observation and from reports of people who live to a healthy old age, it appears that most have or have had deep interests, and continue with what are often considered youthful doings throughout their lives. The implication of such observations is that health can be enhanced if people hold aspirations and allow these to inspire, guide, and assist the utilization of capacities in ways that keep them exercised and working well.

Wilcock AA, Hocking C.
An Occupational Perspective of Health, Third Edition (pp 238-271).
© 2015 Taylor & Francis Group.

Becoming: Explaining the Concept

Ah, but a man's reach should exceed his grasp/

Or what's a heaven for?[2]

Earlier, it was postulated that individuals and communities are in a constant state of becoming different: changing, developing, and transforming as a result of what they do on a daily or occasional basis. The word derives from the Old English becuman, meaning "to happen,"[3] and is related to the Old High German biqueman, meaning "to come to," as well as to the Gothic biquiman, meaning "to appear suddenly." It is relevant to any process of change, for better or worse, but in Aristotelian philosophy is relevant for any change from the lower level of potentiality to the higher level of actuality.[4]

The theme of this chapter from the Ottawa Charter—"to reach a state of complete physical, mental and social well-being, an individual or group must be able to identify and to realize aspirations"—resonates with the concept of becoming.[1] At every point in their lives and every day, people can either grow or diminish: their becoming can be strengthened, stagnant, or sick. It is an ever-incomplete process. People never become—throughout life they are always becoming different even if they cease trying to become. As Schaef explained:

> *Life is a process. We are a process. Everything that has happened in our lives ... is an integral part of our becoming ... awareness of every aspect of ourselves allows us to become who we are.*[5]

Schaeff discussed a "living, moving, evolving energy" and the way things are done rather than what is done or the results of doing. Play, fantasy, and dreaming are integral to becoming and can be regarded as adaptive behavior aimed at creating new ways forward despite Freud's linking of them with escapism.[7]

Being well, or well-being, is about people identifying and utilizing personal capacities and strengths and being motivated and enabled toward their highest level of personal development and the good of others. Such development is central in the rhetoric of humanist psychologists as influenced by existentialism,[8-11] which has been "equated with productiveness, social adjustment, and contentment—'the good life' itself," extending consideration to the further reaches of the human psyche.[12] The humanist tradition upholds the Renaissance tradition of human achievement and the ideals of the Age of Enlightenment.

Maslow has been identified as a front-runner in this sphere of interest, coining the terms "full humanness" and "self-actualization" to describe a state of becoming. "Self-Actualization is the desire to become more and more of what one is, to become everything that one is capable of becoming." He explained that the characteristics of self-actualizing people are discovered, not invented:

> *These are potentialities, not final actualizations. Therefore they have a life history and must be seen developmentally. They are actualized, shaped, or stifled mostly (but not altogether) by extra-psychic determinants (culture, family, environment, learning, etc).*[13]

Humanist and gestalt psychologists hold that potential to self-actualize is given to all human beings at birth.[14] Maslow observed "that the concept of creativeness and the concept of the healthy, self-actualizing, fully human person seem to be coming closer and closer together, and may perhaps turn out to be the same thing."[15] He reached this conclusion following a study of self-fulfilled, mentally healthy subjects. The aim of his research was to determine the attributes and components of a basically healthy intrinsic nature and to discover how people are enabled toward growth and self-actualization. This represented a major shift in psychology from research into illness to the study of what keeps people well. Maslow described the healthiest and most effective people as transcenders. Such people are responsive to beauty, holistic in their perceptions of humanity, motivated by the satisfaction of being and service values, able to adjust well to conflict situations, and

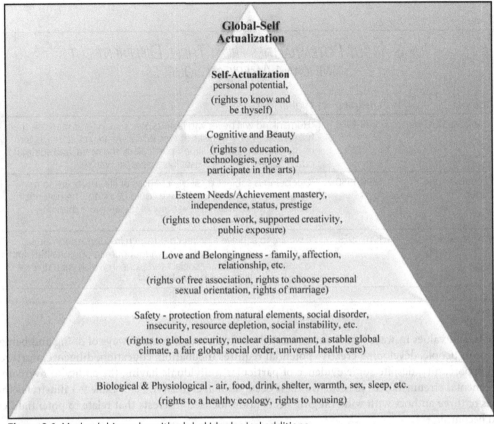

Global-Self Actualization

Self-Actualization
personal potential,

(rights to know and
be thyself)

Cognitive and Beauty

(rights to education,
technologies, enjoy and
participate in the arts)

Esteem Needs/Achievement mastery,
independence, status, prestige

(rights to chosen work, supported creativity,
public exposure)

Love and Belongingness - family, affection,
relationship, etc.

(rights of free association, rights to choose personal
sexual orientation, rights of marriage)

Safety - protection from natural elements, social disorder,
insecurity, resource depletion, social instability, etc.

(rights to global security, nuclear disarmament, a stable global
climate, a fair global social order, universal health care)

Biological & Physiological - air, food, drink, shelter, warmth, sex, sleep, etc.

(rights to a healthy ecology, rights to housing)

Figure 9-1. Maslow's hierarchy with global ideological additions.

more likely to accept others with an unconditional positive regard. They are less attracted by the rewards of money and objects, and work whole-heartedly toward goals and purposes. They tend to fuse work and play, have more peak, creative, or self-actualization experiences and sometimes reach a state of transcendence, described as an increased awareness of self and species potential.[15] The hierarchy has been used for many different purposes, including being adapted to global ideologies.[16] Figure 9-1 depicts Maslow's hierarchy with the global ideological additions. The apex of the triangle represents "global self actualization" that is about a global economy, whole systems design, collective consciousness, achieving resource-based human rights and "awakening to the global brain."[16]

A Gallup poll with 60,865 participants in 123 countries conducted between 2005 and 2010 found universal acceptance of the needs Maslow identified in his theory.[17] However, the order of the needs appeared largely immaterial. Even when the most basic physiological needs, such as food and water, are unavailable, others, such as relationships and self-actualization, remain necessary and imperative. The findings pointed to the primary importance of people as social and self-actualizing beings with a need to fulfill both personal and social goals to achieve happiness.[17] This substantiates the health benefits of the cooperative nature of occupation as a mix of doing, being, belonging, and becoming.

Like Maslow, Carl Rogers proposed that self-growth motivates creativity and that creativity and the achievement of individual potential is synonymous with health. He described "man's tendency to actualize himself, to become his potentialities" as the mainspring of creativity.[18] Aiming toward potentialities provides people with the chance to portray themselves as more than their outward appearance and everyday behavior supposes; it allows the expression of attitudes,

Table 9-1

IDEAS ABOUT POTENTIALITIES FROM THREE DIFFERENT BUT SIGNIFICANT AMERICAN SOURCES

Author	Lifespan	Global Ideology
John Foster Dulles	1888-1959	"Humankind will never win lasting peace so long as men use their full resources only in tasks of war. While we are yet at peace, let us mobilize the potentialities, particularly the moral and spiritual potentialities, which we usually reserve for war."[23b]
Katherine Anne Porter	1890-1980	"Our being is subject to all the chances of life. There are so many things we are capable of, that we could be or do. The potentialities are so great that we never, any of us, are more than one-fourth fulfilled."[23c]
Margaret Mead	1901-1978	"If we are to achieve a richer culture, rich in contrasting values, we must recognize the whole gamut of human potentialities, and so weave a less arbitrary social fabric, one in which each diverse human gift will find a fitting place."[23d]

beliefs, and values in ways that demonstrate self-definition and creative ways of doing and being. For most people, developing creative potential requires incubation, education, diligence, nurture, and opportunity, despite some evidence of particular individuals having the ability to overcome detrimental circumstances to actualize their occupational creativity.[19-23a] Table 9-1 illustrates the ideas of three authors with wide ranging occupation-focused interests that relate to potentialities and becoming.[23a]

Engaging in occupation that people perceive as self-actualizing provides opportunity for self-evaluation and grounds the sense of competency and moral worth. However, becoming is both an agent of self-creation and a product of socializing forces, providing motivation to experience the self as efficacious, competent, and consequential.[24] The latter claim touches on the notion that positive becoming is problematic for people who seek personal isolation or who find close relationships difficult, and points to why such people, if they have a particular talent, may feel compelled to use it to communicate, even if that talent might be, or may appear to be, antisocial. Becoming is an expression of societal values whereas being is intimately related to concepts of the self and is often an expression of autonomy.[25] In a positive sense, it is a way of communicating what people think they are about by allowing them to demonstrate what they can do, what they can contribute to their own growth, and what they can offer the community that is a special gift from them and that, by its provision, their place within the societal structure will alter. In a negative sense, not being able to demonstrate or communicate potential can lead to lack of social acceptance, self-consciousness, inhibition, depression, and anger. Negative becoming is seen here as a precursor to illness and a harbinger of reduced longevity.

The idea of positive becoming is central to an occupational perspective of health and inclusive of those ideas discussed above. That includes the ideas of growing or coming into being; of living, moving, evolving energy; of aiming toward the highest level of personal development and self-esteem; of potentialities; of full humanness; and of self-actualization, which is an ever-incomplete process. Such ideas are seen as integral to the view that people's occupational natures evolved over millennia with structural changes to body and brain in response to changes of environment, habitat, and survival pressures, and as a result of natural selection. It is interesting to compare this with McMichael's description of the inter-related and distinctive features of the history of human ecology and disease found in Chapter 2.[26] Readers may recall that the first two of these addressed the encounters of human societies with new environmental hazards and the recurring tension between biological needs and capacities and changes in living conditions.[26]

Late in the evolutionary chain, as human capacities expanded, the need to keep those of a more diverse intellectual nature exercised for when they were required demanded increased and more flexible patterns of occupation. These patterns were superimposed on and integrated with older activity/rest rhythms. Ornstein and Sobel observed that:

> As the brain evolved, its ability to handle the world became increasingly comprehensive ... The paradox is that as the human brain matures and develops it both enormously increases its ability to find out new things and, at the same time, develops an enormous capacity for getting bored.[27]

The question of boredom is a complex and integral occupational imbalance that is considered a disorder of occupation and a cause of illness.

Becoming: Biological Needs, Natural Health, and Reaching Potential

Once again, it is useful to draw on biological science and history to inform the present and future. As controversial, Chicago-born philosopher, polemicist, and author Francis P. Yockey explained:

> The greatest repository of psychology of all is History. It contains no models for us, since Life is never-recurring, once-happening, but it shows by example how we can fulfill our potentialities by being true to ourselves, by never compromising with that which is utterly alien.[23a]

Some biological needs have been described as the essence of well-being, relating to human health by enabling organisms to flourish and facilitating the fulfillment of potential.[28] In addition, instinctive energy of a primitive nature can be redirected according to choice, enabling the "highest achievements of humanity."[29,30] Maslow described the process as the:

> Development of the biologically based nature of man, [empirically] normative of the whole species conforming to biological destiny, rather than to historically arbitrary, culturally local value models as the terms 'health' and 'illness' often do.[31]

As the Gallup poll mentioned earlier suggests, Maslow's idea of a hierarchy of human needs is more likely to be an assemblage of competing needs rather than a pyramid in which self-actualization forms the apex.[17] Whether or not that is the case, it remains important in understanding the idea of becoming to appreciate the significance to well-being of self-actualization and what Maslow called "growth needs," "being values," or "B-needs." He described how those include needs for justice, truth, beauty, meaning, simplicity, wholeness, and order, in contrast to "deficiency or D needs" that relate to physiological and security requirements, such as for water, air, food, sleep, and safety and that, like the WHO health prerequisites, are vital to survival. Earlier chapters have already discussed the other important social (belonging) needs and esteem (being) needs.[15]

Becoming, in terms of individuals, is the personal outcome aspect of occupation: its fourth dimension or potential purpose. Many people make the mistake of attributing becoming needs only to people who appear gifted with a particular talent such as of an artistic nature (Figure 9-2). However, becoming is a need of all people and can be recognized in many spheres of life while forming the essence of personality. Carl Jung proposed that:

> Personality is the supreme realization of the innate idiosyncrasy of a living being. It is an act of high courage flung in the face of life, the absolute affirmation of all that constitutes the individual, the most successful adaptation to the universal conditions of existence coupled with the greatest possible freedom for self-determination.[32]

Figure 9-2. Becoming Through Artistic Expression. (© Carol Spencer 2012, otspencer@adam.com.au. Used with permission.)

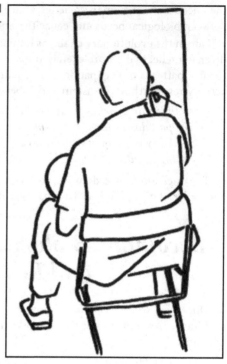

Erik Erikson discussed a further aspect of becoming in the book *Identity*:

> *A man's character is discernible in the mental and moral attitude, in which, when it came upon him, he felt himself to be most deeply and intensely active and alive. At such moments there is a voice inside which speaks and says: "This is the real me."*[33]

Of the numerous hypotheses about a basic need for becoming, another is discussed in Churchill's *Black Dog and Other Phenomena of the Human Mind*.[34] Here, becoming is explained in relation to the need to create order and unity out of complexity and diversity because:

> *Human beings have to order their experience, both spatially and temporally, as part of their biological adaptation to reality, and the forces which impel them to do so are just as "instinctive" as sex.*[34]

In ways that resonate with notions of self-actualization, Storr described the need to discover and to create "new hypotheses which bring order and pattern to the maze of phenomena" as a biological endowment.[7] The everyday search for answers to vexed questions calls on this extraordinary dimension of futurity that is a part of becoming. Building on earlier ideas about how inspiration appears to follow a period of incubation,[35] Storr described how conscious preparation, followed by a stage of apparently doing nothing, leads to the emergence of illumination and inspiration, often overnight following sleep, but sometimes after many years. It can be either an unconscious or conscious process.[7] For instance, Wilcock recalls her father, a builder, sitting quiet and alone, apparently doing nothing, for a day or two before starting any major project. At those times he did not welcome any diversion. Such problem solving is an ongoing creative solution process that triggers becoming activity. Perhaps understandably to those who advocate the remedial nature of occupation, the motivating factor that sets people on the hazardous, often unrewarding task of trying to bring order and meaning to their lives can originate from alienation or despair, as well as joy. Creative endeavor that reconciles disparate elements is essentially integrative and some are driven to it by "a need to prevent their own disintegration."[36]

In Sir Ernst Gombrich's book, *The Sense of Order*, links are also made with exploratory tendencies and the need for "pattern making." By creating order, the need to pay equal attention to every stimulus is reduced, and people only need to take notice of novel stimuli.[37] This explanation meshes with zoologist Watson's determination that, in common with some other species, humans never stop investigating or exploring or adapting. This need or tendency—neophilia—is aimed at thriving, as well as surviving; at becoming, as well as doing. Not without problems, it has been a positive and powerful force in evolution to the current day:

> We create unnecessary problems ... We allow our jobs to become more complex than necessary. We fill our leisure time with more and more elaborate recreations. We tempt fate by courting danger, taking risks ... We look in our own lives, for more complex forms of expression, experimenting with arts and sciences that give free rein to our gigantic brains.[38]

Neophilia "grows from old and well-established roots:"[39] it is a need that is experienced throughout life, not just during childhood and youth. It is easily squashed by external forces of a personal nature, of political initiative or environmental circumstance, or, supposedly, for the safety or health's sake of older people.

While engaged in creative or other demanding occupations, including paid employment, people can live through and seek out what Maslow terms a peak experience[40] and Csikszentmihalyi describes as flow.[41] Those recognized with special talents that require nurture tend either to be seen as exceptionally well-balanced or liable to instability.[7,42] Some creative people, such as Balzac, "keep the devil at bay by manic overwork. Success and public recognition can, in some degree, compensate for inner emptiness by providing recurrent injections of self-esteem from external sources."[43]

Capitalist structures, industrial processes, and emerging electronic technology have narrowed the range of activity of many individuals and reduced the number and variety of peripheral occupations, especially those associated with nature and natural needs or processes. Alexis Carrel, a French-American physiologist who was a Nobel Prize recipient in 1912, called for the scientific study of humankind. He suggested that "it is difficult ... to know exactly how the substitution of an artificial mode of existence for the natural one and a complete modification of their environment have acted upon civilized human beings."[44] People joyfully welcome "modern civilization," adopting new modes of life and "ways of acting and thinking," laying aside "old habits" because these "demand a greater effort."[44] Most accept that technological change is necessarily an improvement and that the reduction of occupational effort is inevitable and desirable. It can be either constructive or destructive in terms of health and well-being. At an ever-increasing rate, new technology leads to massive changes in occupational behaviors, energy expenditure, cultural adaptation, and further technological change so there is scant opportunity to measure health effects over the longer term.

Arthur Penty, a follower of Morris, is credited in the *Fontana Dictionary of Modern Thought* with coining the phrase "postindustrial society" at the turn of the 20th century,[45] but social commentators as diverse as Daniel Bell,[46] Alain Touraine,[47] and Barry Jones[48] give us contemporary descriptions. To them, postindustrial society is characterized by a change from production to service industries, from manual to professional and technical workers, and to decision making based on information technology. Those economic changes are part of "a crisis that is simultaneously tearing up our energy base, our value systems, our sense of space and time, our epistemology as well as our economy" and will result in a "wholly new and drastically different social order."[49] The tension between traditional social forms that are still largely in place and modern postindustrial arrangements has been responsible for a period of unprecedented uncertainty and loss of direction for many people. Jones suggested that, despite "universal literacy, an omnipresent media, and a vast information industry," postindustrial society is threatened by its "preoccupation with materialism, a conviction that national and international salvation is to be found in economic growth alone, and emphasis on externalized (consumption-based) value systems."[50] He predicted that if a new labor-absorbing industry comes into being, as has been the case after earlier economic revolutions, it will turn away from technology. Reintroduced will be labor/time-absorbing work, such as education, home-based industries, craftwork, leisure, tourism, and welfare services that will act as a guard against unemployment, and the concentration of wealth into fewer hands.

A worrying outcome of recent technology is a devaluation of older members of society. Although some elders embrace it, many are confused by the rapid social and technical changes occurring around them. When earlier occupational technologies were dominant, they were often viewed as wise counsellors and spiritual leaders; however, in recent times, their life experiences and even their language are no longer seen as relevant. They have been effectively displaced and are viewed as being part of a "stagnant, marginal social category,"[51] so it is useful to consider their case more fully.

BECOMING AND AN AGING POPULATION

In almost every country, the proportion of people aged over 60 years is growing faster than any other age group, as a result of both longer life expectancy and declining fertility rates.[52]

It is easy to suppose that older people have had their chance to become and can vegetate for their indefinite future. However, if becoming is as important to well-being and health as it appears, it becomes necessary to encourage all people, including those who are older, to do what they can and want to do rather than tell them what they cannot or should not do. The WHO observed that:

Aging of the population is a highly desirable and natural aim of any society. By 2025 there will be 1.2 billion older people in the world, close to three-quarters of them in the developing world. But if aging is to be a positive experience, it must be accompanied by improvements in the quality of life of those who have reached—or are reaching—old age.[53]

To ensure that aging is a positive experience, it is imperative that occupations provide people with sufficient meaningful physical, mental, and social exercise and opportunities to meet their unique becoming needs. Without ongoing or new interests that provide as much purpose and meaning as careers or caring for a family once did and the potential to continue the self-actualization process, some people are unable to thrive. The many stories of individuals who have been committed to careers of great interest dying shortly after retirement support that notion.

At the United Nation's first World Assembly on Aging in 1982, recognition was accorded to the accumulated wealth of knowledge and experience that makes the aged an asset rather than a liability to society. At that time, the World Assembly reaffirmed that the Universal Declaration of Human Rights should:

Apply fully and undiminished to the aging and recognized that the quality of life was no less important than the longevity, and that the aging should therefore, as far as possible, be enabled to enjoy in their own families and communities a life of fulfillment, health, security and contentment, appreciated as an integral part of society.[54]

The United Nations' support of older people needing and being enabled to continue to enhance their occupational capabilities and growth was developed further in 1999 when the International Year of Older People was celebrated. Nations were petitioned to establish or strengthen policies aimed at meeting the changing potential of the aged, as well as their humanitarian needs.[55,56] In 2001, governments were urged to promote healthy, active aging through the development of programs that ensure quality of life,[57] and in the International Plan of Action on Aging produced the following year was another call for the enormous potential of aging to be fulfilled in the 21st century.[58] That same year, the WHO developed a Policy Framework for the second World Assembly on Aging held in Madrid. Based on recognition of the United Nations' principles of "independence, participation, dignity, care and self-fulfillment,"[59] it was recommended that policies and programs for older people need to both enable those who are able to continue to contribute to society in important ways, and prevent discriminatory action that can be counterproductive to well-being. The need to facilitate becoming is clearly articulated as enabling "people to realize their potential for physical, mental and social well-being throughout the life course and to participate in society according to their needs, desires and capacities."[60] The policy of active aging centers older people firmly within the postmodern vision of fair, ethical, and moral societies. Regardless of age, as well as class, income, race, gender, disability, or health status but as a matter of social justice, people should be able to enact aspirations and use their talents, as well as engage in daily life tasks. The civic principles of such advance both freedom of expression and liberty for all people.[61,62] An encouraging example is provided by the publication of *Active, Engaged, Valued: Older People and NSW Public Libraries* nearly a decade ago, during which time many Baby Boomers reached retirement age.[63] Library services have been extended to include staff specializing in senior's requirements, active aging festivals, programs focusing on health and wellness, and exploration of technology services to facilitate access to and use of broadband, Internet, audio, and e-books.[63]

Examples of the call for active and inclusive societies, in which rights carry responsibilities and individuals experience opportunities to realize potential, can be found in legislation throughout the western world. Discussion in such legislation mainly focuses on people of working age despite the growing numbers of older citizens. Rather, their place in the brave new scheme of things was and is as passive clients of welfare systems, and comments are often concentrated on economic concerns, such as the provision of pensions and services.[64-68] Perhaps this is a reflection of the youth culture of postindustrial societies where everything old is disregarded and thrown away and people spend fortunes on looking young. It is even being said that the sale of antiques is decreasing, so generalized is the trend. Commonly and patronizingly, active aging as it pertains to the becoming wants and needs of people beyond "paid employment" years is marginalized. This is often in the name of risk management, particularly for those who come into contact with medical, health, and social welfare services. Risk management strategies fail, in many respects, to recognize that externally imposed strategies can disempower recipients and lead to illness of a kind less obvious in cause than hazards like slipping on mats or rugs. Widespread too is discouragement by family members and caregivers of older people engaging in pursuits of their own choice that are deemed too active. Although apparently altruistic and due to fear of detrimental effects on health that may lead to increasing dependence or of their relative's death, such discouragement can be viewed as discriminatory, whether institutionally or privately constituted.[69]

It is ironic that such outdated attitudes prevail as "the world as a whole, and industrialized countries in particular, are moving through a demographic transition to 'greyer' societies."[70] Taking the view that aging is a natural part of the life course (a transition rather than a crisis) appears to pose a challenge for people or places where services are well developed for older people as disabled and needy adults. It is not uncommon that concerns about increasing public expenditure are therefore attributed to rising numbers, and a tendency to "blame rather than congratulate" older people for living longer:

> The challenge is to promote healthy and productive aging in these added later years of life, and to adjust societal practices and structures to include older people as contributors to society ... They do have the ability, given the opportunities, to work for longer to help fund a comfortable standard of living in retirement.[70]

Meeting that challenge might not only enable older people to improve the quality of their lives in ways that enable them to keep on growing, it might also reduce the numbers it is generally feared will clog the beds available in institutional care. Therefore, not only is it a humanitarian act, it is an economic one.

Boxed Dialogue 9-1:
Excerpts and stories from "A Good Age." Alex Comfort; 1977.[71]

"Agism is the notion that people cease to be people, cease to be the same people or become people of a distinct and inferior kind, by virtue of having lived a specified number of years... Like racism, which it resembles, it is based on fear, folklore, and the hang-ups of a few unlovable people who propagate these. Like racism, it needs to be met by information, contradiction and, when necessary, confrontation. And the people being victimized have to stand up for themselves in order to put it down."

At 64, Maggie Kuhn organized an American network of highly vocal older people, dedicated to fighting agism. They were known as the Gray Panthers. A firm believer in experimenting with new life styles, she claimed: "the old are isolated by government policy."

Italy's great nineteenth-century composer, Giuseppe Verdi, was 73 when he completed Otello, approaching 80 when he composed Falstaff, a scintillating comedy, very different from his previous works. He retired after completing Stabat Mater, an inspired choral work at 84.

Golda Meir resigned as Israel's Prime Minister at the age of 75. She had held the post for five years through two Middle East wars. The following year she was asked to head a committee to rejuvenate the Labour Party.

In Helena Rubinstein's memoirs, "My Life for Beauty," written when she was in her nineties, she told of creating a beauty business over seven decades that crossed six continents. Claiming work had been her beauty treatment she explained her belief that hard work keeps the wrinkles out of the mind and the spirit, helping to keep a woman young and alive.

Duncan MacLean was 90 when he won a silver medal at the 1975 World Veterans' Olympics by running 200 metres in 44 seconds. A sprinting champion of South Africa from 1905 to 1907 he continued sprinting after his retirement at 80. Prior to that he had toured the world with a comedy song-and-dance act and, in his sixties, took up house painting. His future goal was to run a hundred metres on his hundredth birthday.

Charlie Smith who was officially recognized as the oldest person in the United States in 1972 had been made to retire from his work on a citrus farm when he was 113 because he was considered too old to be climbing trees. For twenty years after that he ran a small store in Florida, until he was 133, living alone at the back of his store, when, on medical advice, he moved into a retirement home.

Comfort A. *A Good Life.* Melbourne: Macmillan Company of Australia; 1977:35,82.

Alex Comfort, in a remarkable book that pre-empts WHO active aging initiatives, explained that:

> *Aging has no effect upon you as a person. When you are "old" you will feel no different and be no different from what you are now or were when you were young, except that more experiences will have happened.*[71]

He supplied an extremely useful definition of agism and some prime examples of older people continuing to become what they had the potential to become (Boxed Dialogue 9-1).[71]

The current aging of populations is a "pervasive, unprecedented and enduring process with profound social and economic implications."[72] To create societies in which all older people can continue to contribute according to their capacities is not without difficulty. Despite rhetoric to the contrary even post-industrial economies driven by monetary considerations embrace actions that sustain inequalities rather than the enabling or enhancement of human becoming.[69]

LACK OF UNDERSTANDING THE BIOLOGICAL NEED FOR OCCUPATION

The current driving force of technology-affluent societies is economics rather than human nature and needs. Similar to the difficulties being experienced by the elderly, when technology-affluent societies interact with those that are technology-poor, there appears to be a lack of understanding of the biological need for occupation. The absence of recognition of occupation's relationship with health has contributed to people allowing technological development to drive them, rather than the other way around. Countering this could be possible if all people had a better understanding of the purpose and meaning of occupation in a generic sense and of occupation encompassing the idea of growth, development, and self-actualization "so that we can collectively decide which kinds of work and which kinds of leisure are appropriate to a good life and create the opportunities for those to be realized."[73] From the time when industry began to dominate human endeavour, occupation for its own sake appears to have lost its efficacy and value, perhaps because, for most people, it is no longer tied to self-sustaining natural ways of life and some biological needs that are germane to species' survival are obscured. It is somewhat ironic that the need to use human capacities in a creative, problem-solving, inventive, or adaptive way has led to the domination of occupational technology. That raises queries about the survival of the species in the long term if disuse, or perhaps misuse, of personal capacities causes failure to meet biological requirements.

Some commentators argue that when humans become sufficiently focused on such culturally created problems, the same drive that created them will be able to counteract the ill effects. This could already be in process. Indeed, Toynbee suggested that even though "in making ... tools progressively more effective" and the "misuse of them progressively more dangerous" the "[w]orld's most powerful nations and governments have shown an uncustomary self-restraint on some critical occasions" demonstrating an "advance in social justice" and an increase in humanitarianism.[74] Currently, there is widespread questioning of the wisdom of continuing with economic policies that place technological development and the expansion of trade before human well-being and diminishing natural resources. Robertson called for people to reject a future of technological determinism in which technology, rather than value systems, dictate choice;[75] and Jones suggested that "the most appropriate analogies for economic processes are to be found in biology—with growth, maturation, nourishment, excretion, and decline—rather than physics."[50]

The biological needs associated with becoming are part of human's inheritance, along with capacities, talents, personalities, and biological characteristics. The needs are weak, in terms of how easy it is for them to be overcome by societal, cultural, and environmental expectations and much of people's inner nature is repressed or unconscious, though they rarely disappear. Maslow predicted that if this inner nature is "frustrated, denied or suppressed, sickness results" in some form or other, sooner or later.[76] In their exploration of autonomy as a key human need alongside health, Doyal and Gough identified three major variables:

1. The level of self-understanding and cultural expectations.
2. The capacity to formulate options.
3. The opportunities enabling action.[77]

"People consist of more than the deterministic relationships between their bodily components" because they have the "ability to formulate consistent aims and strategies which they believe to be in their interests and ... to put them into practice in the activities in which they engage."[77]

Becoming: Its Place in Population Health

> *Population aging can be seen as a success story for public health policies and for socioeco-nomic development, but it also challenges society to adapt, in order to maximize the health and functional capacity of older people as well as their social participation and security.*[52]

Despite the WHO's optimistic claims and inspirational rhetoric, becoming is only minimally recognized as part of the health-illness complex. Its place in population health relates, theoreti-cally, to acceptance that health promotion should be aimed toward all people being able to achieve physical, mental, and social aspirations. That aim draws on the holistic vision of the Ottawa Charter that highlights becoming as a health issue[1] and encapsulates it in regional health propa-ganda. The Australian Aboriginal definition of health provided earlier required health services "to achieve that state where every individual can achieve their full potential as human beings."[78] Public health and occupational therapy certainly espouse the need to aim toward similar outcomes but to enact them in the daily scheme of things is difficult, especially as resources are scarce, and becoming is seldom recognized as a medical priority despite the well-being rhetoric. However, well-being depends on the meeting of individual potential, of people striving to become according to their particular genes and interests by doing what they are "suited for and capable of."[79]

There are many sources relating to the belief that health and personal growth are entwined. For example, Carrel, when contemplating the benefits and drawbacks of the "modern society" of his era, concluded:

> *It is a primary datum of observation that physiological and mental functions are improved by work. Also, that effort is indispensable to the optimum development of the individual. Like muscles and organs, intelligence and moral sense become atrophied for want of exercise … the physiological and mental progress of the individual depends on his functional activ-ity and on all his efforts. We become adapted to the lack of use of our organic and mental systems by degenerating … In order to reach his optimum state, the human being must actualize all his potentialities.*[80]

Maslow's ideas echoed these earlier thoughts when he observed "capacities clamor to be used, and cease their clamor only when they are well used. That is, capacities are also needs. Not only is it fun to use our capacities, but it is also necessary for growth."[31] Some empirical research points to the truth of such assertions. For example, in a large, population-based, longitudinal study, Glass et al found "enhanced social activities may help to increase the quality and length of life," and "social and productive activities are as effective as fitness activities in lowering the risk of death."[81] The study corroborates findings from other earlier research,[82,83] supporting the idea that becoming can be intimately related to positive health outcomes. Csikszentmihalyi found that an optimal state relating to health and well-being occurs when individuals are challenged by their occupations and have the personal capacities to meet the challenge.[84] The antithesis is that if this does not occur, ill health may be a consequence.

Not developing and using capacities or skills is detrimental to health, with Maslow claiming that "the unused skill or capacity or organ can become a disease center or else atrophy or disap-pear, thus diminishing the person."[31] Certainly, inactivity, and an associated lack of becoming opportunity, has been found to be associated with several risk factors associated with the likeli-hood of cardiovascular disease[85-88] and with other disorders such as type 2 diabetes and some cancers, as well as "strong emerging evidence that activity delays cognitive decline and is good for brain health."[89]

However, the concept of becoming poses a particular challenge to health workers engaged in institutional or community care or in politically or economically struggling programs for people living in poverty. Often, they feel obliged to overlook people's potential growth or possible future ill-health and simply help them cope with the here and now. The people they work with in that way

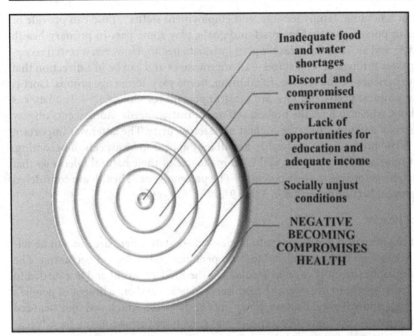

Inadequate food
and water
shortages

Discord and
compromised
environment

Lack of
opportunities for
education and
adequate income

Socially unjust
conditions

**NEGATIVE
BECOMING
COMPROMISES
HEALTH**

Figure 9-3. Lack of prerequisites leading to negative becoming and ill-health, particularly in developing countries.

can be unable to see what they have the capacity to be and how they might go about it. As Kubler Ross reportedly explained about her workshops with the dying:

> We have learned from the dying patient who has been our teacher ... things that regrettably no one helped them accomplish earlier so that they would have been able to say, "I have truly lived."[5]

The question can be asked whether health practitioners compromise their own professional becoming when they concentrate on coping services to the neglect of positive becoming services or on risk elimination instead of encouraging and enabling managed risk taking. It is hypothesized that professional groups, as any other community, will be less effective and will become ill and die a little if the potential and scope of their work is restricted to a great extent by an outside force. This conjecture is applicable to both practitioners in affluent countries and to those working with many populations in the developing world. Practitioner and community alike frequently experience governance that curtails expression of inherent capacities. Many in socially disadvantaged, war-torn, or ecologically devastated countries are unable to meet even the prerequisites of health because of human enterprise, as well as natural causes. Population health intervention for such situations usually meets life-threatening needs first. If possible, practitioners bear in mind and then attend to the being and becoming needs of whole communities that may assist in the future because, as Diener found, all needs are important all the time.[17,90] The latter thought points to becoming as an idea that links personal health with community development. It suggests how significant partnerships with groups in the wider community provide opportunities to promote population health or prevent disasters from being ongoing.

As a Prerequisite of Health

Becoming can be a negative, as well as a positive, experience closely related to health. Indeed, a lack of well-being associated with negative becoming due to a lack of the prerequisites is not uncommon, particularly in war-torn countries, where peace is a priority, and in developing countries (Figure 9-3.) Deprivation or limited access to food and shelter affects health in harmful and direct ways and can lead to early death. As mortality statistics reveal, life expectancy also varies directly with amount of schooling, family income, and employment status. Those can provide or support opportunities to pursue personal interests and goals; play some part in primary health status and in longevity;[91] and are in some measure prerequisite to health. However, it is well recognized that becoming passes through several stages—all are transient and can be in a direction that improves the human experience or the reverse. In addition, needs vary across age groups. Goebel and Brown found that physical needs and love are most important for children.[92a] The latter is shared with young adults, who also have the highest self-actualization needs. Adolescents display the highest need for esteem, and the elderly the highest need for security. The latter was important for all groups. Of the WHO prerequisites for health, not all may appear to be aspects of becoming, but all play some part in establishing people's ability to make use of their natural talents so that they are enabled to become according to their potential. The prerequisites of health are considered (in this instance, in terms of becoming needs) in Table 9-2.

Becoming and Peace

Peace is an ideal. It has been and is still a state to be desired—a state where dreams can be followed and becoming is ongoing. It can be related to both personal and collective becoming. The Nobel Peace Prize is, arguably, the most coveted accolade in the modern world and is awarded to individuals who have truly sought to improve the likelihood of peace and enrichment of people's lives by their own strivings and self-actualization. Recipients of the prize, which was first awarded in 1901, have been involved in occupations such as peace movements and arms control, the advocacy of human rights, humanitarian efforts, and the mediation of international conflicts. According to Alfred Nobel's will, it was to be given to:

> The person who shall have done the most or the best work for fraternity between nations, the abolition or reduction of standing armies and for the holding and promotion of peace congresses.[93]

Most have received the award for courageous and peaceful efforts toward civil and political human rights, with the first two recipients being Henry Dunant, the founder of the Red Cross, and Frédéric Passy, an international pacifist.[93] The decision to award the Nobel Peace Prize for humanitarian aid work was initially controversial, but is now universally applauded because such activity is a fundamental prerequisite of peace, embodying not only its ideals but also its reconciliation.[94] Jane Addams was a recipient of the award in 1931. She provides an example of the interface between individual and collective striving toward healthful becoming. Elected president of the Women's International League for Peace and Freedom, she held what has been described as the "Victorian belief in women's special mission to preserve peace." She headed a commission for the first significant international effort to end World War I, meeting with leaders in countries at war or neutral to discuss mediation.[95] Such early initiatives were forerunners to the United Nations and the 1948 Declaration of Human Rights, which holds that "the inherent dignity and the equal and inalienable rights of all members of the human family is the foundation of freedom, justice and peace in the world."[96] United Nations' missions can support people's activities that assist peace through multidimensional peacekeeping operations, including economic development projects. Those can be particularly helpful in decreasing further conflict and are most effective in the first few years after war.[97] However, war does not always prevent all people from meeting their becoming needs. Some people thrive in times of conflict, whereas others are unable to follow their dreams because of physical restrictions, societal pressures, military rule, or mental trauma. For example, when Tang et al explored the satisfaction of needs for citizens of the Middle East and the United States at the time of the Persian Gulf War, they found cross-cultural variation—the importance given to specific needs and levels of satisfaction differed across the two cultures; and the needs varied from peacetime to wartime. They concluded that human needs are unique, dynamic, and changing.[98-100]

Table 9-2

BECOMING AS A PREREQUISITE OF HEALTH FOR INDIVIDUALS, COLLECTIVES, AND GLOBALLY

WHO Prerequisites of Health	"Becoming" to Meet the Prerequisites: Positive and Negative Examples
Becoming and Peace	**Positive** • Peaceful environment /personal, communal or national circumstances encourage continuance of occupational interests • Lack of conflict enables occupational growth and development **Negative** • Inter-personal, communal or national conflict prevents, inhibits, or discourages continuance of occupational interests • War prevents occupational growth and development
Becoming and Shelter	**Positive** • Shelter appropriate for occupation requirements and aspirations • Accessible to prerequisites needed to meet potential/interests • Sociocultural support for shelter suitable for everyone to become **Negative** • Shelter inappropriate for occupation requirements and aspirations • Not accessible to prerequisites needed to meet potential/interests • Little or no support for suitable shelters • Large populations of refugees remain in camps with limited opportunities to improve their lives. In • 2009, 42 million people had been displaced by conflict or persecution particularly in developing countries.[92b]
Becoming and Education	**Positive** • The same range of education available to all people regardless of age, gender, race, social standing, • cultural or religious norms • Development /access to education for varied occupational needs **Negative** • Education not available to all people • Restricted or no access to education • Lack of education to meet for different occupational needs • "In the world 130 million children do not have a primary education of that 130 million two thirds of them are females"[92c]

(continued)

Becoming and Shelter

It has already been noted that shelter is a primary health requirement because it provides necessary protection from the elements. The simple protection sought by early and nomadic humans

Table 9-2 (continued)

BECOMING AS A PREREQUISITE OF HEALTH FOR INDIVIDUALS, COLLECTIVES, AND GLOBALLY

WHO Prerequisites of Health	"Becoming" to Meet the Prerequisites: Positive and Negative Examples
Becoming and Food	**Positive** • Sufficient food available for occupation requirements • Access to/knowledge of appropriate foods for occupational needs Preparation skills applying knowledge of basic nutrition and care **Negative** • Paucity of food. Insufficient for occupational requirements • Lack of knowledge of relationship between activity and food • Eating the wrong foods for achievement of occupational goals • The number of people who are undernourished has continued to grow, while slow progress in reducing the prevalence of hunger stalled-or even reversed itself-in some regions between 2000-2002 and 2005-2007. About one in four children under the age of five are underweight, mainly due to lack of food and quality food, inadequate water, sanitation and health services, and poor care and feeding practices.[92d]
Becoming and Income	**Positive** • Sufficient income available for occupation requirements • Access to training/jobs that meet occupational potential/interests • Sociocultural support for the achievement of aspirations **Negative** • Insufficient income available for occupation requirements • Limited access to training/jobs that meet potential/interests • Limited sociocultural support for goal development/ achievement • An estimated 1.4 billion people were still living in extreme poverty in 2005. Moreover, the effects of the global financial crisis are likely to persist: poverty rates will be slightly higher in 2015 and even beyond, to 2020, than they would have been had the world economy grown steadily at its pre-crisis pace.[92e]
Becoming: A Stable Ecosystem and Sustainable Resources	**Positive** • Encouragement of occupational interests that reflect personal, communal or global environmental concerns • Environmental programs recognize, reflect and enable occupational growth and development **Negative** • Inter-personal, communal or national interests permit continuance of occupations that are detrimental to environments • Occupational growth and development ignores future environmental needs

(continued)

Table 9-2 (continued)	
BECOMING AS A PREREQUISITE OF HEALTH FOR INDIVIDUALS, COLLECTIVES, AND GLOBALLY	
WHO Prerequisites of Health	*"Becoming" to Meet the Prerequisites: Positive and Negative Examples*
Becoming: Social Justice and Equity	**Positive** • Social environment encourages the development of personal, communal or national occupational interests • Occupational justice enables occupational growth/development **Negative** • Lack of understanding or commitment to the development of personal or communal occupational needs Occupational injustice inhibits occupational growth/development

has, for most people, been superseded by more complex structures, which has been ever changing since sedentism emerged with agriculture. In that way, shelter itself can be seen to have undergone a becoming process as people, their ways of living, and their occupational development escalated. Income is directly related to shelter.[101] Those able to command "big money" may have several shelters in different places and of differing types. The poor and the out of work may be shelterless or dependent on charitable and transient protection from the elements. In the latter case, becoming is likely to be reduced to basic physiological needs that, in some ways, mirror early human experience. Creative skills usually associated with self-actualization may be redirected toward the manufacture of temporary shelter in the spirit of nomadic ways of life. Such shelter often accords with sustainable environment principles. Many believe the future should be aimed toward healthy or ecological cities in which people can:

> Discover and activate their true creative selves for the common good ... The era of the mansion and the private yacht is over! We have to think in terms of rehousing everyone in ecological city designs.[16]

Becoming and Education

John Dewey believed that education should combine personal and social visions of becoming. It should focus "the full and ready use of a person's capacities" toward the acquisition of potential and skill that can be utilized toward social change and reform for the greater good. To prepare people for future life requires participation, adjustment of individual activity, and the development of "social consciousness" as the "only sure method of social reconstruction."[102] Maslow's ideas were not dissimilar, based as they were on the study of social icons such as Jane Addams, Albert Einstein, and Eleanor Roosevelt,[103] and the healthiest 1% of the college student population.[104] More recent deliberations concur. For example, self-determination theory discusses "the adaptive design of the human organism to engage in interesting activities, to exercise capacities, to pursue connectedness in social groups, and to integrate intrapsychic and interpersonal experiences into a relative unity."[105] In specific application to educational objectives, ideas such as preparing the young to be active and reflective citizens, for community, economic, and political life; for confident engagement with other cultures at home and abroad; for participation in work; and for the development of lifelong learning in the midst of constant change are not uncommon.[106] In terms of health, life expectancy varies directly with amount of schooling,[91] and the higher the education levels achieved, the higher the income and the lower the unemployment.[107] Both of those factors, as noted above, also relate to lifespan. Based on the belief that all children possess innate abilities that can be nurtured if they are provided with a rich, experiential learning environment combined with a vision of globally conscious local activism, Lashbrook and Alvarez-Ossa proposed:

> An online global collaboration education network that will tap into the power of youth, with a cross-curricular focus on self-actualization, character development, social justice, equity and global conscience, thus collectively shifting the education paradigm and changing the world for the better ... one child at a time.[108]

In places where educational opportunities are few or missing altogether, such becoming opportunities are absent, although for people currently living a mixed hunter-gatherer-agrarian lifestyle, self-actualization scenarios may be many and varied as people meet the daily occupational challenges, with health and longevity only compromised by disease beyond the sphere of local expertise.

Becoming and Food

Along with water and sanitation, the WHO names three pillars of food security that link food to illness and death, as well as to self-actualization. These are:

1. Availability of food.
2. Access to appropriate foods for nutritional needs.
3. Use of food and knowledge of basic nutrition and care.[109]

Becoming depends on access to food that meets nutritional needs and dietary preferences that enable people to live actively and healthily[109,110] and to work toward personal dreams and aspirations. It has already been noted that in recent decades in affluent countries, food production has exceeded population growth, leading to excess, over consumption, and obesity.[111] The latter may be due in part to boredom; long-standing activity-food patterns of many people changing with the growth of technology, new business and corporate initiatives; or political greed. Conversely, it might be a result of overlegislation that, while providing self-actualizing opportunities for legislators and high flying business executives, limits participation for the masses in as wide a range of occupations as in previous times. In the multitude of articles and texts about diets apart from physical exercise regimens, there is limited reference to the development of self-growth as a motivator for increased activity levels. Much more could be done to highlight the many widely differing circumstances associated with occupation that affect the prevalence of weight disorders, such as the need to vary nutritional intake when occupations change to prevent imbalance between energy input and output.[112-114] A comprehensive study of workers aged 18 years or older, from the U.S. National Health Interview Surveys of 1986 to 1995 and 1997 to 2002 collected information on self-reported weight and height from workers aged 18 years or older. Caban et al found that it is, in part, because of the increasing trend toward automation and other labor-saving strategies that there is a growing epidemic of obesity:

> Primary and secondary prevention of obesity in occupational settings must therefore take into account the many societal and occupational factors that influence energy imbalance via multifaceted interventions.[115]

Occupation in the sense used in that example refers to paid employment but is applicable to the whole range of activity. It is claimed here that a reduction in challenge and satisfaction from occupational achievements because of societal restrictions, technological developments, and political legislation prevents many people from doing what they are most suited to, especially if they are more than adequately fed.

By contrast, in many parts of the world, there has been a dearth of adequate food supplies. The unequal distribution of food, with shortages especially apparent in Africa and Afganistan,[116] has led to common health problems, such as debilitating malnutrition and food-borne diarrhea, that directly affect and reduce what people can do in several ways. A variety of societal occupational factors, such as poor production methods, political action, war, or transport disruptions, may be causative factors, in addition to economic instability, droughts, or fuel shortages. For people experiencing extreme hunger, "utopia can be defined simply as a place where there is plenty of food."[117] In such cases, becoming is equated with primary rather than higher level factors, illustrating that, when people are "dominated by a certain need," their becoming or future needs tend to change.

Becoming and Income

There is a three-fold link between occupation, mortality, and income. Opportunity to engage in occupations of choice for self-growth is often dependent on availability of time and resources but also on income—life expectancy varies according to physical, social, and productive activities,[81] and with family income.[91] In places where failing economies are common, employment opportunities are limited and precarious and unemployment is rife. Unemployment reduces the chances of self-actualization, which is further compromised by limited prospects of wide ranging choices of fulfilling occupations away from the sphere of work. In advanced economies, people are often required to retire from work at a certain time. Superannuation funds have flourished in recent years to provide opportunity for retirement security and the financial means to continue with or engage in new becoming occupations. However, in uncertain economic climates, superannuation funds can deteriorate overnight, leaving many dependent on social welfare. Steven Podnos suggested that when money savings are secure enough for basic survival and safety, people "turn to freedom money, which enables us to do those things outside of work that we find enjoyable and fulfilling," then to "gift money" and finally to "dream money." He described the latter as "having enough financial security to make changes in lifestyle that bring new levels of meaning and personal fulfillment."[118] Becoming is most probable in states where freedom, gift, and dream money prevail or when people believe what they are doing is important to some degree. It has been suggested that earned income may be considered a "lubricant that gets the cogs of life moving," but of itself is insufficient to help people reach a "place of actualization."[119] Alderfer's Existence, Relatedness, and Growth theory, like Maslow's, was hierarchically ordered, but he argued that the order of needs may differ between people and that different levels of need can be worked at concurrently.[120] In addition, crises such as unemployment "can switch the emphasis to a lower level need."[79] This explains why poorly paid lower-level workers appear more motivated by money than the opportunity to be creative in their employment.[101] In such cases, it can be argued that positive self-actualizing health is compromised, and the risk of illness and shorter life-span increased.

Becoming: A Stable Ecosystem and Sustainable Resources

Democracy is not about the private accumulation of wealth; it is about the wise use of the collective wealth for the common good. Ultimately, democracy is about global self-actualization.[16]

Becoming is a global, as well as a personal and communal, matter. The Earth is naturally in a state of constant change, but the development goals of people (individually, collectively, and politically) can also be agents of such change. As people have sought enrichment through the intensification of agriculture, their ability to engineer and fabricate and the all-embracing greed of some corporate endeavors have also changed the environment, often in a way harmful to the stability of the ecosystem and the sustainability of resources. Land has become degraded through "deforestation, overgrazing, unplanned land management, firewood harvesting and urbanization, and encroachment of wetlands and rangelands for cultivation."[121] Degradation of the earth and poverty for large sections of the Earth's peoples has occurred as a result of such socioeconomic, institutional, and technological occupations. Those have also led to the emergence of mega-cities and the expansion of urban slums, increased energy use, and a lack of opportunities for gainful employment in villages across the world.[121] Aspects of health through becoming are closely linked to globalization, a stable ecosystem, and sustainable resources, not least in respect to food security and international agricultural agreements. Globalization may lead to the continuation of food insecurity and poverty in some nations and communities.[109]

> *... One only can be sobered by the awesome manifestations of human greed and destructiveness that largely have been enabled by advances in technology. The same machines and chemical processes that have increased productivity have played havoc with environmental conditions and the health of the natural world.[122]*

Global self-actualization depends on sustainable economic development, environment, and trade, as well as community action and individual commitment to engage in ecologically sustaining occupations.[109] Advocating for protection and conservation of natural environments and resources as integral to health promotion strategies, the Ottawa Charter called for "systematic assessment of the health impact" of ever-changing "technology, work, energy production and urbanization" to address the overall ecological issue of our ways of living.[1] There is discord between the Earth's becoming needs and those of humankind.

Becoming: Social Justice and Equity

The promotion of health for all people is a matter of equity, and justice is the "the key to achieving liberty and domestic tranquility."[16] Action to enable all people to achieve their fullest occupational and health potential requires opportunities and resources to be equally available to all people, as it is not possible for the prerequisites to be ensured by the health sector alone. All individuals must be able "to address and control phenomena that determines health outcomes" so that they have the opportunity to engage in activity that enables them to work toward their becoming. The Ottawa Charter noted that such phenomena includes "a secure foundation in a supportive environment, access to information, life skills and opportunities for making healthy choices," as well as meeting local needs according to "differing social, cultural and economic systems" (Figure 9-4).[1]

Negative Becoming as a Factor in Illness: Occupational Alienation

Occupational alienation is the antithesis of becoming. It can result from particular circumstances in which people find themselves manifesting deep feelings of incompatibility with the occupations associated with a place, situation, or others to the extent that basic needs and wants appear impossible to attain or maintain. It results in feelings of despair, and inability to participate in or even to consider possible alternatives or ways to overcome the feelings that prevent self-actualization, pleasurable or even essential occupations. Experienced as both an individual and a population phenomenon, it can incur aggressive occupations associated with social unrest and unhealthy behaviors, such as participation in regular drunkenness, that are prevalent in postindustrial modern societies.

Alienation has been the subject of debate of several classical and contemporary theorists. Essentially, it is a sociological concept that has captured the attention of philosophers and is particularly associated with Karl Marx, who saw it as "the separation of things that naturally belong together, or antagonism between things that are properly in harmony."[123] The word alienation comes from the Latin alieno, meaning to make strange, and from alius, meaning "other" or "another." It is used to describe feelings of estrangement and a lack of familiarity or comfort in thoughts, environments, situations, or with people. It can refer to a psychological state and a type of social relationship, and has many discipline-specific uses. Although much of the dialogue and argument appears not to include practical application to the world of health, it does appear in medical dictionaries, but mainly in association with mental health. In that context, it can refer both to a psychological state and a type of social relationship. It is described as "a condition

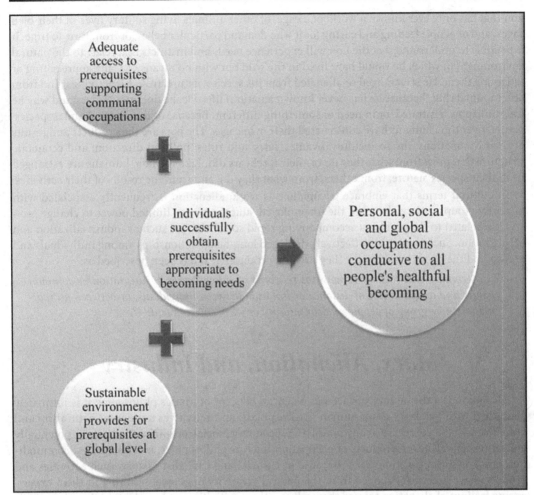

Figure 9-4. Occupational alienation as lack of meaningful relations with others leading to estrangement and exclusion from their occupations.

characterized by lack of meaningful relationships with others, sometimes resulting in depersonalization and estrangement from others"[124] as "a state of estrangement between the self and the objective world or between different parts of the personality;[125] as "estrangement from society; feelings of being an outsider, foreigner, or outcast; estrangement from one's self"; as "feelings of unreality or depersonalization"; and, in terms of "affect," includes "isolation of ideas from feelings, avoidance of emotional situations, and other efforts to estrange one's self from one's feelings."[126] In Ancient Greco-Roman times, physicians referred to disturbed, difficult, or abnormal mental states as *alienatio mentis*, or mental alienation. This was attributed to a physiological imbalance in most cases.[127,128]

Since the time when people lived in harmony with the natural environment, with only the simplest of technology to assist them in meeting their occupational needs, humankind has sought to challenge and master nature. It has done so by developing more sophisticated technology and social structures to meet occupational needs and wants, to conquer ill health, and to delay death by ever-increasingly sophisticated medical science. Such technological change can be described as potentially alienating, even if at the time it seems to be a good thing.

Occupational alienation combines many of those ideas and, because it is a concept far from easy to understand, it is useful to consider the analogy of an animal born in captivity. Think about a lion that has only ever known a world of a cage, of other animals living solitary lives in their own cages, and of people feeding and caring for it who demand particular behavior from time to time. It is possible to understand that the lion will experience needs and instincts that relate to the natural environment in which he would have lived in the wild but with no means of really appreciating or satisfying them. He is estranged or alienated from his species' nature, from his activities, and from other animals but, because he has never known a natural lifestyle, he does not understand why he feels unhappy, frustrated, or in need of something different. Because of their occupational species' nature, over time humans have constructed their own cages. The bars are the products and results of their occupations; the sociocultural values, laws, and rules; political direction; and economic structure that grew from what they do or their forebears did. Like the lion, humans are estranged from their species' nature, from others, from what they do, and from the results of their activities.

In cultural terms that embrace occupation as work, alienation is frequently associated with minority groups such as the poor, the unemployed, and those with limited power to change society. It is related to the problems accompanying rapid social change, such as industrialization and urbanization. Such change has effectively damaged long-held relationships among individuals and groups and the goods and services they use and produce.[125] It has been described as:

> ... A condition in social relationships reflected by a low degree of integration or common values and a high degree of distance or isolation between individuals, or between an individual and a group of people in a community or work environment.[129]

Marx, Alienation, and Industry

Alienation is a theme that surfaced as a central concept of Marx's philosophy: it is intimately connected with his views about human nature, praxis, and activity as a union of naturalism and humanism.[130-132] He regarded any productive, economic, social, or spiritual activity as potentially alienating, as well as the products of occupation, such as philosophies, morals, money, commodities, laws, or social institutions.[130] Because of cultural and capitalist history, such activities and products have become estranged from the natural creativity of people, resulting in them experiencing feelings of alienation toward themselves, others, activities, and products. Alienating activities, such as the division of labor, are "forced upon individuals by the society which they themselves create"[133] and as long as occupation "is not voluntary ... man's own deed becomes an alien power opposed to him, which enslaves him instead of being controlled by him."[134] Marx suggested a direct illness connection with the processes of industrialization because:

> Factory work exhausts the nervous system to the uttermost, it does away with the many sided play of the muscles, and confiscates every atom of freedom, both in bodily and intellectual activity.[135]

Essentially, Marx's ideas about alienation focus on two aspects of human nature. The first contention is that people can become alienated in the quest to stay alive through what are now called the prerequisites of health, such as obtaining necessary food and shelter. His second contention refers to alienation that occurs because of people's tendency to develop more needs or desires after satisfying basic prerequisites. That type of alienation can be a result of an individual seeking out more extreme occupational challenges that fail to satisfy in a deep self-actualizing way. Marx regards the consequential cycle of ever changing and never-ending wants as a self-alienating process.[136] His theories about alienation occur in his early anthropological humanist works. Later, he interpreted from a structural-historical perspective that resulted in a change from internal individual alienation to economic and social alienation. In many ways, that relates to the division apparent between individual aspects of occupation on the one hand and population, corporate, and political aspects on the other, as discussed throughout this text. For Marx, exploitation and people becoming the instruments of machines and production systems epitomized the change. It was particularly related to occupations that emerged with industry and capitalism, in which workers had little control over what they did and in the process lost their sense of self. The owners of industry also experienced alienation through the exploitation process and resultant, ongoing competition.[137]

Industrialization was once the epitome of human becoming. The conditions relating to it are now regarded as so unhealthy that it is difficult to appreciate why people made the mass exodus from country to town. "The move from farm to factory" was based on a ground swell of wanting to be part of the exciting new world, economic need, and "social trends that the individual could not control."[138] Huge numbers of the population changed not only their habitats, but also the structure of their social networks from small, cohesive groups working and playing together to large populations where individuals knew or were close to few people. Work separated men and women, altering the value of their occupations and experiences of social and mental well-being; it separated adults from children, altering teaching and learning roles; and children, unless engaged in child labor with their parents, no longer observed or participated with them as they engaged in the daily round of socially valued roles and skills. Instead, they learned from strangers.

Alienation continues to increase as production and service jobs become "deskilled" and lose their capacity to interest those doing them[139] because "many jobs that have been transformed by new technology are characterized by high levels of boredom."[140] For those employed in intellectual occupations, such as educators, administrators, scientists, and health professionals, stresses caused by what Naisbit called the "chaos of information pollution" are frequently described as overwhelming.[141] For some whose occupations are not personally associated with industry, a source of alienation is often found in corporate and political decisions or policies that fail to meet personal or community occupational becoming needs. For others, the alienation resulting from the dehumanizing process of manufacturing still holds true.

Alienation as
Social, Mental, and Physical Illness

Sociologists from the late 19th century on have identified that collective decisions do not take into account the unique needs and purposes of people and that even in postmodern, consumption-capitalist societies people are required to sell their personality in addition to their work.[142] Concern was expressed in the early 20th century about the alienating effects of modernization in which relationships were increasingly moderated by money.[143] This remains evident today when money rather than occupational capacities is often the over-riding factor in choosing or rejecting a job, especially when there is little difference between social benefits and work remuneration. Today, prominent features of alienation are said to be exhibiting or expressing feelings of powerlessness, meaninglessness, normlessness, isolation, and self and cultural estrangement that were identified by Seeman[144] half a century ago. Powerlessness is about an individual's perception of not having the means to achieve goals, when there appears to be an insurmountable gap between what a person would like to do and the capability to do it.[145] According to Geyer, alienation is linked with globalization, the information explosion, and increased awareness of ethnic conflicts.[146] It is also about the complexity of environments and "overchoice"; being unable to choose between alternative activities or the consequences of the choice, as well as powerlessness from delayed feedback. As a consequence of the latter, the rewards or punishments for what people do are obscured by "time-lag," resulting in apathy and/or alienation. In addition, the overload of unnecessary information that bombards people on a regular basis leads to feelings of meaninglessness.[146]

Social isolation is typically experienced as a form of personal stress, with its sources deeply embedded in the social organization of the modern world. Many people from developing countries have uprooted themselves in search of a better life in postindustrial parts of the world, where many experience restricted ongoing social relationships, and fail to achieve integration or even daily interactions with others.[145,147] Such changes to basic human relationship patterns may affect some of the family and social alienation problems common in the modern world that lead directly or indirectly to ill health.

Mijuskovic puts forth a case that alienation and individual loneliness are more pronounced and prevalent in postindustrial "atomistic societies" than in "organic communities." In the latter, natural functions, role perspectives, mutual interdependence, and intrinsic relations are stressed in contrast to individual freedom, external connections, causal and reductionist explanations, rule orientation, and artificial frameworks.[148] His view has some merit when it is observed how current postindustrial values and changing occupational structures, language, and technologies can reduce freedom of action by ever-increasing rules, regulations, and bureaucracy; replace ongoing human endeavor with labor-saving technology, which often creates work of a mundane variety; reduce the availability of paid employment that holds interest and meaning and meets individual needs for growth and challenge; and create a materialistic way of life out of step with sustaining the natural world of which humans are a part. All such changes have the potential to create environments that are alienating enough to spawn discontent and disease.

Although technological change in itself (unless toxic) is unlikely to cause illness, the effects on people's engagement in occupations and their reaction to the changes can lead to illness, even in high-demand jobs.[149] Justice argued that when work is perceived as stressful, boring, or meaningless, the likelihood of "mass illness" is increased.[150] A review of material from 16 epidemics of illness at various workplaces and schools supports this contention.[151] There is convincing evidence that the health benefits of paid employment depend on its quality,[152-156] and those who are dissatisfied with work experience numerous symptoms and stress and tend to drink or smoke more than those who are satisfied.[157] Social alienation can contribute to people experiencing long-term disorders of mental health. Living in the community, they can continue to experience alienation because of their own negative self-attitudes and other people's response to odd behavior.[158] It has even been argued that self-estrangement in modern societies could be driven by the repressive and potentially alienating injunction to "enjoy."[159] Phillippe Pinel, the French instigator of "moral treatment for the insane," espoused a new understanding of mental alienation in the late 19th century. People experiencing such problems could feel like a stranger—an alien in the world of the sane. In moral treatment, occupation was used to reduce alienation or prevent people becoming alienated from reason by assisting emotional states and improving social conditions.[160] In the mid-20th century, schizoid clinical states were considered broadly in terms of alienation, and currently alienation is recognized in mental health when there are disturbances in relationships or those that relate to self-estrangement.

Aging and physical disability can be causes of alienation because of experiences in which individuals appear to be invisible to other members of society. People disadvantaged in such ways can be talked about or talked over, and their needs and futures can be decided on as if they were not present or able. For example, a study by Susan Foster found that among adults who are deaf, the theme of social rejection and alienation experienced as a result of reactions from the hearing community emerged consistently across all categories of life experience. Such interactions establish the potential marginalization and social meaning of deafness.[161] Numerous other investigations link the notions of alienation with illness and health-risk behaviors for individuals and societies, particularly for those disadvantaged by unsatisfactory occupational opportunities.[162-170] Miller suggested that even the status given to the medical profession and its scientific values can be alienating factors in the way that they exert control over the procedures aimed at rapid repair of body parts decontextualized from the recipient's mental or social needs.[171]

Becoming: Early and Current Guidelines for Health

For millennia, the characteristics and capacities that form the basis of the human need to strive toward becoming were the foundation of creative ways to survive healthily in disparate ecosystems. Selection favored the adaptive and creative. As Dubos explained:

Adaptive patterns of behavior become, of course, increasingly important as one ascends the scale of living things. In higher animals, and more so in man, adaptation expresses itself in instincts, tastes, and habits which help the group and the individual in making use of available resources and in avoiding sources of danger.[172]

Becoming remains a primary mechanism for survival and is important to health and well-being despite changing occupational structures commensurate with technological advancement and urbanization. Currently, change and innovation are evident everywhere and often centered in urban development. The Greeks were among the earliest major urban developers, and their cities were complex, innovative, and beautiful, but for health purposes contained no more than 10,000 people. Medieval and Renaissance cities were also small, yet are said to have been "architecturally, economically, and intellectually satisfactory and satisfying social entities, even though their hygiene was poor and their infant mortality high."[173] With the rise of industry, the picture changed dramatically as paid employment for the masses became segregated from family life and home base and urbanization escalated. From approximately 1730 until the turn of the 20th century, urban conditions were appalling.[174] Workers were too crowded, tired, and sick to have any chance of meeting positive becoming needs. Death rates increased alarmingly.[175] Although as late as 1800, only 3% of the world's population were city residents; currently 51% live in urban areas.[176]

Some people appear to thrive in crowded cities. There may be truth in the claim that city living "provokes to activity those attributes of the brain which are essentially human, namely the capacity to devote major resources of human endeavor to pursuits and goals that are not material."[177] Dubos claimed to "love crowds and cities … All over the world the largest and most polluted cities are also the ones with the greatest appeal even though their inhabitants uniformly complain of congestion and pollution."[178] Currently, they certainly offer the most varied opportunities for people to try out new occupations. However, they may not provide all people with the chance to become according to their particular strengths and interests. Lorenz described how:

Exhaustion of interhuman relationships occur when a superabundance of social contacts forces every one of us to shut himself off in an essentially "inhuman" way and, because of the crowding of many individuals into a small space, elicits aggression.[179]

Currently, the natural health needs of people pale in significance beside the drive to create more sophisticated technology. Technological progress has altered the character of many personal and shared occupations, including entertainment and sport for which chemical potions, as well as mechanical, biophysical, and electronic apparatus, have been developed and marketed so that individuals may achieve previously unrealized feats. Such technology subtly reduces the use of human energies, creativity, and potentials; alters the elements of human toil, the pure skill, and the mental and social exercise components of occupations; and can be alienating to individual growth. Because the technology is primarily used to meet market purposes rather than human needs, it is alienating. Nearly half a century ago, Lorenz saw that the acquisition of assets becoming a primary need was reaching a pathological state with the potential to cause mental and social disruption that he deemed to be symptoms of cultural ill health.[179]

Another major and potentially alienating change that goes along with rapid occupational advances has been a marked increase in the urge to accumulate material goods and property, without a thought for the potential of materialism to destroy the ecosystem. Many erroneously equate material wealth with happiness and health, mistaking the means for the ends. By the mid-20th

Biological Needs Human Characteristics	Underlying Determinants	State/Public Institutions and Utilities	WHO Directive	Positive or Negative Consequences	Health/ Illness Outcomes
Requirements for Survival	Eco-systems and weather patterns	Environmental Management		Doing or opportunities for doing do not provide for becoming according to potential	Disease, Disability, Death
e.g. *Clean air & fresh water shelter,*	Economy Type e.g. *Industrial, agrarian, hunter-gatherer*	Division of labor, work opportunities, technology	*To reach a state of complete physical, mental and social well-being, an individual or group must be able to identify and to realize aspirations*		
sustenance, safety, support, physical, mental & social exercise	National Policies & Priorities e.g. *War/peace, eco-sustainable development*	Armed forces, legislation, fiscal, social, employment, health		Doing or opportunities for doing allow, provide for and encourage becoming according to potential	Absence of illness
Species Features and Capacities e.g. *Language, cerebral capacity*	Cultural & Spiritual Values e.g. *Justice*	Education, Religion, laws & ethics			Physical, mental & social well-being

Figure 9-5. Determinants of illness or well-being through doing, being and belonging to become.

century, Mumford was obviously alienated by "over-charges of empty stimuli, ... materialistic repletion, ... costly ritual of conspicuous waste, ... and highly organized purposelessness" as part of the "clinical picture of the cultural disease from which the world suffers."[180] He went as far as to assert that:

> *The supernatural theology of the Middle Ages was closer to reality than the crass materialism of an age which fancies that the achievement of an 'economy of abundance' will automatically ensure a maximum of human felicity.*[181]

Human characteristics and biological needs are the foundation stones of becoming, just as they are of the foundation of health and cultural evolution. These have furthered the establishment of different and creative economies, political systems, and national values, policies, and priorities. They erect, often by default, division between classes, genders, and age groups in opportunities for engagement in occupation and division based on attitudes, relationships, and occupations within communities. If state and public institutions and utilities do not restrict opportunities for people to engage in activity that nourishes and challenges the mind, body, and spirit, communities are likely to demonstrate increased energy, interest, contentment, and commitment and an increased life expectancy.[81] If not, preclinical global, social, and mental illness, such as war, social unrest, antisocial behavior, increased institutionalization, substance abuse, stress, boredom, and depression, or preclinical physiological signs, such as decreased fitness, increased blood pressure, and changes in sleep patterns and emotional state, can occur. All can ultimately result in disease, disability, or premature death. Figure 9-5 depicts the complex relationship affecting people's becoming capacities and the possible health or illness outcomes.

Since the 1940s, medicine and public health have affected major worldwide changes in the prevalence and outcomes of illness. Some types of infection have become rare and some extinct, and epidemic diseases have declined in importance, where they were previously common and serious. It is hard to exaggerate the impact of those changes on human health and outlook.[182] Such advances ensure that more people are provided with a stable base from which to experience positive health and well-being through becoming what they have the potential to become. However, in many parts of the world, health and well-being seem to sit uneasily amid the rush and stresses of current-day occupational structures that humans have constructed over the years, and it is here that public health intervention is required, not least in more thoroughly addressing how people can aim toward their potential. Morbidity and mortality can result from a lack of individual, community, or social awareness about the relationship between what people do, how they feel about it, and whether they can self-actualize, and from an understanding of the nature of stress or feelings of alienation that can be an outcome of occupational frustration.

Conclusion

People who are able and in a position to follow a regular path toward developing their interests and potential are more likely to experience positive feelings, such as satisfaction, happiness, and commitment. There is compelling evidence that people who are happy and experience life satisfaction, the absence of negative emotions, optimism, and subjective well-being enjoy better health and live between 4 to 10 years longer. Diener and Chan suggested that it is timely to add improvement of subjective well-being to society-wide population health and organizational interventions, as well as those aimed at individuals.[183] It would also be timely to consider the alienating effects of reduced opportunity to experience subjective well-being through the pleasures of appropriate occupational challenges.

Humans have used and continue to use their "becoming capacities" so effectively that population growth is a major concern for the future health of the earth itself. Becoming is, perhaps, a concept almost as difficult as being for people to accept as relevant in the relatively concrete world of health care. However, authorities from various disciplines across time, as well as the WHO, have recognized that for people to achieve physical, mental, and social well-being, they need to have the opportunity to use their particular capacities and to aim at becoming what each person, family, community group, or nation has the potential to be. Societies as a whole can become healthier through their everyday activities that are inclusive of more than the few occupations currently at the forefront of medical prescription. As communities grow, so too does the social, political, and natural environment. As people grow and change throughout life, body, mind, and spiritual well-being are in a state of continual becoming. The opposite is also true. Becoming can be negative particularly if doing, being, or belonging through occupation is restricted or compromised. It is a fundamental need of all people.

For those who have little hope of using their potentialities in a meaningful way, the lack of recognition of becoming needs can lead to physical, as well as mental and social, ill-health. A serious aspect of occupation, becoming is frequently disregarded, and is less and less considered in medical, or health fields of practice. The notion of helping people with medical problems to have some future aim on which to pin their hopes was an understandable focus of occupational therapy from its foundation early in the 20th century, but has been much overlooked in recent decades when immediate functional activities have become the major concern. Despite that, anecdotal instances of reemerging self-actualizing opportunities or amazing cures are not uncommon, if such aims are relevant to some personal purpose or great interest. In addition, it is useful to bear the WHO directive in mind: "to reach a state of complete physical, mental and social well-being, an individual or group must be able to identify and to realize aspirations ..."[1]

References

1. World Health Organization, Health and Welfare Canada, Canadian Public Health Association. *Ottawa Charter for Health Promotion*. Ottawa, Ontario, Canada 1986.
2. Browning R. *Andrea del Sarto*: lines 97-98. Original work published 1855. http://en.wikisource.org/wiki/Andrea_del_Sarto.
3. Becoming. *The American Heritage Dictionary of the English Language*. 4th ed. Boston: Houghton Mifflin Company; 2009.

4. Become. *Collins English Dictionary*. HarperCollins Publishers; 2003.
5. Wilson Schaef A. *Meditations for Women Who Do Too Much*. San Francisco: Harper Collins; 1990.
6. Wilson Schaef A. *Living in Process: Basic Truths for Living the Path of the Soul*. The Ballantyne Publishing Group; 1999.
7. Storr A. *Churchill's Black Dog and Other Phenomena of the Human Mind*. Glasgow: William Collins Sons & Co Ltd; 1989.
8. Burnham W. *The Wholesome Personality*. New York, NY: Appleton-Century; 1932.
9. Fromm E. *Man for Himself*. New York, NY: Holt, Rinehart and Winston; 1947.
10. Rogers C. *On Becoming a Person*. Boston, Mass: Houghton Mifflin; 1961.
11. Bullock A. *The Humanist Tradition in the West*. London, England: Norton; 1985.
12. Ingleby D. Mental health. In: Kuper A, Kuper J, eds. *The Social Science Encyclopedia*. London, England: Routledge; 1985.
13. Maslow A. *Toward a Psychology of Being*. 2nd ed. New York: D. Van Nostrand Company; 1968:191.
14. Maslow A. *Motivation and Personality*. New York, NY: Harper and Row; 1954.
15. Maslow A. *The Further Reaches of Human Nature*. New York, NY: Viking Press; 1971.
16. Doctress Neutopia. *Global-Self Actualization and Maslow's Hierarchy of Needs*. http://www.lovolution.net/MainPages/arcology/globalSelfactualization/Global-SelfActualization.htm. Accessed April 19, 2013.
17. Tay L, Diener E. Needs and subjective well-being around the world. *Journal of Personality and Social Psychology*. 2011;101:354-365.
18. Rogers C. Towards a theory of creativity. In: Vernon PE, ed. *Creativity*. London, England: Penguin Books; 1970:140.
19. Amabile T. *The Social Psychology of Creativity*. New York, NY: Springer Verlag; 1983.
20. Gardner H. *Creating Minds: An Anatomy of Creativity Seen Through the Lives of Freud, Einstein, Picasso, Stravinsky, Eliot, Graham, and Gandhi*. New York, NY: Basic Books; 1993.
21. Stein M. *Stimulating Creativity*. Vols 1 and 2. New York, NY: Academic Press; 1974 and 1975.
22. Golann S. Psychological study of creativity. *Psychological Bulletin*. 1963;60:548-565.
23a. Yockey FP. *Imperium: The Philosophy of History and Politics*. Self published;1948.
23b. Dulles JF. *War or Peace*. University of Michigan; 1957.
23c. Porter KA. In Plimpton G, ed. *Interviewing Writers at Work*. Second Series ed. New York: Viking Press, 1963.
23d. Mead M. *Sex and Temperament in Three Primitive Societies*. New York: Harper Collins; 1935;332.
24. Gecas V. Self concept. In: Kuper A, Kuper J, eds. *The Social Science Encyclopedia*. London, England: Routledge; 1985:739-740.
25. Doyal L, Gough I. *A Theory of Human Need*. London: Macmillan; 1991.
26. McMichael T. *Human Frontiers, Environments and Disease: Past Patterns, Uncertain Futures*. Cambridge: Cambridge University Press; 2001.
27. Ornstein R, Sobel D. *The Healing Brain, A Radical New Approach to Health Care*. London, England: Macmillan; 1988:207,214.
28. Watts E. Human needs. In: Kuper A, Kuper J, eds. *The Social Science Encyclopedia*. London, England: Routledge; 1985:367-368.
29. Knight R, Knight M. *A Modern Introduction to Psychology*. London, England: University Tutorial Press Ltd; 1957:56-57.
30. Lorenz K. *Civilized Man's Eight Deadly Sins*. Latzke M, trans. London, England: Methuen and Co Ltd; 1974:3-5,12-13.
31. Maslow A. *Toward a Psychology of Being*. 2nd ed. New York, NY: D Van Nostrand Co; 1968:201.
32. Jung C. The development of personality. In: Read H, Fordham M, Adler G, eds. *Collected Works 1953-79*. Vol 17. Hull RFC, trans. London: Routledge and Kegan Paul;1981:paragraph 289.
33. Erikson E. *Identity*. London: Faber and Faber; 1958:19.
34. Storr A. *Churchill's Black Dog and Other Phenomena of the Human Mind*. Glasgow: William Collins Sons & Co Ltd; 1989:168-9.
35. Wallas G. *The Art of Thought*. London: Cape, 1926.
36. Storr A. *Churchill's Black Dog and Other Phenomena of the Human Mind*. Glasgow: William Collins Sons & Co Ltd; 1989: 172-3.
37. Gombrich E. *The Sense of Order: A Study in the Psychology of Decorative Art*. Oxford: Phaidon, 1979.
38. Watson L. *Neophilia: The Tradition of the New*. Great Britain: Hodder and Stoughton Ltd; 1989:13.
39. Watson L. *Neophilia: The Tradition of the New*. Great Britain: Hodder and Stoughton Ltd; 1989:180.

40. Maslow A. *Religion, Values and Peak Experiences.* New York: Viking; 1964.

41. Csikszentmihalyi M. Activity and happiness: towards a science of occupation. *Journal of Occupational Science: Australia.* 1993;1(1):38-42.

42. Jamison K. Mood disorders and seasonal patterns in top British writers and artists. Unpublished data in: Storr A. *Churchill's Black Dog and Other Phenomena of the Human Mind.* Glasgow: William Collins Sons & Co Ltd; 1989:254.

43. Storr A. *Churchill's Black Dog and Other Phenomena of the Human Mind.* Glasgow: William Collins Sons & Co Ltd; 1989:265.

44. Carrel A. *Man, the Unknown.* London, England: Burns and Oates; 1935:24-25.

45. Bullock A. Post industrial society. In: Bullock A, Stalleybrass O, Trombley S, eds. *The Fontana Dictionary of Modern Thought.* 2nd ed. London, England: Fontana Press; 1988:670.

46. Bell D. *The Coming of Post Industrial Society: A Venture in Social Forecasting.* New York, NY: Basic Books; 1973.

47. Touraine A. *Post Industrial Society.* London, England: Wildwood House; 1974.

48. Jones B. *Sleepers, Wake! Technology and the Future of Work.* Melbourne, Australia: Oxford University Press; 1995.

49. Toffler A. *The Eco-Spasm Report.* New York, NY: Bantam Book Inc; 1975:3.

50. Jones B. *Sleepers, Wake! Technology and the Future of Work.* Melbourne, Australia: Oxford University Press; 1995:43-44.

51. Hazan H. Gerontology, social. In: Kuper A, Kuper J, eds. *The Social Science Encyclopedia.* London, England: Routledge; 1985:337.

52. World Health Organization. *Health Topics: Aging.* Available at: http://www.who.int/topics/aging/en/. Accessed June 9, 2013.

53. World Health Organization. Fact sheet N°220. *Mental Health: Strengthening our Response.* Updated April 2014. http://www.who.int/mediacentre/factsheets/fs220/en/. Accessed on May 17, 2014.

54. Department of Public Information. *Yearbook of the United Nations 1982.* New York: United Nations; 1982:1186.

55. Flynn-Connors E, ed. *Yearbook of the United Nations 1989.* The Hague: Martinus Nijhoff Publishers, 1989:688-689.

56. Gordon K, ed. *Yearbook of the United Nations 1999.* New York: United Nations; 1999.

57. Gordon K, ed. *Yearbook of the United Nations 2001.* New York: United Nations; 2001.

58. United Nations. *Madrid International Plan of Action on Aging.* UN Department of Economic and Social Affairs; 2002. http://undesadspd.org/Aging.aspx. Accessed May 26, 2014.

59. World Health Organization. *Active Aging: A Policy Framework.* Second United Nations World Assembly on Aging. Madrid, Spain: WHO; 2002:13. http://www.who.int/aging/publications/active_aging/en/. Accessed May 26, 2014.

60. World Health Organization. *Active Aging: A Policy Framework.* Second United Nations World Assembly on Aging. Madrid, Spain: WHO; 2002:12. http://www.who.int/aging/publications/active_aging/en/. Accessed May 26, 2014.

61. Botes A. A comparison between the ethics of justice and the ethics of care. *Journal of Advanced Nursing.* 2000:20:55-71.

62. Metz T. Arbitrariness, justice, and respect. *Social Theory and Practice.* 2000:26:24-45.

63. State Library New South Wales. *Active, Engaged, Valued: Older People and NSW Public Libraries Revisited.* Public Library Services Blog. Posted 12th June 2011. http://blog.sl.nsw.gov.au/pls/index. cfm/2011/6/12/active-engaged-valued-older-people-and-public-libraries-revisited. Accessed August 1, 2013.

64. Gilbert N. *Welfare Justice: Restoring Social Equity.* New Haven and London: Yale University Press; 1995.

65. Commission on Social Justice. Social Justice: Strategies for National Renewal. *The Report of the Commission on Social Justice.* London: Vintage; 1994.

66. Organization for Economic Cooperation and Development. *The Future of Social Protection.* Paris OECD, 1988.

67. Kalisch D. The active society. *Social Security Journal.* 1991:August:3-9.

68. Department of Health and Aging. *Australian Government Response Productivity Commission's Caring for Older Australians Report.* Canberra; May, 2012.

69. Wilcock A. Older people and occupational justice. In: McIntyre A, Atwal A, eds. *Occupational Therapy and Older People.* Oxford, UK: Blackwell Publishing; 2005:14-25.

70. Healy J. *The Benefits Of An Aging Population.* Discussion Paper Number 63. The Australia Institute. Australian National University; March 2004: 40.

71. Comfort A. *A Good Life.* Melbourne, Australia: The Macmillan Company of Australia; 1977:28.

72. Gordon K, ed. *Yearbook of the United Nations 2001.* New York: United Nations; 2001:1002.

73. Parker S. *Leisure and Work.* London, England: George Allen and Unwin; 1983:119.

74. Toynbee A. A study of history. Vol XII. Reconsiderations. In: Kohn H, ed. *The Modern World.* New York, NY: Macmillan; 1963:303-304.

75. Robertson J. *Future Work.* England: Gower Publishing Co; 1985.

76. Maslow A. *Toward a Psychology of Being.* 2nd ed. New York, NY: D Van Nostrand Co; 1968:193.

77. Doyal L, Gough I. *A Theory of Human Need.* London: Macmillan; 1991:59-60.

78. Agius T. Aboriginal health in Aboriginal hands. In: Fuller J, Barclay J, Zollo J, eds. *Multicultural Health Care in South Australia.* Conference proceedings. Adelaide: Painters Prints; 1993:23.

79. Zastrow C, Kirst-Ashman K. *Understanding Human Behavior – The Social Environment.* 8th ed. Belmont, CA., Brooks/Cole; 2010:449.

80. Carrel A. *Man, the Unknown.* London, England: Burns and Oates; 1935:178-179.

81. Glass T, Mendes de Leon C, Marotolli R, Berkman L. Population based study of social and productive activities as predictors of survival among elderly Americans. *British Medical Journal.* 1999:319:478-483.

82. House J, Robbins C, Metzner H. The association of social relationships and activities with mortality: prospective evidence from the Tecumseh community health study. *American Journal of Epidemiology.* 1982;116:123-140.

83. Welin L, Larrsen B, Svardsudd K, Tibblin B, Tibblin G. Social network and activities in relation to mortality from cardiovascular diseases, cancer and other causes – a 12 year follow up of the study of men born in 1913-1923. *Journal of Epidemiological Community Health.* 1992;46:127-132.

84. Csikszentmihalyi M. *Flow: The Psychology of Optimal Experience.* New York, NY: Harper and Row; 1990.

85. Kannel W, Belanger A, D'Agostino R, Israel I. Physical activity and physical demand on the job and risk of cardiovascular disease and death: The Framingham study. *American Heart Journal.* 1986;112:820-825.

86. Paffenburger R, Hyde R, Wing A, Lee I, Jung D, Kampert J. The association of changes in physical activity and its correlates: associations with mortality among men. *New England Journal of Medicine.* 1993;328:538-545.

87. Kaplan G, Strawbridge W, Cohen R, Hungerford L. Natural history of leisure time physical activity and its correlates: associations with mortality from all causes and cardiovascular disease over 28 years. *American Journal of Epidemiology.* 1996;144:793-797.

88. Simonsick E, Lafferty M, Phillips C, et al. Risk due to inactivity in physically capable older adults. *American Journal of Public Health.* 1993;83:1443-1450.

89. Blair S. Physical inactivity: the biggest health problem of the 21st century. *British Journal of Sports Medicine.* 2009;43:1-2.

90. Villarica H. Debunking Maslow's hierarchy of needs. *Tall Tales, Short Stories and Modest Musings.* September 14, 2011. http://www.hongkonggong.com/notebook/?p=272. Accessed February 2, 2013.

91. Rogot E, Sorlie P, Johnson N. Life expectancy by employment status, income, and education in the National Longitudinal Mortality Study. *Public Health Rep.* 1992;107(4):457-461.

92a. Goebel B, Brown D. Age differences in motivation related to Maslow's need hierarchy. *Developmental Psychology.* 1981;17:809-815.

92b. United Nations High Commissioner for Refugees. *UNHCR Annual Report Shows 42 Million People Uprooted Worldwide.* [Press release]. UNHCR; 2009. Available at: http://www.unhcr.org/4a2fd52412d. html. Accessed September 7, 2014.

92c. United Nations Population Fund. *Population Issues 1999: Empowering Women.* Available at: https:// www.unfpa.org/6billion/populationissues/empower.htm. Accessed September 7, 2014.

92d. United Nations. *The Millenium Development Goals Report.* New York: United Nations; 2010;4. Available at: http://www.un.org/millenniumgoals/pdf/MDG%20Report%202010%20En%20r15%20 -low%20res%2020100615%20-.pdf. Accessed September 7, 2014.

92e. United Nations. *The Millenium Development Goals Report.* New York: United Nations; 2010;7. Available at: http://www.un.org/millenniumgoals/pdf/MDG%20Report%202010%20En%20r15%20 -low%20res%2020100615%20-.pdf. Accessed September 7, 2014.

93. Excerpt from the will of Alfred Nobel. "The Nobel Peace Prize." Nobelprize.org. http://www.nobel-prize.org/nobel_prizes/peace/. Accessed January 18, 2013.

94. Lundestad G. *The Nobel Peace Prize, 1901-2000*. http://www.nobelprize.org/nobel_prizes/peace/articles/lundestad-review/index.html. Accessed January 18, 2013.

95. *Jane Addams*. Available at: http://en.wikipedia.org/wiki/Jane_Addams. Accessed May 27, 2014.

96. United Nations. *The Universal Declaration of Human Rights*. UN:1948. http://www.un.org/en/documents/udhr/index.shtml. Accessed January 20, 2013.

97. Doyle M, Sambanis N. *Making War and Building Peace: United Nations Peace Operations*. Princeton University Press; 2006.

98. Tang T, West W. The importance of human needs during peacetime, retrospective peacetime, and the Persian Gulf War. *International Journal of Stress Management*. 1997;4(1):47-62.

99. Tang T, Ibrahim A. Importance of human needs during retrospective peacetime and the Persian Gulf War: Mid-eastern employees. *International Journal of Stress Management*. 1998;5(1):25-37.

100. Tang T, Ibrahim A, West W. Effects of war-related stress on the satisfaction of human needs: The United States and the Middle East. *International Journal of Management Theory and Practices*. 2002;3(1):35-53.

101. Beck R. *Motivation Theories and Principles*. 5th ed. New Jersey: Pearson Prentice Hall; 2004.

102. Dewey J. My pedagogic creed. *The School Journal*. Jan 16, 1897;LIV(3):77-80.

103. Maslow A. *Motivation and Personality*. New York, NY: Harper; 1954:236.

104. Mittelman W. Maslow's study of self-actualization: A reinterpretation. *Journal of Humanistic Psychology*. 1991;31(1):114-135.

105. Deci E, Ryan R. The "what" and "why" of goal pursuits: human needs and the self-determination of behavior. *Psychological Inquiry*. 2000;11:227-268.

106. Schofield K. *The Purposes of Education 3: A Contribution to the Discussion on 2010: Queensland State Education*. September 1999. http://education.qld.gov.au/corporate/qse2010/pdf/purposesofed3.pdf. Accessed January 19, 2013.

107. Infoplease. *Wealth and Poverty: Why Incomes are Becoming more Unequal*. Available at: http://www.infoplease.com/cig/economics/incomes-becoming-more-unequal.html. Accessed January 19, 2013.

108. Lashbrook S, Alvarez-Ossa D. *Harnessing Existing Technologies for Local and Global Educational Collaboration*. Futures Conference. 2012. www.tdsb.on.ca/microsites/futures/seminars.asp. Accessed January 12, 2013.

109. World Health Organization. *Food Security. Trade Foreign Policy, Diplomacy and Health*. WHO; 2013. Available at: www.who.int/trade/glossary/story028/en/. Accessed January 4, 2013.

110. Food and Agriculture Organization of the United Nations: Agricultural and Development Economics Division. *Food Security. Policy Brief*. UN; 2006;Volume 2. ftp://ftp.fao.org/es/ESA/policybriefs/pb_02.pdf. Accessed October 7, 2012.

111. World Resources Institute. *Food Security*. http://www.wri.org/tags/food-security. Accessed January 29, 2013.

112. Passmore R, Eastwood M. *Davidson and Passmore, Human Nutrition and Dietetics*. Edinburgh: Churchill Livingstone; 1986.

113. Garrow J. *Treat Obesity Seriously*. Edinburgh: Churchill Livingstone; 1981.

114. Hafen B, ed. *Overweight and Obesity: Causes, Fallacies, Treatment*. Provo, Utah: Brigham Young University Press; 1975.

115. Caban A, Lee D, Fleming L, Gomez-Marin O, LeBlanc W, Pitman T. Obesity in US workers: The National Health Interview Survey, 1986 to 2002. *American Journal of Public Health*. 2005;95(9):1614-1622.

116. Maplecroft.Global Risk Analytics. *'Extreme' Food Insecurity Map for 2010*. Available from: Maplecroft.com/about/news/food-security. Accessed January 13, 2013.

117. Maslow A. *Motivation and Personality*. 3rd ed. London: University of Santa Clara;1987:17.

118. Podnos S. *Building and Preserving Your Wealth, A Practical Guide to Financial Planning for Affluent Investors*. Bath, UK: Oakhill Press; 2010.

119. 119. Lerotholi B. *Income and its Influence Towards Self-Actualization: Can Employment Help Us Realize Our True Self*. Brain Digital Esoteric Nonsense: 2012. Available at: http://braindigital.wordpress.com/tag/self-acualization/. Accessed January 30, 2013.

120. Alderfer C, Guzzo R. Life experiences and adults' enduring strength of desires in organisations. *Administrative Science Quarterly*. 1979;24:347-357.

121. Mureithi. Functional Ecosystems. *Environmental Degradation - Root Causes*. Posted Monday, May 30, 2011. http://thedrystreams.blogspot.com. Accessed January 15, 2013.

122. Gibbons J. Were Eiseley and Sweitzer correct? *American Scientist*. 2001;89(2):1. http://www.americanscientist.org/issues/pub/2001/2/were-eiseley-and-schweitzer-correct. Accessed January 25, 2013.
123. *Alienation*. Wikipedia. http://en.wikipedia.org/wiki/Alienation. Accessed August 11, 2013.
124. Alienation. *Medical Dictionary for the Health Professions and Nursing*. Farlex; 2012.
125. Alienation. *The American Heritage Medical Dictionary of the English Language*. 4th ed. Boston: Houghton Mifflin Company; 2009.
126. Miller-Keane. *Encyclopedia and Dictionary of Medicine, Nursing, and Allied Health,* 7th ed. Philadelphia: Saunders Elsevier, Inc; 2003.
127. Regis E. *A Practical Manual of Mental Medicine*. 2nd ed. Bannister H, trans. Philadelphia: Blakiston. (Originally bound and printed by "the insane" of Utica Asylum.) 1895.
128. Ladner G. Homo and viator: medieval ideas on alienation and order. *Speculum*. 1967;42(2):233-259.
129. Ankony RC, Kelly TM. The impact of perceived alienation on police officer's sense of mastery and subsequent motivation for proactive enforcement. *Policing: An International Journal of Police Strategies and Management*. 1999; 22(2): 120-134.
130. Marx K. Economic and philosophical manuscripts, 1844. In: Livingstone R, Benton G, trans. *Karl Marx: Early Writings*. New York: Penguin Classics; 1992. Original work published 1932.
131. Marx K. *Grundisse*. New York: Penguin Classics; 1970. Original work published 1857.
132. Petrovic G. Alienation. In: Bottomore T, ed. *A Dictionary of Marxist Thought*. 2nd ed. Oxford, UK: Blackwell; 1991:11-16.
133. Mohun S. Division of labour. In: Bottomore T, ed. *A Dictionary of Marxist Thought*. 2nd ed. Oxford, UK: Blackwell; 1991:155.
134. Marx K, Engels F. *The German Ideology*. London, England: Lawrence and Wishart; 1964. Original work published 1845-46.
135. Fischer E. *Marx in His Own Words*. London, England: The Penguin Press; 1973:43-44.
136. Axelos K. *Alienation, Praxis, and Techne in the Thought of Karl Marx*. Austin, Texas: University of Texas Press; 1976.
137. Ollman B. *Alienation: Marx's Conception of Man in Capitalist Society*. Cambridge: Cambridge University Press; 1976.
138. Triplett T. Hebrides women: a philosopher's view of technology and cultural change. In: Wright BD, Ferree MM, Mellow GO, et al, eds. *Women, Work and Technology*. Ann Arbor, MI: The University of Michigan Press; 1987:147.
139. Farnworth L. An exploration of skill as an issue in unemployment and employment. *Journal of Occupational Science: Australia*. 1995;2(1):22-29.
140. Adler P. Technology and us. *Socialist Review*. 1986;85:67-96.
141. Naisbitt J. *Megatrends; Ten New Directions Transforming Our Lives*. New York, NY: Warner Books; 1982:24.
142. Wright Mills C. *White Collar. The American Middle Classes*. Oxford: Oxford University Press: 1951.
143. Simmel G. *The Philosophy of Money*. 2nd ed. Leipzig: Duncker & Humblot; 1907.
144. Seeman M. On the meaning of alienation. *American Sociological Review*. 1959;24(6):783-791.
145. Kalekin-Fishman D. Tracing the growth of alienation: enculturation, socialization, and schooling in a democracy. In: Geyer F, ed. *Alienation, Ethnicity, and Postmodernity*. Connecticut: Westwood; 1996:107-120.
146. Geyer C. Estimation and optimization of functions. In: Gilks W, Richardson S, Spiegelhalter J, eds. *Markov Chain Monte Carlo in Practice*. London: Chapman and Hall; 1996:241-258.
147. *Social Alienation*. Wikipedia. en.wikipedia.org/wiki/Social_alienation. Accessed August 11, 2013.
148. Mijuskovic B. Organic communities, atomistic societies, and loneliness. *Journal of Sociology and Social Welfare*. 1992;19(2):147-164.
149. Haynes SG. Type A behavior, employment status, and coronary heart disease in women. *Behavioural Medicine Update*. 1984;6(4):11-15.
150. Justice B. *Who Gets Sick: Thinking and Health*. Houston, TX: Peak Press; 1987:179.
151. Colligan MJ, Murphy LR. Mass psychogenic illness in organizations: an overview. *Journal of Occupational Psychology*. 1979;52:77-90.
152. Warr P. Twelve questions about unemployment and health. In: Roberts R, Finnegan R, Gallie D, eds. *New Approaches to Economic Life*. Manchester: Manchester University Press; 1985.
153. Warr P. *Work, Unemployment and Mental Health*. Oxford, UK: Oxford Science Publications; 1987.
154. Winefield A, Tiggerman M. A longitudinal study of the psychological effects of unemployment and unsatisfactory employment on young adults. *Journal of Applied Psychology*. 1991;76(3):424-431.

155. Winefield A, Tiggerman M, Winefield H. Unemployment distress, reasons for job loss and causal attributions for unemployment in young people. *Journal of Occupational and Organizational Psychology.* 1992;65:213-218.

156. Winefield A, Tiggerman M, Winefield H, Goldney R. *Growing Up with Unemployment.* London, England: Routledge; 1993.

157. Verbrugge LM. Work satisfaction and physical health. *Journal of Community Health.* 1982;7(4):162-283.

158. Erdner A, Magnusson A, Nystrom M, Lutzen K. Social and existential alienation experienced by people with long-term mental illness. *Scandinavian Journal of Caring Sciences.* 2005;19(4):373-380.

159. Zizek S. *Mapping Ideology.* London: Verso; 1994.

160. Pinel P. *A Treatise on Insanity 1801.* Davis D, trans. London: Cadell and Davis; 1806.

161. Foster S. Social alienation and peer identification: a study of the social construction of deafness. *Human Organization.* 1989;48(3):226-235.

162. Fromm E. *The Sane Society.* New York, NY: Rinehart; 1955.

163. Burke RJ. Career stages, satisfaction, and well-being among police officers. *Psychological Reports.* 1989;65(1):3-12.

164. Winefield HR, Winefield AH, Tiggemann M, Goldney RD. Psychological concomitants of tobacco and alcohol use in young Australian adults. *British Journal of Addiction.* 1989;84(9):1067-1073.

165. Nutbeam D, Aaro LE. Smoking and pupil attitudes towards school: the implications for health education with young people: results from the WHO study of health behaviour among schoolchildren. *Health Education Research.* 1991;6(4):415-421.

166. Mosher A, Pearl M, Allard MJ. Problems facing chronically mentally ill elders receiving community based psychiatric services: need for residential services. *Adult Residential Care Journal.* 1993;7(1):23-30.

167. Nah KH. Perceived problems and service delivery for Korean immigrants. *Social Work.* 1993;38(3):289-296.

168. Semyonova ND. Psychotherapy during social upheaval in the USSR. Special section: in times of national crisis. *Group Analysis.* 1993;26(91):91-95.

169. Hammarstrom A. Health consequences of youth unemployment: review from a gender perspective. *Social Science and Medicine.* 1994;38(5):699-709.

170. Rodenhauser P. Cultural barriers to mental health care delivery in Alaska. *Journal of Mental Health Administration.* 1994;21(1):60-70.

171. Miller D. Dissociation in medical practice: social distress and the health care system. *Journal of Social Distress and the Homeless.* 1993;2(4):243-267.

172. Dubos R. *Mirage of Health.* New York: Harper & Row Publishers, inc; 1959:43.

173. Gordon D. *Health, Sickness and Society: Theoretical Concepts in Social and Preventive Medicine.* St. Lucia, Queensland: University of Queensland Press; 1976:311.

174. Mumford L. *The Culture of Cities.* New York, NY: Harcourt, Brace; 1938.

175. Bryant JH. Public health: National developments in the 18th and 19th centuries. *Encyclopædia Britannica.* http://global.britannica.com/EBchecked/topic/482384/public-health/35547/National-developments-in-the-18th-and-19th-centuries. Accessed January 27, 2013.

176. Population Reference Bureau. *World Population Data Sheet 2012.* http://www.prb.org/Publications/Datasheets/2012/world-population-data-sheet/data-sheet.aspx. Accessed January 20, 2013.

177. Gordon D. *Health, Sickness and Society: Theoretical Concepts in Social and Preventive Medicine.* St. Lucia, Queensland: University of Queensland Press; 1976:337.

178. Dubos R. In: Hinrichs N, ed. *Population, Environment and People.* New York, NY: McGraw-Hill; 1971:xi.

179. Lorenz K. *Civilized Man's Eight Deadly Sins.* Latzke M, trans. London, England: Methuen and Co Ltd; 1974:8-9,76.

180. Mumford L. *The Condition of Man.* London, England: Heinemann; 1963:380.

181. Mumford L. *The Condition of Man.* London, England: Heinemann; 1963:148.

182. McNeill WH. *Plagues and People.* London, England: Penguin Books; 1979.

183. Diener E, Chan M. Happy people live longer: subjective well-being. *Applied Psychology: Health and Well-Being.* 2011;3(1):1-43.

Section III

Occupation in Illness and Health

Theme 10

"Changing patterns of life, work and leisure have a significant impact on health. Work and leisure should be a source of health for people."

WHO: Ottawa Charter for
Health Promotion, 1986[1a]

Chapter 10

DISORDERS OF OCCUPATION

This chapter addresses:
- Misunderstanding Occupation Can Trigger Illness
- Medically Recognized Occupational Disorders
  - Related to Work
  - Related to Mental Determinants
  - Related to Sleep
- Occupational Deprivation
  - Ideologically Driven Occupational Deprivation
  - Lack of Citizenship and Occupational Deprivation
  - Abuse as Occupational Deprivation
  - Discrimination and Occupational Deprivation
  - Resource-Based Occupational Deprivation
  - Economic Causes of Occupational Deprivation
- Conclusion

Earlier chapters have briefly discussed how difficulties in experiencing a life filled with occupations that meet population, familial, and individual doing, being, belonging, and becoming needs can lead to medically recognized disorders, such as noncommunicable diseases. This differs from place to place, economy to economy, and according to particular circumstance.

Occupation's relationship to illness and positive health is explored more fully in this third section of the book. This chapter focuses on negative aspects of occupation as bases of disorders of health. Some of those are medically recognized, but the occupational causative, predisposing, or precipitating factors are not always identified, except perhaps as a secondary factor. They are not formally acknowledged as illnesses in their own right. One of those—occupational alienation—was identified in the last chapter, and two other such disorders—occupational imbalance and occupational stress—will be discussed in the next; occupational deprivation will be considered later in this chapter. All could be described as illnesses in their own right, if an occupational perspective of health was to be accepted by the WHO and other international and national health authorities.

Wilcock AA, Hocking C.
An Occupational Perspective of Health, Third Edition (pp 274-301).
© 2015 Taylor & Francis Group.

Whether that eventuates or not, the problems are common, relate to, and are precursors to medically defined illness, a few examples of which will be examined. All require serious consideration and research that might be assisted by a lifelong, 24-hour, day-night occupational perspective. Not only are occupations essential to survival, but it is also clear that they are invaluable in the maintenance and creation of health and well-being, and when that fact is misunderstood the result may lead to illness and even death.

Misunderstanding Occupation Can Trigger Illness

That people need to engage in a variety of occupations to exercise all parts of their bodies and minds to maintain health and fitness is not well understood. Rather, for many, the doctor's surgery is thought to be where health happens. Any understanding that is held of needing to exercise inbuilt capacities gets lost in keeping going in the economic rat race, suggesting that it is chance or a particular interest rather than design that leads to personal lifestyles that provide physical, mental, and social health. There is an even greater lack of appreciation of communities, corporate, and political organizations as occupational entities. A void in health-focused research is created by such a lack of understanding and appreciation of the causes of the widespread failure to address occupation as a central health issue at individual, familial, social, corporate, national, and international levels.

Interest in the occupational illnesses occasioned by paid employment is perhaps the only exception and because paid work is a necessity for most people, such concentration is understandable. This interest centers more on the workers than on the employers or corporate activities, with the exception of unions trying to better the employment conditions for their members. Unions mostly focus on pay, conditions of work, and safety, which is not surprising when it is often income considerations rather than aptitude or interest that determines choice of work in the present day. That is important in terms of being able to attain the basic requirements for health, but work as more than income is also an essential aspect of occupation in the prevention of illness. The lack of understanding of occupation encompassing all that people do is furthered by the social value given to particular paid employment in both postindustrial cultures and many others striving to emulate postindustrialism.

Societal pressure to pursue particular types of work may impose on communities or individuals the apparent need to do more than they are capable of or to do less than they can achieve meaning or satisfaction from. Some people take on any work to obtain pay and the prerequisites for health despite their skills and interests. Sometimes employment of any kind is scarce or unavailable and sometimes opportunities for jobs that meet people's occupational needs are limited or poorly paid. Other issues, such as social environments and political agendas, can also affect choice. Aspects like those that determine people's work choices can cause psychological stress, such as frustration and anger, as well as social and mental illness, such as violence, illegal occupations, or depression.

Within paid employment, there is little commonality in the range and extent of physical, mental, and social doing, and many people have few opportunities to engage in the health enhancing, balanced yet stimulating and challenging use of capacities that appear to be associated with reducing the incidence of illness. For example, where working in the garden was once an outlet for the stress of work and a way to provide food for the table (Figure 10-1), opportunities have been considerably reduced with intensive urbanization and reduction in the size or number of gardens. Such changes can add to the number of people who seek enjoyment in unhealthy personal and social occupations, such as alcohol, drug, and tobacco use; those who become depressed, inactive, or engaged in abusive activity; or those who feel fatigue that prevents them from regular physical

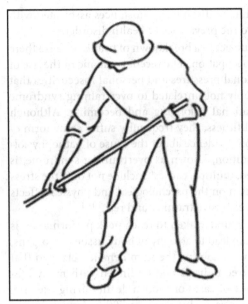

Figure 10-1. Working in the garden to relieve work stress and provide food for the table. (© Carol Spencer 2012, otspencer@adam.com.au. Used with permission.)

activity, leading to disorders associated with obesity. However, specific occupational causes and unhealthy occupational behavior are seldom teased out from other social determinants of health.

When illness occurs, the usual course of action, at least for people in advanced societies, is to seek medical reasons. Thagard contended that within medicine there are two kinds of important explanations. The first of these is a physician's judgment of the cause for the presenting symptoms: a diagnosis. The second is usually the job of medical researchers; they seek explanations for the causes of illness.[1b] In the field of population health, that is mainly the role of epidemiologists. Present research is vigilant, but because of the dominance of quantitative methodologies, holistic and complex mechanisms are often reduced in ways that make it hard for people to consider total lifestyle effects. Although the research is valuable, the concentration on the benefits of physical exercise in both professional and popular media leads to the assumption that other types of doing are of less value. That results in research about the effects of occupations considered to be frivolous or unimportant to health being reported in other than gold standard journals and not adequately considered. It is hardly surprising that people hearing this type of rhetoric do not equate their health status with their everyday doings, as a small retrospective study demonstrated.[2] The majority of 100 people older than age 60 years did not associate their life's occupations with their health. This finding appears to be indicative of the medicalized understanding of health by the general public alluded to earlier, which is, perhaps inadvertently, being reinforced by health education strategies, the media, and the limited direction of occupation-focused research.[3]

Physiological imbalance and illness can result from individual responses to, and coping with, the vicissitudes of everyday life, which are closely tied to what people do or do not do and how they feel about such doings. Because they relate to people's different natures and needs being met through what they do, simply recommending an exercise regime that meets predetermined health criteria is not effective for everybody. Occupation in the past met many physiological, psychological, and societal needs and values; what is recommended to replace superseded physically, mentally, and socially demanding occupations in the current age has got to meet similar basic needs and values and appeal to human neophilic nature.[4] This requires vigilance in terms of health requirements and research, as societal values will continue to alter with the impact of continual change and development while basic biological needs remain constant. For example, when considering the activity-rest nexus, modern reductionism contrasts with the holistic nature of earlier lifestyles in which active or restful doing was often associated with day and night or food and nutrition as part of an ecological healthy whole.[5] Currently, many widely differing circumstances associated with what people do and what they eat have contributed to the prevalence of health disorders.

Even those committed to physical excellence are subject to a breakdown of health because there is insufficient understanding of the complexities of occupation. The recent epidemic of the use of performance-enhancing drugs is related to occupational pressures and personal insecurities that are themselves a form of occupational illness, probably not unrelated to overtraining syndrome and the need for psychosocial approval of occupational belonging and becoming. Although athletes generally experience a high level of physical fitness, they frequently suffer some form of breakdown of health at the time of major competition. Evidence about the cause of pathophysiology of the physical, behavioral, and emotional condition, known as overtraining syndrome, is limited. However, it has been suggested that integrated, multiple causes[6] include not only the stress of training,[7] but also the chemical addiction or fixation on the psychological and physical effects of exercise and fitness[8,9] and the imbalance between excessive training and rest.[10,11]

This gives rise to the notion that too much exercise, undertaken to reach peak performance, is detrimental to health, as is too little exercise, which can lead to atrophy of body tissue and organs, as well as obesity. Kenneth Cooper, who is credited with coining the term *aerobics*, claimed that overexercising could trigger the overproduction of free radicals and be linked with many lifestyle disorders and even death.[12] Indeed, from a study of cases of sudden death during exercise, Siscovick et al found that the risks of death during exercise are increased by 700%, despite the fact that men who exercise have a death rate that is half of those who do not exercise.[13] It is now largely understood that "the reality is that people who die during exercise have some underlying, probably undetected condition that predisposes them to a cardiac event during exercise … [T]here are conditions that predispose us to sudden cardiac death, and exercise can bring this out."[14] It is clear that the benefits outweigh the dangers but require a protective level of regular vigorous activity and careful screening beforehand to check for any predisposing conditions that might result in sudden death.[15]

Sleep disorders are recognized within mainstream medicine and will be discussed later in this chapter. In preparation for that discussion, a few thoughts about emerging theories that point to a complex relationship between sleep and what people do during waking states will be mentioned. Theories suggest that recuperation, information processing, energy conservation, and self-preservation are important aspects of the relationship. As earlier chapters revealed, Kleitman found sleep to be complementary to wakefulness, the day/night sequence providing for the "basic rest activity cycle."[16] A biological clock controls the cycle and, although best observed in stages of sleep, is apparent throughout day and night as differing levels of excitement and rest occur over an 80- to 120-minute period (usually described as approximately 90 minutes).[17] Leger suggested that "just as musicians' pauses are a component of the performance, pauses from the stream of behavior are a component of the repertoire. The organism 'doing nothing' is doing something."[18] Blessing et al recently incorporated Kleitman's theory into a behavioral hypothesis that takes a coherent integrative view of organism function. Based on their laboratory findings about "heating and eating" and the daily activity of rats, they proposed that the thermogenic activity of brown adipose tissue acts as a key determinant in setting levels of activity, with the brain requiring warming to engage well in an activity over a long period of time.[19] Future research that considers human occupation in terms of such physiological research might suggest practical applications that are helpful in terms of preventing the occurrence of illness because of ill-timed activity or rest.

The impact of the activity-rest continuum on health is not considered in social welfare programs that provide money rather than opportunities for occupational involvement, particularly for people who are older or have a recognizable disability. Such decisions put risk elimination before reasonable challenge to capacities, and favor keeping people breathing rather than living in a way that promotes what limited capacities they may have. Consider the rows of older, well, rugged and drugged people in some nursing homes, seated day after day in warm and sanitary conditions but without stimulation to enable continued achievement, however small that may be. In such situations, maybe there is an unstated, unrecognized form of euthanasia or even murder through lack of activity that is practiced on a daily basis and applauded as kindly. Certainly, occupational therapists report as a fact that occupational programs have been reduced in long-term care institutions, in the name of health and safety but perhaps more influenced by fear of financial losses through insurance, claims should any mishap occur.

However, as noted earlier, physical inactivity is one of four common occupational risk factors that result in the world's foremost causes of death—cancer, cardiovascular diseases, chronic obstructive pulmonary disease, and diabetes. The WHO describes these disorders as "the leading threat to human health and development," as well as "causing an estimated 35 million deaths each year—60% of all deaths globally—with 80% in low- and middle-income countries."[20] Research considering such detrimental behaviors in occupational terms and according to occupational circumstances might be useful in the discovery of occupational antidotes and deterrents.

The other three extensively researched risk factors are unhealthy diets, tobacco use, and excessive use of alcohol.[21] All are forms of occupation—they are what people do to feel a certain way, to belong, and to become temporarily happy. Those occupations have been brought about by changes in what people do in their daily lives to satisfy appetites, to meet social norms, and to feel good, and are responses to the pressures created by contemporary forces, such as the media, fashion, conformity, and corporate bodies whose occupation is aimed at making money by selling addictive products. Where once all people engaged in communal occupations that met healthy physical activity requirements to obtain and prepare food and drink that was, on the whole, fresh and nutritious, they can now indulge in new oral experiences, taste sensations, rapid gratification, and "feel good" moments to instantly satisfy some of their doing, being, belonging, and becoming needs.

An approach offered in *The Lancet* by Geneau et al suggests the use of an adapted political process model to:

> Reframe the debate to emphasize the societal determinants of disease and the inter-relation between chronic disease, poverty, and development; mobilize resources through a cooperative and inclusive approach to development and by equitably distributing resources on the basis of avoidable mortality; and build on emerging strategic and political opportunities.[22]

They add a cautionary note:

> Until the full set of threats—which include chronic disease—that trap poor households in cycles of debt and illness are addressed, progress towards equitable human development will remain inadequate.[22]

This suggests yet again the closeness of fit between illnesses; discrepancies in what people are able to do according to the circumstances of what, where, and how they live; and the impact of communal, commercial, corporate, and political occupations.

A critical review of research from 22 studies in the health and social sciences literature to specifically examine the relationship supports the view that occupation is an important influence on health and well-being.[23] Despite that, it has not necessarily followed that authorities have sought to provide structures that encourage all people to engage in a variety of occupations to exercise their particular capacities to attain healthy balance. Rather, a limited understanding of exercising inbuilt capacities suggests that it is chance rather than design that leads to lifestyles that provide for physical, mental, and social well-being.

Many authorities, employing bodies, and health professionals fail to consider the impact that variation throughout the day, and over the recognized periods of lowered activity levels within each approximate 90-minute period, might have on occupational productivity, effectiveness, and safety. For instance, the drudgery of domestic work, with its potential for subsequent neglect of some women's occupational capacities and interests, can lead to mental and social breakdowns (Figure 10-2). As an aspect of that, lack of consideration of the arbitrary dividing of occupation into socially determined categories of paid or unpaid employment and leisure or play makes it

Figure 10-2. Unequal opportunities for occupation beyond the home (woman doing domestic work). (© Carol Spencer 2012, otspencer@adam.com.au. Used with permission.)

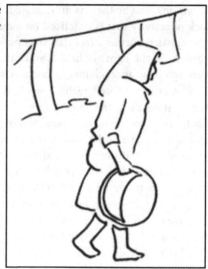

possible to appreciate some of the impediments to understanding the need to balance mental, physical, social, solitary, spiritual, rest, chosen, and obligatory occupations as integral aspects of health.

Occupational balance is important because if capacities are overused, people feel fatigue, stress, and burnout, which can lead to increased susceptibility to accident and illness. People who overdo occupations can also increase the experience of pain that leads to enforced rest and subsequent avoidance of particular or most activity.[24] If capacities are underused, they will atrophy, cause a disturbance to equilibrium, and can result in depression, sleeping problems, stress, decreased strength and fitness, and a decline in physical health. People may experience a loss of confidence in their ability to perform occupations; a "loss of role at work or at home as they do not do the activities expected of them;" or may overdo, it if they do try, because of a lack of fitness.[25] Stovitz and Johnson suggested that current health terminology puts too much emphasis on overuse and too little on underuse, and that this precludes accurate investigations and recommendations.[25]

Except in terms of physical/aerobic exercise, the balanced use of personal capacities to enable the maintenance and development of the organism is perhaps the most primary and least appreciated function of people's occupations. Some authorities throughout the 20th century have been exceptions. Meyer considered "it is the use that we make of ourselves that gives the ultimate stamp to our every organ."[26] In a similar spirit, Sigerist proposed that occupation is essential to the maintenance of health:

> ... because it determines the chief rhythm of our life, balances it, and gives meaning and significance. An organ that does not work atrophies and the mind that does not work becomes dumb.[27]

Medically Recognized Occupational Disorders

RELATED TO WORK

Within the broad field of occupation, work-related disorders have been studied most extensively and are the occupational matter that largely concerns corporate and political authorities, particularly with regard to insurance, compensation, and the legal aspects of health and safety legislation.

Such disorders have generated medical interest for centuries, with the most comprehensive account emanating from the pen of Ramazzini,[28] as mentioned in earlier chapters. He is known as the father of occupational medicine, with his opus magnum *A Treatise of Diseases of Tradesman* published in 1705 addressing 54 illnesses associated with particular work occupations, from sewers to the desks of scholars.[28] It has been noted that interest in occupational illness increased as the industrial revolution evolved. Industrialization resulted in overcrowded and unsanitary working and living conditions that were large factors in population illness, as was the continual exposure to dangerous and unprotected machinery and toxic materials by men, women, and children.[29,30]

Work-related diseases include compensable and non-compensable occupational diseases. Chronic disease that occurs as a result of work is described as occupational disease. It is typically identified when an increased prevalence is demonstrated in comparison to other work populations or in general community, such as when orthopedic surgeon Sir Percival Potts singled out squamous cell carcinoma of the scrotum in boys who worked as chimney sweeps.[31] Occupational disease is distinguished from occupational hazards that cause trauma.

There are many work-related disorders recognized by the medical fraternity as occupational disease:

- Lung diseases particularly, but not exclusively, associated with mining, such as asbestosis, silicosis, "black lung," or coal worker's pneumoconiosis.
- Asthma associated with a wide range of occupations.
- Skin conditions usually caused by chemicals or hands being wet for long periods in jobs such as hairdressing, catering, motor vehicle repair, printing, or metal machining, and those that involve long exposure to the sun, such as building construction or horticulture.
- Diseases such as "computer vision syndrome" and carpal tunnel syndrome associated with information processing.

RELATED TO MENTAL DETERMINANTS

Current mass occupational changes can lead to unexpected occupation associated illness. One example is related to the common activity of television viewing, and the extensive media coverage of the 9/11 terrorist attacks of 2001. Adults and children who had no direct exposure to the attack watched the coverage and were assessed for symptoms of post-traumatic stress disorder. One hundred and sixty-six children were found to identify with victims of the attack, and the amount of television viewing predicted an increased risk of post-traumatic stress disorder symptoms for younger children.[32]

In the field of psychiatry, current research is demonstrating that without sufficient physical occupation people can be subject to common mental illnesses, such as depression and anxiety disorders. The opposite (increased physical activity promoting mental well-being) proves the case; data from the U.S. National Comorbidity Survey[33] was used to compare the prevalence of mental disorders among 8098 adults between ages 15 and 54 years according to their reporting of regular physical activity. For slightly more than 60% of those surveyed, regular physical activity was self-reported. This was found to be associated with a "significantly decreased prevalence of current major depression and anxiety disorders," such as panic attacks, as well as social, specific, or agoraphobias. It was "not significantly associated with other affective, substance use, or psychotic disorders."[33] Another study of 40,401 Norwegian residents explored the bidirectional relationship, context, and social benefits of exercise to determine the "antidepressant and/or anti-anxiety effects" and the "type and intensity of activity" that is required. The purpose was to "explain why individuals who engage in regular leisure-time activity of any intensity are less likely to have symptoms of depression." The study demonstrates that physical activity "may have antidepressant and/or anti-anxiety effects." An inverse relationship was found between the amount of leisure-time physical activity and case-level symptoms of depression. Interestingly, this was not associated with work occupations and was independent of the intensity of activities undertaken.[34]

In line with such findings, and despite all of the mechanisms responsible for improvements not being known, it has been reasoned that the most likely explanation is a complex underlying, mediating, or moderating interaction of psychological and neurobiological mechanisms.[35] This suggests that physical activity can be used for the treatment of depression and anxiety disorders,[36a] which occupational therapists have long known from practice in the field of mental health. However, research over the past two decades has added recommendations collected in a range of fields such as sport and exercise psychology, exercise science, community medicine, general medicine, human kinetics, psychiatry, and behavioral epidemiology. A collection is shown in Table 10-1.

RELATED TO SLEEP

Sleep and sleep disorders are another aspect of occupational illness recognized by medical authorities. Most experts agree that different age groups need different amounts, that sleep needs are individual, and that there is no definitive number of hours to ensure best functional capacity. There are some generally accepted guidelines, such as those of the National Sleep Foundation in the United States. Those recommend that babies up to the age of 2 months require 12 to 18 hours daily, and this figure reduces gradually to adulthood, when 7 to 9 hours of sleep is accepted as a normal range each day.[37] However, sleep researchers tend to vary in their recommendations, according to study findings.

There has been a gradual reduction in the average amount of sleep people get in postindustrial societies, with shortened sleep patterns being more common among people who work full-time.[38] Current reduction in sleep hours may be indicative, in part, of occupational factors such as increased television and Internet use, longer commute times, or manufacturing and service sectors requiring increased numbers of people to work at night or on shifts.[39,40] A 2010 study of 3000 people in the United Kingdom found an average nightly sleep pattern of just 6 hours,[41] and according to the National Sleep Foundation, approximately one-third of adults in the United States reported sleeping an average of less than 6 hours.[42,43] Data collected over 25 years in 16 studies with a total population of more than 1.3 million people across three continents confirm that consistent short times of sleep of 6 hours or less are related to a range of medical disorders and premature death.[44] A multi-ethnic study of 30,000 adults in the United States found that people who sleep less than 5 hours per day were twice as likely as those getting 7 hours of sleep to experience cardiovascular disease, including stroke, heart, and angina attacks.[45,46]

In addition to those already mentioned, the neurobehavioral and physiological disorders associated with short sleep duration, sleep deprivation, or frequent disturbance includes high blood pressure, artery damage due to reduced glucose tolerance, obesity, diabetes, depression, substance abuse, Alzheimer's disease, and metabolic and hormone dysfunction that can make people hungrier and fatter.[47-49] Short sleep can also cause occupational disorders of mood, alertness, and performance; a decreased ability to pay attention, to react to warning signs, to remember new or associated information; and an increased risk of inhibited productivity or accidents.[43]

A study in which people were allowed only a few hours of sleep each night for a week immediately followed by 3 days of 8 hours sleep demonstrated that measurable declines in performance remained.[50] Similar results were found in a Swedish study in which healthy adults experienced three pre-deprivation days that were followed by three nights without sleep, and 4, 6, or 8 hours in bed per night randomized over 14 consecutive days, followed by three recovery days. Sleep restricted to 6 hours or less a night produced cognitive performance deficits equivalent to a maximum of two nights of total sleep deprivation, although subjects were largely unaware of cognitive deficits. The researchers concluded that even relatively moderate sleep restriction weakens neurobehavioral functions in healthy adults.[51] The outcomes were better for people who took long sleeps of 10 hours for one week before another week of little sleep, with subjects recovering normal abilities sooner

Table 10-1

Recommendations Regarding Physical Activity in the Treatment of People With Mental Disorders

Researcher	Recommendations
Dishman and Buckwort: 1996[36b]	Moderate intensity activities such as walking are more successful than vigorous activity programs
Marcus et al: 1998[36c] Marcus and Forsyth: 1998[36d] Strecher et al: 2002[36e] Segar et al: 2002[36f]	Interventions targeting specific groups or individually tailored are more effective than more generic interventions
Swinburn et al 1998[36g] Smith et al: 2000[36h]	Computer-accessed or printed exercise prescription or motivational messages appear to be more effective than face-to-face counseling alone
Broocks et al: 1998[36i] Strohle: 2009[36j]	People with major depression that includes diurnal changes should exercise later in the day. Those with panic disorders or panic attacks should be informed that despite an anxiolytic activity of acute and long-term exercise, in rare cases, activity associated with bodily sensations may trigger panic attacks
Otto et al: 2007[32]	Strategies used in cognitive behavioral therapy such as goal setting, self monitoring, homework, and supportive follow-up may support compliance with exercise regimes and help achieve and maintain a new behavior Some people experiencing severe forms of major depression require prior improvement of symptoms before participating in physical activity programs Subjects with barriers to traditional medical or psychological treatment approaches, such as minority women, may especially benefit from exercise training

than if the different patterns are reversed.[52] Such findings have implications for the occupational performance and health of shift workers, or the regular late night revelers of today's postindustrial youth culture, among many others.

Too much sleep may also be harmful, indicative of illness and responsible for some premature deaths. In two surveys of 1.1 million adult respondents conducted by the American Cancer Society, it was found that "those who said they slept 6.5 to 7.5 hours lived a bit longer than people who slept 8 hours or more."[53,54] Youngstedt and Kripke's review of the study showed that sleeping more than 7.5 hours per night was associated with approximately 5% of the total mortality of those sampled "even after controlling for 32 potentially confounding risk factors."[55] Spending an excessive time in bed can also exacerbate sleep fragmentation and create a vicious cycle of daytime lethargy. They claimed that there was sufficient evidence to test the benefits of restricting sleep as a potential aid to longer survival of regular long sleepers, and that restricting sleep might be used as treatment for people experiencing depression or primary insomnia.[55] Several studies suggest that rather than a risk, per se, oversleeping or sleep durations of 9 or more hours may point to underlying problems or undiagnosed illness, especially as deterioration of health is often associated with extended sleep time, as are depression and low socioeconomic status.[44]

The duration of sleep patterns that appear to be injurious to health should be regarded as behavioral risk factors that are influenced by familial, communal, social, and work environments. Population health practitioners from a range of disciplines need to be cognizant of how sleep variations affect morbidity, mortality, and occupation so that public awareness can be increased and measures can be taken to modify behaviors, working environments, corporate expectations, and public legislation. The slight variations between study findings suggests that consistently managing to sleep for 7 to 8 hours on a regular basis appears necessary for optimal performance and health.

Taking a nap in the middle of the day has also been found to be effective in consolidating recent memories and skills and giving the brain a chance to reorganize itself, whereas sleep within 12 hours of learning new activities by watching others enhances learning and improves performance. The final couple of hours of sleep appear to play a special role that is vital to occupational performance. Learned material or skills are committed to memory banks through sleep spindle activity of very high intensity, but only during the last 2 of 8 hours sleep. This enhances wide-ranging and skilled occupational behaviors that are dependent on the procedural memory system, such as working on a computer, using a musical instrument, or playing sport.[56] After a comparatively brief nap, people improve on declarative memory activities more than those who stay awake. Although in the past daytime napping has been discouraged in occupations where mental acuity and substantial memory capacity is required, the opposite may be the case.[57-59]

Disorders of sleep have been identified in numerous studies as an unmet population health problem, hindering the daily functioning, quality of life, safety, health and longevity of possibly 50 to 70 million Americans.[60-65] Emphasizing the societal impact of sleep disorders, Colten and Altevogt point to performance deficits such as decreased attention, vigilance, cognition, memory, and complex decision making as partially responsible for some of the most devastating disasters to have impacted human and environmental health.[66] Sleep loss–induced neurobehavioral effects, which often go unrecognized, can extend to complex errors in judgment and decision making.[67] A report from the Institute of Medicine estimated that as many as 98,000 deaths occur annually in U.S. hospitals because of medical errors due to sleep loss and shift duration.[68] Sleep disorders disrupt families and the wider community. They are common in adolescence, attributable in part to occupational factors such as increased academic demands, social and recreational opportunities, after school employment, TV viewing, and Internet access.[69] Sleep disorders are serious contributors to motor vehicle accidents independent of the effects of alcohol,[70] independent risk factors in work-related injury and death,[71,72] and increase the risk of older people experiencing falls.[66,73,74]

The activity-rest continuum is not given sufficient attention, despite it being one of the ancient rules of health, and despite substantial exploration of sleep patterns over recent decades. Sleep provides the natural mechanism to prevent activity overuse and a time for repair. Because sleep deprivation results in symptoms such as decreased coordination and reaction times, irritability, and blurred vision,[75] sleep appears to be necessary for effective doing, being, belonging, and becoming. For example, although fatigue is acknowledged as a factor in unsafe driving, it is significantly underreported in official crash statistics, and a high-priority safety issue for the transport industry.[76] A case in point is provided by a study of *Fatigue, Work-Rest Cycles, and Psychomotor Performance of New Zealand Truck Drivers*.[77] A high level of fatigue was found in the sample, with fatigue being understood as a generalized subjective state resulting from "a combination of task demands, environmental factors, arrangement of duty and rest cycles, and factors such as drivers' consumption of alcohol and medications." One in 4 drivers rated themselves in the tired range, even if at the start of their shift, and 24% failed the psychomotor performance criteria:

> Amount of rest and sleep, shift length, and number of driving days per week were all significantly related to psychomotor performance ... There was significant correspondence between drivers' self-ratings, psychomotor performance, and daytime sleepiness fatigue measures.[77]

Neither the effect of sleep on occupation nor occupation's effect on sleep can be considered apart from the other. Because sleep impacts almost every aspect of life, it is central to the occupation–health nexus. Occupation and lifestyle directly impact sleep. Considering the quality and quantity of sleep across the 24-hour continuum against what people do and how it interacts with how they feel, relate, and develop is important. Changes to sleep patterns may call for increased understanding of the relationship between regular daytime occupations that exercise and challenge the mind and body; establishing a pattern of relaxing occupations before bedtime while avoiding food, caffeine, and alcohol; and developing more consistent sleep-wake schedules.[78]

Stressful experiences and even minor variations that cause interruption during the day can be strongly linked to interrupted sleep on previous nights.[79] In addition, stress associated with time pressure, when people work shifts or long hours or experience a feeling of always being in a hurry, imprint on people's pattern of daily occupation, constituting an increased risk of sleep disturbance.[80] For example, in line with those ideas, Erlandsson and Eklund discussed sleep in relation to the levels of complexity in women's patterns of daily occupations. They point to the dual obligations of mothers who often experience interruptions at night to attend to the needs of young children. Those become a health issue when the mothers end up with too little sleep or if their sleep is interrupted more than five times a night over long periods. The complex occupation of motherhood, like many other occupational roles, is too seldom considered in terms of health and the basic rest activity cycle interacting with the 24-hour role of doing, being, belonging, and becoming.[81]

Apart from medically recognized disorders of occupation, there are some that are precursors to them or that are considered here to be disorders of health. These can derive from availability and aspects of, or responses to, physical, mental, and social occupation across the active rest continuum throughout life. With that in mind, occupational deprivation is an important disorder to consider.

Occupational Deprivation

Deprivation implies being denied something that is considered essential—a necessity is removed or withheld, causing damage. Although usually associated with material goods, such as food and shelter, the term is also used to refer to removal from office, or a loss of dignity or beneficence. In medical contexts, deprivation is directly linked with a loss of mental or physical well-being, as in sleep deprivation or being deprived of oxygen.[82] Broader definitions encompass dispossession, divestment, confiscation, or taking from, as well as the influence of an external agency or circumstance that keeps a person from "acquiring, using, or enjoying something."[83] Whatever the context, announcing a situation to be one of deprivation is to signal that something serious is awry.

Occupational deprivation contains all of those meanings, as being occupied is considered to be an innate need, an essential aspect of being human, and the basis of health, development, and well-being. Although seldom meant to imply a complete absence of occupation, invoking occupational deprivation signals a serious absence, causing an actual and consequential reduction in well-being. It might be characterized by a restricted range of occupations, so that development is stunted or capacities are unused, or by an insufficiency of occupation, having too little or nothing of value to do.

Occupational deprivation comes in many guises. Its causes might be global, such as the recent economic recession, and at other times localized. The external agency or circumstance that denies, withholds, or removes access to occupation may be deep-seated within a culture, such as the division of labor, including class and caste systems and cultural values that sustain gender, ethnic, and other forms of discrimination, such as those that operate to exclude people with leprosy, mental illness and dementia. Equally, occupational deprivation may be caused by progress, the advances in technology that replace human labor and render skills redundant, or by loss of employment opportunities due to economic restructuring, corporate decisions about relocating its manufacturing arm, exhaustion of natural resources, or environmental degradation. Poverty or affluence, limitations imposed by social services and education systems, and local regulations may also act as barriers to occupation significantly enough to warrant a claim of occupational deprivation. In all cases, in making that judgment, a substantial health impact must be evident and, because deprivation is relative, the historic, cultural, economic, societal, and geographic context must be considered.

Bringing those thoughts together, occupational deprivation is defined as "a state of prolonged preclusion from engagement in occupations of necessity and/or meaning due to factors beyond the control of the individual,"[84] or the community to which they belong. It is the resultant impact on health that perhaps most distinguishes occupational deprivation from occupational disruption. Although the latter also refers to the loss of valued activities and routines, there is an expectation that the situation will resolve with time, as in recovering from a short-term illness or a relationship breakup or returning to a familiar living situation. That is not to say that an occupational disruption will not be distressing and bewildering, or that it will be chosen and under the individual's control. Many disruptions are both predicable and normative, such as the transition from school to employment, single to married status, and childless to being a parent. However, with these and other sorts of disruptions, there is an expectation that things will resolve or be better than before, and that no long-term harm will be done to health and well-being.

In emphasizing the external causality of occupational deprivation, consideration must be given to the nature of those causes. In the discussion that follows, both malevolent and focused, and diffuse causes are considered.

IDEOLOGICALLY DRIVEN OCCUPATIONAL DEPRIVATION

In some instances, occupational deprivation is a deliberate measure, designed to exert control or inflict harm. There is an ideological stance that those who are deprived of valued activities or anything to do are unworthy of humane treatment or deserve to be punished. That sentiment may be endemic within a culture, such as the distrust of the Jews that sparked pogroms, the violent massacres of Jewish people, and the destruction of their synagogues and businesses that recurred over centuries in Europe. Hitler capitalized on that latent prejudice in his plans to force Jewish people into labor camps and to exterminate them. For prisoners in Nazi concentration camps, finding meaning through occupation was an important factor in their survival odds. In a study of the coping behavior of survivors, purpose was identified as essential to who would survive: one prisoner found this by focusing on "where I could find a blanket, something to chew, to eat, to repair a torn shoe, an additional glove."[85] Frankl, an existential psychiatrist, observed about his own concentration camp experiences that mortality rates were highest among those unable to find purpose.[86]

The forced relocation of American Indians to reservations and the South African apartheid era are additional examples of political regimes that enacted legislation that, along with the loss of civil liberties, inflicted occupational deprivation. In both cases the segregation of sectors of a population was along racial lines, with whole communities stripped of their homes, livelihood, and resources and forced to live in defined areas. For the Navajo people, that involved a 2-year forced march (1864-1866) that took them from Arizona to Bosque Redondo in New Mexico. In addition to the loss of life along the way and dislocation from ancestral lands, there was a massive disruption of culturally significant occupations, such as their weaving traditions.[87] In South Africa, relocation meant living in remote areas without infrastructure but with overcrowding, poor quality housing, and a lack of access to social services and recreational facilities.[88] Pointing to the restrictions placed on Black and "colored" people's access to education, work, sport, and cultural activities, the term occupational apartheid was coined (Figure 10-3). It is defined as "the restriction or denial of access to dignified and meaningful participation in occupations of daily life on the basis of race, color, disability, national origin, age, gender, sexual preference, religion, political beliefs, status in society, or other characteristics. Occasioned by political forces, its systematic and pervasive social, cultural, and economic consequences jeopardize health and wellbeing as experienced by individuals, communities, and societies."[89]

Apartheid policies continue to exist and, tragically, such repressive regimes have a long legacy. For example, almost 20 years from the end of apartheid in South Africa, the occupational choices of youths growing up in a "colored" residential area are powerfully shaped by that sociopolitical

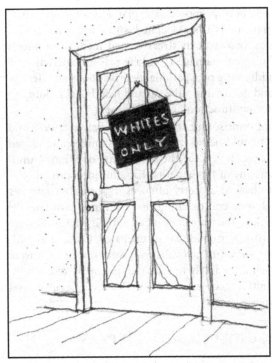

Figure 10-3. Apartheid restrictions placed on black and colored peoples' access. (© Trevor Bywater 2013. Used with permission.)

history and the patterns of marginalization, low educational attainment, manual labor, gang violence, and substance abuse it spawned.[88] In situations such as this, occupation itself can be the vehicle that reproduces social inequalities and systems of oppression. However, accusations of occupational apartheid must be made with due respect for the power of such labeling; false allegations can destroy collaborative efforts to improve conditions, falsely misrepresent ignorance as willful harm, and entrench the attitudes that create occupational injustice.[90]

Ideologically driven occupational deprivation is also sometimes intended to produce a deterrent effect. One example is prison regimes, which are caught between conflicting philosophies of retribution for wrongdoing and rehabilitating prisoners to make them fit to rejoin society.[91] Retribution is enacted through depersonalization, a stark and harsh environment, and cutting inmates off from their social networks. In addition, occupations are both limited and performed under surveillance. Choices about when and how to do things may be nonexistent. Because occupation is considered a privilege, access can be withdrawn as punishment for misdemeanors. Solitary confinement demonstrates the intention to inflict punishment in its extreme form—in combining occupational deprivation with social isolation. Some hostages endure similar levels of deprivation, but with even less surety of avoiding harm and eventual release. Among such accounts are examples of lessening the impact of deprivation by engaging in self-constructed occupations, such as reading, doing mental arithmetic, planning one's autobiography or elaborate fantasies, and maintaining a strict hygiene and exercise routine.[92] Perhaps jail inmates also employ occupational strategies, which go unreported because they are not greeted as heroes upon release.

In jails, states of occupational deprivation have been linked with both community and individual disorders, such as prison riots[93] and suicide while in custody.[94] The opposite is the case where structured occupations are provided. For example, a 1995 study of 371 US state prisons found that those with a large percentage of prisoners involved in educational, vocational, and prison industry programs, as opposed to 'keep busy' assignments, reported lower rates of violence against other inmates and warders. That association held true even after other characteristics of the prison were controlled for[95] and has been supported by numerous other studies.[96,97] Both the lack of employment and more time being idle have been proposed as explanations for such find-ings. Lacking access to meaningful occupation in prison is also associated with fewer social bonds, negative self-image,[98] dysphoric emotional states, increases in stress-related medical problems and disciplinary incidents,[99] and greater psychological damage from the prison experience.[100] Although there is ample evidence that actively addressing occupational deprivation is an effective approach to both managing prisoner behavior and decreasing survival and health risks, doing so is contrary to the retributive philosophy and deterrent function of imprisonment.

It is hard to imagine the deprivation effects of imprisonment on children. Between 1979 and 1990, Brazilian minors found roaming the street could be taken from their families and placed in dreary places known as Funamen (National Foundation for the Well-being of Minors) until they were aged 18 years. There, they were without any of the benefits that education provides.[101] Imprisonment of children, with most instances charged as petty offences, reportedly continues to be a significant problem in the Philippines, despite contravening that country's own laws.[102] Although the outcomes for those children are unclear, the impact of incarceration on 35,000 juve-nile offenders jailed in the United States over a 10-year period was investigated. Compared with those who committed similar crimes but did not serve time, youths who were imprisoned were much less likely to complete high school and much more likely to return to prison as an adult.[103] That outcome suggests that in addition to the health outcomes, early experiences of occupational deprivation make people vulnerable to repeat experiences.

LACK OF CITIZENSHIP AND OCCUPATIONAL DEPRIVATION

In addition to the ideologically driven occupational deprivation of criminals and prisoners of war, states can withhold access to occupation from outsiders. Typically, this relates to the right to work. In Western societies, where work is the primary measure of an adult's worth,[104] being excluded reinforces outsiders' lack of political, civil, and social rights.[105] Discourses that promote the value of working further serve to emphasize the deviance of not working.[106] By preventing foreigners from participating in the formal economy, the intent appears to be to deter them from entering the country or perhaps, to ring fence those opportunities for those who are citizens. Examples of those legally barred from working include asylum seekers[107,108] and people applying for refugee status.[109,110] Determining refugee status can be a protracted process, extending over many years, and the emotional distress, loss of identity, sense of hopelessness, and longing to work are palpable in documented accounts. Although a few find work within the camps or centers they are allocated, in general those roles are neither full-time nor commensurate with their qualifica-tions and skills.

Undocumented migrants and over-stayers, people who remained in a country after their visitor, student, or temporary work visa has expired, are other groups who do not have the right to sign on for paid employment. Those who do secure a job are at high risk of exploitation, with employers hiring whoever is prepared to work for the lowest hourly pay rate[111] or demanding that they work excessive hours or in poor conditions. This is occupational deprivation of a different kind, in that while their time is occupied, the work is unlikely to be secure or to satisfy the need to belong and become. Furthermore, the low remuneration and high work hours may preclude satisfying engage-ment in other family, social, religious, or recreational occupations. Examples include the many undocumented Latino migrants seeking work in the United States and many of the seasonal work-ers in market gardens in New Zealand. Among the undocumented workers are foreigners assisted to travel to a foreign country by their own countrymen, with the specific intent of removing their passports and forcing them to work in sweatshops, restaurants, or prostitution.

Another example are Turkish guest workers in Germany, who were encouraged to come to take up low-paid factory work but denied citizenship. Their jobs were generally the first to be displaced in economic downturns so that, in 2006, the unemployment rate among Turkish men living in Berlin was 40% compared to 8% of Germans. Furthermore, because they were not citizens, they were not protected by antidiscrimination legislation. This means that German shopkeepers and restaurateurs could deny them entry, and the education system was not obliged to provide language support or appropriate religious education for their Turkish-speaking children.[112] The legal situation was exacerbated by attitudinal barriers to occupation, with many Germans believing the Turks should be banned from political activities and from marrying Germans. Thus, their occupational deprivation extended well beyond paid employment and was intergenerational.

ABUSE AS OCCUPATIONAL DEPRIVATION

All types of biological and social deprivation have been associated with a failure to provide occupational opportunities for any age group.[113-115] That failure, framed here as abusive, encompasses neglect of a duty of care; corrupt or unjust practices; and outright maltreatment, such as the sustained physical and psychological violence inflicted by a parent, partner, or captor; as well as sexual abuse. Although such abuse may be systemic, as in the Catholic priests who abused children in their care over decades, it may also occur within the family home or workplace. The abuse may be to deprive victims of occupation, or the trauma may render victims unable to engage in occupation.

Infants deprived of the opportunity for learning through doing because of a lack of sensory stimulation within their environments fail to develop normally or to thrive.[116-120] In extreme examples, where abused children have been left alone in almost empty rooms and provided with only food and a place to sleep, they have failed to develop even basic skills of walking and self-care. The classic example of childhood deprivation is the "wild boy of Aveyron" who appeared from the woods of Caune, in France, in the late 18th century, after living at least 7 of his 12 years alone. Despite five years of experimental education by Jean Itard, he never attained normal language or robust health, although he did develop in many ways.[121]

The prolonged deprivation experienced by children in Romanian orphanages is a more recent example. Every child in these institutions for more than six months showed significant developmental delays.[122] Infants were initially found to be functioning at a level between the at risk and deficiency categories of the total Test of Sensory Functions.[123] Following a 6-month program within an enriched environment, children improved in all but adaptive motor functions.[124] Where that deprivation was institutionalized, there are also documented cases of infants growing into adolescence in situations of prolonged sexual abuse. One such describes a boy kept apart from other children and away from school, with the exception of being taken out to be traded among pedophiles, whose occupational deprivation extended well into adulthood.[125]

Although seldom framed as abuse, older people in residential care settings are routinely deprived of occupation. Since Townsend's study of care homes in the United Kingdom,[126] persistently high levels of inactivity have been reported, with observational studies finding that residents just sit or lie down 50% to 60% of the time. Moreover, there is evidence that lack of occupation has health consequences, with opportunities for occupation and experiencing satisfaction from doing things shown to be powerful predictors of survival among residents without severe cognitive impairment.[127] One contributing factor to their occupational deprivation is the misguided assumption that caring for older adults means doing things for them. In Western societies, the dominant discourse about ensuring safety and the widespread practice of overmedication compound the issue.[128,129]

DISCRIMINATION AND OCCUPATIONAL DEPRIVATION

In addition to the occupational deprivation directly imposed by identifiable individuals, such as prison guards, police officers, and abusive carers, the discriminatory attitudes commonly held by members of society also bring about situations that bar others from occupation. At times, the intention might appear to be to right past wrongs. For example in 1968-1969, Australia's Pastoral

Award forced station owners to pay equal wages to Aboriginal stockmen. Until that time, their remuneration had been clothing, board, and lodgings for themselves and their families, and a ration of tobacco, perhaps supplemented by a pittance in cash. In addition to paying slave wages, many pastoralists misappropriated the old-age pensions paid by the Commonwealth Government to aboriginal elders, using it as an extra source of income to supplement their profits. The justification advanced for that feudal relationship was Aboriginal people's alleged inability to handle money, such that giving them access to it would be dangerous. That system of exploitation had a long history. In the language of the day, the Australian Workers Union in 1910 had condemned the conditions imposed on aboriginal workers in Western Australia as worse than those endured by Negro slaves working in the cotton fields of America before the Civil War.[130]

The Pastoral Award resulted in mass evictions, described as "a refugee crisis of enormous proportions."[131] Being kicked off the stations meant not just loss of work. It also indicated loss of skills, community, and aspects of their culture that access to their ancestral lands had enabled them to retain. Most migrated to the fringes of rural communities, seeking education, housing, and jobs, but their narrow range of vocational skills, limited English language, and poor educational background worked against them. Among Indigenous populations, the occupational deprivation caused by unemployment and the loss of traditions is associated with "self-destructive activities such as drinking [and] violence" and poor health.[132] Aboriginal elders who were disturbed by the phenomenon, particularly those from remote areas, "asked that 'sit-down' money be replaced by money for work done by those who were unemployed" (sit-down money is welfare or dole money).[132] When the Community Development Employment Project Scheme came into being, it provided "an increase in the health of communities, ... more people involved in physically active tasks, a decrease in alcohol consumption, an increase in cleanliness, and better nutrition."[133] Leaders of other tribal groups, such as the Windjingare in Western Australia, found ways to pool their resources to buy land and support socially useful activities consistent with tribal beliefs.[134] These are rare examples of occupational initiatives being implemented for combined health, social, and economic benefits.

Women, too, have generally suffered occupational deprivation, with Mackie and Pattullo describing its effects as destroying women's vitality.[135] Women and girls have enjoyed some respite during particular eras, when more equal opportunity between men and women is apparent, but still subject to subservience to fathers or husbands, and not extending to economic or political equality. In the Medieval period, women in towns were able to engage in many trades, as the number of medieval English words ending in "ster" or "ess" attests, such as "webster" (woman weaver), "baxter" (woman baker), and "seamstress" (woman sewer).[136-139] In fact, the *Book of Trades*, written by the mayor of Paris, Etienne Boileau, records that women there worked in 86 of 100 trade and professional guilds. Although accepted as of lesser value than the roles men undertook, women's occupations, which were often "gruelling and virtually unending," were also productive; rich in variety, self-expression, responsibility, achievement, and satisfaction; and were not "compartmentalized, isolated, or solitary."[135] Unmarried women from the upper and merchant classes could receive a better education and the chance to engage in a greater range of occupations by entering a nunnery.

The restricted occupational role of affluent Western women in the 19th century was hazardous to health because their physical activity was slight, the use of their mental capacities restricted, and their "social usefulness was never recognized or recompensed."[140] Florence Nightingale, at the age of 26 years, said that she knew of some women who had gone mad for lack of things to do, observing that many "don't consider themselves as human beings at all."[141] Similarly, in 1874, Elizabeth Garrett Anderson suggested that "there is no tonic in the pharmacopoeia to be compared with happiness, and happiness worth calling such is not known where the days drag along filled with make-believe occupations and dreary sham amusements."[142]

The strong preference for women to follow domestic and child-raising occupations in the home in Victorian times was linked with infant health.[143] It was thought that if married women undertook paid employment outside the home, it could be at the cost of infants' lives.[144] Criticism of this conclusion was linked with statistics providing evidence that overcrowding and insanitary conditions were more crucial variables, and that some children might benefit from better food and conditions provided by the mother's wages.[145] The 1893-1894 Royal Commission on Labour, which investigated the conditions of women's work, including "the effects of women's industrial employment on their health, mortality, and the home," found the association between women's employment and infantile mortality was imprecise and impressionistic.[146] However, as recently as 1976, in the field of social health, Gordon expressed occupational gender bias:

> It is said that a man's job provides him with a means to satisfy his ego by preserving his personal integrity and by maintaining his place in the world. On average a man's occupation is more important to his mental health than is outside occupation to a woman. She gains status as a wife and mother and from her home ... Some women need to work outside: a lot do not wish to do so. At least that is what they say.[147]

The inequality of opportunity that has characterized women's occupations for thousands of years is still evident today, particularly in developing countries. However, even in affluent countries, delayed motor development among girls aged 3 to 5 years who live in deprived neighborhoods has been reported.[148] Increased opportunity for women in Westernized contexts to exercise their capacity and develop their potential has contributed to remarkable improvements in women's morbidity and mortality since the 19th century. The improvement is multifactorial, including the effects of reduced birth rate, greater understanding of obstetrics and gynecology, emancipation, and changed attitudes. Through to the 1980s, research into the relationship between women's occupations and health continued to be limited, on the whole, to job stress,[149-152] reproductive hazards,[152-156] and the threat to family function and maternal responsibilities.[157] Moreover, biological determinism, which rests on the assumption that women are physiologically inferior to men and incapable of strenuous activities, such as running a long distance, continues to influence social attitudes about activities suitable for women and girls. Against that social background, women's participation in physical activities is directly limited by the attitudes of their fathers, husbands and sons, and by harassment from sports coaches. Recognizing the health consequences, a 2012 UNESCO advocacy brief argues that the physical, psychological, and health benefits of well-planned physical education and sports programs in schools, promoting them as tools to empower girls born into the poorest communities.[158]

Immigrants are also subject to occupational deprivation, with detrimental health impacts. For example, in many English-speaking nations, immigrant doctors and other health professionals who have English as a second language struggle to have their qualifications recognized, despite worldwide shortages in the health workforce. Regulatory bodies are charged with the responsibility to protect the public from dangerous, unscrupulous, and incompetent doctors, yet in discharging that duty they have been accused of "social closure." That is, rather than taking reasonable measures to ensure non-native English speakers are trained to a suitable standard and have opportunities to develop language skills, they are perceived to be actively excluding foreigners from the benefits and status accrued by health practitioners, and inculcating public anxiety about the perils of registering them.[159] Other people who are at risk of illness from occupational deprivation include disadvantaged groups within the community, such as the poor and ethnic minorities,[160] with the WHO noting "the remarkable sensitivity of health to the social environment."[161] Occupational deprivation might also be the social impact (or external circumstance) of being excluded from everyday life activities[162] or confined to a bed or wheelchair because of illness or physical handicap. Illness or disability itself is an example favored by occupational therapists, perhaps because of its familiarity. However, Whiteford, who is a leader in exploring occupational deprivation,[163-166] claims that it is the "external, socially constructed phenomenon based on cultural values that creates exclusion," rather than illness or disability itself.[166] Therefore, the deprivation associated with illness or mobility issues must be considered as societal failures to provide appropriate support, to enable participation, to implement universal design principles,[167,168] or

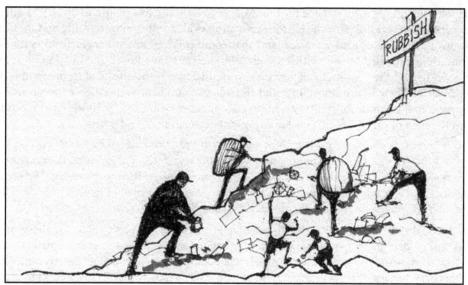

Figure 10-4. Picking through garbage to support the family's income. (© Trevor Bywater 2013. Used with permission.)

to challenge the attitudinal barriers that allow people to presume that those who are ill or have impairments are less able or less worthy to participate.

RESOURCE-BASED OCCUPATIONAL DEPRIVATION

In addition to the occupational deprivation associated with the discriminatory attitudes of members of the public, other instances hinge, in an immediate sense, on a lack of available resources. For the millions of people living in abject poverty, those resources begin with access to adequate food, clothing, and housing. Securing those can facilitate access to other resources (most importantly, education and health). Without food security, in particular, parents cannot free their children from contributing to the household income, however dirty or dangerous the options available to them (Figure 10-4). Otherwise described, the occupational deprivation that is part and parcel of extreme poverty is alleviated by individuals or households acquiring the capacities to not be deprived of resources, capabilities, choices, security, or power.

The key to achieving that is two-fold: first working with people living in poverty to generate solutions sensitive to their specific context and second, to their finances. That might be microloans, subsidies, or cash transfer programs that have been implemented in Latin America, Africa, and South Asia, and take the form of noncontributory old age pensions, child support grants, widow's grants, and the like.[169] Often, with the intention of breaking the cycle of intergenerational poverty, recipients become co-responsible with fund providers to ensure that children attend school or attend scheduled health checkups. Although discussed here as an example of resource-based occupational deprivation, failure to alleviate the situation of the poorest of the poor can also be viewed as a failure of political will, generated by discrimination against those least able to claim a political voice.

Another instance of occupational deprivation grounded in the lack of resources are the camps, often quickly established, to house forcibly displaced people. One such group is the internal refugees from the conflict in Northern Uganda. The dearth of occupation available to men in particular is a culmination of multiple factors, including the imminent risk of violence if they venture outside the camp; dislocation from their traditional farmland; lack of resourcing from the government and aid agencies; overcrowding; poverty; and the availability of alcohol.[170] Geographic isolation might also be considered to be a form of resource-based occupational deprivation, in that people are located at such a distance from necessary resources that participation is rendered occasional or impossible. Whiteford provided a poignant example of a woman residing at a remote farm, whose yearning for female company pervades every moment of an infrequent trip into town.[165]

ECONOMIC CAUSES OF OCCUPATIONAL DEPRIVATION

Many people experience reduced options to do, be, belong, and become because they are deprived of paid employment. In Western countries, decades of research has established without doubt that being unemployed is associated with increased stress, health-risk behavior, ill-health, and suicide rates. However, there are gender differences. Among women, unemployment is associated with suboptimal self-rated health; among men, it is more strongly associated with high alcohol consumption. Financial stresses partially explain the relationship of unemployment to ill-health for both men and women but have stronger explanatory power for women, who are more likely to have dependent children in their care and, as a result of the gendered division of labor, be less financially secure.[171]

For both sexes, pessimism about the future is also influential, as the current economic recession means diminished work prospects and thus limited ability to make choices about employment. The value placed on paid employment by society increases the potency of the deprivation by making people feel powerless, although that seems to be more true of unemployed women who, like other women, are commonly excluded from power and decision making.[171] Unemployed women with weak social networks report worse health status, but the protective role of being socially connected is decreased if the majority of those people are also unemployed so that their ability to provide emotional, financial, and social support is also compromised.[172]

The causes of unemployment and underemployment are various, including structural factors, such as an enforced retirement age, or the lack of regulation of banking that brought about the current economic recession. Those deprived of occupation by such processes include reluctant retirees, middle-aged process workers facing factory closures, or school leavers joining the burgeoning ranks of other unemployed school leavers. The numerous individuals who have little respite from unpaid caregiver duties can also be viewed from an economic perspective, in that women's role in providing care to children, the sick, and the elderly members of the family and local community remains outside the economic fabric of society.

When profit and mechanization took precedence over creativity and craftsmanship, corporate practices dating from the industrial revolution robbed many of the satisfaction derived from work in earlier times. The quest for improved productivity continues the trend toward tightly controlled work processes and workplace engineering to minimize workers' ability to waste time interacting on the job (Figure 10-5). Where unionization moderates the worst abuses in Western societies, the possibility of resisting inhumane work demands and unsafe conditions are beyond the reach of workers in off-shore factories, whose corporate managers can decide to relocate the work to countries with a lower paid and more compliant workforce. Neither is it available to workers in repressive regimes or situations of high unemployment, where bosses have abundant replacements for injured, ill, aging, or despondent workers.

The push toward cost efficiency also favors technological advances, which displaces people from work, with the possibility of more radical changes resulting in serious health consequences. Half a century ago, Dubos warned that although humans may appear to adapt to new environments, their biological inheritance only enables adaptation up to a point and that chronic disease states can develop over time.[173] Maslow too was concerned that humankind was "at a point in history unlike anything that has ever been before" with "huge acceleration in the growth of facts, of knowledge, of techniques, of inventions, of advances in technology." He suggested that the rapidity of the changing world calls for "a different kind of human being...who is comfortable with change," because "societies that cannot turn out such people will die."[174] That might be responsible for much of the

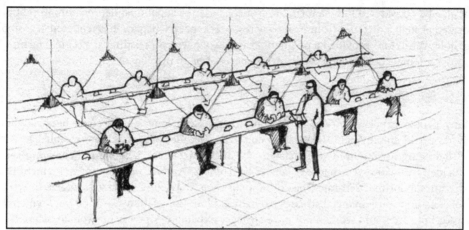

Figure 10-5. Tightly controlled work processes as sites of occupational deprivation. (© Trevor Bywater 2013. Used with permission.)

occupational illness in modern societies. Uncovering the range of reasons for occupational stress, imbalance, and the deprivation of populations, as well as individuals, is a matter of urgency.

Conclusion

The Ottawa Charter holds that

> *"professional and social groups, and health personnel, have a major responsibility to mediate between differing interests in society for the pursuit of health. Health promotion strategies and programs should be adapted to the local needs and possibilities of individual countries and regions to take into account differing social, cultural and economic systems."[1]*

As the discussion of occupational deprivation and alienation reveals, societal interests serve many purposes—from punishing and excluding those perceived to pose a threat to following the prevailing economic rationale of increasing productivity to bolster gross national product. Where the result is occupational disorder, whether of citizens, criminals, the poor and elderly, foreigners, or workers, health suffers as a consequence. In making evident the link between disorders of occupation and health, the concepts of occupational deprivation and alienation, as well as stress and imbalance, considered in the next chapter, point the way to creating fairer, more enabling societies. That discussion is also picked up in Chapter 14, which addresses the issue of occupational justice.

Throughout the text it has been suggested that occupation has rarely been considered as a holistic entity in relation to health. Instead, segments of occupation are researched and addressed separately by several health professions. It is mentioned in WHO directives such as the Ottawa Charter, that addresses occupational issues with terms such as "learning, loving, work and play,"[175] and the *Social Determinants of Health* with other terms such as life's experiences, "education, economic status, employment and decent work."[176] Instead of regarding all of the things that people do as an interactive whole, segmentation by occupation-based health professions has led to a poor understanding of the interactive nature of the brain-body-social environment-occupation-health nexus. That, in turn, prevents changing patterns of life, work and leisure from having a significant impact on maintaining and improving health. Work and leisure should be a source of health for people, but inadequate recognition or understanding of the total picture of people's doing, being, belonging, and becoming in terms of population health prevents that from eventuating.

The next chapter continues the investigation of occupational disorders of health focusing on occupational imbalance and stress that, like occupational deprivation, should be understood as illnesses in their own right.

References

1a. World Health Organization, Health and Welfare Canada, Canadian Public Health Association. *Ottawa Charter for Health Promotion.* Ottawa, Canada; 1986.

1b. Thagard P. *How Scientists Explain Disease.* Princeton, NJ: Princeton University Press; 1999.

2.   Wilcock AA, et al. *Retrospective Study of Elderly People's Perceptions of the Relationship Between Their Lifes, Occupations and Health.* Unpublished material, University of South Australia, 1990.

3.   Glass TA, Mendes de Leon CF, Marotolli RA, Berkman LF. Population based study of social and productive activities as predictors of survival among elderly Americans. *British Medical Journal.* 1999:319:478-483.

4.   Watson L. *Neophilia: The Tradition of the New.* Great Britain, Hodder and Stoughton Ltd; 1989.

5.   King-Boyes MJE. *Patterns of Aboriginal Culture: Then and Now.* Sydney, Australia: McGraw-Hill Book Co; 1977:17,155.

6.   Roose J, de Vries W, Schmikli S, Backx, F, van Doornen L. Evaluation and opportunities in overtraining approaches. *Research Quarterly for Exercise and Sport.* 2009;80(4):756-64.

7.   Budgett R. Overtraining syndrome. *British Journal of Sports Medicine.* 1990;24(4):231-236.

8.   Draeger J, Yates A, Crowell D. The obligatory exerciser: assessing an overcommitment to exercise. *The Physician and Sportsmedicine.* 2005;33(6):13-23.

9.   Adams J, Kirkby R. Exercise dependence: A review of its manifestation, theory and measurement. *Research in Sports Medicine.* 1998;8(3):265-76.

10. Bresciani G, Cuevas M, Molinero O, Almar M, Suay F, et al. Signs of overload after an intensified training. *International Journal of Sports Medicine.* 2011;32(5):338-343.

11. Baldwin D. Exercise motivational triggers. *iUniverse*; 2002-03-27:53.

12. Cooper K. *Dr Kenneth Cooper's Antioxidant Revolution.* Melbourne, Australia: Bookman; 1994.

13. Siscovick DS, Weiss NS, Fletcher RH, Lasky T. The incidence of primary cardiac arrest during vigorous exercise. *New England Journal of Medicine.* 1984;311:874-877.

14. Tucker R, Dugas J. Sudden death during exercise: The media, risk and running. *The Science of Sport. Scientific Comment and Analysis of Sporting Performance.* Thursday, October 22, 2009. http://www.sportsscientists.com/2009/10/3-runners-die-in-detroit-safety-of.html Accessed July 10, 2013.

15. Leong K. Sudden death during exercise: are you more likely to die while you're working out? *Yahoo! Contributor Network.* Sept 8, 2011.

16. Kleitman N. *Sleep and Wakefulness.* Chicago, Ill: University of Chicago Press; 1963:188. Reprint 1987.

17. Kleitman N. Basic rest-activity cycle—22 years later. *Journal of Sleep Research & Sleep Medicine.* 1982;5(4):311-317.

18. Leger DW. *Biological Foundations for Behavior: An Integrative Approach.* New York, NY: Harper Collins Publishers; 1992:374.

19. Blessing W, Mohammed M, Ootsuka Y. Heating and eating: brown adipose tissue thermogenesis precedes food ingestion as part of the ultradian basic rest-activity cycle in rats. *Physiology and Behavior.* 2012;105(4):966-74.

20. World Health Organization. *2008-2013 Action Plan for the Global Strategy for the Prevention and Control of Noncommunicable Diseases.* WHO; 2009. http://whqlibdoc.who.int/publications/2009/9789241597418_eng.pdf?ua=1. Accessed July 12, 2013.

21. World Health Organization. *United Nations High-level Meeting on Noncommunicable Disease Prevention and Control.* September 2011.

22. Geneau R, Stuckler D, Stachenko S, NcKee M, Ebrahim S, Basu S, et al. Raising the priority of preventing chronic diseases: a political process. *The Lancet.* 376;9753:1689-1698, 13 November 2010.

23. Law M, Steinwender S, Leclair L. Occupation, health and well-being. *Canadian Journal of Occupational Therapy.* 1998;65:81-91.

24. The Physiotherapy Site. *The Over/Under Activity Cycle.* http://www.thephysiotherapysite.co.uk/physiotherapy/pain-management/over-under-activity-cycle. Accessed February, 2013.

25. Stovitz S, Johnson R. "Underuse" as a cause for musculoskeletal injuries: is it time that we started reframing our message? *British Journal of Sports Medicine.* 2006, September;40(9):738-739.

26. Meyer A. The philosophy of occupational therapy. *Archives of Occupational Therapy.* 1922;1:1-10.

27. Sigerist HE. *A History of Medicine. Vol 1. Primitive and Archaic Medicine.* New York, NY: Oxford University Press; 1955:254-255.

28. Ramazzini B. *A Treatise of Diseases of Tradesmen.* Printed for Andrew Bell et al, London; (English edition) 1705.

29. Pott P. *Chirugical Observations.* London: Hawes, Clarke and Collins; 1775.

30. Thackrah C. *The Effects of the Principal Arts, Trades and Professions, and of Civic States and Habits of Living, on Health and Longevity.* Longman, Rees, Orme, Brown, & Green; 1831.

31. Gordon R. *The Alarming History of Medicine.* New York, St Martin's Press; 1994.

32. Otto M, Henin A, Hirshfeld-Becker D, Pollack M, Biederman J, Rosenbaum J. Posttraumatic stress disorder symptoms following media exposure to tragic events: Impact of 9/11 on children at risk for anxiety disorders. *Journal of Anxiety Disorders.* 2007; 21(7)888-902.

33. Goodwin R. Association between physical activity and mental disorders among adults in the United States. *Preventive Medicine.* 2003;36(6):698-703.

34. Harvey S, Hotopf M, Overland S, Mykletun A. Physical activity and common mental disorders. *British Journal of Psychiary.* 2010;197(5):357-364.

35. Cotman C, Berchtold N. Exercise: a behavioral intervention to enhance brain health and plasticity. *Trends in Neurosciences.* 2002;(6):295-301.

36a. Strohle A. Physical activity, exercise, depression and anxiety disorders. *Journal of Neural Transmission.* 2009;116:777-784.

36b. Dishman R, Buckworth J. Increasing physical activity: A quantitative synthesis. *Medical Science Sports Exercise.* 1996;28(6):706-719.

36c. Marcus B, Bock B, Pinto B, et al. Efficacy of an individualized, motivationally-tailored physical activity intervention. *Ann Behav Med.* 1998;20:174-180.

36d. Marcus B, Forsyth L. Tailoring interventions to promote physically active lifestyles in women. *Womens Health Issues.* 1998;8:104-111.

36e. Strecher V, Wang C, Derry H. Tailored interventions for multiple risk behaviours. *Health Educ Res.* 2002;17:619-626.

36f. Segar M, Hankon J, Jayaratne T, et al. Fitting fitness into women's lives: effects of a gender-tailored physical activity intervention. *Women's Health Issues.* 2002;12:338-347.

36g. Swinburn B, Walter L, Arroll B, et al. The green prescription study: a randomised controlled trial of written exercise advice provided by general practitioners. *Am J Public Health.* 1998;88:288-291.

36h. Smith B, Bauman A, Bull F, et al. Promoting physical activity in general practice: a controlled trial of written advice and information materials. *Br J Sports Med.* 2000;34:262-267.

36i. Broocks A, Bandelow B, Pekrun G, et al. Comparison of aerobic exercise, clomipramine, and placebo in the treatment of panic disorder. *American Journal of Psychiatry.* 1998;155(5):603-609.

36j. Strohle A. Physical activity, exercise, depression and anxiety disorders. *Journal of Neural Transmission.* 2009;116:777-784.

37. National Sleep Foundation. *How Much Sleep Do We Really Need?* Available at: http://sleepfoundation. org/. Accessed May 3, 2013.

38. Cappuccio F, D'Elia L, Strazzullo P, Miller M. Sleep duration and all-cause mortality: a systematic review and meta-analysis of prospective studies. *Sleep.* 2010;33(5):585-592.

39. Institute of Medicine. *Sleep Disorders and Sleep Deprivation: An Unmet Public Health Problem.* Washington, DC; The National Academies Press. 2006.

40. Malik S, Kaplan J. Sleep deprivation. *Primary Care.* 2005;32:475-490.

41. Donnelly L. Seven hours sleep is the recipe for health. *The Telegraph.* 01 Jul 2010. http://www.telegraph.co.uk/health/healthnews/7920197/Seven-hours-sleep-is-the-recipe-for-health.html.

42. National Sleep Foundation. *Sleep in America Poll 2009.* Washington, DC; 2009. www.sleepfoundation org/article/sleep-america-polls/2009-health-and-safety. Accessed August 2013.

43. Bonnet M, Arand D. We are chronically sleep deprived. *Sleep.* 1995;18:908-911.

44. Cappuccio F, Cooper D, D'Elia L, Strazzullo P, Mille M. Sleep duration predicts cardiovascular outcomes: a systematic review and meta-analysis of prospective studies. *European Heart Journal.* 2011;32(12):1484-1492.

45. Sabanayagam C, Shankar A. Sleep duration and cardiovascular disease: results from the National Health Interview Survey. *Sleep.* 33(08). http://www.journalsleep.org. Accessed August 7, 2013.

46.   Shankar A, Syamala S, Kalidindi S. Insufficient rest or sleep and its relation to cardiovascular disease, diabetes and obesity in a national, multiethnic sample. *PLoS ONE*. 2010;5(11):e14189. doi:10.1371/journal.pone.0014189

47.   Knutson K, Ryden A, Mander B, Van Cauter E. Role of sleep duration and quality in the risk and severity of type 2 diabetes. *Archives of Internal Medicine*. 2006;166:1768-1774.

48.   Knutson K, Van Cauter E, Rathouz P, Yan L, Liu K, Lauderdale D. Association between sleep and blood pressure in mid life: the CARDIA Sleep Study. *Archives of Internal Medicine*. 2009;169(11):1055-1061.

49.   Knutson K. Sociodemographic and cultural determinants of sleep deficiency: implications for cardiometabolic disease risk. *Social Sience and Medicine*. 2013;79:7-15.

50.   Rupp T, Wesensten N, Bliese P, Balkin T. Banking sleep: realization of benefits during subsequent sleep restriction and recovery. *Sleep*. 2009;32(3):311-321.

51.   Van Dongen H, Maislin G, Mullington J, Ginges D. The cumulative cost of additional wakefulness: dose response effects on neurobehavioral functions and sleep physiology from chronic sleep restriction and total sleep deprivation. *Sleep*. 2003;(26)2:117-126.

52.   Szalavitz M. Healthy sleep: new research on memory, fat, golf. *Time*. 2009. Available at: http://healthland.time.com/2009/11/03/healthy-sleep-new-research-on-memory-fat-timing/. Accessed August 7, 2013.

53.   Kripke D, Garfinkel L, Wingard D, Klauber M, Marler M. Mortality associated with sleep duration and insomnia. *Archives of General Psychiatry*. 2002;59(2):131-136.

54.   Kripke D. *Mortality and Cancer Risks, Which Pills to Avoid & Better Alternatives*. http://www.darksideofsleepingpills.com/all.html#dsch3. Last Revised March 2013. Accessed August 16, 2013.

55.   Youngstedt S, Kripke D. Long sleep and mortality: rationale for sleep restriction. *Sleep Medicine Reviews*. 2004;8(3):159-174.

56.   Tamminen J, Payne J, Stickgold R, Wamsley E, Gaskell M. Sleep spindle activity is associated with the integration of new memories and existing knowledge. *Journal of Neuroscience*. 2010;30(43):14356-14360.

57.   Tucker M, Hirota Y, Wamsley E, Lau H, Chaklader A, Fishbein W. A daytime nap containing solely non-REM sleep enhances declarative but not procedural memory. *Neurobiology of Learning and Memory*. 2006;86(2):241-247.

58.   Takahashi, M. The role of prescribed napping in sleep medicine. *Sleep Medicine Reviews*. 2003;7(3):227-235.

59.   Mednick S, Nakayama K, Stickgold R. Sleep-dependent learning: a nap is as good as a night. *Nature Neuroscience*. 2003; 6(7): 697–698.

60.   Baldwin C, Griffith K, Nieto F, O'Connor G, Walsleben J, Redline S. The association of sleep-disordered breathing and sleep symptoms with quality of life in the Sleep Heart Health Study. *Sleep*. 2001;24(1):96-105.

61.   Baldwin D Jr, Daugherty S. Sleep deprivation and fatigue in residency training: results of a national survey of first- and second-year residents. *Sleep*. 2004;27(2):217-223.

62.   Hasler G, Buysse D, Gamma A, Ajdacic V, Eich D, Rossler W, Angst J. Excessive daytime sleepiness in young adults: A 20-year prospective community study. *Journal of Clinical Psychiatry*. 2005;66(4):521-529.

63.   Kuppermann M, Lubeck D, Mazonson P, Patrick D, Stewart A, Buesching D, Fifer S. Sleep problems and their correlates in a working population. *Journal of General Internal Medicine*. 1995;10(1):25-32.

64.   Simon G, VonKorff M. Prevalence, burden, and treatment of insomnia in primary care. *American Journal of Psychiatry*. 1997;154(10):1417-1423.

65.   Rosen C, Palermo T, Larkin E, Redline S. Health-related quality of life and sleep-disordered breathing in children. *Sleep*. 2002;25(6):657-666.

66.   Colten H, Altevogt B, eds. *Sleep Disorders and Sleep Deprivation: An Unmet Public Health Problem*. Washington, DC, National Academies Press (US); 2006.

67.   Durmer J, Dinges D. Neurocognitive consequences of sleep deprivation. *Seminars in Neurology*. 2005;25(1):117-129.

68.   Institute of Medicine. *To Err Is Human: Building a Safer Health System*. Washington, DC: National Academy Press; 2000.

69.   Wolfson A, Carskadon M. Sleep schedules and daytime functioning in adolescents. *Child Development*. 1998;69(4):875-887.

70.   Connor J, Norton R, Ameratunga S, Robinson E, Civil I, Dunn R, Bailey J, Jackson R. Driver sleepiness and risk of serious injury to car occupants: population-based case control study. *British Medical Journal*. 2002;324(7346):1125.

71. Akerstedt T, Fredlund P, Gillberg M, Jansson B. A prospective study of fatal occupational accidents–relationship to sleeping difficulties and occupational factors. *Journal of Sleep Research.* 2002;11(1):69-71.

72. Swaen G, Van Amelsvoort L, Bultmann U, Kant I. Fatigue as a risk factor for being injured in an occupational accident: results from the Maastricht Cohort Study. *Occupational and Environmental Medicine.* 2003;60(suppl 1):88-92.

73. Brassington G, King A, Bliwise D. Sleep problems as a risk factor for falls in a sample of community-dwelling adults aged 64-99 years. *Journal of the American Geriatrics Society.* 2000;48(10):1234-1240.

74. Avidan A, Fries B, James M, Szafara K, Wright G, Chervin R. Insomnia and hypnotic use, recorded in the minimum data set, as predictors of falls and hip fractures in Michigan nursing homes. *Journal of the American Geriatrics Society.* 2005;53(6):955-962.

75. Horne JA. A review of the biological effects of total sleep deprivation in man. *Biological Psychology.* 1978;(7):55-102.

76. Moore B. An integrated approach to the regulation of heavy vehicle driver fatigue. *Fifth International Heavy Vehicle Safety Symposium.* Knoxville, Tennessee; November 2001.

77. Charlton S, Baas P. Fatigue, work-rest cycles, and psychomotor performance of New Zealand truck drivers. *New Zealand Journal of Psychology.* 2001;30(1):32-39.

78. Division of Sleep Medicine, Harvard Medical School. *Twelve Simple Tips to Improve Your Sleep.* Produced in partnership with WGBH Educational Foundation. Last reviewed December 2007. Available at: http://healthysleep.med.harvard.edu/healthy/getting/overcoming/tips. Accessed August 12, 2013.

79. Åkerstedt T. Återhämtning/sömn (Recovery/sleep). In: Theorell T, ed. *Psykosocial Miljö Och Stress.* Lund, Sweden: Student litteratur. 2003:77-95.

80. Ribet C, Derriennic F. Age, working conditions, and sleep disorders: a longitudinal analysis in the French cohort ESTEV. *Sleep.* 1999; 22:491-502.

81. Erlandsson L, Eklund M. Levels of complexity in patterns of daily occupations: Relationship to women's well-being. *Journal of Occupational Science.* 2006; 13(1): 27-36.

82. Deprivation. *Merriam-Webster Inc:* 2013. http://www.merriam-webster.com/dictionary/deprivation. Access August 15, 2013.

83. *Funk & Wagnall's Standard Desk Dictionary.* Vol 1 A-M. New York, NY: Harper and Row; 1984:172.

84. Whiteford G. Occupational deprivation: global challenge in the new millennium. *British Journal of Occupational Therapy.* 2000;63:201.

85. Dimsdale, JE. The coping behavior of Nazi concentration camp survivors. *American Journal of Psychiatry.* 1974;131(7):795.

86. Frankl VE. *Man's Search for Meaning.* Boston, Mass: Beacon Press; 1962.

87. Frank G. The transactional relationship between occupation and place: indigenous cultures in the American Southwest. *Journal of Occupational Science.* 2011;18(1):3-20. doi:10.1080?1442759.2011.562874

88. Galvaan R. Occupational choice: the significance of socio-economic and political factors. In: Whiteford GE, Hocking C, eds. *Occupational Science: Society, Inclusion, Participation.* Oxford, UK: Wiley-Blackwell; 2012:152-162.

89. Kronenberg F, Pollard N. Overcoming occupational apartheid: a preliminary exploration of the political nature of occupational therapy. In: Kronenberg F, Simo Algado S, Pollard N, eds. *Occupational Therapy without Borders: Learning from the Spirit of Survivors.* London: Elsevier Ltd, 2005;67.

90. Thibeault R. Occupational justice's intents and impacts: from personal choices to community consequences. In: Cutchin MP, Dickie VA, eds. *Transactional Perspectives on Occupation.* Dordrecht: Springer; 2013;245-256.

91. Pollock JM. The rationale for imprisonment. In JM Pollock, ed. *Prisons Today and Tomorrow.* 2nd ed. Boston: Jones and Bartlett Publishers. 2006;3-21.

92. Alexander DA, Klein S. Kidnapping and hostage-taking: a review of effects, coping and resilience. *Journal of the Royal Society of Medicine.* 2009;102(1):16-21. doi:10.1258/jrsm.2008.080347.

93. Useem B. Disorganization and the New Mexico prison riot of 1980. *American Sociological Review.* 1985;50(5):677-688.

94. Liebling A. Suicides in young prisoners: a summary. *Death Studies.* 1993;17(5):381-409.

95. McCorkle RC, Miethe TD, Drass KA. The roots of prison violence: a test of the deprivation, management, and not so total institution models. *Crime and Delinquency.* 1995;41(3):317-331.

96. Gerber J, Fritsch EJ. Adult academic and vocational correctional programs: a review of recent research. *Journal of Offender Rehabilitation.* 1995;22(1-2):119-142.

97. Perez DM, Gover AR, Tennyson G, Santos SD. Individual and institutional characteristics related to inmate victimization. *International Journal of Offender Therapy and Comparative Criminology.* 2010;54(3):378-394.

98. Hassine V. *Life without Parole: Living and Dying in Prison Today.* 5th ed. New York: Oxford University Press; 2010.

99. Zamble E. Behavior and adaptation in long term prison inmates: descriptive longitudinal results. *Criminal Justice and Behavior.* 1992;19(4):409-425.

100. McCorkle RC. Fear of victimization and symptoms of psychopathology among prison inmates. *Journal of Offender Rehabilitation.* 1993:19(1/2);27-41.

101. Bomfim V. Once a street kid, now a citizen of the world. In: Kronenberg F, Pollard N, eds. *Occupational Therapy without Borders: Learning from the Spirit of Survivors.* London: Elsevier Ltd; 2005.

102. Children in Jail in Philippines. Wikipedia. 2013. http://en.wikipedia.org/wiki/Children_in_jail_in_Philippines. Accessed June 12, 2012.

103. Aizer A, Doyle JJ. *Juvenile Incarceration, Human Capital and Future Crime: Evidence from Randomly-Assigned Judges.* National Bureau of Economic Research Working Paper No. 19102; 2013. Available at: http://nber.org/papers/w19102

104. Beck U. *The Brave New World of Work* (P Camiller, translator). Cambridge: Polity; 2000.

105. Barnes C, Mercer G. Disabilty, work, and welfare: challenging the social exclusion of disabled people. *Work, Employment & Society.* 2005;19(3):527-545.

106. Riach K, Loretto W. Identity work and the unemployed worker: age, disability and the lived experience of the older unemployed. *Employment & Society.* 2009;23(1):102-119.

107. Burchett N, Matheson R. The need for belonging: the impact of restrictions on working on the well-being of an asylum seeker. *Journal of Occupational Science.* 2010;17:85-91. doi:10.1080/14427591.2010.9686679.

108. Horghagen S, Josephsson S. Theatre as liberation, collaboration and relationship for asylum seekers. *Journal of Occupational Science.* 2010;17:168-176. doi:10.1080/14427591.2010.9686691

109. Steindl C, Winding K, Runge U. Occupation and participation in everyday life: women's experiences of an Austrian refugee camp. *Journal of Occupational Science.* 2008;15(1):36-42. doi:10.1080/14427591.2008.9686605.

110. Morville A-L, Erlandsson L-K. The experience of occupational deprivation in an asylum centre: the narratives of three men. *Journal of Occupational Science.* 2013;20(3):212-223. doi:10.1080/14427591.2013.808976.

111. Bailliard AL. Laying low: fear and injustice for Latino Migrants to Smalltown, USA. *Journal of Occupational Science.* 2013;1-15. doi:10.1080/14427591.2013.799114

112. Mueller C. Integrating Turkish communities: a German dilemma. *Population Research and Policy Review.* 2006;25:419-441.

113. Mackie A. Social deprivation and the role of psychological services. *Educational and Child Psychology.* 1992;9(3):84-89.

114. Townsend P, Simpson D, Tibbs N. Inequalities in health in the city of Bristol: a preliminary review of statistical evidence. *International Journal of Health Services.* 1985;15(4):637-663.

115. Mechanic D. Adolescents at risk: new directions. *Journal of Adolescent Health.* 1991;12(8):638-643.

116. Gilfoyle EM, Grady AP, Moore JC. *Children Adapt.* Thorofare, NJ: Charles B Slack; 1981.

117. Short MA. Vestibular stimulation as early experience: historical perspective and research implications. *Physical and Occupational Therapy in Pediatrics.* 1985;5:135-152.

118. Drotar D. Failure to thrive and preventive mental health: knowledge gaps and research needs. In: Drotar D, ed. *New Directions in Failure to Thrive.* New York, NY: Plenum Press; 1985:27-44.

119. Provence S, Lipton RC. *Infants in Institutions.* New York, NY: International Universities Press; 1962.

120. Day S. Mother-infant activities as providers of sensory stimuation. *American Journal of Occupational Therapy.* 1982;36:579-589.

121. Itard J. The wild boy of Aveyron. In: Malson L, ed. *Wolf Children and the Problem of Human Nature.* New York, NY: Monthly Review Press; 1972.

122. Bascom B. Program summary, projects and descriptions. In: *Brooke Foundation Annual Report.* Washington, DC: Brooke Foundation; 1993:12.

123. DeGangi GA, Greenspan SI. *Test of Sensory Functions in Infants (TSFI) Manual.* Los Angeles, CA: Western Psychological Services; 1989.

124. Haradon G, Bascom B, Dragomir C, Scipcaru V. Sensory functions of institutionalized Romanian infants: a pilot study. *Occupational Therapy International.* 1994;1:250-260.

125. Lentin P. The human spirit and occupation: surviving and creating a life. *Journal of Occupational Science.* 2002;9(3):143-152.

126. Mozley CG. Exploring connections between occupation and mental health in care homes for older people. *Journal of Occupational Science.* 2001;8(3):14-19.

127. Mozley CG, Sutcliffe C, Bagley H, Cordingley L, Huxley P, Challis D, Burns A. *The Quality of Life Study: Outcomes for Older People in Nursing and Residential Homes.* Final Report to the NHS Executive 2000.

128. Dennhardt S, Laliberte Rudman D. When occupation goes 'wrong': a critical reflection on occupation. In: Whiteford G, Hocking C, eds. *Occupational Science: Society, Inclusion, Participation.* Oxford, UK: Wiley-Blackwell; 2012;117-136.

129. Smith BL. Inappropriate prescribing. American Psychological Association. *Monitor on Psychology.* 2012;43(6):36. http://www.apa.org/monitor/2012/06/prescribing.aspx. Access August 17, 2013.

130. Skyring F. Low wages, low rents, and pension cheques: the introduction of equal wages in the Kimberley, 1968-1969. In: Fijn N, Keen I, Lloyd C, Pickering M, eds. *Indigenous Participation in Australian Economies II: Historical Engagements and Current Enterprises.* Canberra: Australian National University E Press; 2012. http://epress.anu.edu.au/apps/bookworm/view/Indigenous+Participation+in+Australian+Economies+II/9511/ch08.html. Access August 1, 2013.

131. Yu P. Aboriginal peoples, federalism and self-determination. *Social Alternatives.* 1994;13(1):19.

132. Jensen H. What it means to get off sit-down money: community development employment projects (CDEP). *Journal of Occupational Science: Australia.* 1993;1(2):12-19.

133. Aboriginal and Torres Strait Islander Commission. *No Reverse Gear: A National Review of the Community Development Projects Scheme.* 1993.

134. Shaw K, Dann J. Work is sacred: the journey out of welfare. *Journal of Occupational Science.* 1999;6(2):80-87.

135. Mackie L, Pattullo P. *Women at Work.* London, England: Tavistock Publications; 1977:10.

136. Stavrianos LS. *The World to 1500: A Global History.* 4th ed. Englewood Cliffs, NJ: Prentice Hall; 1988:273-275.

137. Boileau E. *Livre de Metiers (Book of Trades).* 13th century.

138. Power E. The position of women. In: Crump CG, Jacob EF, eds. *The Legacy of the Middle Ages.* Oxford, UK: Clarendon Press; 1926:401-434.

139. Gross SH, Bingham MW. *Women in Medieval-Renaissance Europe.* St. Louis Park, Minn: Glenhurst; 1983.

140. Rowbotham S. *Hidden from History.* London, England: Pluto Press; 1973:58.

141. Woodham-Smith C. *Florence Nightingale.* London, England: The Reprint Society; 1952:71.

142. Anderson EG. *Fortnightly Review.* London, England; 1874:590.

143. Jones H. The perils and protection of infant life. *Journal of the Royal Statistical Society.* 1894;1(vii):1-98.

144. Hewitt M. *Wives and Mothers in Victorian Industry.* London, England: Rockcliff; 1958.

145. Dyhouse C. Working class mothers and infant mortality in England, 1895-1914. *Journal of Social History.* 1978;xii:248-267.

146. Collett CE. The collection and utilization of official statistics bearing on the extent and effects of the industrial employment of women. *Journal of the Royal Statistical Society.* 1898;219-261.

147. Gordon D. *Health, Sickness and Society: Theoretical Concepts in Social and Preventive Medicine.* St. Lucia, Queensland: University of Queensland Press; 1976:378.

148. Goodway JD, Robinson LE, Crowe H. Gender differences in fundamental motor skill development in disadvantaged preschoolers from two geographical regions. *Research Quarterly for Exercise and Sport.* 2010;81(1):17-24.

149. Waldron I. The coronary-prone behavior pattern, blood pressure, employment and socio-economic status in women. *Journal of Psychosomatic Research.* 1978;22:79-87.

150. Lemkau JP. Women and employment: some emotional hazards. In: Beckerman CL, ed. *The Evolving Female.* New York, NY: Human Sciences Press; 1980.

151. Haw MA. Women, work and stress: a review and agenda for the future. *Journal of Health and Social Behavior.* 1982;23:132-144.

152. Lewin E, Olesen V. Occupational health and women: the case of clerical work. In: Lewin E, Olesen V, eds. *Women, Health and Healing: Toward a New Perspective.* New York, NY: Tavistock Publications; 1985.

153. Bell C. Implementing safety and health regulations for women in the workplace. *Feminist Studies.* 1979;5(2):286-301.

154. Hunt VR. A brief history of women workers and hazards in the workplace. *Feminist Studies.* 1979;5(2):274-285.

155. Petcheky R. Workers, reproductive hazards, and the politics of protection: an introduction. *Feminist Studies.* 1979;5:233-245.

156. Wright MJ. Reproductive hazards and "protective" discrimination. *Feminist Studies.* 1979;5(2):302-309.

157. Fogarty MP, Rapoport R, Rapoport RN. *Sex, Career, and Family.* Beverly Hills, CA: Sage Publications; 1971.

158. Kirk D. *UNESCO Advocacy Brief: Empowering Girls and Women through Physical Education and Sport.* Bangkok: UNESCO; 2012.

159. Mpofu C, Hocking C. "Not made here": occupational deprivation of non-English speaking background immigrant doctors and dentists in New Zealand. *Journal of Occupational Science.* 2013;20:131-145. doi:10.1080/14427591.2012.729500

160. Marmott M, Wilkinson RG, eds. *Social Determinants of Health.* Oxford, UK: Oxford University Press, 1999.

161. World Health Organization. *International Centre for Health and Society Social Determinants of Health: The Solid Facts.* World Health Organization, Europe. 2003.

162. World Health Organization. *World Report on Disability.* WHO; 2011. Retrieved from www.who.int/disabilities/world_report/2011/report/en/.

163. Whiteford G. Occupational deprivation and incarceration. *Journal of Occupational Science.* 1997; 4:126-130.

164. Whiteford G. Occupational deprivation: global challenge in the new millennium. *British Journal of Occupational Therapy.* 2000;63:200-204.

165. Whiteford G. Occupational deprivation: understanding limited participation. In: Christiansen CH, Townsend EA, eds. *Introduction to Occupation: The Art and Science of Living.* Second ed. Upper Saddle River, NJ: Prentice Hall, 2010;303-328.

166. Whiteford GE. Understanding the occupational deprivation of refugees: a case study from Kosova. *The Canadian Journal of Occupational Therapy.* 2005;72(2):78-88.

167. Ostroff E. Universal design: an evolving paradigm. In: Preiser WFE, Smith KH, eds. *Universal Design Handbook,* 2nd ed. New York, NY: The McGraw-Hill Companies; 2011:1-3.

168. Steinfeld E, Maisel JL. *Universal Design: Creating Inclusive Environments.* Hoboken, NJ: John Wiley & Sons; 2012.

169. Carmona MS. *Promotion and Protection of all Human Rights, Civil, Political, Economic, Social and Cultural Rights, Including the Right to Development.* Report of the Indepentent Expert on the Question of Human Rights and Extreme Poverty. United Nations General Assembly. A/HRC/11/9; 2009.

170. McElroy T, Muyinda H, Atim S, Spittal P, Backman C. War, displacement and productive occupations in northern Uganda. *Journal of Occupational Science.* 2012:19(3);198-212. doi:10.1080/14427591.2011.614681

171. Reine I, Novo M, Hammarström A. Unemployment and ill health – a gender analysis: results from a 14-year follow-up of the northern Swedish cohort. *Public Health.* 2013;127(3):214-222. doi:10.1016/j.puhe.2012.12.005

172. Kroll LE, Lampert T. Unemployment, social support and health problems: results of the GEDA study in Germany, 2009. *Deutsches Arzteblatt International.* 2011;108:47-52.

173. Dubos R. Changing patterns of disease. In: Brown RG, Whyte HM, eds. *Medical Practice and the Community: Proceedings of a Conference Convened by the Australian National University, Canberra.* Canberra: Australian National University Press; 1968:59.

174. Maslow A. *The Farther Reaches of Human Nature.* Viking Press; 1971.

175. World Health Organization. *Social Determinants of Health.* Available at: http://www.who.int/social_determinants/en/. Accessed July 6, 2013.

Theme 11

"Health promotion is the process of enabling people to increase control over their health and its determinants, and thereby improve their health. It ... contributes to the work of tackling communicable and noncommunicable diseases and other threats to health."

WHO: Bangkok Charter for Health Promotion in a Globalized World, 2005[1]

Chapter 11

OCCUPATION AS A DYNAMIC IN HEALTH AND ILLNESS

The chapter addresses:
- Understanding Occupational Balance
- Health-Giving Balanced Lifestyles
  - Work-life Balance, Lifestyle Balance, and Life Balance
    - Work-life Balance
    - Lifestyle Balance and Life Balance
  - Occupational Balance
    - Balance of Physical, Mental, Social, and Rest Occupations
    - Balance of Doing, Being, Belonging, Becoming, and Rest Occupations
- Occupational Imbalance and Stress as Disorders of Occupation
  - Occupational Imbalance
  - Occupational Stress
- Conclusion

Consideration of other disorders of occupation will be the focus of this chapter, namely occupational imbalance and occupational stress. However, to begin the exploration of occupational imbalance, it is necessary first to reflect on the idea of occupational balance that is central in both preventing occupational disorders and in maintaining the well-working of populations and individual human organisms. That leads to the consideration of unhealthy states of balance, and sets the scene to think about occupation as an agent of population health in the following chapter.

Understanding Occupational Balance

So, what is balance? The word derives from the Latin bilanx. In Middle English, it was used in offsetting or comparing the value of one thing with another. Currently, in a health context, balance is defined as "a situation in which different elements are ... in the correct proportions," such as keeping a balance between work and relaxation, "work and family life," and "mental or emotional

Wilcock AA, Hocking C.
An Occupational Perspective of Health, Third Edition (pp 302-332).
© 2015 Taylor & Francis Group.

stability."[2] It does not necessarily relate to equal amounts of time, but rather to the combined effects of people's occupations to support feelings of health and well-being. Recently, Lipworth et al identified 170 studies relevant to balance in health-related contexts. They found that balance has profound effects on the ways in which people view, experience, and respond to their health-related circumstances, and that balance and imbalance are culturally recognized concepts that can refer to either a state or a process with either an internal or external orientation.[3]

The concept of balance can be found across the world in Eastern philosophies and in the cultural and religious traditions of Native Americans, Africans, and Australians[4]; and despite a paucity of current medically initiated research, the idea of balance within the health fraternity is long-standing. For example, in Classical Greek medicine, a physician's job was to advise on due proportion, to "restore a healthy balance," and to aid "the natural healing powers believed to exist in every human being."[5] Plato advocated avoiding "exercising either body or mind without the other" in order to maintain "an equal and healthy balance between them." He advised those engaged in "strenuous intellectual pursuit" to exercise the body, and those interested in physical fitness to develop "cultural and intellectual interests."[6]

> For Hippocrates and Galen, a life in balance was not a determinant of health, a sign or symptom of health, or even a cause of health. Rather, balance was health and well-being.[7]

Outside the home, the principle venue for the Greek citizen to engage in balanced occupations on a daily basis was the social environment of the gymnasia. This was necessary because the more mundane (yet health providing) physical activities of living had been handed over to enslaved peoples of conquered territory. In current-day affluent societies, gymnasia are once more necessary because mundane physical activities are, increasingly, the domain of clever tools and machines. Such examples demonstrate how individual or population occupational balance can alter as technology changes and as social and environmental circumstances vary, and as changes in doing, being, belonging, and becoming are necessitated as people grow and age. In Chapter 1, Howard's ideas of balance in relation to health were outlined in terms of work, play, rest, nutrition, physical, psychological, intellectual, and spiritual capacities, and self, environment, and culture.[8]

Health-Giving Balanced Lifestyles

Some discussion of the terms *work-life balance, lifestyle balance,* and *life balance* is an important starting point, because it assists in understanding occupational balance to promote health, as well as to prevent occupational imbalance as a health disorder in its own right. Some researchers use the terms interchangeably, and all maintain concepts common to the view held here. However, most, but not all, are more applicable to individuals in postindustrial environments than populations in differing circumstances across the globe. Work is also required to understand corporate or political occupations that drive individual occupational balance experiences, and more discussion is needed about occupation's day-night continuum within the basic rest activity cycle.

WORK-LIFE BALANCE, LIFESTYLE BALANCE, AND LIFE BALANCE

Work-life Balance

As early as 1951, and revisited in 2006, Kathleen Hall used the term *work-life balance* to challenge people about the health dangers of modern life, particularly in a spiritual sense. She claimed that:

- "Our lives are out of balance."
- People are "seeking to reclaim balance and order" in their lives.

- "The first word people say when asked how they are is 'busy.'"
- "We do more, go more, and buy more."
- "We have overstretched our personal boundaries and forgotten that true happiness comes from living an authentic life fuelled with a sense of purpose and balance."[9]

It was not until the 1970s that the phrase *work-life balance* became common,[10] and its popularity, as well as individual perspective, continues to provide valuable insights.

By including the word *work* and placing it first, emphasis is given to it as the primary factor in balance. This reflects the place of and importance given to paid employment as it has been understood since the industrial revolution in the western world. With that orientation, work is an important aspect of occupation's relationship with health, having the capacity to bore "people to death" and to "develop as human beings. Work both destroys people physically and helps people build physical health."[11] As Sigerist advised more than half a century ago, work may:

> ... be harmful to health, may become a chief cause of disease, when there is too much of it, when it is too hard, exceeding the capacity of an individual, when it is not properly balanced by rest and recreation, or when it is performed under adverse circumstances.[12]

The model of work-life balance reflects the modern preoccupation that paid employment is the focus of life. Leisure is recognized as the opposite of work but often of lesser value, rather than a complementary and equally important aspect of healthy living. In past or current preindustrial societies, leisure is not separated from work arbitrarily. Common practice for workers included celebration of many different aspects of local, national, and religious occasions with festivals, as well as informal and irregular breaks from obligatory occupations, at convenient or special times. Burke argued, with some justification, that the modern division between work and leisure did not manifest until the mid-19th century and the industrial revolution.[10]

To highlight the corporate and political nature of occupational balance and the need to raise its profile and importance, it is useful to outline the long process of legislation required to attain some work-life balance following the advent of industry. At that time, family and leisure were disregarded, partly because people spent long hours at work separated from other aspects of life, leaving little time for other occupations, and because fatigue and overwork made it too hard. Even then, there was some understanding that this was far from healthy, and it was certainly not balanced. *The Federation of European Employers in Labour Relations: The History of Working Time*[13] records major changes aimed at correcting work-time imbalance. It was as early as 1784, in England, that a proposal was put forward at the Manchester Quarter Sessions that work should be restricted to a 10-hour working day. This was not achieved until 1847, and it was only 3 years earlier that the maximum working hours of 6.5 a day was made mandatory for children.

In the United States, the New England Association of Farmers, Mechanics and Other Workingmen had condemned child labor in 1832, resolving that "children should not be allowed to labor in the factories from morning till night, without any time for healthy recreation and mental culture," because it "endangers their ... well-being and health."[14] In 1836, Massachusetts required children younger than age 15 years working in factories to attend school at least 3 months each year, and 6 years later limited children's work to 10 hours a day.[15] Although other states passed similar laws, enforcement was inconsistent.[14] The National Child Labor Committee was formed in 1904 to abolish all child labor and gradually led to regulation,[16] but it was not until 1938 that Federal regulation enacted laws regarding minimum ages and hours of work. However, currently, children can work at any age on a small farm, and on any farm when they reach 12 years.[17]

According to a 2009 petition by Human Rights Watch:

> Hundreds of thousands of children are employed as farmworkers in the United States, often working 10 or more hours a day. They are often exposed to dangerous pesticides, experience high rates of injury, and suffer fatalities at five times the rate of other working youth.[18]

In Europe, resolutions about night work for women and children were passed at the Berlin Conference in 1890; however, "working time" lingered on agendas at the 1905 and 1913 Berne Conventions. Demonstrating a growing awareness of the importance of work-life balance, late 19th century advances in the social sciences had begun to query the impact of long hours on both productivity and worker's physical and mental health. In New Zealand, the first strike for an 8-hour day was held in 1840, and in 1899 an 8-hour day for government workers was adopted in Puerta Rico. In 1916, the Eight Hours Act was passed in Australia; in 1917, the new revolutionary government in Russia ordered an 8-hour day; and, in 1919, the International Labor Organization agreed to a maximum 8-hour day/48-hour week at its first meeting. The International Labor Organization, established in Paris as part of the Peace Conference following World War I, was later incorporated into the United Nations.[13]

As that major imbalance was amended, another emerged. The 1920s in the United States saw the beginning of what would later be described as the "gospel of consumption." This was activated when advertisers started persuading readers that happiness results from purchasing commodities rather than enjoying leisure.[19] The commercialization of happiness triggered a new work ethic of consumerism that now persists globally.[20] In the United States, work is still seen as the means of acquiring goods that are touted as desirable,[21] and as employers are not legally required to provide any paid annual leave, Americans experience longer working hours and less vacation time than many other advanced countries.[22]

The 2000 Lisbon European Council called for an integrated approach to achieve economic and social renewal outlined in strategies toward "employment, economic reform, and social cohesion."[23] Work-life balance, as outlined in the Strategic Objectives 2000-2005,[24] requires "more balanced ways of combining working life with personal life" and a "dynamic job-creating Europe that delivers on both economic and social objectives," but also "more and better employment."[24] The European Employment Commission (EEC) urges member states to achieve a better work-life balance for families, but also, perhaps ironically, to make it "attractive for older workers to remain employed" because "more people are needed to work and for longer."[25] An emphasis on work is similarly strong in the United Kingdom's work-life balance campaign that commenced in 2002,[26] with both British and European strategies aimed at return to work after a period of absence and aspiring to reconcile work and private life principally through childcare facilities.[27]

Perhaps signaling the emphasis on work rather than other aspects of life, and despite apparent population focused intent, Caproni contended that the well intentioned discourse on work-life balance "reflects the individualism, achievement orientation, and instrumental rationality that is fundamental to modem bureaucratic thought and action." Indeed, it "may further entrench people in the work/life imbalance that they are trying to escape," undermining efforts toward fulfilling lives.[28]

Further consideration of the discourse on work-life balance within four major Canadian newspapers published between 2003 and 2005 forms the basis of another exploration. The analysis suggests that environmental expectations, as well as individual practices and perceptions, were both the process and reason for balance or imbalance. That is despite the depiction of work-life balance not providing a broad representation of the multiple realities that all Canadians face. Obtaining balance was portrayed as an ongoing process during which individuals "negotiate and sacrifice" in attempts to achieve ideal levels.[29]

In contrast to the over-emphasis on work and in line with other ideas about healthy balance, some ideas about work-life balance include the following:

- "Having enough time and energy for work and enough for other important aspects of lives.[30]
- "Proper prioritizing between work, including career and ambition on the one hand, and other aspects of life, including health, pleasure, leisure, family, and spiritual development on the other"[31]

- "A range of practices designed to improve the balance between the demands of an employee's work and personal life"[32]
- A "lifestyle that maintains an equilibrium between professional, familial, and personal pursuits"[33]
- A state or goal of attainable well-being that allows a person to manage multiple responsibilities at work, at home, and in the community. Work-life balance is different for everyone.[34]
- Having a measure of control over the when, where, and how of work, enabling the ability to enjoy an optimal quality of life.[35]

Lifestyle Balance and Life Balance

Lifestyle balance and *life balance* are terms often used interchangeably and are principally related to the health needs of individuals, particularly for those living in technologically advanced societies. In a recent study using grounded research with a small group of Swedish workers, balance was regarded as individualistic, contextual and dynamic, advanced by a sense of security, and health related. The study identified four interrelated dimensions: activity balance, a balance of body and mind, a balance in relation to others, and time balance.[36]

The individualistic bias predominates in the literature, despite recognition that balance is influenced by external, as well as intrinsic, factors and can be a population issue. A *Lifestyle Balance Sheet* used in the "Exposure, Response, Prevention (ERP) Therapy Center for Substance Abuse" recognizes the value of balance in health intervention. Its checklist provides insight into many aspects of lifestyle that primarily refer to a range of occupations:

> *Lifestyle is composed of everything you do. It is a collection of all the activities and places that define who you are as a person. Your lifestyle has a strong emotional impact on you. If your lifestyle's net effect leaves you feeling bad about yourself then changes in it are needed. If your lifestyle leaves you feeling good, then all is right in the world ... Your lifestyle is composed of several major parts: work, family, friends, intimate relationships, recreational activities (and energy boosters), self-development, money, future plans, spiritual connections, and values.*[37]

The Lifestyle Balance Sheet includes a multipaged questionnaire about activities with either the major or sole focus of one of the following:
- Improving psychological functioning, such as understanding personal development, reducing stress levels, "soothing past psychological trauma, or developing new behavioral skills."[37]
- Improving physical functioning, such as exercising more, losing weight, managing heart disease or diabetes better, or "giving up an addictive activity."[37]

One of many other sources addressing the idea of lifestyle balance is the Millton's Health Pages. These discuss six interactive areas of lifestyle balance: social, physical, intellectual, spiritual, emotional, and financial (Figure 11-1).[38]

According to this model, social balance is described as "non-dependent interaction with friends, family, neighbors, and associates," with opportunity for time out to recharge the batteries.[38] Physical balance involves eating patterns and habits, exercise, and activity to meet daily energy demands. Intellectual balance is acquiring and understanding knowledge pertinent to self and community. Spiritual balance is about finding meaning to connect the various activities and aspects of human existence. Emotional balance is about learning to understand the true cause of human happiness and unhappiness. Financial balance involves living within means, while preparing for the unexpected and the future.[38]

A life balance model was developed by Matuska and Christiansen from earlier work on occupational balance and lifestyle balance,[39] a synthesis of related research about need-based theories,[40] and the earlier explorations of Maslow,[41,42] Ryff,[43-45] and Deci and Ryan.[46] They use the terms *life*, *lifestyle*, and, sometimes, *occupational balance*, interchangeably, arguing that life patterns must:

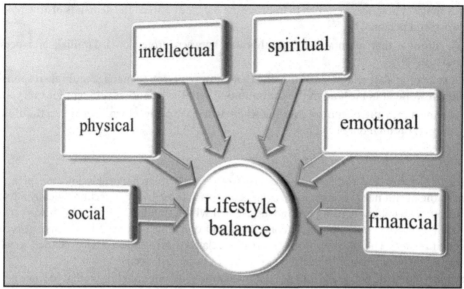

Figure 11-1. Interaction of social, physical, intellectual, spiritual, emotional, and financial in lifestyle balance.

- Meet basic biological and safety needs
- Embrace rewarding and self-affirming relationships
- Engage, challenge, and promote competence
- "Create meaning and a positive personal identity"
- Enable important goals and renewal to be met through the organization of time and energy.[40]

Meeting those five requirements would be important to individuals and populations in whatever environment, but are far from possible in many parts of the world. Illness abounds, often unchecked by initiatives aimed at change to lifestyle/occupation opportunities across populations. Such interventions are often piecemeal and far from adequate because of lack of resources and inability to effect social change.

Matuska and Christiansen's 2009 textbook *Life Balance: Multidisciplinary Theories and Research*[39] draws together a wealth of ideas from the variously named forms of balance, and from different disciplines covering historical, theoretical, empirical, and practical perspectives.[47-52] For example, sociologist Ruut Veenhoven, director of the World Data Base of Happiness, described life-balance as:

- Meeting preconceptions of what a balanced life is
- Thinking one leads a balanced life
- Leading a life that is apparently balanced, because one thrives well.[53]

He related balance to happiness and happiness to four qualities of life, described as "livability of the environment," "life ability of the person," "utility of life," and "satisfaction with life." Life balance denotes "the degree of aptness, which can vary from inapt (imbalanced) to optimal (balanced)" with the habitual activities that make up lifestyles.[53] Other authors extend those ideas, with Pentland and McColl[54] discussing how occupational integrity is an essential precondition of life balance because it extends doing into the realms of personal values, strengths, and identity, with the capacity to enable satisfaction and meaning in life.

In her later exploration of life balance, Wagman[55] added financial security, self-security, and having secure relationships to Matuska and Christiansen's[39] five dimensions. In her thesis, Wagman describes life balance as dynamic in nature, nondualistic, multidimensional, subjective, and affected positively or negatively by the environment. It is influenced by personal strategies and apparent within "short-term time" and "the overall life course," while going beyond occupational balance.[55]

OCCUPATIONAL BALANCE

Some investigators, such as Wagman,[55] regard occupational balance as a subset of work-life balance, life balance, or lifestyle balance or have chosen to adopt those more common alternatives so that occupation becomes recognized as an important entity in the balance debate. Because occupation is integral to lifestyle, work-life, and life balance, occupational balance is inclusive of many of the ideas discussed above. That includes the inextricable link between balance, health, and well-being that has been recognized for millennia. It builds on and extends the concepts from the particular perspective of people as occupational beings. It can refer to an individual, as well as a population perspective, with a wealth of variation between studies demonstrating the complexity of the concept. Occupational balance may manifest in entirely different forms according to natural and sociocultural environments and particular circumstances, and is inclusive of corporate and political initiatives and the differing nature and capacities of people both individually and collectively. Ideas about it differ because of the orientation of those who seek to understand it and who apply it to their own terms of reference.

Occupational therapists have been at the forefront of exploring occupational balance. Several studies have concentrated on the relationship of health to work, rest (including self-care), and play (or leisure); that is, perhaps, the most common description of occupational balance.[56-58] This has a long history, dating from when Adolph Meyer addressed the fledgling profession in the United States in 1922, using the term "work and play and rest and sleep." "Our organism," he said, must be able to balance "the larger rhythms of night and day ... of sleep and waking ... of hunger and its gratification" even under difficulty.[59]

Some such ideas have already been discussed in relation to life balance, such as the lifestyle balance and life balance models developed by Matuska and Christiansen. They defined occupational balance as "a satisfying pattern of daily occupation that is healthful, meaningful, and sustainable to an individual within the context of his or her current life circumstances."[40] Further clarification of the definition explains that:

- Satisfying denotes congruence between the amount of time actually spent "participating in activities and the amount of time one would like to spend"
- Meaningful denotes that the activities are "valued and important"
- Healthful denotes that the activity contributes to "physiological and mental health"
- Sustainable denotes "the activity configurations can be maintained over the long term."[60]

Their definition was derived from a review of pertinent literature about time use, social roles, psychological needs, and chronobiology applicable to individuals. That revealed balance differs from person to person and between environments, and that particular configurations of occupation are more likely than others to result in better health and well-being.[61-64] It focuses on how basic human needs are met and supported through a total configuration of occupation over time.

Christiansen has been particularly active over many years, exploring the concept and nature of occupational balance. At the 1992 University of Southern California Occupational Science Symposium, he outlined his thoughts, describing three differing concepts, time-use, chronobiological rhythms, and relationships among life tasks.[58] He pointed to Meyer's early influence and emphasis on people deriving meaning and maintaining well-being through their organization of time in the daily occupations of work, play, rest, and sleep[59]; to Reilly's occupational therapy program for patients with disturbed mental health that drew on economics, existence tasks such as "eating, sleeping, and hygiene," subsistence tasks such as work and income, and choosing time tasks for leisure and recreation[65]; and to Backman's more recent view of balance as "a perceived state of satisfactory participation in valued, obligatory and discretionary activities" occurring "when the impact of occupations on one another is harmonious, cohesive and under control."[66] In earlier definitions, Christiansen described occupational balance as "a belief, not substantiated by research, that a general configuration of daily occupations can contribute to health and well-being,"[67] Recently, although not specifically referring to political or corporate occupations or the day-night, active-rest continuum considered important here, Christiansen and Townsend's definition of occupational balance is useful in relation to the potential causes of imbalance, as well as alienation, stress, and deprivation. They see it as:

> *A concept referring to the distribution of time for engagement in the habits and routines of everyday occupations; an interpretive concept for assessing time use with reference to health, well-being, and quality of life when the patterns of occupation are taken into account for individuals, groups, and communities; perceived state of satisfactory participation in valued, obligatory, and discretionary activities; occurs when the impact of occupations on one another is harmonious, cohesive and under control.*[68]

Over the years, other occupational therapists have defined occupational balance in a variety of ways. For example:

- Reed and Sanderson, 1992: Occupational balance facilitates maintenance of health and a satisfying life, provides for basic needs and permits leisure pursuits. Balance does not imply an equal amount of time in self-maintenance, productivity, and leisure, but does imply some time on a regular occurring basis.[69]

- Yerxa, 1998:Occupational balance is achieved when the time a person spends in rest, self-care, work, and play/leisure is adequate for health, well-being, and life satisfaction.[70]

- Backman, 2010: Occupational balance depends on the extent to which people are able to organize and participate in occupations in a manner congruent with their aspirations and values.[71]

- Wagman, 2012: Occupational balance is "having the right amount and variation of occupations in relation to occupational categories, occupations with different characteristics and time spent in occupations." Those included balancing work and private life, body and mind, food and drink, exercise and sleep, feeling control over time, and being stimulated and finding meaning through occupations.[55]

Hakansson et al found that meaningful occupation "appears to be the mechanism that enables people to achieve balance in their everyday life."[72] They determined that both occupational balance and occupational overload are complex and multidimensional concepts that are not only the result of occupational repertoires, but also the result of people's occupational experience, image of occupational self, and strategies to manage and control everyday life. The participants in their study experienced pleasure, enjoyment, satisfaction, and self-improvement when engaged in occupations that "challenged their limits." Such occupations were described as "important, challenging and intrinsically gratifying," "extrinsically rewarding," and "sources of energy."[72] Another study found gender differences within a random sample of 2286 women and 397 men working in human service departments. In a 2-year longitudinal study, the men appeared to experience a better balance between employment, domestic work, leisure, and health than the women, who, perhaps, had less regular opportunity for leisure. The demands of work were the largest predictor of health for men.[73]

Occupational balance stands in its own right because what people do across the rest-activity cycle is the historical and ever present factor in survival. It can be considered from population, corporate, communal, and individual health perspectives and relates to any or all ways of life, while being inclusive of the conceptual understanding of balance inherent in other models. It does not give presumptive bias to work as opposed to other occupations or suggest that some preconceived lifestyles are better than others in terms of health outcomes. For example, there is little proof that long work hours toward the acquisition of material possessions central in many postindustrial

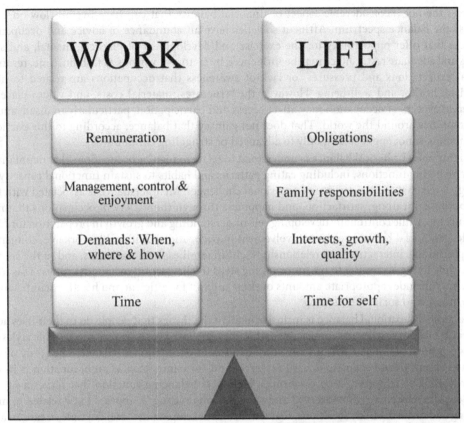

Figure 11-2. Occupational balance: when different elements are in the correct proportions.

societies provides a healthier balance than simpler, more natural ways of living that are the foundation of people's occupations in many other communities around the world.

Occupational balance is a major concern applicable not only to an individual way of life in more developed parts of the world, but also a foundation for global health and well-being along with increased understanding of the following:

- The range of economic structures and corporate and political occupations throughout the world that have somehow escaped major attention in the accumulating balance literature and are integral to health of people in the postmodern and developing world
- The range and structures of occupations integral to survival, particularly in preindustrial and industrial societies, as well as the impact of economic, political, and corporate structures that determine what people living in them can or cannot do.

It is implicit that occupational balance is, in many ways, dependent on the natural environment and sociocultural, religious, corporate, and political norms of particular places in the daily lives of communities. It is also implicit that a healthy balance may differ from person to person because of differing genes, circumstances, and environments, but it will reflect when the different elements are in proportions suited to communal and individual need (Figure 11-2).

Balance of Physical, Mental, Social, and Rest Occupations

Various theories address aspects of a balance between physical, mental, social, and rest occupations. For example, *Millton's Health Pages* addressed physical, intellectual, emotional, social, financial, and spiritual balance.[38] That equates to the physical, mental, and social dimensions of the WHO definition of health, and although it does not address the rest activity continuum, it does address the not inconsiderable aspect of financial balance that can have overall flow-on effects across the balance spectrum. Affluent societies have an abundance of advice and occupational choices that offer opportunity for the exercise and development of physical, mental, and social skills and adequate rest. Choice may be influenced by factors as various as fashion, time, resources, social expectations and pressures, or lack of awareness that occupations are related to needs, survival, health, and well-being. However, the structures, material costs, and values placed on different aspects of occupation may affect access and participation, particularly in disadvantaged communities around the world. That does not gainsay that balance, according to this particular orientation, is not applicable equally to advanced or struggling communities.

In this model, physical balance is understood to relate to regular occupations that maintain and exercise bodily functions, including eating patterns and habits to sustain functional capacity and energy levels that meet every day or occasional challenges. Mental balance is associated with finding purpose, meaning, satisfaction, and happiness through the variety of occupations that make up daily life, while continually developing self-understanding and growth in preparation for future challenges. Social balance requires involvement in occupations that enable workable, compatible, and pleasurable interaction and relationships within families, with associates, and in the community, while living according to means or taking steps to alleviate financial difficulties. This model of balance includes appropriate amounts of sleep and rest for efficient and healthy maintenance of body, mind, and social functioning.

Because occupational balance is inclusive of all of the things that people do in their lives across the basic 24-hour rest-awake continuum and is not segmented in the way of modern life styles, rest and sleep must be integral within any consideration of occupational balance. The study of sleep is often absent from occupation based research, and "to name sleep as an occupation is in itself controversial."[74] However, sleep performs a biological balancing function that serves a survival purpose whereby energy is conserved and stored during resting; it appears to be related to maintaining and restoring body functions, regulation, and development;[75] and daytime stress can affect REM sleep,[76,77] whereas disturbed sleep leads to daytime difficulties.[78]

In evolutionary terms, the cycle is related to differential brain hemisphericity. Its 90-minute rhythm is found not only in heart rate, oxygen consumption, gastric contractibility, vigilance or alertness, perception of motion and eye movements, but also in behavioral task performance, eating, drinking, smoking, daydreaming, and physical activity.[79] In western society, the instinct for recreational inactivity as a natural means of resting or conserving energy remains, although the need for it has been largely eliminated.[80] Resting, as well as contributing to the other purposes of sleep, provides a time for watchfulness that provides data in readiness for action should a need arise. Although its original survival function is obscured, watchfulness remains sometimes under the sociocultural guise of entertainment. For example, watching television is a common resting occupation of current times and provides a time for watchfulness, but also a time for people to learn about and reflect on their world for similar survival reasons to ages past. Despite such purposes, it is universally reported that watching television involves practically no challenges or skills, does not provide flow experiences,[81-83] and may lead to "a progressive atrophy of the desire for new challenges."[84]

Researchers in Sweden have taken a lead role in exploring occupational balance that includes rest. For example, one group of researchers found that the central temporal balance issue was harmony between work and self-maintenance versus rest and enjoyable occupations.[72] Others used the phrase "pattern of daily occupations" to refer to all of the "main, hidden, and unexpected" occupations performed by an individual during a 24-hour period, including sleep.[85,86] In Erlandsson and Ekland's study of the everyday occupations of 100 women who worked at home and in the paid workforce, increasing complexity was found to be associated with lower levels of self-rated health, but not with lower levels of well-being.[87] Persson et al described how occupational balance is dependent on differences over 24 hours per day and lifetime periods in what they describe as micro-, meso-, or macro-perspective. Although a micro-perspective is relevant to a single action and has little impact on overall healthy balance, a meso-perspective applies to all of the occupations performed during 24 hours through "days, weeks and months." The macro-perspective totals all patterns of "daily occupations performed in an individual's lifetime."[88] The differing perspectives are important to balance because they vary between people because of age, gender, time, and place and "individual repertoires."[89]

A pilot study exploring the perceptions of occupational balance and its relationship to health found that, for the respondents, ideal occupational balance was approximately equal to involvement in physical, mental and spiritual, social, and rest activities. A significant relationship using one-way analysis of variance (P = .0001) was found between the closeness of current occupational patterns to those perceived by respondents as ideal and their reported health. Each of the 12.3% of respondents who had identical current and ideal balances reported their health to be fair or excellent, whereas none who reported poor health rated their current balance as identical to their ideal.[90] Similar studies in the United Kingdom and Europe largely support these findings.[72,91] According to those outcomes, occupational balance can be simply defined as "A regular mix of physical, mental, social, and rest occupations that provide an overall feeling of well-being."[92]

Although it is essential to understand balance in terms that relate to the physical, mental, and social categories of the WHO definition of health, it is also important to relate it to occupation as doing, being, belonging, and becoming as discussed throughout this book.

Balance as Doing, Being, Belonging, Becoming, and Rest Occupations

Occupational balance, at an individual, corporate, or population level, can be considered in several different and valid ways, such as between occupations that are strenuous or restful; chosen or obligatory; personal or communal; corporate or political; extrinsic or intrinsic; exciting or boring; romantic or rational; isolating or inclusive; fulfilling or frustrating; or simply being able to meet basic prerequisites for health, such as food and shelter, or having an excess of choice. Any or all of those can be considered aspects of balance in terms of doing, being, belonging, and becoming. Heeding such aspects of balance is seldom, if ever, the primary concern of medical science, political planning, or corporate structures, and the mechanisms for ensuring a balance of occupations throughout the age span remain elusive despite a growing awareness of the concept. However, it should be the serious concern of those working in the health field with commitment toward uncovering the occupational determinants of disease distribution, such as where and when occupational imbalances are occurring.

In preindustrial or war-torn communities where even the basic requirements of life itself are difficult to attain or maintain, occupational balance is often an undreamed of possibility, and imbalance can lead to occupational alienation, stress, and deprivation that in themselves are rife. In postindustrial societies, an imbalanced lifestyle may be simply due to a lack of understanding, a matter of choice, a matter of economy, or a matter of political, corporate, or social disease. Not surprisingly, there is void of research about occupational balance between individual requirements and corporate and or political endeavors. Occupational imbalance will be discussed within the next section of the chapter, which begins to explore further disorders of occupation.

Occupational Imbalance and Stress as Disorders of Occupation

The exploration of medically recognized disorders of occupation and occupational deprivation in the previous chapter demonstrates some of the complexity and seriousness of the relationship between health and what people do. It is apparent that disorders of occupation can be individual or collective. Currently, the phrase "social determinants of health" is the popular and accepted theory source for research and discussion that is about the diverse range of factors that affect health apart from mainstream medical science. Occupational disorders are largely considered under that umbrella. Because of the different orientation, they have not been recognized sufficiently as important in their own right. They are certainly part of the social context, and often the result of unequal power relations, and that is why the terms *corporate* and *political occupations* have been introduced in this edition.

Another phrase that relates to occupation used currently and prevalently in the population health field is physical activity. This is often taken to refer to exercise, but is inclusive of all or any activities or occupations of a physical nature. Research adopting exercise terminology is increasing and is pertinent to occupation. Cotman and Berchtold described exercise as a behavioral intervention to enhance brain health and plasticity. They suggested that physical activity could "have benefits for overall health and cognitive function, particularly in later life," pointing to how recent animal studies have clearly demonstrated that voluntary occupations can increase, improve, provide, stimulate, or mobilize:

- Levels of brain-derived neurotrophic and other growth factors
- Neurogenesis
- Resistance to brain insult
- Learning and mental performance
- "Gene expression profiles" predicted to benefit brain plasticity processes
- Maintenance of brain function and promotion of brain plasticity.[93]

Such positive attributes and potentials can be seen in reverse. To follow the WHO guidelines, it is essential to take into account disorders of occupation that are recognized as social disorders within the WHO definition of health. In many parts of the world, these are essentially political in nature and manifest because "participation in occupations is barred, confined, restricted, segregated, prohibited, undeveloped, disrupted, alienated, marginalized, exploited, excluded or otherwise restricted."[94] Although occupation can have particular meanings in different socio-cultural-political contexts, occupational disorders may persist to different degrees in different parts of the world according to the availability of the prerequisites of health and sociocultural, corporate, political, and environmental factors.

When there is too much or too little choice, growth, interest, complexity, necessity, demand, pressure, or inclusion in patterns of daily occupations that suit health and relationship needs, a whole range of problematic occupational states of illness can result. They are often connected. That is true of disorders, such as occupational alienation and deprivation discussed in previous chapters, and imbalance and stress that will be considered next.

OCCUPATIONAL IMBALANCE

Complexity is a factor in occupational imbalance that can result from community and individual responses to, and ways of coping with, the vicissitudes of everyday life. Those are closely tied to aptitudes, opportunities, and freedoms to do, be, belong, and become according to occupational natures and needs across the sleep-wake continuum and natural, social, and economic environments. Because internal balance is essential to health and survival, physiological imbalance is an underlying factor in disorders of occupation, as well as medically recognized illness. Occupational imbalance extends to that within and between groups and conglomerates of people and is dependent on communal, corporate, and political authorities. Currently, such authorities appear to give limited attention to constituents and groups of people achieving balanced occupational lifestyles. An example is provided in a special edition of *Gender, Work and Organization* in which the editors seek to address the question of whether a balanced lifestyle is "freely determined by individuals or whether it is constrained by a wide range of factors operating at a micro (individual), meso (organizational) and macro (national) level."[95]

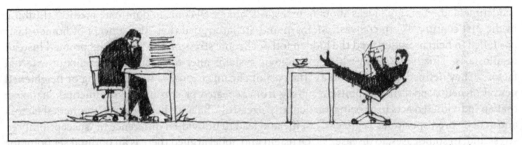

Figure 11-3. Imbalance because of being over or under-occupied. (© Trevor Bywater 2013. Used with permission.)

It is clear that occupational imbalance occurs when there is incompatibility or mismatch between occupational requirements and time, talent, or skill; when there is occupational overload or scarcity; and when there is lack of opportunity, resources, or encouragement. Imbalance is linked with situations in which the balance between things is unequal or unfair, such as disparity of access to the prerequisites of health, community opportunities, or power, or between sexes, family members, and age groups.[96] It is associated with an imbalance between energy expenditure and food intake that leads to obesity. It is associated with a loss of equilibrium attributable to unstable situations in which some forces outweigh others,[97] as well as ideas about disparity, instability, mismatch, strain, stress, tension, and even lunacy. Such ideas resonate with problems encountered when people experience imbalance associated with occupation—with what they do, how they feel about it, relate to others, and change through what they do. Occupational imbalance has been described as:

- "An individual or group experience in which health and quality of life are compromised because of being over-occupied or under-occupied" (Figure 11-3).[98]
- Work-life conflict such as:
  - Role overload—having too much to do in too short a time
  - Feeling time crunched
  - A misfit between personal, family, and work-life demands[99]
- Role strain—distress due to excessive demands or insufficient knowledge, skills, or financial, educational, and/or social resources or support[100]
- Being unable to make sense of life; too busy to enjoy relationships or the many other important aspects of life; and low life satisfaction due to sacrificing purpose, depth, and meaning,[101]
- A pattern of incompatible or overabundant occupations at odds with people's life. Disharmony or lack of congruence across life's activities or between occupations and personal core values.[71]
- Occupational patterns that "… limit or compromise participation in valued relationships; are incongruent for establishing or maintaining physiological health and a satisfactory identity; or are mundane, uninteresting or unchallenging."[102]

In the last of those, Matuska links life imbalance with negative health, arguing that imbalance occurs if people are stressed or dissatisfied with the amount of time they spend on occupations or if they are unable to meet health, relationship, challenge, and identity needs.[103,104]

Imbalance is closely associated with internal body systems, such as homeostasis: the balance the body must maintain to ensure health. Cells, organs, and systems rely on a stable environment to function requiring specific amounts of fluids and biochemicals, as well as the body temperature maintained within a limited range. The body becomes stressed when imbalance occurs from any cause.[105] Friedman suggested that because "the interdependence of the internal bodily systems is revealed, and as the role of harmony between the person and the environment is documented," Cannon's ideas about homeostasis "may well come to dominate medical thinking in the 21st century."[106] In contrast, McEwen and Stellar argued that "the concept of homeostasis has failed to help us understand the hidden toll of chronic stress on the body," and pointed instead to allostasis. This is a state in which physiologic systems alter to meet requirements of external factors. They defined allostatic load as "the cost of chronic exposure to fluctuating or heightened neural or neuroendocrine response resulting from repeated or chronic environmental challenge that an individual reacts to as being particularly stressful." Balance between environmental factors and genetic predispositions begin early in life and lead to individual difference in "susceptibility to stress and, in some cases, to disease."[107] Ornstein and Sobel argued there is an optimal set point for stimulation "in the middle of an organism's response level" that is maintained "through feedback processes similar to the homeostatic mechanisms of the body" and that when there is either "too much or too little, instability results and disease may follow."[108]

Such lack of balance can result in boredom or burnout, which are forms of stress linked with illness. Burnout is the widely reported emotional response to overstimulation, inappropriate occupation, and too much to do, leading to an increase in associated fatigue-related disorders.[109] It can result from various factors in addition to fatigue, such as lack of control, interest, or skill; monotony; isolation; dysfunctional workplace dynamics, such as bullying, mismanagement, a mismatch of values, unclear expectations; or work demands that limit participation in other aspects of life. The consequences may include medically recognized disorders, such as insomnia, depression, anxiety, alcohol or substance abuse, high cholesterol, heart disease, stroke, obesity, or type 2 diabetes.[110] Burnout as a result of increasingly stressful, frenetic, and fast-paced lifestyles in many parts of the world is reaching epidemic proportions throughout the adult population. However, Glouberman argued that it can provide the impetus to redirect lives.[111]

Although overload has received more attention than insufficient occupation as a cause of illness, if energy systems are not used, they deteriorate. Boredom is the most common emotional response to lack of occupation. Imbalance through boredom occurs when people are prevented from engaging in wanted occupations, forced to engage in unwanted occupations, or unable to maintain engagement in any occupation.[112] Ardell claimed that "boredom is the arch-enemy of wellness" and that "it is the leading cause of low level worseness." He argued that it can be held responsible for health risk behaviors, such as smoking, drug and alcohol abuse, and "a failure to take the positive initiatives associated with potent lifestyles."[113] Imbalance and boredom are prevalent for "highly conditioned endurance athletes who go through a period of detraining" and people who are bedridden. Both can experience huge "decreases in the oxygen energy system in relatively short periods of time"[114] that can decrease immune responses and increase susceptibility to illness.[115-118] Work, leisure, or family roles and routines that are imbalanced often result in boredom, anxiety, or fears about future occupational competence. In addition, they can result in overload for those assuming a supporting role on top of established life roles.[71] A recent national survey in the United States considered work-family imbalance along with job stress, bullying, and job insecurity. It found that workers in legal occupations demonstrated the highest prevalence rate of work-family imbalance.[119] It is apparently an issue of growing concern in that field.[120]

There is widespread acknowledgement of an association between occupational imbalance and medically recognized illness particularly in relation to stress from overwork.[121] Indeed, imbalance is a well-recognized aspect of occupational health and safety, although it has not attracted widespread study in mainstream medicine apart from that specialty. Research in medicine has tended to concentrate more on overcoming illness through anatomical, physiological, and psychological explorations than investigating environmental, social, and occupational factors, such as imbalance.

Occupational health psychologists have considered various aspects of occupational imbalance in the workplace, including those of a corporate nature between a worker's efforts and rewards, such as pay, recognition, status, and promotion prospects. Siegrist described how imbalance between high effort and low reward is maintained when people are over-committed to the job, perceive some future advantage, or have little choice of alternative work.[122] Imbalance might also manifest in psychological distress, such as burnout or depression,[123] or be carried over into worker's homes,[124] whilst an imbalance between low decision making and high workload described as job strain has been related to cardiovascular disease.[125-130]

When people are ill, hospitalized, or recovering, the experience of imbalance is not uncommon. For example, Stamm et al discussed how balance is affected by illness or disability of self or others, and caring for self or others. Subjects suffering a health condition and mothers of children with a disability identified occupational balance as multidimensional.[131] For several reasons, occupational balance can be difficult to achieve or maintain for carers or for people with disabilities.[72,131-134] Table 11-1 reveals how lifestyle balance and imbalance is experienced by two groups of women: the first group with multiple sclerosis[135] and a second when recovering from a stress-related disorder.[136]

A survey of 239 adults (81% female) with rheumatoid arthritis was designed in consultation with them, to uncover their experiences of perceived imbalance between paid and unpaid occupations.[137] The latter included household activities, home maintenance, caregiving, studying, and volunteering. More hours worked "were associated with psychologically demanding work, higher social function, less pain, being male, managerial job type, and lower ratings of occupational balance." More time spent on other occupations "were associated with more children in the household, greater perceived physical and psychological demand of the work, social support from family, and having a post-secondary education. Seventy-three respondents reported limitations associated with lower functional status, more pain, and less psychologically demanding work. Factors associated with greater participation in paid work differed from those associated with unpaid work; however, work limitation affects both paid and unpaid workers.[137]

Erlandsson and Eklund argued that higher level of stress experienced in everyday life mirrors higher levels of complexity in the pattern of daily occupations.[87] Their study seeking evidence of what constitutes a healthy, balanced pattern of occupations investigated Meyer's[59] and later Wilcock's core assumption that people need a daily balance of occupations to maintain health.[138] (In the first edition of this text, occupational imbalance was described as too much or too little complexity in patterns of occupation with either of those being responsible for possible decreases in health and well-being.) Women's and men's use of time is different. The well-being of a group of women with a complex load comprising household, child care, and remunerative work was sought to test the premise that "higher complexity in patterns of daily occupations was related to a reduction in experienced health." A lack of control and frequent experiences of hassles in daily occupations were found to be risk factors for experiencing lower quality of life and lower self-rated health. Multiple obligations, too little sleep, and time pressure constitute phenomena that result in occupational imbalance and a form of occupational disorder: the experience of health and well-being should differ between groups of women or men when occupational patterns differ in levels of complexity.[87]

The relationship between food and activity is another aspect related to occupational imbalance; people who do less than their food intake would fuel, risk becoming overweight or obese in the longer term. Obesity is a health concern that makes a frequent appearance in popular media of affluent countries and can be directly linked to imbalance in the energy expenditure of daily occupations. For example, according to Garrow's obesity index, and based on the ratio W/H^2, an individual will expend approximately 1.5 calories per minute per 121 pounds of body weight who is employed as a typist, in contrast to 3.5 if engaged in domestic work.[139,140] Although the index is the source of endless debate, it is still being used.[141] However, in the multitude of articles and texts about diets, there is only limited reference to the range and type of people's occupations as opposed to exercise. Many widely differing occupational circumstances affect the prevalence of weight disorders, including the need to vary nutritional intake when occupations change, to overcome any resultant imbalance between energy input and output.

Occupational imbalance has and will manifest differently in different times and different places. It can be a precipitating factor or the root cause of noncommunicable diseases or other internal

Table 11-1

COMPARISON OF LIFESTYLE BALANCE AND IMBALANCE FOR WOMEN WITH MULTIPLE SCLEROSIS AND WOMEN RECOVERING FROM STRESS-RELATED DISORDERS

Health and Occupation/ Lifestyle Requirements	Group 1: Multiple Sclerosis		Group 2: Stress-Related Disorders	
	Balance	**Imbalance**	**Balance**	**Imbalance**
Meet basic biological and safety needs	Through: healthier occupations and environmental adaptation	Through: stress; an "unknown health future"; and needing improved medical management, information, and support	Through: Adequate rest; regular exercise; and use of stress-reducing strategies	Through: stress, anxiety, and feeling overloaded; Insufficient sleep; and insufficient exercise
Embrace rewarding and self-affirming relationships	Through: acceptance of their situation and help from others, and valuing time with others	Through: trying to maintain social roles; frustration at being misunderstood; and needing to seek help from others	Through: prioritizing important close and reciprocal relations; and being assertive about relationship needs	Through: Not prioritizing relationship needs; feeling misunderstood; and social isolation
Engage, challenge, and promote competence	Through: maintaining some enjoyable occupations and compromising with others	Through: depression and having to make choices between occupations	Through: choice of occupation; variety and challenge, and stimulation through doing	Through: over focus on obligatory occupations; daily occupations cheerless and unenjoyable
Create meaning and a positive personal identity	Through: acceptance	Through: loss of meaningful occupations	Through: occupation that is personally meaningful and congruent with values	Through: occupation not meeting personal needs; focused on others expectations and maintenance of previous occupation-identity; intolerant of imperfection
Enable important goals; renewal through organization of time and energy	Through: changing standards, simplifying, planning ahead, changing the environment, and resting	Through: fatigue, depression, and guilt over not managing to get things done	Through: making business choices about time-use; time for rest and renewal; and being willing to change standards or level of ambition	Through: Self identity focused on one occupational role; work too demanding of time and energy; and difficulty saying "No"

Adapted from Matuska and Erickson[135] and Håkansson and Matuska.[136]

dysfunction. As McKeown maintained, most classes of noncommunicable diseases "have environmental origins and are potentially preventable by changes in living conditions and behavior."[142] When "our responses to problems in life are excessive or deficient, ... the balance is upset between us and our resident pathogens"[143] because "the central nervous system and hormones act on our immune defenses in such a way that the microbes aid and abet disease."[144] For example, imbalance

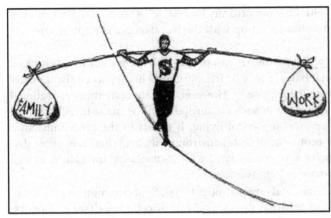

Figure 11-4. Occupational imbalance between work and home. (© Trevor Bywater 2013. Used with permission.)

can cause the production of "excessive stress hormones—cortisol and catecholamines—which can lead to artery damage, cholesterol build-up, and heart disease."[145]

Although the physiological mechanisms and outcomes of occupational imbalance are common to humans, it can be experienced differently throughout the world according to sociocultural norms, pressures, or circumstances. For example, in Europe, where the employment of mothers of young children has increased rapidly in recent years, employers and governments have needed to make policy adjustments, whilst families have needed to make occupational change. Comparative analysis of different countries demonstrate that trends for occupational imbalance are not only shaped by state policies, but also by embedded gender norms relating to the division of labor between men and women that differ from place to place.[146-148] In the United Kingdom, reader in social policy at the London School of Economics and Political Science, Hartley Dean attempted to "locate the contested notion of work–life balance within the context of global trends and recent policy developments" using a small-scale qualitative study within a low-income neighborhood.[149] Recent alterations in social and labor market policy have imposed calculative responsibilities on many working parents that have left them feeling powerless to adequately accommodate family life (Figure 11-4). Recommendations to policymakers seek to change the occupational balance from "the current preoccupation with business interests in favour of wider social responsibility concerns."[149]

Earlier, it was discussed how postindustrial cultures exist around work-based occupational concepts, such as the 8-hour day, 5-day working week and shift work. Despite the energy and effort that has been expended on such constructs, they may have little to recommend them in terms of occupational balance, as the study of more natural balance between the activity and rest of earlier cultures illustrates. For example, numerous studies have found that shift work, which disrupts sleep-wake patterns, can lead to irritability, malaise, fatigue, stomach complaints, diminished concentration, diminished functional capabilities, mood changes, and increased susceptibility to accidents.[150-152] It can also be suggested that the amount of time people have available for restful occupations, intellectual or spiritual reflection, may not meet healthy balance requirements. It is probable that people are required to attend to much more routine but demanding paper or electronic work. A common complaint is that people lack energy and are tired by the mental and social demands of what they have to do.

Occupational imbalance is not only the case in postindustrial societies; for example, African women have a triple workload as biological, social, and economic producers, which is deleterious to their health.[153,154] In a marginal area of Kenya, the demands of women's many occupations are acerbated by poor nutrition, high fertility rates, and limited access to health care.[155] Equally, Galvaan's description of the experience of South African women's live-in domestic work describes how their accommodation ensures they are available to work whenever their employer demands.

The workload is unreasonably heavy, with little opportunity for rest, self-chosen activities, or even self-chosen food. They have little choice but to put up with the imbalance and ensuing stress to ensure family survival.[156]

Whiteford argued, in a discussion about South African people who are grossly disadvantaged by poverty and AIDS, that occupational balance may be irrelevant or a luxury when fiscal, material, education, and health resources are inadequate.[157] However, that suggests that occupational imbalance is an ongoing fact of life for people in such circumstances. It is made invisible by the challenges to obtain and maintain the prerequisites of living. It points to the gross imbalance between peoples from differing socio-economic-political environments, and that those most disadvantaged will be at risk of experiencing illness associated with occupational imbalance, as well as disorders associated with their particular circumstances.

The imbalance in health-giving occupational opportunities throughout communities is a cause for concern. It affects sociocultural and spiritual values, political direction, welfare economics, and community history. In some form, it is a common topic of conversation in many community venues and is a constant theme in popular media. There is occupational imbalance between and within postindustrial, industrial, and developing nations in terms of the prerequisite occupations of life. Individual choice is constrained by prevailing national, sector-specific, and organizational cultures that thrive within them, labor market opportunities and expectations, gender, and individual preferences and constraints within socioeconomic groups.[94] For example, in terms of paid employment, at one extreme are the unemployed and at the other the overemployed. Both have decreased opportunity to maximize their occupational potential but for different reasons. Organizations play a central role in the complex and dynamic nature of occupational imbalance. An article addressing the continuing overwork evidence from several major postindustrial nations suggests that many people in paid employment are now expected to take on increased duties, to spend longer hours on work tasks without extra rewards, and that health breakdowns from this cause are increasing.[158,159] In addition, new corporate practices, national organizations, and cultures continue to show gender bias and occupational imbalance of opportunity.[94] Women are particularly vulnerable, as increasingly more must maintain domestic occupations in addition to reentering the sphere of paid employment.

Communities in the developing world are now faced with the same industrial environments that were depriving, imbalanced, and alienating 100 years or so ago in Europe. Not surprisingly, workers are experiencing similar health problems even though, outside work, many live more natural lifestyles than postindustrial affluence permits. Those without work face poverty and lack of opportunity to meet even the prerequisites of health. Both experience occupational imbalance. Occupational imbalance occurs because of failure to meet not only natural health requirements for physical, social, and mental exercise and rest, but also unique doing, being, belonging, and becoming needs. Personal and communal experiences of occupational imbalance include individuals or collectives of people not being able to do, be, belong, or become through:

- Not meeting the needs for basic survival; the prerequisites of health
- Not balancing activity, rest, and sleep to meet biological needs
- Not being able to fulfil the promise of genetic inherence
- Not being able to forge satisfactory and lasting relationships
- Not being able to respond appropriately to the positives and negatives of environments
- Not being able to make best use of opportunities
- Not being able to develop opportunity toward the attainment of aspirations because of physical, mental, social, cultural, corporate or political restrictions
- Not being able to meet the needs for healthy living and well-being.

These will differ from person to person, community to community, population to population, and from one historical time to another, but the differences do not gainsay their importance, nor are they an artifact of recent years.

Occupational imbalance can be a form of stress, be a stressor that could result in either improved or worsened occupational outcome, or lead to stress related disorder. Computers and the Information Age have exacerbated the problems of balancing work-life and family-life, especially for dual-earner families.[160] High stress level, otherwise known as hurry sickness, is common to workaholics, who have insufficient relaxation or friendships.[161,162] At home, they may experience problems related to an increase of obligatory non-work occupations that can contribute to the perception of a chronic lack of time. This may cause people to engage in unhealthy occupations, such as drinking excessively, overeating, smoking, weight problems, or gambling.[163]

OCCUPATIONAL STRESS

Stress is a regular component of occupational alienation, deprivation, and imbalance. It can be conceptualized as responses to events that disturb the usual pattern of a person's life. The events may be no more than daily hassles, such as forgetting an essential ingredient for a meal, losing the car keys, or missing school assignment or work deadlines. Stressors may be isolated occurrences, such as failing an examination, moving homes, dealing with divorce or death in the family, or more ongoing factors, such as living in a war-torn state, caring for family members with HIV/AIDS, being unable to find work or being bored by it, being bullied at school, looking after a child with a long-term illness, or ongoing relationship problems. Stress refers to whatever disrupts a person's psychological equilibrium.[164]

Stress is a basic phylogenic mechanism that, under normal circumstances, works to maintain physiological equilibrium in times of physical and emotional pressure. If prolonged at an unacceptable level, susceptibility to illness is increased. Meyer is credited with recognizing that disease appeared to occur when this regulatory system became subjected to overload,[165] and Selye described the "general adaptation syndrome" in which he hypothesized that the adaptive response can break down due to "innate defects, understress, overstress, or psychological mismanagement."[166] Common stress diseases include "high blood pressure, heart accidents, and nervous diseases."[167] Currently, it is probable that nutritional disorder might join that list. Selye argued that the type of illness experienced as a result of stress expresses an individual's weakest points.[168] This suggests that genetic or familial predisposition, such as mental breakdown, arthritis, or cardiac failure, can be activated by prolonged stress.[169] Work based on Selye's hypothesis has largely sustained it, but there is still no definitive proof.

A well-publicized 1970s study by French and Caplan linked stress with coronary heart disease,[170] and other studies about that time associated it with depressive illness and disorders of the musculoskeletal, digestive, and immune systems.[171] A decade later, Roskies and Lazarus put forward that the inability to cope with everyday stress has more effect on physical, mental, and social health than stress episodes themselves,[172] and similarly, Moore argued that:

> Long-term chronic stress and especially chronic unpredictable stress can result in an earlier demise or long-term disability (mental and/or physical), unless therapeutic intervention can reverse the individual's way of coping and/or reverse the situations which are causing the stress.[173]

She listed some effects of chronic unpredictable stress as increased heart rate, respiration, muscle tension, and blood-glucose levels and decreased peristalsis, lymphocytes, T and B cells, immune response, destabilization of lyosomes, and hyper-alert states, as well as blood pressure. Although Temoshok argued that there is little empirical evidence either "to support or refute potential biological pathways linking stress factors and disease initiation or progression for any disorder," he suggested that this reflects the complexity of the connections. Those probably include personal and situational variables, physiological and psychological predispositions, as well as social, cultural, economic, and political contexts.[174]

Cohen et al, in a continuation of decades-long searches for answers about stress and its contribution to a variety of disease processes, have recently found that specific biochemical pathways link stress and health. Stress reduces the sensitivity of the receptors (that are, in effect, chemical switches) that are supposed to control the level of inflammation in the body. In addition, part of the explanation is probably behavioral. People who are stressed often sleep badly, take less exercise, and smoke and drink more than others, all of which can harm health. Although there is no definitive proof, the consistency of research findings strongly supports a causal link between stress and clinical depression, cardiovascular disease, cancer, and HIV/AIDS.[175]

Both stressful experiences and feeling stressed can affect health.[176,177] In earlier chapters, stress has been discussed as a natural biological mechanism that can be both helpful in getting things done or, if overwhelming, informs that there is something amiss through the mechanism known as the fight-or-flight response. Physical changes occur, such as an increase in blood pressure and heartbeat, tightening of muscles, quickening of breath, and a sharpening of senses to increase strength, stamina, speed of reaction time, and ability to focus in preparation for action. Although the body is relatively proficient at dealing with acute stressors, chronic stress can produce a "variety of adverse effects."[178] When threatened, deregulation of an interconnected network of physiologic command terminals known as the hypothalamic-pituitary-adrenal axis occurs, releasing a flood of stress hormones, including adrenaline and cortisol to incite emergency action. Cortisol operates as an adaptation hormone, as well as having anti-inflammatory, blood glucose modulating, and immune modifying functions, and its receptors are expressed throughout the body, including in the brain. It breaks down tissue, so "when out of balance and unregulated, can have detrimental effects on body composition."[179] Depending on the amounts of stress, activity, food, or time of day, levels of cortisol can vary. Too much can suppress the immune system and, if in the bloodstream for too long, a variety of responses can occur, such as anxiety, depression, impaired cognitive performance, dementia, high blood pressure, increases in abdominal fat,[178,179] and some types of cancer.[180-183] Too little can result in autoimmunity and rheumatologic disorders and disrupt many physiologic systems.[184-187]

The consequences of stress can be deadly because it can lead to a spontaneous weakening of the heart, known as stress cardiomyopathy, which can lead to arrhythmia and sudden cardiac arrest.[188,189] It has been estimated that more than 10,000 deaths per year occurred in Japan after World War II as a result of overwork and were attributed to chronic, unremitting stress known as Karoshi, with high-level executives suffering heart attacks and strokes at a relatively young age because of severe physical and emotional stress.[190,191] Reportedly, in both the US and Russia, nearly two-thirds of doctor's office visits relate to stress.[192] Occupational signs of chronic stress can include difficulty waking up, even following adequate sleep; excessive fatigue after little exertion; perceived bursts of energy in early evening; being overwhelmed by relatively trivial tasks; feeling hazy; poor memory; decreased sex drive; and little appetite with cravings for sugar and salty foods, caffeine, and energy drinks.[192]

The diathesis-stress model is a major psychological theory explaining behavior and disorders of mental health that emerged in the 1960s.[193,194] The model explores how nonbiological or genetic traits (described as diatheses) interact with life experience and environmental stressors. The term *diathesis* derives from the Greek word for disposition or vulnerability, so from this perspective stress may be related to genetic, psychological, biological, or situational factors, as well as variability between people's vulnerability to stress experiences.[195-197] Precipitating factors are events in an individual's life that may be neither good nor bad, but are deemed stressful because people experience and interpret them differently. Commonly, change of any kind causes stress whether large or small, desirable or undesirable. "An accumulation of small changes can be just as powerful as one major change."[198]

Although direct links between stress and disease probably have physiological foundations, there remains support for the theory proposed here that it is the complex relationship between physiological mechanisms, all parts of the brain, and the outside world that are involved in both

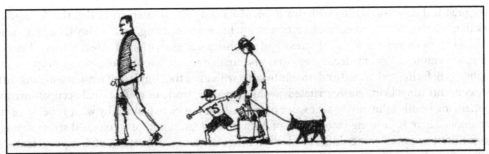

Figure 11-5. Stress-related Illness as a result of daily pressures. (Artwork: © Trevor Bywater 2013. Used with permission.)

the maintenance of health and occupation that can lead to stress. Stress-related illnesses as a result of finding little meaning or purpose in doing (occupational alienation), not having opportunities to aim to meet the prerequisites of living and life satisfaction (occupational deprivation), and doing too much or too little (occupational imbalance) have undoubtedly increased during evolution.[199-203] Figure 11-5 depicts a not uncommon situation of daily pressures on a woman experiencing stress-related illness as a result of overload, lack of occupational satisfaction, and little meaning. Such unhealthy outcomes occur regularly despite the obvious benefits of living in today's postindustrial world rather than that of hunter-gatherers, and despite the longer life expectancy, lower infant mortality, and miraculous advances in technological and pharmaceutical medicine for those living in postindustrial societies.

Stress can be either problematic or therapeutic. When the body's stress response is working well, it improves the ability to perform under pressure, helping to increase alertness and energy to meet challenging situations. Ongoing stress that persists can prevent people doing the occupations they need and want to do. It can leave them feeling overwhelmed or underwhelmed, unable to cope with challenges they need to overcome. It can result in not being able to call on the resources or people who might help. It prevents achieving self-actualization, health, or well-being.

The most common form of stress is known as *acute stress*. It is experienced as people meet the demands of everyday and occasional occupations and can be exciting or taxing and exhausting if it challenges the limits of occupational competencies. Overdoing short-term stress can lead to accidents and cause acute distress and physiological symptoms, such as upset stomachs or tension headaches. If people are disturbed to the extent that they unable to organize or order their activities and take on too much, what is known as episodic acute stress takes over: things go wrong; they rush or are always late and breathless. When stress becomes continuous and chronic, people are often unable to meet the prerequisites of life through what they do or can afford to do. In places where there are advanced social services, they may become habitual users. Chronic stress is experienced as feeling anxious, even when not facing difficult situations, and feeling trapped by "unrelenting demands and pressures for seemingly interminable periods of time. With no hope, the individual gives up searching for solutions."[204]

Some individuals appear more vulnerable than others to medically recognized disorders triggered by stress, such as depression. A disorder may only develop when exposed to a specific stressor, and may be aggravated by significant personal loss or life change, or stimulants and recreational drugs.[205] Not all individuals who are stressed, or experience stressful life events, develop a psychological disorder.[197,206] However, whether a medically recognized outcome occurs or not, occupational stress may be considered a disorder of occupation that prevents people experiencing health and well-being from satisfying doing, being, belonging, or becoming through such engagement.

Occupational stressors might include problems at work or no work; boredom with having too little to do; responsibilities that bombard and overwhelm; unrealistic expectations; demanding families, friends, or cultural activities; difficulties at school or with examinations; moving homes;

or the practical issues of dealing with death. Matuska and Christiansen argue that the demands of work in modern economies encroach on non-work, health-enhancing, and quality time. This leads inevitability to increasing levels of stress and a subsequent escalation of stress-related illness.[40] Common symptoms include feeling anxious and unable to "switch off"; not eating properly; not sleeping well; feeling exhausted and unable to cope with even the simplest of requests; having difficulty concentrating; being easily irritated; avoiding people, work, or recreational occupations; and experiencing bodily ailments or aches and pains that cannot be explained by what is being or has been done. There is growing recognition of both physiological and psychological stress that can also manifest in poor coping skills, headaches, binge drinking and eating, and, if persistent, can result in a weakening immune system and cardiovascular disease.[207] If occupational stress occurs it can be relieved by occupational anti-stressors. Perhaps the most important of those is physical activity, such as "walking, jogging, gardening, housecleaning, biking, swimming, weightlifting or anything else that gets you active" as recommended in the Mayo Clinic's "tips for stress relief."[208] Those explain how physical occupations refocus the mind on body movements and inflate "feel-good endorphins and other natural neural chemicals" that enhance a sense of well-being and improve mood. Other Mayo Clinic recommended occupations to relieve stress are reading or telling jokes, hanging out with fun friends or watching a comedy to the point of laughter; emailing, talking to or having coffee with someone; volunteering for a charitable group; and learning to say no or to delegate.[208] Symptoms of stress can be eased by modifications to occupation, use of relaxation, yoga, music therapy, and owning a pet,[209-214] as well as avoiding stressful situations,[185,215-217] alcohol, and caffeine before bedtime.[218,219]

Conclusion

The second of three chapters to deliberate on occupation as a dynamic in population health and a potential source of illness has considered the opposing effects of occupational balance and imbalance. The latter has been identified as a disorder of occupation that is largely outside the field of medicine, although many of the consequential illnesses are recognized. The case of occupational stress is similar. Both imbalance and stress are physiological mechanisms that can effect autonomic change within the human organism or inform the mind that action—occupations—need to change. Change may be outside of an individual's control, and modification may be needed at community, corporate, or political levels.

Both the world and the people in it are experiencing occupational disorder. As "health promotion is the process of enabling people to increase control over their health and its determinants" to improve them, an occupational view of order and disorder could be useful in "the work of tackling communicable and non-communicable diseases and other threats to health" of an occupational nature.[1]

References

1. World Health Organization. *Bangkok Charter for Health Promotion in a Globalized World.* 2005.
2. Balance. *Oxford Dictionaries: English (UK).* Oxford, Britain: Oxford University Press; 2014. http://oxforddictionaries.com/definition/balance. Accessed June 20, 2014.
3. Lipworth W, Hooker C, Carter S. Balance, balancing and health. *Qualitative Health Research.* 2011;21(5):714-725.
4. Sheldon K. Defining and validating measures of life balance: suggestions, a new measure, and some preliminary results. In: Matuska K, Christiansen CH, eds. *Life Balance: Multidisciplinary Theories and Research.* Thorofare, NJ: Slack Inc and AOTA Press; 2009:62.
5. Risse GB. History of Western medicine from Hippocrates to germ theory. In: Kiple KF, ed. *The Cambridge World History of Human Disease.* New York, NY: Cambridge University Press; 1993:11.

6. Plato. *Timaeus*. Lee HDP, trans. Penguin Classics; 1965:116-117.
7. Bichenbach J, Glass T. Life balance: the meaning and the menace in the metaphor. In: Matuska K, Christiansen CH, eds. *Life Balance: Multidisciplinary Theories and Research*. Thorofare, NJ, Slack Inc and AOTA Press; 2009:62.
8. Howard R. Wellness: obtainable goal or impossible dream. *Post Graduate Medicine*. 1983;73(1):15-19.
9. Hall K. *A Life in Balance: Nourishing the Four Roots of True Happiness*. New York: AMACON; 1951, 2006.
10. Burke P. The invention of leisure in early modern Europe. *Past and Present*. 1995;146:136-150.
11. Jonsson H. A new direction in the conceptualization and categorization of occupation. *Journal of Occupational Science*. 2008;15(1):3-8.
12. Sigerist HE. *A History of Medicine. Vol 1. Primitive and Archaic Medicine*. New York, NY: Oxford University Press; 1955:254-255.
13. Federation of European Employers. The International HR Think Tank. Labour Relations: History of Working Time. *The History of Working Time Regulation 1784-2002*. Available at: http://www.fedee.com/labour-relations/history-of-working-time/. Accessed June 14, 2012.
14. Child Labor Public Education Project. *Child Labor in U.S. History*. Available at: http://www.continuetolearn.uiowa.edu/laborctr/child_labor/about/us_history.html. Accessed July 16, 2013.
15. Child Labor Coalition. *Timeline of Child Labor Developments in the United States*. October 20, 2010. Available at: http://stopchildlabor.org/?p=1795. Accessed May 29, 2014.
16. National Child Labor Committee. *About Us*. http://www.nationalchildlabor.org/history.html. Accessed May 29, 2014.
17. U.S. Department of Labor. *Child Labor Requirements in Agricultural Occupations under the Fair Labor Standards Act*. http://www.dol.gov/whd/regs/compliance/childlabor102.pdf. Accessed May 29, 2014.
18. Human Rights Watch. *Fields of Peril: Child Labor in US Agriculture*. http://www.hrw.org/news/2010/05/05/us-child-farmworkers-dangerous-lives. Accessed July 18, 2013.
19. Barker J. Tightening the iron cage: concertive control in self-managing teams. *Administrative Science Quarterly*. 1993;38:408-437.
20. Boswell W, Olson-Buchanan J. The use of communication technologies after hours: the role of work attitudes and work-life conflict. *Journal of Management.*2007;33(4):592-608.
21. Reynolds J. When too much is not enough: Actual and preferred works hours in the United States and abroad. *Sociological Forum*. 2004;19(1):89-120.
22. Ray R, Schmitt J. European Economic and Employment Policy Brief No. 3 – 2007. *No Vacation Nation USA - A Comparison of Leave and Holiday in OECD Countries*. http://www.law.harvard.edu/programs/lwp/papers/No_Holidays.pdf 5. Accessed May 29, 2014.
23. *Presidency Conclusions*. Lisbon European Council 23 and 24 March 2000. http://www.europarl.europa.eu/summits/lis1_en.htm. Accessed May 27, 2014).
24. *Council Decision of 22 July 2003 on Guidelines for the Employment Policies of the Member States* (COM2003/578/EC). http://europa.eu.int/comm/employment_social/employment_strategy/prop_2003/adopted_guidelines_2003_en.htm. Accessed February 16, 2004.
25. Time to Move up a Gear. *President Barroso Presents Annual Progress Report on Growth and Jobs Brussels, January 25, 2006*. http://europa.eu/rapid/press-release_IP-06-71_en.htm?locale=en. Accessed May 1, 2014.
26. Department of Trade and Industry. *Work-life Balance*. 2002. http://www.dti.gov.uk/work-lifebalance/index.html. Accessed February 4, 2014.
27. Commission of the European Communities. *Communication from the Commission: Strengthening the implementation of the European Employment Strategy*. Brussels; 7.4.2004, COM(2004) 239 final; 10. http://www.rreuse.org/t3/fileadmin/editor-mount/documents/000/00049-Strenghtening-the-Implementation-of-the-EES-(2004)-239-Final.pdf. Accessed February 4, 2014.
28. Caproni P. Work life balance: what do you mean? The ethical ideology underpinning appropriate application. *Journal of Applied Behavioral Science*. 2007;43:273-294.
29. Reece K, Davis J, Polatajko H. The representations of work-life balance in Canadian newspapers. *Work*. 2009;32:431-42.
30. Heathfield SM. *Basics of Work-Life Balance*. http://humanresources.about.com/od/glossaryw/g/balance.htm. Accessed June 2, 2014.
31. Mageswari U, Prabhu NRV. A conceptual study on stress and work-life balance. *Discovery Science*. 2012;1(3):50-53. http://www.discovery.org.in/PDF_Files/ds_20120902.pdf. Accessed June 3, 2014.

32. Work-life balance. *Resources and Downloads: HR Glossary.* Hrcouncil.ca/hr-toolkit/HRToolkitGlossary. cfm. Accessed February 4, 2014.

33. Work-life balance. *Elearning Glossary.* Elearners.com; 2012. www.elearners.com/guide/faq-glossary/ glossary/. Accessed February 4, 2014.

34. *Work-life Balance.* wmhp.cmhaontario.ca/glossary. Accessed February 4, 2014.

35. Stredwick J. *An Introduction to Human Resource Management.* 3rd ed. Students: Glossary. Work-life balance. Oxon, UK: Routledge; 2013. http://www.routledge.com/cw/stredwick-9780415622295/s1/ glossary/. Accessed February 4, 2014.

36. Wagman P, Bjorklund A, Hakansson C, Jocobsson C, Falkmer T. Perceptions of life balance among a working population in Sweden. *Qualitative Health Research.* 2011;(21)3:410-418.

37. ERP Therapy Centre. *Lifestyle Balance Sheet.* http://www.erptherapy.com/lifestylebalance.asp Accessed February 14, 2014.

38. Milltons Health Pages. *Lifestyle Balance.* http://www.milltonshealthpages.com.au/. Accessed September 23, 2013.

39. Matuska K, Christiansen CH, eds. *Life Balance: Multidisciplinary Theories and Research.* Thorofare, NJ: Slack Inc and AOTA Press; 2009.

40. Matuska KM, Christiansen CH. A proposed model of lifestyle balance. *Journal of Occupational Science.* 2008;15(1):9-19.

41. Maslow A. A theory of human motivation. *Psychological Review.* 1943;50:370-396.

42. Maslow A. 1970. *Motivation and Personality.* 2nd ed. New York: Harper and Row; 1970.

43. Ryff C. Happiness is everything or is it? Explorations on the meaning of psychological well-being. *Journal of Personality and Social Psychology.* 1989;57:1069-1081.

44. Ryff C, Singer B. Psychological well-being: Meaning, measurement, and implications for psychotherapy research. *Psychotherapy and Psychosomatics.* 1996;65:14-23.

45. Ryff C, Singer B. The contours of positive human health. *Psychological Inquiry.* 1998;9:1-28.

46. Deci E, Ryan R. The "what" and "why" of goal pursuits. Human needs and the self determination of behavior. *Psychological Inquiry.* 2000;11:227-268.

47. Bickenbach J, Glass T. Life balance: the meaning and the menace in a metaphor. In: Matuska K, Christiansen CH, eds. *Life Balance: Multidisciplinary Theories and Research.* Thorofare, NJ: Slack Inc and AOTA Press: 2009:13-22.

48. Marks S. Multiple roles and life balance: an intellectual journey. In: Matuska K, Christiansen CH, eds. *Life Balance: Multidisciplinary Theories and Research.* Thorofare, NJ: Slack Inc and AOTA Press; 2009:43-58.

49. Sheldon K. Defining and validating measures of life balance: suggestions, a new measure, and some preliminary results. In: Matuska K, Christiansen CH, eds. *Life Balance: Multidisciplinary Theories and Research.* Thorofare, NJ: Slack Inc and AOTA Press; 2009:61-72.

50. Cummins R. Measuring life balance through discrepancy theories and subjective well-being. In: Matuska K, Christiansen CH, eds. *Life Balance: Multidisciplinary Theories and Research.* Thorofare, NJ: Slack Inc and AOTA Press; 2009:73-94.

51. Harvey A, Singleton J. Time use and balance. In: Matuska K, Christiansen C, eds. *Life Balance: Multidisciplinary Theories and Research.* Thorofare, NJ: Slack Inc and AOTA Press; 2009: 95-114.

52. Zuzanek J. Time use imbalance: development and emotional costs. In: Matuska K, Christiansen CH, eds. *Life Balance: Multidisciplinary Theories and Research.* Thorofare, NJ: Slack Inc and AOTA Press; 2009: 207-222.

53. Veenhoven R. Optimal lifestyle mix: an inductive approach. In: Matuska K, Christiansen CH, eds. *Life Balance: Multidisciplinary Theories and Research.* Thorofare, NJ: Slack Inc and AOTA Press; 2009:33-42.

54. Pentland W, McColl M. Occupational integrity: another perspective on "life balance." *Canadian Journal of Occupational Therapy.* 2008;75(3):135-138.

55. Wagman P. *Conceptualizing Life Balance from an Empirical and Occupational Therapy Perspective.* Dissertation Series No. 25. School of Health Sciences, Jönköping University; 2012.

56. Rogers J. Why study human occupation? *American Journal of Occupational Therapy.* 1984;38:37-49.

57. Spencer E. Toward a balance of work and play: promotion of health and wellness. *Occupational Therapy in Health Care.* 1989:5(4);87-99.

58. Christiansen C. Three perspectives on balance in occupation. In: Zemke R, Clark F, eds. *Occupational Science: The Evolving Discipline.* Philadelphia, PA: F.A. Davis; 1996:431-451.

59. Meyer A. The philosophy of occupational therapy. *American Journal of Occupational Therapy.* 1978;31:639-642.(Reprinted from Archives of Occupational Therapy. 1922;1(1).)

60. Matuska K. *Validity Evidence for a Model and Measure of Life Balance.* Minnesota: Doctoral thesis University of Minnesota; 2010.

61. Christiansen C, Matuska K. Lifestyle balance: a review of concepts and research. *Journal of Occupational Science.* 2006;13(1):49-61.

62. Walker S, Sechrist K, Pender M. The health promoting lifestyle profile: development and psychometric characteristics. *Nursing Research.* 1987;36:76-81.

63. Camporese R, Freguja C, Sabbadini l. Time use by gender and quality of life. *Social Indicators Research.* 1998;44:119-144.

64. Zuzanek J. Time-use, time pressure, personal stress, mental health and life-satisfaction from a life cycle perspective. *Journal of Occupational Science.* 1998;5:26-39.

65. Reilly M. A psychiatric occupational therapy program as a teaching model. *American Journal of Occupational Therapy.* 1966;22:61.

66. Backman C. Occupational balance: Measuring time-use and satisfaction across occupational performance areas. In: Law M, Baum C, Dunn W, eds. *Measuring Occupational Performance: Supporting Best Practice in Occupational Therapy.* Thorofare, NJ; Slack, Inc. 2005:287-300.

67. Christiansen C, Baum C, eds. *Occupational Therapy: Enabling Function and Well-being.* Thorofare, NJ: Slack Inc.; 1997:592.

68. Christiansen C, Townsend E, eds. *Introduction to Occupation: The Art and Science of Living.* 2nd ed. Upper Saddle River, NJ: Pearson; 2010: 420.

69. Reed K, Sanderson S. *Concepts of Occupational Therapy.* 3rd ed. Baltimore: Williams and Wilkins; 1992:75.

70. Yerxa E. Health and the human spirit for occupation. *American Journal of Occupational Therapy.* 1998;52(6):412-418.

71. Backman C. Occupational balance and well-being. In: Christiansen C, Townsend E, eds. *Introduction to Occupation: The Art and Science of Living.* 2nd ed. Upper Saddle River, NJ; Pearson; 2010.

72. Håkansson C, Dahlin-Ivanoff S, Sonn U. Achieving balance in everyday life. *Journal of Occupational Science.* 2006;13(1):74-82.

73. Håkansson C, Ahlborg Jr G. Perceptions of employment, domestic work, and leisure as predictors of health among women and men. *Journal of Occupational Science.* 2010;17(3):150-157.

74. Christiansen C, Townsend E, eds. *Introduction to Occupation. The Art and Science of Living.* 2nd ed. Upper Saddle River, NJ: Pearson; 2010: 17.

75. Hobson J. *Sleep.* New York: Scientific American Library; 1995.

76. Horne J, Minard A. Sleep and sleepiness following a behavioral active day. *Ergonomics.* 1985;28:567-575.

77. Meguro K, Ueda M, Yamaguchi T, et al. Disturbance in daily sleep/wake patterns in patients with cognitive impairment and decreased daily activity. *Journal of American Geriatrics Society.* 1990;38(11):1176-1182.

78. Aronoff M. *Sleep and its Secrets: The River of Crystal Light.* Los Angeles, CA: Insight Books; 1991.

79. Backon J, Matamoros N, Ticho U. Changes in intraocular pressure induced by differential forced unilateral breathing, a technique that affects both brain hemispherically and autonomic activity: A pilot study. *Graefe's Archive of Clinical and Experimental Opthalmology.* 1989;227:575-577.

80. Hetzel BS, McMichael T. *L S Factor: Lifestyle and Health.* Ringwood, Victoria: Penguin; 1987:186-187.

81. Kubey R, Csikszentmihalyi M. *Television and the Quality of Life.* Hillsdale, NJ: Erlbaum; 1990.

82. Csikszentmihalyi M, Larson R, Prescott S. The ecology of adolescent activity and experience. *Journal of Youth and Adolescence.* 1977;6:281-294.

83. Larson R, Kubey R. Television and music: contrasting media in adolescent life. *Youth and Society.* 1983;15:13-31.

84. Csikszentmihalyi M. Activity and happiness: towards a science of occupation. *Journal of Occupational Science: Australia.* 1993;1(1):38-42.

85. Erlandsson L-K. *101 Women's Patterns of Daily Occupations: Characteristics and Relationships to Health and Well-being.* Doctoral Thesis. Department of Clinical Neuroscience, Division of Occupational Therapy, Lund University; 2003.

86. Erlandsson L-K, Rögnvaldsson T, Eklund M. Recognition of similarities (ROS): an attempt to analyse and characterise patterns of daily occupations. *Journal of Occupational Science.* 2004;11(1):3-13.

87. Erlandsson L-K, Eklund M. Levels of complexity in patterns of daily occupations: Relationship to women's well-being. *Journal of Occupational Science.* 2006;13(1):27-36.

88. Persson D, Erlandsson L-K, Eklund M, Iwarsson S. Value dimensions, meaning and complexity in human occupation: a tentative structure for analysis. *Scandinavian journal of Occupational Therapy.* 2001;8:7-18.

89. Erlandsson L-K, Håkansson C. Aspects of daily occupations that promote life balance among women in Sweden. In: Matuska K, Christiansen CH, eds. *Life Balance: Multidisciplinary Theories and Research.* Thorofare, NJ: Slack and AOTA Press: 2009.

90. Wilcock AA, Hall M, Hambley N, et al. The relationship between occupational balance and health: a pilot study. *Occupational Therapy International.* 1997;4(1):17-30.

91. Lovelock L, Bentley J, Dunn T, Wallenbert I. Occupational balance and perceived health: a study of occupational therapists. Conference Abstracts, World Federation of Occupational Therapists Congress. Stockholm; 2002.

92. Wilcock A. Relationship of occupations to health and well-being. In: Christiansen C, Baum C, eds. *Occupational Therapy: Performance, Participation and Well-being.* Thorofare, NJ: Slack; 2005:134.

93. Cotman C, Berchtold N. Exercise: A behavioral intervention to enhance brain health and plasticity. *Trends in Neurosciences.* 2002;6:295-301.

94. Townsend E, Wilcock A. Occupational justice and client-centred practice: A dialogue-in-progress. *Canadian Journal of Occupational Therapy.* 2004;71:75-87.

95. Gregory A, Milner S. Editorial: Work–life balance: a matter of choice? *Gender, Work and Organization.* 2009;16 (1):1-13.

96. Imbalance. *Macmillan Dictionary.* Available at: http://www.macmillandictionary.com/dictionary/british/imbalance. Accessed August 5, 2013.

97. Equilibrium. *The Free Online Dictionary.* www.thefreedictionary.com/equilibrium. Accessed August 9, 2013.

98. Townsend E, Wilcock A. Occupational justice. In: Christiansen C, Townsend E, eds. *Introduction to Occupation: The Art and Science of Living.* Upper Saddle River; NJ: Prentice Hall; 2004:243-273.

99. Duxbury L, Higgins C, Coghill D. Voices of Canadians: Seeking Work-life Balance. Catalogue RH54-12/2003. Montreal, Quebec: Human Resources Development Canada; 2003.

100. Erdwins C, Buffardi L, Casper W, O'Brien A. The relationship of women's role strain to social support, role satisfaction and self efficacy. *Family Relations.* 2001;50:230-238.

101. Amundson N. Three dimensional living. *Journal of Employment Counseling.* 2001;38:114-127.

102. Matuska K, Christiansen C. *Life Balance: Multidisciplinary Theories and Research.* Slack. and AOTA Press: 2009.

103. Matuska K, Barrett K. Patterns of occupation. In: Boyt Schell B, Gillen G, Scaffa M, Cohn E, eds. *Willard and Spackman's Occupational Therapy.* 12th ed. Philadelphia, PA: Wolters Kluver/Lippincott Williams and Wilkins; 2014: 170.

104. Matuska K. Validity evidence for a model and measure of life balance. *Occupational Therapy Journal of Research.* 2012;32(1):229-237.

105. Busch S. *What Does Homeostatic Balance Mean?* http://www.livestrong.com/article/77571-homeostatic-balance-mean/#ixzz2bihKMgJE. Accessed May 4, 2011.

106. Friedman H, ed. *Personality and Disease.* New York, NY: John Wiley and Sons; 1990:7,11.

107. McEwen B, Stellar E. Stress and the individual mechanisms leading to disease. *Arch Intern Med.* 1993;153(18):2093-2101.

108. Ornstein R, Sobel D. *The Healing Brain, A Radical New Approach to Health Care.* London, England: Macmillan; 1988:206-207,213-217.

109. Cox D. *Occupational Therapy and Chronic Fatigue Syndrome.* London: Whurr; 2000.

110. Mayo Clinic. *Job Burnout: How to Spot It and Take Action.* http://www.mayoclinic.com/health/AboutThisSite/AM00057. Accessed August 24, 2013.

111. Glouberman D. *The Joy of Burnout.* London: Hodder and Stoughton; 2002.

112. Cheyne J, Carriere J, Smilek D. Absent mindedness: lapses in conscious awareness and everyday cognitive failures. *Consciousness and Cognition.* 2006;15(3):578-592.

113. Ardell D. *High Level Wellness.* 2nd ed. Berkeley, CA: Ten Speed Press; 1986.

114. Williams M. *Lifetime Fitness and Wellness: A Personal Choice.* 2nd ed. Dubuque: Wm. C. Brown Publishers; 1990:9,27.

115. Geschwind N, Galaburda A, eds. *Biological Foundations of Cerebral Dominance.* Cambridge, Mass: Harvard University Press; 1984.

116. Andervont H. Influence of environment on mammary cancer in mice. *Journal of National Cancer Institute.* 1944;4:579-581.

117. Achterberg J, Collerrain I, Craig P. A possible relationship between cancer, mental retardation and mental disorder. *Social Science and Medicine.* 1978;12:135-139.

118. de la Pena A. *The Psychobiology of Cancer.* New York, NY: Praeger Publishers; 1983.

119. Alterman T, Luckhaupt S, Dalhamer J, Ward B, Calvert G. Job insecurity, work-family imbalance, and hostile work environment: Prevalence data from the 2010 National Health Interview Survey. *American Journal of Industrial Medicine.* 2013;56(6):660-669.

120. McCaffery E. *Conversations with the Dean: Balancing Work and Life: Is it Possible?* Gould School of Law. March, 2007. weblaw.usc.edu/news/article.cfm?newsID=370. Accessed August 15, 2013.

121. World Health Organization. *The Burden of Occupational Illness: UN Agencies Sound the Alarm.* 1999. Available at: http://who.int/inf-pr1999/en/pr99-31.html. Accessed February 6, 2004.

122. Siegrist J. Adverse health effects of high effort-low reward conditions at work. *Journal of Occupational Health Psychology.* 1996;1:27-43.

123. Hakanen J, Schaufeli W, Ahola K. The job demands-resources model: a three-year cross-lagged study of burnout, depression, commitment, and work engagement. *Work and Stress.* 2008;22(3):224-241.

124. Haines V, Marchand A, Harvey S. Crossover of workplace aggression experiences in dual-earner couples. *Journal of Occupational Health Psychology.* 2006;11:305-314.

125. Fredrikson M, Sundin O, Frankenhaeuser M. Cortisol excretion during the defence reaction in humans. *Psychosomatic Medicine.* 1985;47:313-319.

126. Belkić K, et al. Psychosocial factors: review of the empirical data among men. *Occupational Medicine: State of the Art Reviews.* 2000;15:24-46.

127. Johnson J, Hall E. Job strain, workplace social support, and cardiovascular disease: a cross-sectional study of a random sample of the Swedish working population. *American Journal of Public Health.* 1988;78:1336-1342.

128. Belkic K, Landsbergis P, Schnall P, Baker D. Is job strain a source of major cardiovascular risk? *Scandinavian Journal of Work, Environment, and Health.* 2004;30:85-128.

129. Siegrist J, Peter R. Job stressors and coping characteristics in work-related disease: issues of validity. *Work & Stress.* 1994;8:130-140.

130. Landsbergis P, et al. The workplace and cardiovascular disease: relevance and potential role for occupational health psychology. In: Quick J, Tetrick L, eds. *Handbook of Occupational Health Psychology.* Washington, DC: American Psychological Association. 2003:265-287.

131. Stamm T, Lovelock L, Stew G, Nell V, Smolen J, Machold K, et al. I have a disease but I am not ill: a narrative study of occupational balance in people with rheumatoid arthritis. *Occupation, Participation and Health (OTJR).* 2009;29(1):32-39.

132. Forhan M, Backman C. Exploring occupational balance in adults with rheumatoid arthritis. *Occupation, Participation and Health (OTJR).* 2010;30(3):133-41.

133. Bejerholm U. Occupational balance in people with schizophrenia. *Occupational Therapy in Mental Health.* 2010;26(1):1-17.

134. McGuire B, Crowe T, Law M, VanLeit B. Mothers of children with disabilities: occupational concerns and solutions. *Occupation, Participation and Health (OTJR).* 2004;24(2):54-63.

135. Matuska K, Erickson B. Lifestyle balance: how is it described and experienced by women with multiple sclerosis. *Journal of Occupational Science.* 2008;15(1):20-6

136. Håkansson C, Matuska KM. How life balance is perceived by Swedish women recovering from a stress-related disorder: a validation of the life balance model. *Journal of Occupational Science.* 2010;17(2):112-9.

137. Backman C, Kennedy S, Chalmers A, Singer J. "How satisfied are you with the balance of time you spend on work, self-care, leisure and rest?" Participation in paid and unpaid work by adults with rheumatoid arthritis. *Journal of Rheumatology.* 2004;31:47-57.

138. Wilcock AA. *An Occupational Perspective of Health.* Thorofare, NJ, Slack Inc; 1998.

139. Passmore R, Eastwood M. *Human Nutrition and Dietetics.* Edinburgh: Churchill Livingstone; 1986.

140. Garrow J. *Treat Obesity Seriously.* Edinburgh: Churchill Livingstone; 1981.

141. Stephenson W. *BMI: Does the Body Mass Index Need Fixing?* BBC News. 29 January 2013.

142. McKeown T. *The Origins of Disease.* Oxford, UK: Basil Blackwell, 1988:1-2.

143. Justice B. *Who Gets Sick: Thinking and Health.* Houston, Texas: Peak Press; 1987:28-29,31-32,179.

144. Wolf S, Goodell H. *Behavioural Science in Clinical Medicine.* Springfield, Ill: Charles C Thomas; 1976.

145. Price V. *Type A Behaviour Pattern: A Model for Research and Practice.* New York, NY: Academic Press; 1982.

146. Crompton R. *Employment and the Family: The Reconfiguration of Work and Family Life in Contemporary Societies.* Cambridge: Cambridge University Press. 2006.

147. Windebank J. Dual-earner couples in Britain and France. *Work Employment and Society.* 2001;15 (2):269-290.

148. Gregory A, Windebank J. *Women's Work in Britain and France.* Houndmills: Macmillan; 2000.

149. Dean H. Tipping the balance: the problematic nature of work–life balance in a low-income neighbourhoods. *Journal of Social Policy.* 2007;36(4):519-537.

150. Monk T. Coping with the stress of shift work. *Work and Stress.* 1988;2:169-172.

151. Dinges D, Whitehouse W, Carota-Orne E, Orne M. The benefits of a nap during prolonged work and wakefulness. *Work and Stress.* 1988;2:139-153.

152. Rosa R, Colligan M. Long workdays versus restdays: assessing fatigue and alertness with a portable performance battery. *Human Factors.* 1988;5:87-98.

153. Barrett H, Browne A. Workloads of rural African women: the impact of economic adjustment in Sub-Saharan Africa. *Journal of Occupational Science: Australia.* 1993;2:3-11.

154. Barrett H. Women, occupation and health in rural Africa: Adaptation to a changing socioeconomic climate. *Journal of Occupational Science: Australia.* 1997;4(3):93-105.

155. Ferguson A. Women's health in a marginal area of Kenya. *Social Science and Medicine.* 1986;23:17-29.

156. Galvaan R. Domestic workers narratives: transforming occupational therapy practice. In: Kronenberg F, Algado S, Pollard N, eds. *Occupational Therapy without Borders: Learning from the Spirit of Survivors.* Edinburgh: Elsevier Churchill Livingstone; 2005:429-439.

157. Whiteford G. Problemizing life balance: difference, diversity and disadvantage. In: Matuska K, Christiansen CH, eds. *Life balance: Multidisciplinary Theories and Research.* Thorofare, NJ: Slack Inc. and AOTA Press; 2009:23-31.

158. Gare S. The age of overwork. *The Weekend Australian Review.* 1995;April 8-9:2-3.

159. Schor J. *The Overworked American: The Unexpected Decline of Leisure.* New York, NY: Basic Books; 1991.

160. Simon R. The joys of parenthood, reconsidered. *Contexts.* 2008; 7:41-48.

161. Karasek R, Theorell T. *Healthy Work.* New York: Basic Books; 1990.

162. Friedman M, Rosenman R. *Type A Behavior and Your Heart.* New York: Knopf; 1974.

163. *Stress.* Better Health Channel. Available at: http://www.betterhealth.vic.gov.au/bhcv2/bhcarticles.nsf/pages/Stress?open. Accessed August 12, 2013.

164. Oatley K, Keltner D, Jenkins J. *Emotions and Mental Health in Childhood. Understanding Emotions.* 2nd ed. Oxford, UK: Blackwell Publishing; 2006.

165. Adams JD, ed. *Understanding and Managing Stress: A Book of Readings.* Calif: University Associates Inc; 1980.

166. Selye H. A syndrome produced by diverse nocuous agents. *Nature.* 1936;138:32.

167. Selye H. In: Monat A, Lazarus RS, eds. *Stress and Coping: An Anthology.* 2nd ed. New York, NY: Columbia University Press; 1985:25.

168. Selye H. *The Stress of Life.* New York, NY: McGraw-Hill; 1976.

169. Kobasa SC, Maddi SR, Courington S. Personality and constitution as mediators in the stress-illness relationship. *Journal of Health and Social Behavior.* 1981;22:368-378.

170. French JRP, Caplan RD. Organizational stress and individual strain. In: Marrow AJ, ed. *The Failure of Success.* New York, NY: Amacon; 1972:30-66.

171. McQuade W, Aikman A. *Stress.* New York, NY: EP Dutton and Co; 1974.

172. Roskies E, Lazarus RS. Coping theory and the teaching of coping skills. In: Davidson PO, Davidson SM, eds. *Behavioural Medicine: Changing Health Lifestyles.* New York, NY: Brunner/Mazel; 1980.

173. Moore JC. *Neurosciences and Their Application to Occupational Therapy.* Unpublished lecture notes. Neuroscience Conference, Adelaide, 1989:185.

174. Temoshok L. On attempting to articulate the biopsychosocial model: psychology-psychophysiological homeostasis. In: Friedman HS, ed. *Personality and Disease.* New York, NY: John Wiley and Sons; 1990:211.

175. Cohen S, Janicki-Deverts D, Miller G. Psychological stress and disease. *Journal of the American Medical Association.* 2007;298(14):1685-1687.

176. Steptoe A. The links between stress and illness. *Journal of Psychosomatic Research.* 1991;35:633-644.

177. Hallman T. *Gender Perspectives on Psychosocial Risk Factors: Conditions Governing Women's Lives in Relation to Stress and Coronary Heart Disease.* Doctoral thesis. Stockholm, Sweden: Dept. of Clinical Neuroscience, Karolinska Institutet. 2003.

178. Stress Management. *Life Extension.* http://www.lef.org/protocols/emotional_health/stress_management_01.htm. Accessed August 12, 2003.

179. Jameson L, Jameson B. *Brain Injury Survivors Guide: Welcome to our World.* Outskirts Press. 2007.

180. Thaker P, Lutgendorf S, Sood A. The neuroendocrine impact of chronic stress on cancer. *Cell Cycle.* 2007;6(4):430-433.

181. Eiland L, et al. Early life stress followed by subsequent adult chronic stress potentiates anxiety and blunts hippocampal structural remodeling. *Hippocampus.* 2010;Sep 16.

182. Saul A, et al. Chronic stress and susceptibility to skin cancer. *Journal of the National Cancer Institute.* 2005;97(23):1760-1767.

183. Liu R, et al. Stress generation in depression: a systematic review of the empirical literature and recommendations for future study. *Clinical Psychology Review.* 2010;30(5):582-93.

184. Chrousos G. The stress response and immune function: clinical implications. *Ann N Y Acad Sci,* 2000;917:38-67.

185. Tak L. Meta-analysis and meta-regression of hypothalamic-pituitary-adrenal axis activity in functional somatic disorders. *Biol Psychology.* 2011;87(2):183-194.

186. Sapolsky R. Endocrinology of the stress-response. *Behavioral Endocrinology.* 2nd ed. Cambridge, MA: MIT Press: 2002:409-450.

187. Wu J. Adrenal insufficiency in prolonged critical illness. *Crit Care.* 2008;12(3):R65.

188. Sakihara S, et al. Ampulla (Takotsubo) cardiomyopathy caused by secondary adrenal insufficiency in ACTH isolated deficiency. *Endocr J.* 2007;54(4):631-636.

189. Korlakunta H, et al. Transient left ventricular apical ballooning: a novel heart syndrome. *International Journal of Cardiology.* 2005;102(2):351-353.

190. Mechanic D. Effects of psychological distress on perceptions of physical health and use of medical and psychiatric facilities. *J Human Stress.* 1978;4:26-32.

191. Saleeby JP. *Wonder Herbs: A Guide to Three Adaptogens,* Xlibris: 2006.

192. Life Extension: Foundation for Longer Life. *Health Concerns: Stress Management.* http://www.lef.org/protocols/emotional_health/stress_management_01.htm. Accessed May 30, 2014.

193. Bleuler M. Conception of schizophrenia within the last fifty years and today. *Proceedings of the Royal Society of Medicine.* 1963;56:945-952

194. Rosenthal D. A suggested conceptual framework. In: Rosenthal D, ed. *The Genian Quadruplets.* New York: Basic Books; 1963:505-516.

195. Ingram R. Luxton D. Vulnerability-stress models. In: Hankin B, Abela J, eds. *Development of Psychopathology: A Vulnerability Stress Perspective.* Thousand Oaks, CA; Sage: 2005:32-46.

196. Prevention Action. *Diathesis-Stress Models.* http://www.preventionaction.org/reference/diathesis-stress-models. Accessed August 23, 2013.

197. Lazarus R. From psychological stress to the emotions: A history of changing outlooks. *Annual Review of Psychology.* 1993;44:1-21.

198. Newton C. *Understanding Mental Disorders.* Available at: http://www.clairenewton.co.za/understanding-mental-disorders.html (accessed August 23, 2013).

199. Smith LA, Roman A, Dollard MF, Winefield AH, Siegrist J. Effort reward imbalance at work: the effects of work stress on anger and cardiovascular disease symptoms in a community sample. *Stress and Health.* 2005;21:113-128.

200. Dollard MF, Dormann C, Boyd CM, Winefield HR, Winefield AH. Unique aspects of stress in human service work. *Australian Psychologist.* 2003;38:84-91.

201. Winefield AH, Gillespie NA, Stough C, Dua J, Hapuarachchi J, Boyd C. Occupational stress in Australian university staff: results from a national survey. *International Journal of Stress Management.* 2003;10:51-63.

202. Dollard MF, Winefield AH, Winefield HR, eds. *Occupational Stress in the Service Professions.* London: Taylor and Francis; 2003.

203. Winwood PC, Winefield AH, Lushington K. The role of occupational stress in the maladaptive use of alcohol by dentists: a study of South Australian general dental practitioners. *Australian Dental Journal.* 2003:48:102-109.

204. Mindhealthconnect. *Stress. Types of Stress.* http://www.mindhealthconnect.org.au/stress Accessed June 3, 2014.

205. Nolen-Hoeksema S. *Suicide. Abnormal Psychology.* 4th ed. New York, NY: McGraw-Hill; 2008.

206. Monroe S, Simons A. Diathesis-stress theories in the context of life stress research: implications for depressive disorders. *Psychological Bulletin.* 1991;110:406-425.

207. Livestrong.com. *Common Stress Related Medical Conditions.* http://www.livestrong.com/article/95992-common-stressrelated-medical-conditions/. Accessed May 30, 2014.

208. Mayo Clinic staff. Stress getting to you? Try some of these tips for stress relief. Stress relievers: Tips to tame stress. *Mayo Clinic: Health Information.* http://www.mayoclinic.com/health/stress-relievers/MY01373. Accessed August 22, 2013.

209. Hanley J, Randomised controlled trial of therapeutic massage in the management of stress. *The British Journal of General Practice.* 2003;53:20-25.

210. Field T. Cortisol decreases and serotonin and dopamine increase following massage therapy. *The International Journal of Neuroscience.* 2005;115 (10):1397-1413.

211. Dixit S. Executive fatigue and its management with Mentat. *Pharmacopsychoecologia.* 1993;6:7-9.

212. Barker S, Wolen A. The benefits of human-companion animal interaction: a review. *Journal of Veterinary Medical Education.* 2008;35(4):487-95.

213. Friedmann E, Son H. The human-companion animal bond: how humans benefit. *Veterinary Clinics of North America: Small Animal Practice.* 2009;39(2):293-326.

214. Allen K, et al. Pet ownership, but not ace inhibitor therapy, blunts home blood pressure responses to mental stress. *Hypertension.* 2001;38(4):815-20.

215. Kalaitzakis E. Is fatigue related to suppression of hypothalamic-pituitary-adrenal axis activity by bile acids in chronic liver disease? *Medical Hypotheses.* 2011;77(3):464-465.

216. Head K. Nutrients and botanicals for treatment of stress: adrenal fatigue, neurotransmitter imbalance, anxiety, and restless sleep. *Alternative Medicine Review.* 2009;14(2):114-140.

217. Wirth M. Shiftwork duration and the awakening cortisol response among police officers. *Chronobiology International.* 2011;28(5):446-457.

218. Ping J, et al. Inheritable stimulatory effects of caffeine on steroidogenic acute regulatory protein expression and cortisol production in human adrenocortical cells. *Chemico-Biological Interactions.* 2012;195(1):68-75.

219. Lovallo W. Cortisol responses to mental stress, exercise, and meals following caffeine intake in men and women. *Pharmacology Biochemistry and Behavior.* 2006;83(3):441-447.

Theme 12

"The enjoyment of the highest attainable standard of health is one of the fundamental rights of every human being without distinction of race, religion, political belief, economic or social condition."

WHO: Rio Political Declaration on Social Determinants of Health, 2011

Theme 12

"The enjoyment of the highest attainable standard of health is one of the fundamental rights of every human being without distinction of race, religion, political belief, economic or social condition"

WHO: Rio Political Declaration on Social Determinants of Health, 2011[1]

Chapter 12

OCCUPATION AS AN AGENT OF POPULATION HEALTH

This chapter addresses:
- Historical Overview of Occupation-Focused Directives for Population Health
  - Prehistory to Modern Medicine
- An Interpretation of Population Health
- Occupation, Population, Natural Health, and Biological Needs
  - Role of Occupation in Terms of Natural Health and Survival
  - Occupation and Current Health Practices
- Population Health Through Doing, Being, Belonging, and Becoming
  - Meeting the Prerequisites
    - Collective, Corporate, and Organizational Occupation
  - Achieving Physical, Mental, and Social Well-Being
- United Nations and World Health
- Conclusion

In this chapter, ideas that have been discussed previously about occupation as a potential agent of population health will be drawn into an occupational perspective. The focus will be on both the positive and the negative; people doing, being, belonging, and becoming well, or doing, being, belonging, and becoming ill. The chapter begins with a summary of the gradual development of modern views of health, so that the useful advice about creating or maintaining health that has surfaced throughout human history can be borne in mind. However, because we live in the present, ideas that are in line with WHO directives and have provided chapter themes will be the major guides. The discussion leads naturally to the last section of the book that brings together occupation-focused ideas to improve population health.

Wilcock AA, Hocking C.
An Occupational Perspective of Health, Third Edition (pp 334-366).
© 2015 Taylor & Francis Group.

Historical Overview of Occupation-Focused Directives for Population Health

To consider 21st century directions, it is necessary to pull together the part played by changing global and national politics, spiritual beliefs and philosophical mores, sociocultural contexts, and changing technologies. Histories of health and disease,[2-4] and of occupational therapy[5-8] have traced developments in occupation's connections to health from the earliest times. These suggest the intimacy of the relationship.

PREHISTORY TO MODERN MEDICINE

At first, occupation was driven by biological need and natural health that gradually coexisted with concepts of spirit or magic. During that time and for millennia, health was dependent on occupation: what and how people went about their lives, what they did alone and with others, how they felt about what they did, and continual exploration to improve their experiences. In terms of illness, a seeking out of shelter, food, or environment that appeared to reduce both symptoms and course of illness is likely, along with rest, support from community members, and possibly advice from spiritual leaders or those seen to have special healing skills. In China, rules of health were linked to a belief that all creation emanates from the relationship of the polar opposites (Yin and Yang) connected via a circular harmony. Examples are night and day, cold and hot, wet and dry, body and mind, and, in terms of health, harmony and health or disharmony and disease. The latter required restoration of harmony through acupuncture, herbs, and food.[9] In the West, throughout Arabia and Europe, what was originally based on common sense, trial and error, and folklore resulted in the long-used Classical Greek rules of health. Based on naturalistic observation, it has already been observed that the four elements of air, fire, water, and earth that are the foundation stone of the rules are closely related to the four basic requirements of life itself—oxygen, warmth, water, and food—the four humors being determined as "the things that make up its (the human body) constitution, and causes its pains, and health."[10] Treatment was aimed at correcting imbalance.

Within those explanations, occupation, as related to everyday aspects of life, was recognized for its potential as exercise and interwoven with ideas about healthy rest, nutrition, personality type, environment, and emotional tone. The rules were particularly useful across the ages when medicine had no sophisticated tools to aid recovery. An example is provided by St Benedict's 6th century interpretation that labor is necessary for a healthy soul, and that a healthy soul is essential for a healthy body and mind. The inclusion of occupation as a curative agent was embedded in medical practice for millennia. No clear-cut difference was made between social, mental, and physical health. People were much more holistic in their views enmeshing "body and soul, flesh and spirit, mind and matter," and bodily condition and the fluctuations between health and sickness interlocked with social ideas about identity, destiny, moral, and spiritual well-being.[11]

As germ theories arose in the 19th century, health became understood as more complex than the absence of disease and living wisely according to a set of rules, yet the natural truths that formed the basis of the earlier theories have been revisited to some extent by the WHO's directives. These offer an overarching picture that is inclusive of physical, mental, and social well-being, as well as medical explanations of infectious, autoimmune, genetic, noncommunicable, nutritional, social, and behavioral disease.[12] The WHO has sought to rectify how the health and well-being lifestyle factors encompassing what people do in their daily lives were initially overlooked in favor of communal, economic, and sociopolitical gains. However, the call for policy makers of all kinds to recognize the health consequences of their courses of action remains problematic despite directives of the WHO about the social determinants of health and the call for the development of healthy cities.

Table 12-1

ABBREVIATED HISTORY OF THE USE OF OCCUPATION FOR POPULATION HEALTH AND WELL-BEING

Activists	Occupation-Focused Initiatives
Hippocrates and Galen, Physicians	Activity and rest, food and drink, sleep and waking, evacuation and repletion, affections of the soul
St. Benedict and Monastic Rule	Spiritual health through labor, prayer, good works, and pilgrimage
More, Philosopher/Statesman	Utopianism
Pare and Mercurialis, Physicians	Occupation as exercise
Ramazzini, Physician	Occupational health and safety
Howard, Philanthropist	Hospital and prison research, environmental and social conditions
Pinel, Tuke, Browne, Moral Treatment	Justice, benevolence, and occupation
Owen, Industrialist/Socialist	Education, community development, housing, industrial reform
Ruskin and Morris, Arts and Crafts Philosophers	Nature of doing, social and communal reform
Chadwick, Lawyer/Politician	Industry, sanitation, public health
Southwood-Smith, Physician	Happiness and longevity, housing, mines, industry, public health
Octavia Hill, Social Environmentalist	Housing, environment, doing
Jane Addams, Social Settlements	Community and community development, women's suffrage, social health

The new public health ambitions to reduce the social determinants of illness and to create healthy cities might be considered utopian. Utopia was the name given by Sir Thomas More[13] to his vision of an ideal environment in which all people lived free, simple, and natural lives without the excesses of affluence on the one hand or deprivation, alienation, or imbalance on the other. At an international conference on utopian thought and communal experience, Hardy and Davidson recognized "the idea of contemplating the perfect society and of seeking to create it in practice has roots that run deep in human history."[14] It is apparent in work of philosophers like John Locke, who anticipated the need for a science of occupation,[15] and philanthropists like John Howard[16] who recognized that people were turned out of hospital "unfit to work, or the common mode of living." It is manifest in work of physicians such as Pare's[17] and Mercurialis'[18] therapeutic and preventive approach to using occupation as exercise, Ramazzini's recognition of the need to include occupational reform to prevent disease,[19] and in moral treatment.[20-22] It is also apparent in the work of a large group of utopian social activists during the late 18th and 19th centuries whose occupation-focused population health initiatives are catalogued in Table 12-1.

Currently, because the concept of individualism dominates postindustrial economies, health services are largely driven by individualistic research and practice, as was the case in the 1960s when Paul Shepard became the world's first professor of human ecology. At that time, he claimed:

> Many educated people today believe that only what is unique to the individual is important or creative, and turn away from talk of populations and species ... worried that ... concepts of communities and systems seemed to discount the individual ... looking instead ... to the profit motive and capitalistic formulas, in terms of efficiency, investment, and production.[23]

Ways of thinking about population health grew as views of the relationship between well-being, health, and health care systems evolved through the latter half of the 20th century. Defining population health is a fairly recent activity and definitions vary according to particular interests. However, there is growing understanding that health and well-being is influenced by human activity and the way societies are organized. Population health is concerned with the determinants of health and is, potentially, an all-encompassing field of "virtually everything that medical care aimed solely at treating illness is not."[24] If all "economic and social activity has the capacity to influence health outcomes," then population health is to do with every activity that bears on a population's well-being.[24]

The first international framework to enshrine the enjoyment of the highest attainable standard of health as a fundamental right of everyone was the Constitution of the WHO. It is an inclusive right applying to populations, as well as individuals—it encompasses the underlying determinants of health; timely and appropriate health care; and the guarantee that health care will "be exercised without discrimination of any kind."[25] For each country, there is an "obligation to take deliberate, concrete and targeted steps" toward the full realization of health for all of its people. However, the right "acknowledges resource constraints" and is "subject to progressive realization."[25]

That overview clearly shows that as human occupations and lifestyles changed so too did the ways to explain health. These were dependent on lifestyle, cultural beliefs, and scientific expertise at the time. A diagrammatic representation of two of those views indicates how aspects of doing, being, belonging, and becoming mesh with the core ideas of each model (Figure 12-1).

The first explanation of health grew from observation and knowledge as biological needs were met through accessing water, food and shelter. Individual and group occupations that were dependent on understanding the natural environment in which they lived, were made sense of by theories about psychological and physical inter-relationships and according to spiritual or mythical suppositions. Wise selection of food and habitat were paramount. That wisdom was drawn from practical knowledge of the benefits or dangers of particular environmental features and behaviour of predators, along with advice from those understood to have spiritual or healing powers.

The second explanation is current. It began with germ theories that arose in the 19th century but is now multi-factorial because health is understood to be more complex than the absence of disease. The WHO offers the overarching picture that is inclusive of physical, mental, and social well-being, as well as medical explanations of infectious, autoimmune, genetic, noncommunicable, nutritional, social, and behavioral disease.[12] Lifestyle factors based on what people do in their daily lives that are determinants of positive or negative health experiences are easily overlooked in favor of economic gains in sociopolitical or environmental planning and resource allocation. The call for policymakers of all kinds to recognize the health consequences of their decisions remains elusive.

An Interpretation of Population Health

The *Rio Political Declaration on Social Determinants of Health*[1] is the source of the chapter theme: the heart of the ideology surrounding population health. It describes how "the enjoyment of the highest attainable standard of health is one of the fundamental rights of every human being without distinction of race, religion, political belief, economic or social condition." In line with that, what people do, how they think and feel about what they do, how it connects them to others, and how they grow or diminish through the doing is intimately connected to population health, especially as much of what people do is done within communal, socioeconomic, commercial, corporate, and organizational domains. The Australian Institute of Health and Welfare explained:

> *The study of population health is focused on understanding health and disease in community, and on improving health and well-being through priority health approaches addressing the disparities in health status between social groups. There are a number of population*

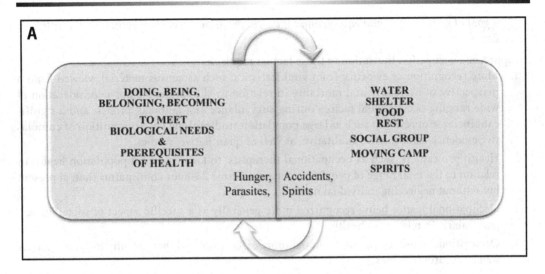

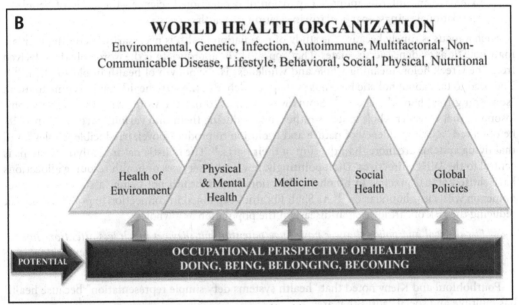

Figure 12-1. (A) Ancient and (B) modern explanations of health.

subgroups who do not enjoy the same level of health as the general population and identified as priority population groups.[26]

Focusing on issues beyond the individualistic emphasis of mainstream medicine and traditional public health approaches toward particular illness in specific groups, population health addresses "the capacity of people to adapt to, respond to, or control life's challenges and changes."[27] It focuses on factors that affect health on a population-level, such as social structures and determinants, environment, and resource distribution to complement and extend "the relatively minor impact that medicine and healthcare have on improving health overall."[28]

Increasingly, population health is a prime objective of the discipline of public health that its founders, "Farr, Chadwick, Virchow, Koch, Pasteur, and Shattuck helped to establish on the basis of four factors":

(1) Decision making based on data and evidence (vital statistics, surveillance and outbreak investigations, laboratory science); (2) a focus on populations rather than individuals; (3)

a goal of social justice and equity; and (4) an emphasis on prevention rather than curative care.[29]

To appreciate occupation in relation to those factors requires:

1. More recognition of evidence from vital statistics, such as census material, viewed from a perspective of morbidity and mortality in relation to all that people do; a consideration of wide ranging occupational factors during surveillance and outbreak probes; and a significant increase of research such as large population studies along with recognition of cumulative evidence from smaller qualitative, as well as quantitative, studies.

2. Health professions, such as occupational therapists, to focus more on population health in relation to the total range of people's occupation across 24-hour continuums than at present but without neglecting individual need.

3. Occupational justice being recognized more generally as a specific aspect of social justice, particularly in relation to health.

4. Occupational issues being incorporated more extensively and thoughtfully in preventive, as well as curative regimes.

5. Extensive and interdisciplinary expansion of occupational science—the study of people as occupational beings—particularly in relation to health.

Such a focus is timely because the study of population health is necessarily becoming increasingly holistic as evidence accumulates. That appears to be appropriate as the word holistic is derived from the Greek holos, meaning whole and wholeness is a synonym of health in old English.[30,31] The need to talk about holistic health is perhaps evidence of the term health having come to mean "something less than wholeness."[32] Smuts was the first to use the word holism to describe philosophies that consider whole systems rather than reducing them into various parts.[33-35] In 1928, he observed "a basic tendency of nature and evolution to produce novel, irreducible wholes," and that living systems are more than the sum of their parts.[36] The holistic nature of living systems is central to the WHO directives. Disappointingly, few health services or health resource allocations have shifted actual practice in a holistic direction despite health not being "a stand-alone phenomenon with clear boundaries."[37] As Shah Ebrahim explained in connection to policies aimed at reducing the risk of cardiovascular disease in the population as a whole:

Fiscal, legal and policy changes have huge potential but they get much less attention than the latest blockbuster statin. It would have much more impact, it is eminently doable today—but it will take another ten years to persuade people to do it.[38]

Pourbohloul and Kieny noted that "health systems defy simple representation" because health has multiple and social causes that are:

Interrelated with nature and nurture, and evolve over time ... Diseases and health conditions are, by and large, studied in separate silos. Policies to reduce morbidity and mortality are developed within each "disease silo."[39]

They recommend the use of new technologies to assist complex systems analysis that allow "the patterns of many real-life phenomena" to be mapped[39] because, as the WHO reminds, health systems are complex global and local networks that permeate all dimensions of human health. "Health is everybody's business."[40] It requires cooperative and collaborative approaches across wide ranging domains,[41] yet "scientific literature has demonstrated very little overlap between disciplines involved in studying complex systems and those concerned with health systems evaluation."[39]

Since Canada hosted the first International Health Promotion Congress in Ottawa in 1986, it has been a leader in the change toward positive holistic health and population wellness models. In 1994, its *Strategies for Population Health: Investing in the Health of Canadians*[42] gave emphasis to uncovering and improving the entire range of factors that determine health, with a key direction being intersectoral action. Inter-sectoral action recognizes crucial factors that determine population health are the province of many sectors. Only through action within and between sectors at

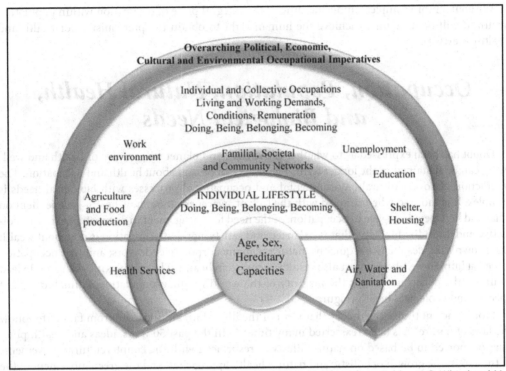

Figure 12-2. Occupational determinants of population health. (Adapted from Dahlgren G, Whitehead M. *Policies and strategies to promote equity in health.* Copenhagen: WHO Regional Office for Europe; 1992.)[43b]

local, regional, provincial, and national levels will it be possible to influence the conditions that enable and support health and well-being (Figure 12-2).[42]

In 2006, Whitehead and Dahlgren put forward 10 population health principles for policy action to the WHO Collaborating Centre for Policy Research on Social Determinants of Health in Europe. These specified that population health policies and action should promote health gains and reduce health inequities in the population as a whole by levelling up rather than down. Actions should be concerned with the social determinants of health, such as inequities, gender differences, ethnicity, geographical, and socioeconomic background and giving "voice to the voiceless."[43a] Not surprisingly, such action is applicable to the occupation-health nexus. There are inequities in people's access to prerequisites for health and health promoting occupations across many domains: between genders; across different ethnic groups; and according to people's different geographical and socioeconomic background and income. Occupationally, many are voiceless.

Ban Ki-moon, Secretary-General of the United Nations, put on record that The *Millennium Declaration* of 2000 aimed at ending poverty by 2015 was a milestone in international cooperation and the utilization of current resources and knowledge. It lead to "inspiring development efforts that have improved the lives of hundreds of millions of people around the world" even in the poorest countries and those held back by disease, geographic isolation, or civil strife.[44] The Millennium Development Goals represent the basic rights and needs of all people and mirror, to a large extent, the prerequisites of health listed in the Ottawa Charter. However, "improvements in the lives of the poor have been unacceptably slow, and some hard-won gains are being eroded by the climate, food and economic crises." Ban Ki-moon added:

> Meeting the goals is everyone's business. Falling short would multiply the dangers of our world—from instability to epidemic diseases to environmental degradation. But achieving the goals will put us on a fast track to a world that is more stable, more just, and more secure.[44]

Without a more complete understanding of the integral place of occupation within population health, it will be difficult to achieve the human right to obtain the prerequisites for health and healthy lifestyles.

Occupation, Population, Natural Health, and Biological Needs

Doubt has been expressed as to whether the species and planet will survive or health and well-being can be sustained in the longer term. The same can be said about health and occupation. The interaction of socio-cultural-environmental and occupational processes with biological needs is complex. It is more so when coupled with the lack of awareness about how health is dependent on what and how people engage in occupation; of the need for engagement in occupation at both a collective and an individual level that is balanced and satisfying; that occupation is not about wealth for its own sake despite the acquisitive nature of many corporate endeavors; and that occupation aimed at human well-being must also result in ecosystem health. The complexities can and do lead to unhealthy consequences for the majority of the world's human population, animal and plant species, and ecological health (Figure 12-3).

From "ancient times, the theory that most of the ills of humankind arise from failure to follow the laws of nature" has been reasserted many times.[45] In the past 50 years, ideas and health practices purported to be based on natural lifestyles resurfaced with the countercultural movements of the 1960s, the growth of holistic and natural health approaches, and the green movement of the present time. It is beyond the bounds of practicability to suggest that modern populations should return to a natural lifestyle based on hunter-gatherer occupations in the cause of health and happiness. However, the repeated interest in the topic suggests that keeping in touch with innate needs is important in refocusing attention on matters relating to healthy survival of the species. Whether people can achieve health through meeting natural laws that ensure health of communities and an individual's mind, body, and spirit is problematic. In many respects, the structure and value systems that determine which, how, and why particular needs can be met and what, how and why people and communities get to do, be, belong and become is socioculturally determined. Added to that is medicine's overwhelming attention to healing and success in counteracting what sometimes appear to be insurmountable odds. That may account for the current fascination with the reversal of illness rather than natural health—with flouting rather than following recommendations for healthy living. Advances in medicine to overcome the effects of illness and disability are indeed remarkable and valuable. They are also expensive and out of the reach of many of the world's populations, making health and well-being from that source an unequal possibility.

The exploration detailed in previous chapters leads to the proposition that all people still need to make use of their biological capacities if they are to enjoy health and well-being, and reduce the need to use medical breakthroughs aimed at the reversal of illness. For people to flourish, they not only need to meet the prerequisites of health, but also an apparent need for action, purpose, meaning, connectedness, and self-actualization. It is the total range of people's physical, obligatory, meaningful, shared, and fulfilling doings that can maintain homeostasis, ensure social connectedness, and provide sufficient exercise to keep communities, bodies, minds, and spirit functioning efficiently. Studies have demonstrated that even older people who lead active lives, continuing with a wide range of occupations, tend to feel better and to require less medical attention than those who are isolated and sedentary.[46,47] "The best sort of exercise in terms of retaining one's powers is the kind you don't call exercise."[48] Doing a multitude of occupations can enhance, or at the very least, maintain joint stability and range, muscle tone, cardiovascular fitness, respiratory capacity, and keep weight in check, without undue consideration of body functioning; provide psychological stimulation and a balance between physical and mental challenges and relaxation; and provide a

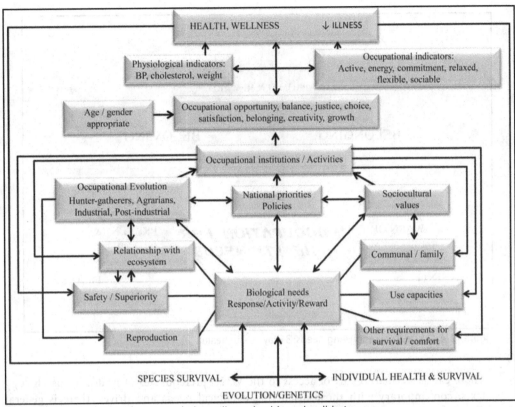

Figure 12-3. Occupational factors underlying illness, health, and well-being.

vehicle that enables socialization and the realization of shared and unique interests, talents, and skills.

In Chapter 4, it was proposed that there is a 3-way link between survival, health, and occupation. This proposal has been supported by the wide-ranging exploration undertaken in this search for an occupational perspective of health. Throughout time, occupation has provided the mechanism for people to fulfill biological needs essential for survival, to adapt to environmental changes, to develop and exercise genetic capacities to maintain health, and, for some populations, communities and individuals to flourish. However, a downside to the mechanism has also been uncovered: it has the capacity to lead to the creation of societies and ways of life that are far from health-maintaining; that increase the health divide between "the haves and the have nots"; and that is so powerful that it could result in the demise of the world as we know it, because of failure to halt occupation that leads to potentially irreversible ecological degradation or to its destruction, through national and religious power plays.

An individual's biological needs were described well by Wolman in the 1970s as "a force in the brain which directs and organizes the individual's perception, thinking, and action, so as to change an existing, unsatisfying situation."[49] From the ideas that have been unearthed, it is also possible to propose that needs, from a homeostatic perspective, have a 3-way role in maintaining the stability and health of the organism through occupation prompted by a specific feeling. Three categories of needs provide both motivation and feedback: they serve to warn when a problem occurs; to protect and prevent potential disorder; and to prompt and reward use of capacities so that the organism will flourish and reach potential (Figure 12-4):

1. To warn and protect, "primary doing needs" are experienced as a form of discomfort that calls for some kind of action to satisfy or assuage the need. Examples of these experiences are cold, hunger, pain, fatigue, fear, boredom, tension, depression, anxiety, anger, or loneliness.

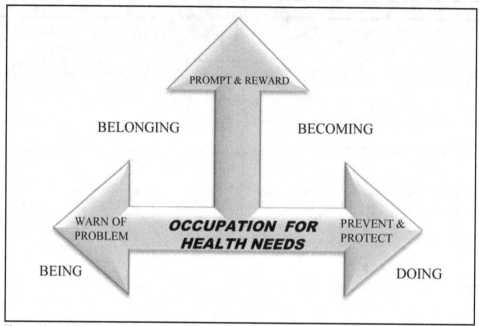

Figure 12-4. Occupation prompting needs: 3-way role in health.

Those can be related to lack of access to the WHO prerequisites of health. In psychology texts, contemporary with those discussing biological needs and drives, there is general acceptance that people engage in some activities that do not involve purposive "foresight" or "distant ends"; that people are inclined toward action, or experience an impulse toward action, that is conducive to biological well-being.[50,51] Csikszentmihalyi[52] uses the term *psychic entropy* when he discusses people's integrated responses to the "self-system," that has a main goal to "ensure its own survival." Many studies have researched these experiences as separate emotions.[53-56] In addition, they have explored whether "psychological well-being and ill-being comprise opposite ends of a bi-polar continuum, or are best construed as separate, independent dimensions of mental health."[57]

2. To prevent disorder and prompt the use of capacities, "doing needs" are experienced in a positive action sense, such as a need to spend extra energy, walk, explore, create, understand or make sense of, use ideas, express thoughts, talk, listen or look, meditate or worship, spend time alone or with others, and so on. This mechanism, in interaction with the first, acts to balance over- or under-use as discussed in Chapter 12.

3. To reward the use of capacities, there are being, belonging, and becoming needs, such as for meaning, purpose, satisfaction, relationships, fulfillment, pleasure, and happiness. Happiness has been recognized as a powerful human need by many writers, from Aristotle more than 2000 years ago, to public health pioneers like Southwood-Smith,[58] to more recent researchers who maintain that pleasure is biologically related to health promoting activity, physically triggered in areas of the limbic system.[52,59-67] This does not mean that pleasure is the ultimate drive of humans, but rather that it forms an integral part of health maintenance.[56,66]

Together, the second and the third categories of needs serve to establish a sense of identity and autonomy, the latter being recognized by Doyal and Gough as one of two universal needs, the other being physical health. In the negative terms of their concept, physical health is the "minimization of death, disability and disease," and autonomy includes minimization of "mental illness, cognitive deprivation, and restricted opportunities."[68]

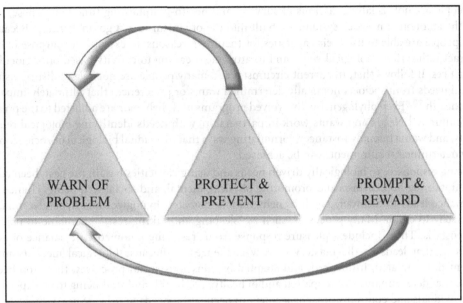

Figure 12-5. Biological–based occupation feedback loop warns of unmet needs.

The proposal that biologically based occupation needs have this 3-way role in maintaining stability and health was tested in a survey of 150 subjects with ages ranging from 6 to 98 years (mean: 35 years).[69] Asked if they had experienced such needs, 99% admitted they had experienced all 3 types and had acted on them. Failure to do so resulted in up to 99% of respondents experiencing the type of discomfort described in the first category. This acts as a feedback warning mechanism. The majority of those surveyed reported that they consider the satisfaction of the three categories of needs to affect their mental, physical, and social health in a positive way (Figure 12-5).

People's intellectual and cognitive capacity, freed by the mechanism of choice, has enabled satisfaction of those needs despite diverse challenges that have been addressed over time. In affluent nations, action to satisfy or assuage discomfort, such as the regulation of temperature, the acquisition of water and a wide range of food, or measures to reduce pain have reached a level of sophistication far beyond the simple methods used by early humans living in natural habitats.

To prevent disorder, people have developed ways of using their capacities in adaptive, inventive, and exploratory fashions to the extent that they can provide meaning and purpose, as well as prompt the pursuit of potential and reward with happiness, self-esteem, and belonging. In fact, these needs have focused human energies toward developing both occupations and sociocultural structures to meet them. Because of this, people have been successful survivors—to the point of overpopulation. There are downsides to the mechanism of choice in that people can "act in ways that [go] against the millennial wisdom that natural selection had built into the biological fabric of the species."[56] The capacity to ignore biological needs in either a general or a particular way enables people to sanction the development of sociopolitical structures and action, or make lifestyle choices, that result in detrimental health consequences for all or some members of the population. War is a prime example. Another is the occupational restrictions that were the common lot of all women until fairly recently, and remain the case for many. Political, social, and occupational gender injustices in advanced economies were only lessened in the 20th century as a result of extreme action taken by women. Women's suffrage is a prime example, when deliberate starvation was a chosen occupation of extremists to force attention to the social and occupational injustices of the system. Currently, starvation to achieve a fashionable appearance is another socially driven occupational option for some, and another example of the possibility for people to make unhealthy choices to the point of untimely death.

People are not usually conscious of survival and health-maintaining functions. These, rather like the autonomic nervous system, are built into the organism to just go on working. Because of this, people are able to use their capacities for their own reasons, to explain the purpose of life in abstract rather than biological ways, and to attribute meaning to activity based on sociocultural influences. It follows that, in current circumstances, many people are not able to distinguish biological needs from socioeconomically determined wants or preferences that ultimately impact on their health.[70] "Even phylogenetically evolved programs of ... behavior are adjusted to the presence of a culture."[71] Needs and wants work in partnership, with needs identifying biological requirements, and wants in many instances, formulating ways that individual biological or socioeconomically determined requirements can be achieved.

Being responsive to biologically driven needs and using capacities has, in the past, been central to maintaining homeostasis and promoting physical, mental, and social well-being. Homeostatic imbalance leads to disorders, such as dehydration, diabetes, hypoglycemia, hyperglycemia, and ultimately to death. Many processes, such as "sleeping and taking rest,"[72] combine to maintain homeostasis. These include a pleasure response from "restoring a homeostatic balance of bodily needs ... that leads to the mastery of new challenges."[73] Because biological mechanisms are informed, stimulated, influenced, and adapted by conscious social processes, these too become influential determinants of occupation and of health. For health and well-being to be experienced by individuals and communities, engagement in occupation needs to provide not only the prerequisites, but also a balanced use of capacities; meaning; a sense of belonging; social credit; optimal opportunity for desired growth toward potential; and flexibility to develop and change according to context, choice, and corporate-political initiatives. Such engagement, if it is in accord with sociocultural values and ecological sustainability, will enable populations, communities, families, and individuals to flourish and the species to survive. However, because needs are not omnipotent, a lack of awareness about health's dependence on engagement in balanced and satisfying occupation can lead to unhealthy consequences because of the complexity of the interaction with medical, political, sociocultural, and economic occupations and processes.

Some of the features of natural health and biological needs as they relate to what people do, be, belong, and strive to become that have surfaced are provided in Table 12-2.

ROLE OF OCCUPATION IN TERMS OF NATURAL HEALTH AND SURVIVAL

The discussion in previous chapters about how humans have evolved over millennia has established that the inbuilt need to engage in occupation is a major biological characteristic enabling survival and natural health. Four major inbuilt functions of occupation have been identified according to past and current research, and the thoughts of scholars and health activists over time. From those sources, occupation as an agent of health is described in this text, in terms of:

1. Doing to provide and develop:
   - The prerequisites of health at a global level—for immediate bodily needs of sustenance, self-care, and shelter of all people
   - Population and collective occupations, skills, political, social, and socioeconomic structures and technology aimed at the maintenance of supportive and caring environments, safety and superiority over dangers, ecological disasters, and predators of any kind
   - Exercise of body, mind, and spirit of individuals and groups though challenge, utilization of capacities, energy, and enjoyment tempered by appropriate rest
2. Being to maintain health through:
   - Contemplation, planning, reflection, and reasoned consideration of what can and needs to be done to meet the prerequisites of health.

Table 12-2

EMERGING FEATURES OF NATURAL HEALTH AND BIOLOGICAL NEEDS RELATING TO DOING, BEING, BECOMING, AND BELONGING

- The links between human biology, human need, the natural environment, social and occupational behaviors, health and illness are dynamic.
- The encounters of human communities with new environmental hazards have led to changes in occupational form and performance and subsequent experience of health and illness.
- There is a recurring tension between biological needs and changes in living conditions that is manifest in both occupation and health and illness.
- The impact of changes from natural, to rural, to urban living along with population aging is manifest in occupational structures, performance and technology and patterns of health and illness.
- Health and illness are products of biological variability coupled with the meeting of biological needs, social and occupational behaviors and relationships, and environmental possibilities or constraints.
- Adaptiveness provides more chance (relative to others) of some individuals or communities surviving and reproducing in given social, occupational and environmental situations.
- Health and illness affect the chances of individuals to survive and reproduce. Those who do are able to extend the social and occupational environment best suited to their needs into the future. In turn this affects the health and survival of future humans.
- Participation in occupations directly related to the health and maintenance of the organism and survival can be in tune with the natural world, and must be so in terms of long-term species survival.
- Occupational behavior that fails to meet biological, social and environmental needs can result in failure to flourish, because of a reduction of physical mental or social well-being, the occurrence of illness, and possibly premature death.
- The complexity of the interaction between occupation and political, sociocultural and economic processes obscures the direct links between the occupations of individuals, families, communities, and populations, and health and illness experiences.

- Occupations that enable individuals, families, and communities to find meaning and purpose; understanding that other people have to meet being needs; encouraging satisfactory and balanced exercise of occupational capacities with rest and relaxation.
- Planning of and reflection on pleasurable or challenging pursuits.

3. Belonging to ensure social well-being through:
    - Occupations undertaken with and for others.
    - The forging of links and bonds in shared interests and pursuits.
    - Supportive social relationships maintained through occupation.
    - Enabling or participating in economic, developmental, and sociopolitical occupations that link and bond people in rich and environmentally friendly ways.

4. Becoming and developing physical, mental and social well-being through:
    - Occupation that enables all people to meet the prerequisites of health.
    - Occupation that enables reaching out toward personal potential and individual improvement.
    - Occupation with and for others so that each person and community can grow stronger and happier.
    - Reflecting and acting on occupational issues so that the population, the species, and the environment will flourish.

OCCUPATION AND CURRENT HEALTH PRACTICES

Previous chapters have identified that engagement in a broad range of occupations is integral to all of the prerequisites needed for people to experience health. In addition, it is central to positive well-being at individual, familial, communal, and population levels. It can also be a negative factor in people's experience of health, if occupational needs are not met adequately.

Occupation, as the total range of activities discussed in this text, is poorly understood. It is researched in a disjointed fashion by different disciplines. The aspects best recognized by medically focused disciplines are "occupation as work" and "occupations as risk factors." That understanding is reflected in the population at large and in media reports. This may be because of the current interest in all things medical and particularly of curative substances or procedures to remedy disorders that are feared as disabling or likely to cause early death, or it may be because occupation as work is central to obtaining income, food, shelter, and community approval.

Public health practitioners are addressing some but not all of the range of occupational needs that have been identified. They, too, focus on work, as well as advocating for physical activity, community development, and sociopolitical changes to promote better health for populations as a whole, but do not necessarily recognize the interactive occupational nature within those components. They demonstrate less interest in research or programs aimed at occupational health through the finding of meaning, satisfaction, purpose, belonging, and becoming through doing. In addition to work and income, they evince separate interest in other occupation-based prerequisites of health, such as food, social justice, and equity, and shelter in terms of "healthy cities." The WHO describes a healthy city as:

> One that is continually creating and improving those physical and social environments and expanding those community resources which enable people to mutually support each other in performing all the functions of life and in developing to their maximum potential.[74]

In 2013, the WHO asserted that the key principles of creating healthy settings include community participation, partnership, empowerment, and equity.[75] Occupation is central in both descriptions, with obvious key words being "performing," "functions," "community participation," "developing to their maximum potential," and "empowerment and equity." These can be met through people being permitted and encouraged to do whatever is required to meet their doing, being, belonging, and becoming needs.

Practitioners in the field of occupational health and safety, on the whole, limit their interest to issues concerned with work as opposed to the total range of people's activities, with the International Labor Organization upholding their early view of occupational health as "the adaptation of work to man and of each man to his job."[76] Similarly, occupational medicine, as described in Chapter 5, is defined as "the prevention and treatment of diseases and injuries occurring at work or in specific occupations."[77] Recognition of the wider picture that includes the impact of work on relationships and other aspects of life is developing gradually in this field, so that the term *life balance* is beginning to supersede the more common work-life balance.[78]

Occupational therapists, who evince interest in the occupational nature of humans as a whole, are addressing some but not all doing, being, belonging, or becoming needs. They demonstrate more concern for the substrata of people who are disadvantaged by physical or mental disability that leaves the great majority of people without access to information that might assist understanding of the health impact of their occupations. Their practice largely relates to individuals rather than community or populations, and to pockets of interest according to the availability of their own employment opportunities. That limits the focus of interventions to directives given by medical or other senior health or community personnel whose requests may mirror their own area of expertise or restrictions imposed by administration, often in the name of economy. In the last decades this has led to more concentration on self-care and functional skills rather than in people finding meaning and self-actualization through what they do. Hammell addressed these issues, suggesting that:

> *Although espousing the importance of meaning in occupation, occupational therapy theory has been primarily preoccupied with purposeful occupations and thus appears inadequate to address issues of meaning within people's lives...the fundamental orientation of occupational therapy should be the contributions that occupation makes to meaning in people's lives, furthering the suggestion that occupation might be viewed as comprising dimensions of meaning: doing, being, belonging and becoming.[79]*

The being, belonging, and becoming aspects of occupation are seldom addressed by occupational therapists in current times except in rhetoric, although earlier approaches had wider purposes. Hammell believed that a greater focus on meaning will more closely align occupational therapists with an "espoused aspiration to enable the enhancement of quality of life."[79] This coincides with Hocking's call for occupational therapists to revisit in practice their earlier focus on Romantic as opposed to rational ideologies:

> *Most pertinent here is the Romantics' belief in self-creation, that each man could invent himself, fashion his own character, or by heroic effort, transform himself. This is achieved, in part, by construing one's world of desires, values, meanings and physical circumstances.[80]*

Some occupational therapists are receptive to the broad ideas of population health articulated by the WHO. The British College of Occupational Therapist's 2002 strategy *From Interface to Integration* that embraces the directives of both the WHO's *International Classification of Functioning (ICF)* and the Ottawa Charter is a case in point (Figure 12-6).

The American Occupational Therapy Foundation also expresses interest in the broader terms of population health on their website, where they draw attention to papers such as the United Nations' *Millennium Development Goals*[44] to do the following:

1. Eradicate extreme poverty and hunger
2. Achieve universal primary education
3. Promote gender equality and empower women
4. Reduce child mortality
5. Improve maternal health
6. Combat HIV/AIDS, malaria, and other diseases
7. Ensure environmental sustainability
8. Develop a global partnership for development.

The interest has not yet manifest in wide ranging, well-recognized programs or multidisciplinary action that address the occupational nature of health and illness. More attention to, or advocacy for, population health approaches to embrace doing, being, belonging, and becoming within health promotion schemes is called for. This also requires advocacy to acquire adequate resources to fund such programs. In current socioeconomic climates that would necessitate attention to how the economic benefits would outweigh the costs of establishing programs.

For any health profession, the teasing out of positive or negative health attributes of occupation is difficult, even though it is relatively easy to see that there is a correlation between health and obvious survival occupations. The correlation between health and the biological need of humans to engage in other types of occupations tends to be obscure, is complex, and is poorly researched. However, because of the variety and complexity of the occupational needs that are prerequisite to meeting the four functions listed in the previous section, alienation, deprivation, imbalance, and occupational stress are possible, as are medically recognized disorders of occupation. These may differ for particular groupings within any given population. In addition, if the needs are not recognized for what they are, political will could establish occupational expectations of a population that are counter to long-term survival of the species and the health of people over a lifetime.

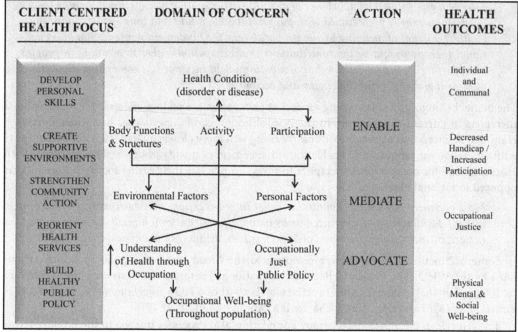

Figure 12-6. College of Occupational Therapists Strategy 2002: A mix of the WHO Ottawa Charter for Health Promotion and International Classification of Function. (Reprinted with permission from the British Association of Occupational Therapists, 2002.)

Population Health Through Doing, Being, Belonging, and Becoming

Over the past two decades renewed attention has been given to the business of improving population health through:
1.   Increasing the number of people able to meet the prerequisites of health
2.   Action toward physical, mental and social well-being.

MEETING THE PREREQUISITES

In the preceding chapters, doing, being, belonging, and becoming have been considered in terms of meeting the prerequisites for health. Not surprisingly, when the fundamental nature of occupation is considered, they are central to all aspects. Food, income, and shelter embrace a large range of daily and occasional occupations that relate to obtaining, preparing, caring for, and using them; formal or informal education is an ongoing occupational process that continually impacts on future lives; peace has to be worked at constantly—personally, communally, and internationally; as does maintaining a stable ecosystem and sustainable resources; and social justice and equity has to be acted on and fought for in almost all fields of human activity.

Although occupation has mostly been viewed in health circles as of individual concern, all human doing relates to health, and the increasingly global nature of living in the world means that collective doings have enormous significance in occupation for health terms. One of the factors emerging from those considerations is that improving population health relates to economic development. Development is the result of occupational forces usually driven initially by individual action and later by corporate and political action. In 2000, the WHO established The Commission on Macroeconomics and Health to "assess the contribution of health to global economic development."[81] Macroeconomics focuses on economic collective forces at a national level, such as national income, monetary policies, total employment, production, consumption, inflation, and international factors, such as trade imports and exports. In its report to the WHO, the Commission pronounced that "health is a creator and pre-requisite of development," arguing that improvement of health could be a stratagem toward poverty reduction and income growth in low- and middle-income countries.[81] In a subsequent report about the impact of health on the economy in the European Union and other high-income countries, the European Commissioner for Health and Consumer Protection proposed that although complex and, perhaps fragile, the relationship between health and the economy is a key to both:

> While it has long been recognised that increased national wealth is associated with improved health, it is only more recently that the contribution of better health to economic growth has been recognised. Yet while this relationship is now well established in low-income countries, the evidence from high-income countries, such as the Member States of the European Union, has been more fragmented.[82]

A main challenge for population health is the significant differences in health that currently exist between socioeconomic groups. Health inequalities, such as higher morbidity and mortality rates due to inequalities in education, job choice, and income, could be lessened by "active engagement of many policy sectors, not only of the public health and health care systems, but also of education, social security, working life, city planning, etcetera ..."[83] In 2004, deaths attributable to health inequalities in the European Union were estimated at 707,000 per year, and the prevalent cases of illness "that can be attributed to health inequalities is estimated to be more than 33 million."[83]

Public policy is important in establishing conditions that assist all people to access the prerequisites of health. There is a tendency, though, in advanced economies to concentrate efforts toward health education, behavioral risk factors,[84] illness imperatives, and reductionism to the exclusion of different viewpoints, such as the one taken here. This is despite the strong social health lobby and rhetoric that espouses learning from multiple disciplines and sources. A greater appreciation and investigation of occupation (as it is defined in this text) undertaken by collectives of people and how that impacts on meeting the prerequisites of health would be timely.

Collective, Corporate, and Organizational Occupation

In most sectors of the health care domain, health and illness are considered from an individual perspective as distinct from population health, public health, and, more recently, social determinant directives that have addressed issues relating to groups of people on a local and global scale. That points the way to considering the relationship to health of collective, corporate, and organizational occupations on a local and global scale. This has already been discussed to some degree throughout the text but appears so important that giving it a name and identifying the dimensions could assist future understanding, research, and action.

As for many other animals, collective occupations have been important in the survival of human populations throughout time. Histories that consider the evolution of the relationship between health and activity have noted the impact of collective occupations.[2-8,12] These tell of how early humans survived and thrived naturally as they met their innate biological needs through what they did with others within communities as an integral part of their ecosystem. For millennia, familial/tribal occupations, such as provision of shelter, food, water, and education, and community actions, such as moving camp, provided the basis for population health. What was originally based on trial and error and what appeared to be common sense gradually became part of folk-lore and, later, in the Western World, the basis of rules of health formulated in the Classical Greek period. Those were transmitted across the centuries through Medieval medicine and in use until recently. For many centuries, spiritual matters reigned supreme not only in religious organizations, but also in political, social, and local communities. What religious leaders decided on local, national, or international policy affected not only what people did on a regular basis, but also the health outcomes that resulted from their occupations. In this way, communal occupations were closely aligned with spiritual health, as well as physical, mental, and social survival. Apart from that organizational input, in the western world, communal occupations such as church attendance, pilgrimages, and physical labor were used for illness prevention, curative medicine, therapy, or health promotion purposes. Even after the demise of monasteries in Britain these health ideals continued. Young King Edward VI's agreement to establish a Hospital of Occupations to overcome the communal occupation deprivation–based illnesses largely caused by closure of the monasteries is a case in point.[5]

A major occupational change in the form of the industrial revolution, in a short period of time, led to a transformation in communal occupations, expanding to include corporate and organizational groupings that now affect the personal occupations of people anywhere in the world. With great rapidity, national and international corporations, institutions and organizations emerged from small local concerns and regional authorities where people engaged in collective occupations to deliver commodities and services to communities and individuals. Regional, national, and international governments and bodies across many occupational domains mushroomed and became powerful entities in terms of what groups of people and individuals do across the globe. The occupational domains formed collectives of occupational beings. Within those collectives, individuals still engage in occupations that together drive policies and initiatives, yet the occupational nature of groups and organizations is largely ignored, as well as the health impact of collective and individual occupations outside the organization that emanate from their activity. Indeed, collective, corporate, and organizational occupations are seldom considered in the same way as individual activity, yet they can have profound effects on the health of the planet, populations, and communities around the world, as well as on individuals and members of the cooperatives.

In today's world, occupational groupings can be held largely responsible for whether individuals and communities can achieve the prerequisites of health. It is occupational collectives at a political level who control the air people breath, their food and water, the nature and availability of shelter, educational opportunities, the type of work and subsequent income, ecological practices, social justice and equity, and whether they are at war or peace.

ACHIEVING PHYSICAL, MENTAL, AND SOCIAL WELL-BEING

Occupational collectives are also powerful in whether people achieve physical, mental, and social well-being. The WHO, itself is a multi-tiered, multi-focused occupational collective, and has drawn on the combined wisdom of experts from around the globe to increase the health of populations everywhere. Advice is given to other occupational collectives, such as political bodies, public agencies, and social planners, so that practitioners working toward population health can attend to the health and illness experiences of communities as a whole. Often, the advice given assists in the recognition of overall trends and problems related to physical, mental, and social health that can be apparent in every sphere of life. Such recognition can enable future policy to address the reduction of illness and premature death more effectively. It also has the potential to increase the experience of social, as well as physical and mental well-being, in a way that is just for people everywhere.

The 2011 *Rio Political Declaration on Social Determinants of Health* confirms population health explanations about external determinants of health and illness that include environmental and sociopolitical causes of illness.[1] The WHO determinants now embrace broad-ranging causal factors. Many are occupationally based. It is within all parts of that expanded field that occupation as a determinant of illness or of well-being can be explored more fully and inclusively. But for this to occur requires recognition of occupation as a total entity that includes all that people do, that it relates to health, and that occupational "inequities within and between countries are politically, socially and economically unacceptable, as well as unfair and largely avoidable."[1] The WHO resolution to actively reduce health inequities notes the three overarching recommendations of the Commission on Social Determinants of Health:

To improve daily living conditions; to tackle the inequitable distribution of power, money, and resources; and to measure and understand the problem and assess the impact of action.[85]

The Declaration maintains "the promotion of health equity is essential to sustainable development and to a better quality of life and well-being for all, which in turn can contribute to peace and security."[1] It also reaffirmed the principles and provisions set out in the Ottawa Charter[86] and in the series of international health promotion conferences that followed.[1] Effective collective action could work toward the Ottawa and Bangkok Charter directives through communal occupation aimed at:

- Building occupationally healthy public policy and civic society by clarifying and encourageing an occupation for health focus among "policy makers at all levels" including "legislation, fiscal measures, taxation, and organizational change,"[86] as well as grass roots community projects and civil society groups. A useful starting point would be recognition of the occupational nature of organizations in which policymakers and well-organized, empowered communities themselves work and the consequent organizational health status and effects would be a useful starting point.

- Creating environments that are occupationally supportive, and conditions that are "safe, stimulating, satisfying, enjoyable,"[86] and provide a positive benefit to health for individuals and communities through doing, being, belonging, and becoming, and working to decrease the "inequalities within and between countries."[86]

- Strengthening community occupations by empowering members to exert ownership, control and action over their own and collective occupational endeavors and destinies, and through assisting them to understand the relationship between occupation and health and to overturn the "vulnerability of children and exclusion of marginalized, disabled and indigenous peoples."[87]

- Developing personal occupation for health skills by providing information that enables the enhancement of life competencies and education about the relationship between doing, being, belonging, and becoming, and collective and individual health.

- Reorienting health services toward an increased focus on the prevention of illness and the facilitation of health through occupation. The responsibility for both occupation and health is "shared amongst individuals, the community, government, institutions and other organisations,"[86] who are charged with working together to achieve this outcome.

The interest in the effects of physical activity on health is a useful starting place, even though it compartmentalizes one aspect of occupation from the total range. The 13-year longitudinal Harvard public health study of mortality published in the *British Medical Journal* in 1999 studied older Americans with regard to their social and productive activities and clearly shows the long-term positive and protective impact of doing more than physical exercise.[46] Its authors argued that "while physical fitness itself is important and clearly related to health and survival, the exclusive focus on physical activity obscures the health benefits that may be associated with other, non-physical activities."

The half-forgotten ways of early in the previous century offer another insight into the connection between occupation and health. The mental hygiene movement was influential in the growth and development of mental health services of the first half of the 20th century.[88] Adolph Meyer held a then-radical viewpoint that life experiences play an important role in the etiology of mental disease.[89,90] His fundamental psychobiological approach reflects the idea of personal and communal occupation in some ways when he conceptualized whole people in action including society as part of the whole.[91] Repudiating reductionist, analytical, and mechanistic views, Meyer took a holistic standpoint influenced by William James' pragmatism[92] and John Dewey's Functionalism.[93,94] He made use of their "concept of habit," arguing that the "cumulative effect of early faulty habit patterns was to produce abnormal or inefficient behavior in later life."[95] Meyer embraced the revolutionary view that the chief purpose of the mind "is to enable individuals ... to

Table 12-3

WORLD HEALTH ORGANIZATION DIRECTIVES FOR WELL-BEING AS DOING, BEING, BELONGING, AND BECOMING

WHO Directives for Well-Being	Doing, Being, Belonging, Becoming
Capacity to change or cope with the environment	Doing to satisfy the prerequisites of health
Capacity to satisfy needs	Being satisfied and finding meaning, and purpose through use of capacities
	Belonging through taking an active and satisfactory part in collective occupations
Capacity to identify and realize aspirations	Becoming according to potential

Abbreviation: WHO, World Health Organization.

pursue specific interests and achieve specific goals" and that its study should consider "the ordinary, practical situations of everyday life."[96] He professed that "doing, action, and experience are being" and that the activities expressed in living demonstrate mind-body synthesis.[34,97] A similar approach might be useful in working toward an increased understanding of an occupational perspective of physical and social aspects, as well as mental health, since people alone or collectively pursue specific interests and goals as part of everyday life, as Meyer suggested.[89] That would have the potential to provide direction on how to maintain health and ensure human survival in economic and self-sustaining ways that meet the biological and sociocultural needs of people and, perhaps, help to reduce ecological degradation. For those committed to understanding people as occupational beings, the challenge is to increase awareness of the connection between how what people do contributes to their being, belonging, and becoming needs and impacts on health and illness.

In recent times, occupation has been overlooked as a holistic phenomenon despite the fact that the WHO rhetoric appears to embrace the whole. The theme of Chapter 6—"health is created and lived by people within the settings of their everyday life; where they learn, work, play and love"—is an example of the latter thought. It is about what people need to be able to do to reach a state of complete physical, mental, and social well-being along with three occupational directives given in the Ottawa Charter (Table 12-3).[86]

There are few venues where doing, being, belonging, and becoming happen effectively for all members of a community, despite many obvious attempts. It may be a utopian vision, but radical improvement requires utopian thought. How health is achieved through what people do, by being true to their nature and needs, by belonging through shared activity, and by striving toward reaching occupational potential requires spelling out. This needs to be done by people who understand, respect, and articulate the power of occupation; include collective occupations; embrace practical, achievable solutions; and facilitate occupation focused health and social policies.

To improve population health through personal, communal, corporate, and organizational occupation requires:

- Occupation-based programs at the forefront of intervention in countries that are striving to meet the fundamental prerequisites for life so that ongoing health benefits accumulate. Prerequisites for sustaining life are attained through people's participation in socially acceptable, personally satisfying, and ecologically sustainable activities. The provision of social welfare should be tied to satisfying occupational requirements whenever possible, to reduce the illness-producing ennui that results from lack of purpose and meaning.

- Fostering understanding of how all and any doing, being, belonging, and becoming through occupation impacts on morbidity, mortality, and well-being. Through research, publishing, advocacy, the seeking out of powerful allies, and media support, spreading the facts about the occupation/health relationship to increase healthy life expectancy and reduce the experience of illness or disability would be invaluable.

- Increasing community, corporate, organizational, and political awareness about fair, meaningful, and challenging communal doing, being, belonging, and becoming that is integral to the prevention of illness and experience of well-being at organizational and personal level.

- Increasing community, corporate, organizational, and political awareness about physical, mental, and social well-being attained through occupation that is personally satisfying, socially valued, sufficiently challenging, and meaningful.

- Encouragement and support of corporate and organizational initiatives that recognize occupation for health criteria and integrate them into work situations and customer/political/population outcomes.

- Encouragement and support of people striving toward a balance of active and rest occupations that maintain physical, mental, and social fitness.

- Increasing awareness of the holistic physical, mental, and social fitness effects of balancing active and rest occupations, food, and activity.

- Advocating for and enabling practical education programs to suit personal and communal occupational interests.

- Availability of opportunity for enhancement of capacities, individual potential, spiritual contentment, and quality of life by actively advocating for public policies that enable rather than restrict a wide range of occupations, to counter risk reducing, litigation-scared policies.

- Advocating for occupationally just social policies that enable and encourage people of all ages without discrimination to actively participate in wide ranging occupations.

- Not necessarily accepting the policies or social conventions of the time if people of any age, in any situation or walk of life, are occupationally alienated, deprived, stressed, or lacking occupational balance.

- Increasing awareness of occupational injustices in the community and at policy level, researching the causes and effects, actively advocating for change, and mediating on behalf of those less able.

- Increasing community cohesion, support, and opportunity.

- Learning to recognize the positive and negative impact of supportive and cohesive or fragmented and isolating communities, and take an enabling approach appropriate to its particular needs and potential, encouraging local participation and leadership, and being ready to advocate and mediate for improvement of occupation for health opportunities.

- Encouragement of occupations that are compatible with a sustainable ecology.

- Recognition that people are an active part of ecosystems and as such their needs are as important, but not more, so than those of any other animate or inanimate species. With that in mind, support occupations that are compatible with ecological sustainability.

- Seeking and advocating for alternative occupational opportunities through legitimate "sought" comment on policies, particularly when communities and political determination appear tied to unsustainable and damaging practices.

There is a lack of widespread implementation of the WHO's population-focused ideas by health professionals, governments, and the wider community. In affluent societies, current-day expectations are that all problems can be solved by medical ingenuity and technological advances. People are excited and absorbed with the treatment of illness in which apparent miracles have overturned the incidence and prevalence of once common diseases. Advanced health technologies and pharmaceuticals are expensive but expected to be available to all people in postindustrial nations.

In contrast, there is a scarcity of funding for the development of population health programs in more needy parts of the world; that makes it more difficult to take appropriate action to address occupation related disorders or to even overcome the lack of understanding or interest in the broad picture of a healthier world. There is also a lack of awareness of the WHO directives and initiatives among the wider population, and even among health workers. This further negates the type of work many thoughtful leaders in the field of population health are keen to implement. It may also be that the directives are not given sufficient emphasis in the education process of health professionals, or that their importance is lost in the acquisition of particular skills for daily practice. Some of the United Nations' and the WHO directives relevant to occupation for health are discussed briefly and displayed collectively in the next section.

United Nations and World Health

The Universal Declaration of Human Rights recognizes, without distinction, the "equal and inalienable rights of all members of the human family" as the "foundation of freedom, justice and peace in the world."[98] In terms of the prerequisites, it calls for a standard of living adequate for health and well-being "including food, clothing, housing and medical care and necessary social services, and the right to security in the event of unemployment, sickness, disability, widowhood, old age or other lack of livelihood in circumstances beyond … control." In terms of occupation for positive health and well-being, the United Nations calls for the free development of personality through respect "for human rights and fundamental freedoms;" education; the free choice of employment with "equal pay for equal work" in just and favorable conditions, such as reasonable working times and "protection against unemployment;" rest and leisure, including periodic holidays from employment with pay; free and full development of personality as a result of "duties to the community;" and the right to participate in cultural life and "to enjoy the arts and to share in scientific advancement and its benefits."[98]

International law, in terms of satisfying the fundamental needs of children and providing assistance for the harmonious development of their personalities, talents, and abilities, the *Convention on the Rights of the Child*, came into force in 1990.[99] The Convention recognizes that society has an obligation to ensure that every child can:

- Survive—by meeting the prerequisites "including nutrition, shelter, an adequate standard of living and access to healthcare"
- Develop—so that they "reach their full potential" through education, play, leisure, and cultural activities
- Be protected from all forms of abuse, neglect, and exploitation but provided with opportunities for rehabilitation if they have "suffered any form of abuse or exploitation"
- Be enabled to take active roles in "decisions affecting their own lives, in their communities and societies in preparation for responsible adulthood."[99]

Those claims closely reflect occupational prerequisites of health. The roots of the Convention can be traced from the work of Eglantyne Jebb,[100] who founded Save the Children in 1923, through the *Universal Declaration of Human Rights*,[98] and the 1959 *Declaration of the Rights of the Child*.[101] Unfortunately, this has not prevented the continued suffering of some children, many homeless, with the number living on the streets being aggravated by war in which many factors affect children's development—physically, mentally, emotionally, and occupationally, accumulating and interacting with each other. As Braveman points out, "in the wake of the first Gulf War" many more deaths occurred as a consequence of "the massive after-shocks resulting from destruction of infrastructure (for example, clean water) critical for survival and health" than as "a direct result of the military action itself."[102]

Table 12-4
WHO: ACTIVE AGEING POLICY: *OCCUPATION FOCUSED POPULATION HEALTH OBJECTIVES*

- Optimize opportunities for health, participation and security to enhance quality of life for individuals and populations

- Recognize the UN principles of independence, participation, dignity, care and self-fulfilment, allowing people to realize their potential for physical, mental and social well-being throughout the life course and to participate in society according to their needs, desires and capacities

- Increase number of people actively participating as they age in the social, cultural, economic and political aspects of society in paid and unpaid roles and in domestic, family and community life

In the particular case of an occupational approach to health, it is worth noting afresh the United Nations' claim that:

> A number of activities have been identified as supporting healing by fostering in children a sense of purpose, self-esteem and identity. These include establishing daily routines such as going to school, preparing food, washing clothes, and working in the fields; providing children with intellectual and emotional stimulation through structured group activities such as play, sports, drawing, drama and story-telling; and providing the opportunity for expression, attachment and trust that comes from a stable, caring, and nurturing relationship with adults.[103]

In addition, the United Nations provides recommendations for action toward enabling the occupation process. For children to experience the least physical, mental, and emotional trauma from the results of war, it is recommended that:

- "Children's well-being is best ensured through family and community-based solutions that draw on local culture and an understanding of child development"

- "Helping war-affected children to build on their own strengths and resilience, in collaboration with trusted caregivers, is an important strategy in the process of healing"

- "Child-focused health needs assessments" should be expedited while taking into account "food, health and care factors and the coping strategies likely to be used by the affected population"

- Education should continue despite difficult circumstances, even in situations of armed conflict. Such was the case in the former Yugoslavia when "classes were held in the cellars of people's homes, often by candlelight" during the height of the fighting, and in Sierra Leone where "non-traditional teachers, including mothers and adolescents, were trained and deployed."[99]

At the other end of the age spectrum, the United Nations' report of the *International Year of Older Persons* stressed the importance of meeting, recognizing, involving, and consulting older people as a potential societal resource, and keeping in mind that stereotyping can lead to discrimination and violations of human rights.[104] Table 12-4 provides examples of occupational population health objectives from the WHO's Active Ageing Policy.

Despite apparent lip service to the notion of Active Ageing, there remains much more media coverage about governmental concerns regarding estimates of the likely soaring health and pension costs. That has not led to better provision of occupation-based services to reduce illness, either in the community or in residential care.

Other long-standing issues are addressed in the United Nations' *Millennium Development Goals*. For example, those of gender equality and the empowerment of women are recognized as being at the heart of the preconditions for overcoming poverty, hunger, and disease. Unfortunately, progress has been slow across all domains from education to access to political decision making.[44] Another issue is the cruelly inequitable and lopsided global economy that Werner[105] argued is the biggest obstacle to health, particularly in the developing world. These are also occupation for health issues at individual and collective levels that require understanding and action from an occupational perspective that must take into account the regulation or transformation of the prevailing market system so that need is put before greed. Werner advised that:

> In such a transition, the World Health Organization and UNICEF need to reclaim their mandate as world coordinators of well-being of the disadvantaged. They need to gain strong enough popular support to stand up to the transnational corporations – the pushers of weapons, cigarettes and infant-formula – without fear of funding cuts by the US Government. Likewise, financial institutions such as the World Bank must be structurally adjusted to place basic human needs before unregulated corporate profits.[105]

The list of inequities and the illness resulting from corporate greed that are rife in poorer countries of the world are horrendous, so it becomes possible to forget that they are also apparent in the postindustrial, more affluent world. In socially- and occupationally-just communities, respect, fairness, and understanding should be explicit in policies, and corporate occupational groups should be engaged in economics, industry, education, social welfare, and health systems that empower what and how other people do, be, belong, and become. Currently, many decisions of these powerful occupational agencies are invisible, and it is possible to experience occupational injustice as a result of taken-for-granted beliefs, values, and assumptions, or power conflicts and tensions between competing interests.[106]

It is useful to be aware of and to use documents such as *The Universal Declaration of Human Rights*[98] and *The Convention on the Rights of the Child*[99] to back-up potential new directions toward occupational approaches to population health to the "powers-that-be." The rights are reflected in WHO initiatives, which are guidelines to workers in the field of population health who could look more widely, inclusively, and extensively at the relationship between health and all of the things that people need, want, or are obliged to do within everyday life and the corporate world. The greater the awareness of rights, as well as the recognition of occupation as both a personal and collective issue, the more of a chance there is of securing them or facilitating change.

Table 12-5 displays a collection of individual and corporate occupation for population health strategies selected from three WHO Health Promotion Congresses at Ottawa,[86] Jakarta,[107] and Bangkok.[87] Table 12-6 displays a collection of population health strategies selected from various other WHO publications, namely the *Global Strategy on Diet, Physical Activity and Health*,[108] *Mental Health Fact Sheet No. 220*,[109] and the *Social Determinants of Health*.[1] Neither Table 12-5 nor Figure 12-6 include all of the relevant directives that could be in the listings. The fact that despite being incomplete they are extensive does more than suggest the importance of actively seeking their implementation.

The relationship between occupation and population health is clearly illustrated and recognized by the WHO in the directives shown in Tables 12-4 and 12-5. For example, the WHO explanation about "appropriate regular physical activity" points to well-chosen occupation as a major component in preventing the "growing global burden of chronic disease."[108] From an economic point of view "inactivity greatly contributes to medical costs - by an estimated $75 billion in the USA in 2000 alone." However, "[i]ncreasing physical activity is a societal, not just an individual problem, and demands a population-based, multi-sectoral, multi-disciplinary, and culturally relevant approach."[108] The same is true of mental and social activity. Imagine the impact of a mix of appropriate physical, mental, and social occupation initiatives at the public policy level for all aspects of prevention and health promotion within the world's population.

Table 12-5

WHO OCCUPATION-FOCUSED DIRECTIVES TOWARD THE ABSENCE OF ILLNESS AND PHYSICAL, MENTAL, AND SOCIAL WELL-BEING

WHO: Ottawa Charter for Health Promotion

- An individual or group must be able to identify and realize aspirations, to satisfy needs, and to change or cope with the environment
- Improvement in health requires a secure foundation in the basic prerequisites
- Good health is a major resource for social, economic and personal development
- Changing patterns of life, work and leisure have a significant impact on health
- Work and leisure should be a source of health for people
- Health promotion generates living and working conditions that are safe, stimulating, satisfying and enjoyable
- Systematic assessment of the health impact of rapidly changing environments is essential particularly in technology, work, energy production and urbanization
- Protection of natural & built environments and conservation of natural resources must be addressed in any health promotion program
- Community development based on self help, social support, local resources, and access to funding are required to encourage effective community action
- Provision of information, health education, enhancement of life skills to increase healthy options
- Enabling life-long learning, facilitated in school, home, work and community settings
- Reorientation of health services beyond the clinical & curative towards health promotion - opening channels to broad social, political, economic & environmental components
- Health is created and lived by people within the settings of their everyday life; where they learn, work, play and live
- Health is created by caring for oneself and others, by being able to take decisions and have control over one's life circumstances
- Focus attention on public health issues such as pollution, occupational hazards, housing and settlements

WHO: The Jakarta Declaration

- Affirmed the Ottawa Charter's five strategies and prerequisites for health and identified poverty as its greatest threat
- Comprehensive approaches that use the five strategies are more effective than single-track approaches
- Urbanization, social, behavioural and biological changes such as increased sedentary behaviour, increased drug abuse, civil and domestic violence threaten health and well-being
- Put people at the centre of health promotion action and decision-making processes to increase community capacity and empower individuals
- Health promotion is carried out by and with people, not on or to people. It improves both the ability of individuals to take action, and the capacity of groups, organizations or communities to influence the determinants of health
- Access to practical education, leadership training, resources and information is essential. Empowering individuals demands more consistent, reliable access to the decision-making process and the skills and knowledge essential to effect change
- New forms of action are required to unlock the potential for health promotion inherent in many sectors of society, among local communities, and within families
- Cooperation is essential, requiring the creation of new partnerships for health, on an equal footing, between the different sectors at all levels of governance in societies

(continued)

Table 12-5 (continued)
WHO OCCUPATION-FOCUSED DIRECTIVES TOWARD THE ABSENCE OF ILLNESS AND PHYSICAL, MENTAL, AND SOCIAL WELL-BEING

WHO: The Bangkok Charter

- Health promotion is a critical human right offering a positive and inclusive concept of health as a determinant of the quality of life and encompassing mental and spiritual well-being
- Factors that influence health include rapid and often adverse social, economic and demographic changes that affect working conditions, learning environments, family patterns, and the culture and social fabric of communities
- Women and men are affected differently. The vulnerability of children and exclusion of marginalized, disabled and indigenous peoples have increased
- Health is influenced by rapid and often adverse social, economic and demographic changes that affect working conditions, learning environments, family patterns, and the culture and social fabric of communities
- Women and men are affected differently. The vulnerability of children and exclusion of marginalized, disabled and indigenous peoples have increased
- Effective mechanisms for global governance for health are required to address all the harmful effects of: trade; products; services, and marketing strategies
- The corporate sector has a direct impact on the health of people and on the determinants of health through its influence on: local settings; national cultures; environments, and wealth distribution

Conclusion

Doing, being, belonging, and becoming in accord with people's occupation-based species' nature is biologically normative of human populations. Although not every disorder or disability can be prevented, population health; physical, mental, and social well-being; and the absence of illness are dependent on occupation. If well chosen, it can provide protection, as well as advantages, toward the promotion of health, even for those with poor health. This is clear in the WHO directives for populations around the world, despite them not identifying occupation as a composite entity encompassing all of life-domains.

Being responsive to biological needs that are, in part, stimulated, influenced, and adapted by conscious social processes, and making use of capacities through engagement in occupation remains central to maintaining homeostasis and the well-working of people. This can be provided, in large part, through engagement in occupation to obtain the prerequisites of population survival and health. In addition, communal and corporate occupations can provide for meaning, purpose, and belonging within populations, as well as affording opportunity toward desired outcomes. On the downside, if corporate, sociocultural, and political occupations and processes continue their current track to economic wealth for a minority, illness will continue to flourish. Apparently generous handouts to the majority of people who live in poverty provide only transient and unsustainable benefits. The United Nations' *Declaration of Human Rights* provides a way forward in terms of research, diagnosis, prescription, and action. However, the implementation of those rights is highly dependent on political will and what populations are allowed, encouraged, or assisted to do. Occupation is a major factor in "the enjoyment of the highest attainable standard of health" being the fundamental right of "every human being without distinction of race, religion, political belief, economic or social condition."[98] Population health can only be achieved if the occupational nature

Table 12-6

WHO OCCUPATION-FOCUSED INDIVIDUAL AND CORPORATE DIRECTIVES TOWARD POPULATION HEALTH

WHO: Mental Health Fact Sheet 220

- Enable people to realize abilities, cope with the normal stresses of life, work productively and fruitfully, and make a contribution to the community.

WHO: Global Strategy on Diet, Physical Activity and Health

- Recognize the need to reduce the major risks resulting from unhealthy diet and physical inactivity, and the largely preventable nature of the consequent diseases
- Physical activity and diet are major behavioural and environmental risk factors amenable to modification through implementation of concerted action
- Create environments that empower and encourage individuals, families and communities to make positive decisions on healthy diet and physical activity
- Recognize the socioeconomic importance and health benefits of traditional dietary and physical-activity practices, including those of indigenous peoples
- Promote lifestyles that include a healthy diet and physical activity and foster energy
- Encourage and foster a favourable environment for the adoption of lifestyles that include a healthy diet and physical activity
- Physical activity is a fundamental means of improving the physical and mental health of individuals, independent of nutrition and diet
- Encourage the development of global, regional, national and community policies and action plans to improve diets and increase physical activity, and actively engage all sectors, including civil society, the private sector and the media
- Physical activity is a key determinant of energy expenditure, and thus is fundamental to energy balance and weight control
- Physical activity reduces risk for cardiovascular diseases and diabetes and has substantial benefits for many conditions, not only those associated with obesity
- Physical activity reduces blood pressure, improves the level of high density lipoprotein cholesterol, improves control of blood glucose in overweight people, even without significant weight loss, and reduces the risk for colon cancer and breast cancer among women
- Strategies need to be consistent with the Ottawa Charter principles and recognize the complex interactions between personal choices, social norms, economic and environmental factors
- It is recommended that individuals engage in adequate levels of physical activity throughout their lives: at least 30 minutes of regular, moderate-intensity physical activity on most days reduces the risk of cardiovascular disease and diabetes, colon cancer and breast cancer. Muscle strengthening and balance training can reduce falls and increase functional status among older adults. More activity may be required for weight control
- Strategies to reduce non-communicable diseases should include requirements for physical activity in working, home and school life, increasing urbanization, and various aspects of city planning, transportation, safety and access to physical activity during leisure
- Priority should be given to activities that have a positive impact on the poorest population groups and communities. Such activities will generally require community-based action with strong government intervention and oversight.
- Health-care providers can play an important part in prevention by providing information and skill-building to change behaviour, taking a life-course approach, can reach a large part of the population and be a cost-effective intervention
- Form networks and action groups to promote the availability of healthy foods and possibilities for physical activity, and advocate and support health-promoting programmes and health education campaigns
- Workplaces are important settings for health promotion and disease prevention. People need to be given the opportunity to make healthy choices in the workplace in order to reduce their exposure to risk

(continued)

Table 12-6 (continued)
WHO OCCUPATION-FOCUSED INDIVIDUAL AND CORPORATE DIRECTIVES TOWARD POPULATION HEALTH

WHO: Social Determinants of Health:

- Social determinants of health and health inequities arise from the societal conditions in which people are born, grow, live, work and age. These include early years' experiences, education, economic status, employment and decent work, housing and environment, and effective systems of preventing and treating ill health

- Improve daily living conditions

- Good health requires a universal, comprehensive, equitable, effective, responsive and accessible quality health system

- Good health, the promotion of health equity and more inclusive and productive societies is dependent on the involvement of and dialogue with wide-ranging sectors in communities

- Collective goals, good health and well-being for all should be given high priority at local, national, regional and international levels

- Comprehensive programs of research and surveys to inform policy and action

- Strengthen occupational health safety and health protection

- Encourage public and private sectors to offer healthy working conditions

- Give special attention to gender-related aspects and early child development in public policies and social and health services

- Empower communities and strengthen civil society contribution to policy-making and implementation to enable their effective participation in decision-making

- Consider the contributions and capacities of civil society to take action in advocacy, social mobilization and implementation on social determinants of health

and needs of all people are met through population-focused policies and corporate activities that address both individual and population occupational requirements.

References

1. World Health Organization. *Rio Political Declaration on Social Determinants of Health*. Rio de Janeiro, Brazil, 21 October 2011. Available at: http://www.who.int/sdhconference/declaration/Rio_political_declaration.pdf

2. McMichael T. *Human Frontiers, Environments and Disease: Past Patterns, Uncertain Futures*. Cambridge: Cambridge University Press; 2001.

3. Porter R. *The Greatest Benefit to Mankind: A Medical History of Humanity*. London: Harper Collins; 1997.

4. McKeown T. *The Origins of Disease*. Oxford, UK: Basil Blackwell, 1988.

5. Wilcock AA. *Occupation for Health. Vol. 1. A Journey from Self Health to Prescription*. London: British College of Occupational Therapists; 2001.

6. Wilcock AA. *Occupation for Health. Vol. 2. A Journey from Prescription to Self Health*. London: British College of Occupational Therapists; 2002.

7. Bing RK. The evolution of occupation. In: Christiansen CH, Baum CM, eds. *Occupational Therapy: Performance, Participation, and Well-Being*. Thorofare, NJ: Slack Inc; 2005.

8. Christiansen CH, Townsend EA, eds. *Introduction to Occupation: The Art and Science of Living*. Upper Saddle River, NJ: Prentice Hall: 2004.

9. Carteret M. *Traditional Asian Beliefs and Healing Practices. Dimensions of Culture*. http://www.dimensionsofculture.com/2010/10/traditional-asian-health-beliefs-healing-practices/. Accessed February 13, 2013.

10. Hippocrates. In: Thagard P. *How Scientists Explain Disease*. Princeton, NJ: Princeton University Press; 1999:22.

11. Porter R. *Disease, Medicine and Society in England 1550-1860*. Basingstoke and London: MacMillan Education; 1987:13-17.

12. Thagard P. *How Scientists Explain Disease*. Princeton, NJ: Princeton University Press; 1999.

13. More T. *Utopia*. Abridged ed. London. UK: Phoenix, 1996. Original work published 1516.

14. Hardy L, Davidson L, eds. *Utopian Thought and Communal Experience*. Middlesex University, UK: Geography and Management Paper No 24; 1989:Introduction.

15. Locke J. *An Essay Concerning Humane Understanding*. London, UK: Printed for Tho. Basset, and sold by Edw. Mory at the sign of the Three Bibles in St Paul's Church-Yard; 1690.

16. Howard J. *An Account of the Principal Lazarettos in Europe; With Varios Papers Relative to the Plague: Together with Further Observations on Some Foreign Prisons and Hospitals; and Additional Remarks on the Present State of Those in Great Britain and Ireland*. Warrington, UK: Printed by William Eyres; 1789:140-142.

17. Pare A. The Authors Dedication to Henry the third, the Most Christian King of France and Poland. 1579. In: Johnson T. *The Workes of that Famous Chirurgion Ambroise Parey. Translated out of Latin and compared with the French*. Printed by Th Cotes and R Young; 1634.

18. Blundell JWF. *The Muscles and Their Story from the Earliest Times (an Adaptation of the 'Ars Gymnastica') including the Whole Text of Mercurialis, and the Opinions of other Writers Ancient and Modern on Mental and Bodily Development*. London, UK: Chapman & Hall; 1864.

19. Ramazzini B. *Of The Diseases Of Tradesmen, Shewing The Various Influence Of Particular Trades Upon The State Of Health; With The Best Methods To Avoid or Correct It,...*London, UK: Printed for Andrew Bell et al; 1705.

20. Pinel P. *A Treatise on Insanity*. Translated from the French by D. D. Davis, MD. Sheffield: Printed by W. Todd, for Messrs Cadell and Davies, Strand London: 1806. Reprinted: Birmingham, Alabama: Classics of Medicine Library, 1983.

21. Tuke S. *Description of the Retreat*. York: Alexander; 1813:141,156.

22. Browne WAF. *What Asylums Were, Are and Ought to Be*. Edinburgh: A. & C. Black; 1837. Reprinted: Classics in Psychiatry: Arno Press Collection. North Stratford, UK: Ayer Company Publishers Inc; 2001:177.

23. Shepard P, McKinley D, eds. *The Subversive Science: Essays Toward an Ecology of Man*. Boston: Houghton Mifflin Company. 1969.

24. Woodley P. *Occasional Papers: Health Financing Series: Volume 7*. National Population Health Planning Branch. Commonwealth Department of Health and Aged Health Financing and Population Health. 2001. Available at: www.health.gov.au/internet/main/publishing.nsf/.../ocpahfsv7.pdf. Accessed March 28, 2013.

25. World Health Organization. *Health Topics: Human Rights*. 2013. http://www.who.int/topics/human_rights/en/. Accessed March 29, 2013.

26. Population Health. *AIHW: Authoritative Information and Statistics to Promote Better Health and Wellbeing*. Canberra: Australian Institute of Health and Welfare; 2012.

27. Frankish C, et al. *Health Impact Assessment as a Tool for Population Health Promotion and Public Policy*. Institute of Health Promotion Research, University of British Columbia, Vancouver: 1996.

28. Population Health. Wikipedia, the free encyclopedia. Accessed February 16, 2013.

29. Koplan JP, Bond TC, Merson MH, Reddy KS, Rodriguez MH, Sewankambo NK, Wasserheit JN. Towards a common definition of global health. Consortium of Universities for Global Health Executive Board. Viewpoint. *The Lancet*. 2009;373:1993-1995.

30. *The Australian Concise Oxford Dictionary of Current English*; 1987.

31. *Funk & Wagnall's Standard Desk Dictionary*. Vol 1. New York, NY: Harper and Row; 1984:296.

32. Boddy J, ed. *Health: Perspectives and Practices*. Palmerston North, New Zealand: The Dunmore Press; 1985:113.

33. Smuts JC. *Holism and Evolution*. London, England: Macmillan and Co Ltd; 1926.

34. Golley FB. *A History of the Ecosystem Concept in Ecology: More Than the Sum of the Parts*. New Haven, Conn: Yale University Press; 1993.

35. Pietroni PC. Holistic medicine. In: Bullock A, Stalleybrass O, Trombley S, eds. *The Fontana Dictionary of Modern Thought*. 2nd ed. London, England: Fontana Press; 1988.

36. Kopelman L, Moskop J. The holistic health movement: a survey and critique. *Journal of Medicine and Philosophy*. 1981;6(2):209-235.

37. Hidalgo C, Blumm N, Barabási A, Christakis N. A dynamic network approach for the study of human phenotypes. *PLOS Computational Biology.* 2009;5:e1000353.

38. Regnier M. Focus on Stroke: Shah Ebrahim – Changing States of Risk. Life from a Wellcome Trust Perspective. *Wellcome Trust Blog.* 11 May 1912. Accessed February 15, 2013.

39. Pourbohloul B, Kieny M. Complex systems analysis: towards holistic approaches to health systems planning and policy. *Bulletin of the World Health Organization.* 2011;89:242-242.

40. World Health Organization. *Everybody's Business: Strengthening Health Systems to Improve Health Outcomes: WHO's Framework for Action.* Geneva: World Health Organization; 2007.

41. Beaglehole R, Horton R. Chronic diseases: global action must match global evidence. *Lancet.* 2010; 376: 1619-21.

42. Federal/Provincial/Territorial Advisory Committee on Population Health; Canada. *Strategies for Population Health: Investing in the Health of Canadians.* Ottawa: Health Canada Communications Directorate; 1994.

43a. Whitehead M, Dahlgren G. Levelling up: a discussion paper on concepts and principles for tackling social inequities in health. *Studies on Social and Economic Determinants of Population Health, No. 2.* WHO Collaborating Centre for Policy Research on Social Determinants of Health, University of Liverpool. 2006.

43b. Dahlgren G, Whitehead M. *Policies and Strategies to Promote Equity in Health.* Copenhagen: WHO Regional Office for Europe; 1992.

44. United Nations. *The Millennium Development Goals Report.* New York: 2010.

45. Dubos R, ed. *Mirage of Health: Utopias, Progress and Biological Change.* New York, NY: Harper and Row; 1959:9.

46. Glass TA, de Leon CM, Marottoli RA, Berkman LF. Population based study of social and productive activities as predictors of survival among elderly Americans. *British Medical Journal.* 1999;319:478-483.

47. Corbin HD. Brighter vistas for senior citizens: salient thoughts. *Journal of Physical Education and Recreation.* 1977;October:52-53.

48. Comfort A. *A Good Age.* Melbourne, Australia: Macmillan Co Pty Ltd; 1977:82.

49. Wolman B, ed. *Dictionary of Behavioral Science.* New York, NY: Van Nostand, Reinold Co; 1973:250.

50. Knight R, Knight M. *A Modern Introduction to Psychology.* London, England: University Tutorial Press Ltd; 1957:56-57,177.

51. McDougall W. *Social Psychology.* 23rd rev ed. London, England; Methuen; 1936.

52. Csikszentmihalyi M. Activity and happiness: towards a science of occupation. *Journal of Occupational Science: Australia.* 1993;1(1):38-42.

53. Izard CE. *Human Emotions.* New York, NY: Plenum; 1977.

54. Izard CE, Kagan J, Zajonc RB. *Emotions, Cognition, and Behavior.* New York, NY: Cambridge University Press; 1984.

55. Frijda NH. *The Emotions.* New York, NY: Cambridge University Press; 1986.

56. Csikszentmihalyi M, Csikszentmihalyi I, eds. *Optimal Experience: Psychological Studies of Flow in Consciousness.* New York, NY: Cambridge University Press; 1988:20-25.

57. Ryff C, Love G, Urry H, Muller D, Rosenkranz M, Friedman E, Davidson R, Singer B. Psychological well-being and ill-being: do they have distinct or mirrored or biological correlates? *Psychotherapy and Psychosomatics.* 2006;75:85-95.

58. Southwood-Smith T. *The Philosophy of Health; or an Exposition of the Physical and Mental Constitution of Man, with a View to the Promotion of Human Longevity and Happiness.* Vol 1. London, UK: Charles Knight;1836.

59. Argyle M. *The Psychology of Happiness.* New York, NY: Methuen and Co; 1987.

60. Leone RE. Life after laughter: one perspective. *Elementary School Guidance and Counselling.* 1986;21(2):139-142.

61. Ornstein R, Sobel D. *Healthy Pleasures.* Reading, Mass: Addison-Wesley Publishing Co Inc; 1989.

62. Simon JM. Humor and its relationship to perceived health, life satisfaction, and moral in older adults. *Issues in Mental Health Nursing.* 1990;11(1):17-31.

63. Southam M, Cummings M. The use of humour as a technique for modulating pain. *Occupational Therapy Practice.* 1990;1(3):77-84.

64. Buxman K. Make room for laughter. *American Journal of Nursing.* 1991;91(12):46-51.

65. Coveney J, Bunton R. In pursuit of the study of pleasure: implications for health research and practice. *Health.* 2003;(7)2:161-179.

66. Mallett J. Use of humour and laughter in patient care. *British Journal of Nursing.* 1993;2(93):172-175.

67. Rose S. *The Conscious Brain*. Rev ed. Harmondsworth, England: Penguin Books; 1976:39,292-293.
68. Doyal L, Gough I. *A Theory of Human Need*. Houndmills, Hampshire: Macmillan; 1991:172.
69. Wilcock A. *Unpublished Survey*. University of South Australia; 1993.
70. Fitzgerald R, ed. *Human Needs and Politics*. Sydney, Australia: Permagon; 1977:153.
71. Lorenz K. *The Waning of Humaneness*. Munich, Germany: R Piper and Co Verlag; 1983:124.
72. Godbole M. *Maintaining Homeostasis*. Buzzle: 9/22/2011. http://www.buzzle.com/articles/maintaining-homeostasis.html. Accessed February 19, 2013.
73. Jackson S, Csikszentmihalyi M. *Flow in Sports: The Keys to Optimal Experiences and Performances*. Champaign, IL: Human Kinetics; 1999:167.
74. World Health Organization. WHO/HPR/HEP/98.1. *Health Promotion Glossary*. Geneva: WHO; 1988. http://www.who.int/healthpromotion/about/HPG/en/. Accessed February 2, 2013.
75. World Health Organization. *Healthy Settings*. Geneva: WHO; 2013. Available at: http://www.who.int/healthy_settings/en/ Accessed February 4, 2013.
76. Coppee GH. World Health Organization, International Labor Organization. *Definition of Occupational Health*. 1950, 1995. In: Occupational Health Services and Practice. http://www.ilo.org/safework_bookshelf/english?content&nd=857170174. Accessed February 17, 2013.
77. Occupational medicine. *American Heritage Dictionary of the English Language*, 4th ed. Houghton Mifflin Co. Available at: http://www.answers.com/library/Dictionary. Accessed May 6, 2012.
78. Edwards G. *Occupation for Population Health*. 6th Australasian Occupational Science Symposium. University of Canberra. December 2012.
79. Hammell KW. Dimensions of meaning in the occupations of daily life. *Canadian Journal of Occupational Therapy*. 2004;71(5):296-305.
80. Hocking C. *The Relationship Between Objects and Identity in Occupational Therapy: A Dynamic Balance of Rationalism and Romanticism*. Unpublished PhD thesis. Auckland University of Technology; 2004:171.
81. World Health Organization. *Trade, Foreign Policy, Diplomacy and Health*. Commission on Macroeconomics and Health. http://www.who.int/trade/glossary/story008/en/. Accessed February 23, 2013.
82. Kyprianou M. (European Commissioner for Health and Consumer Protection). Foreword. In: Suhrcke M, McKee M, Arce R, Tsolova S, Mortensen J, eds. *The Contribution of Health to the Economy in the European Union*. Luxembourg: Office for Official Publications of the European Communities; 2005.
83. Mackenbach J, Meerding W, Kunst A. *Economic Implications of Socio-Economic Inequalities in Health in the European Union*. Health and Consumer Protection Directorate-General; European Communities: July 2007.
84. Bunton R, Macdonald G, eds. *Health Promotion: Disciplines, Diversity, and Developments*. 2nd ed. Philadelphia: Taylor and Francis; 2002.
85. World Health Organization. *Resolution WHA62.14 Reducing Health Inequities Through Action on the Social Determinants of Health*. Rio: 2011.
86. World Health Organization, Health and Welfare Canada, Canadian Public Health Association. *The Ottawa Charter for Health Promotion*. Ottawa: WHO; 1986.
87. World Health Organization. *The Bangkok Charter for Health Promotion in a Globalized World*. 2005. http://www.who.int/healthpromotion/conferences/6gchp/bangkok_charter/en/. Accessed January 30, 2013.
88. Meyer A. The philosophy of occupational therapy. *Archives of Occupational Therapy*. 1922;1:1-10.
89. Leys R, Evans R, Evans B, eds. *Defining American Psychology: The Correspondence Between Adolph Meyer and Edward Bradford Titchener*. Baltimore, MD: The Johns Hopkins University Press; 1990:43-46,59,162.
90. Meyer A. The problems of mental reaction types, mental causes and diseases. In: Winters EE, ed. *The Collected Papers of Adolph Meyer*. Baltimore, MD: The Johns Hopkins Press; 1950-1952:2,598.
91. Muncie W. The psychobiological approach. In: Arieti S, ed. *American Handbook of Psychiatry*. Vol 2. New York, NY: Basic Books; 1959.
92. James W. *Pragmatism: A New Name for Some Old Ways of Thinking*. New York, NY: Longmans, Green and Co; 1907.
93. Dewey J. *Democracy and Education: An Introduction to the Philosophy of Education*. Toronto, Canada: Collier-MacMillan; 1916.
94. Leys R, Evans R, Evans B, eds. *Defining American Psychology: The Correspondence Between Adolph Meyer and Edward Bradford Titchener*. Baltimore, Md: The Johns Hopkins University Press; 1990:59.

95. Leys R, Evans R, Evans B, eds. *Defining American Psychology: The Correspondence Between Adolph Meyer and Edward Bradford Titchener.* Baltimore, Md: The Johns Hopkins University Press; 1990:46.

96. Leys R, Evans R, Evans B, eds. *Defining American Psychology: The Correspondence Between Adolph Meyer and Edward Bradford Titchener.* Baltimore, Md: The Johns Hopkins University Press; 1990:44-45.

97. Breines E. *Origins and Adaptations: A Philosophy of Practice.* NJ: Geri-Rehab, Inc; 1986:46.

98. Office of the High Commission of Human Rights. *Universal Declaration of Human Rights.* United Nations Department of Public Information: 1948. http://www.un.org/en/documents/udhr/. Accesed November 1, 2005.

99. United Nations. *Convention on the Rights of the Child.* Office of the High Commissioner for Human Rights: 1989. http://www.ohchr.org/en/professionalinterest/pages/crc.aspx. Accesed November 1, 2005.

100. Save the Children Norway. *History.* No date. http://www.scnorway.ru/eng/history/. Accesed April 3, 2014.

101. United Nations. *Declaration of the Rights of the Child.* Adopted by UN General Assembly Resolution 1386 (XIV) of 10 December 1959. http://www.un.org/cyberschoolbus/humanrights/resources/child.asp. Accesed November 1, 2005.

102. Braveman PA. Health, equity, human rights, and the invasion of Iraq. *Journal of Epidemiology and Community Health.* 2003;57:593.

103. Machel G. Expert to the Secretary-General of the United Nations. *The Impact of Armed Conflict on Child Development. Promoting Psychological Recovery and Social Reintegration Education: Investing in the Future of Children.* UNICEF and United Nations. http://www.un.org/rights/impact.htm.

104. United Nations Department of Economic and Social Affairs (DESA). *International Year of Older Persons 1999.* http://undesadspd.org/Ageing/Resources/ArchivedResources/InternationalYearofOlderPersons1999.aspx. Accesed November 1, 2005.

105. Werner D. *Health and Equity: Need for a People's Perspective in the Quest for World Health.* Conference: PHC21-Everybody's Business. Almaty, Kazakhstan: November 1998:2.

106. Townsend EA, Wilcock AA. Occupational justice. In: Christiansen CH, Townsend EA, eds. *Introduction to Occupation: The Art and Science of Living.* Upper Saddle River, NJ: Prentice Hall; 2004.

107. World Health Organization. *Jakarta Declaration on Leading Health Promotion into the 21st Century.* Geneva: WHO; 1997.

108. World Health Organization. Global Strategy on Diet, Physical Activity and Health. 2003. www.who.int/dietphysicalactivity/media/en/gsfs_general.pdf. Accesed June 27, 2012.

109. World Health Organization. *Mental Health: Strengthening Our Response.* Fact Sheet No220; Updated April 2004. http://www.who.int/mediacentre/factsheets/fs220/en/. Accessed November 1, 2005.

Section IV

Occupational Perspectives of Health

Theme 13

"To accept the community as the essential voice in matters of its health, living conditions and well-being"

"To recognize health and its maintenance as a major social investment and challenge: and to address the overall ecological issue of our ways of living"

WHO: The Ottawa Charter for Health Promotion, 1986[1]

Chapter 13

OCCUPATION, ENVIRONMENT, AND COMMUNITY DEVELOPMENT

The chapter addresses:
- The Concepts of Occupational Eco-sustainable Community Development
  - Environment and Ecological Sustainability
  - Community Development
- Occupational Eco-sustainable Community Development for Health
  - Why an Occupational Eco-sustainable Community Development Approach Is Necessary
  - Practical Action
- Conclusion

This chapter is the first of four occupational perspectives to be considered for improvement in population health. It combines the concept of community development with that of environmental issues and ecological sustainability. Generally, the latter aspect is poorly understood as a health approach, yet it is possibly the most vital in the long term. The combination of environment and community development is useful because people are integral to ecosystems and, without both being taken into consideration, either could founder. This view is in line with WHO and the United Nations' directives in relation to the promotion of health that recognize:

> ... *The need to encourage reciprocal maintenance—to take care of each other, our communities and our natural environment. The conservation of natural resources throughout the world should be emphasized as a global responsibility.*[1]

In a recent issue of *Canadian Journal of Public Health*, Cole et al argued that practitioners working toward global health "must be committed to improving health equity through global systems changes."[2] Their suggestions are particularly pertinent to occupation-focused environmental community development, especially in disadvantaged parts of the world. Practitioners in this genre must be able "to work responsibly in low-resource settings, foster self-determination in a world rife with power differentials, and engage in dialogue with stakeholders globally." That calls for understanding of "north-south power dynamics, linkages between local and global health problems, and the roles of international organizations," as well as being competent in cross-cultural communication and critical self-reflection.[2] Those skills are required because environmentally sustainable

Wilcock AA, Hocking C.
An Occupational Perspective of Health, Third Edition (pp 368-389).
© 2015 Taylor & Francis Group.

community development aims at balancing development objectives with environmental concerns while enabling social relationships and humane local societies to flourish sometimes in war-torn or politically unstable conditions.

Both environmental and community development issues have escalated since the concept emerged as a popular solution to address growing concerns over the negative consequences of human activities,[3] so that sustainability has become a legitimate component of development rhetoric in various interactive fields including population health.[4-13] Professor of Public Health, Anthony Capon, contended that although it is clear that "occupations affect human health and well-being," for "the first time in history, human occupations are now affecting the health of planetary systems." He called for a widening field of vision toward an occupational perspective that links the health of people, places, climate, and other environmental changes to reshape cities and towns so that they become "healthy places to live, learn, care and play."[14]

The Concepts of Occupational Eco-sustainable Community Development

The 1987 World Commission on Environment and Development defined sustainable development in the Brundtland Report as:

> ... Development that meets the needs of the present without compromising the ability of future generations to meet their own needs.[15]

This highlights that occupational needs loom large among those that will continue to affect the health of people and planet in future generations. In order to further kick-start action toward environmental protection and socio-economic development, when the United Nations convened a further conference in Rio de Janeiro in 1992, more than 100 heads of state attended. At the Earth Summit, as it became known, a plan for achieving sustainable development in the 21st century, known as Agenda 21, was developed.[16] A Commission on Sustainable Development was established to ensure effective follow-through and provide policy guidance to the Johannesburg Plan of Implementation[17] that was adopted at the conclusion of the World Summit on Sustainable Development in 2002.

The Johannesburg Plan provides a framework for action inclusive of participation by civil society and focusing on health, as well as water, energy, agriculture, and biodiversity. Aimed at protecting and managing the natural resource base of economic and social development, it addresses health and sustainable development issues, including poverty eradication, changing unsustainable patterns of consumption and production, implementing the "plan" through trade, finance, technology transfer, the scientific community, education, capacity building, and decision making.[17,18]

ENVIRONMENT AND ECOLOGICAL SUSTAINABILITY

Although Ernest Haekel coined the word *ecology* in 1866 to refer to the interdependency between plants, animals, and their natural environments,[19] it was as recent as the mid-1960s that James Lovelock,[20-24] an atmospheric chemist, formulated the Gaia Hypothesis. He proposed that the Earth is a single living organism that maintains its own conditions necessary for its survival. The hypothesis provided a basis for considering the interaction of the Earth's biosphere, atmosphere, oceans, soil, climate, rocks, and all living things as part of a self-regulating process that constitutes a feedback system seeking an optimal physical and chemical environment for life on the planet. Lovelock's theory stimulated a new awareness of the connectedness of all things on earth and the impact people have on global processes, such as the deforestation or reforestation of trees, the removal or planting of crops, or the increase or decrease of emissions of carbon dioxide.

Table 13-1
CHARACTERISTICS OF THE SCIENCE OF ECOSYSTEM HEALTH
McMichael's Views of Ecosystem Health Science[29]
Diversity, vigor, internal organization, and resilience
Its breadth and holistic vision "is a world of contingent probabilities" lacking specificity, precision of measurement, crispness of definition, and causal inference
Such big questions are not deliberately ignored but are often side-stepped or not asked because they do not fit the accepted template of western science.
"If we do not respond constructively to the ideas of ecology, then we can hardly avoid living in a world of declining natural capital, of persistent poverty for many people, of increasing political tensions, and of increased risks to our health and survival."

Shepard and McKinley,[25] Campbell,[26] and Suzuki[27] provide simple but cogent pointers to the conceptual core of ecology:

- "There is only one ecology; not a human ecology on one hand and another for the subhuman."[25]
- "... the components of the natural world are myriad but they constitute a single living system. There is no escape from our interdependent nature ..."[26]
- "... you and I do not end at our fingertips or skin—we are connected through air, water and soil; we are animated by the same energy from the same source in the sky above. We are quite literally air, water, soil, energy and other living creatures."[27]

At the time of Shepard's professorial appointment in 1973,[28] it was challenging to consider that people were "subject to ecological interdependence and that there were limits to the ecosphere's capacity to supply, replenish and absorb, particularly under the weight of human numbers and economic activities."[29] He explained that from one perspective:

> *the self is an arrangement of organs, feelings, and thoughts—a "me"—surrounded by a hard body boundary: skin, clothes, and insular habits ... conferred on us by the whole history of our civilization.*

> *The alternative is a self ... constantly drawing on and influencing the surroundings ... instead of excluding it.*

> *Both views are real and necessary for healthy societies and human maturity. The second view—that of relatedness of the self—has been given short shift.[30]*

Because scientists have only recently become serious about understanding "human biology, culture, social relationships, health and disease within an ecological framework," McMichael,[29] in line with Lander and Weinberg,[31] calls for a "more integrative systems type of science." He describes the science of ecosystem health as a "relatively novel perspective," with characteristics that differ from the narrowness and specificity of much medical science (Table 13-1).[31]

Although not necessarily accepting all of the Gaia postulates, scientists today generally support the idea that life has a substantial effect on abiotic processes[32] and that ecological investigation covers:

- "The scientific study of the relationships between living things and their environments. Also called bionomics ... A system of such relationships within a particular environment."[33]

- "Individual organisms (for example, behavioural ecology, feeding strategies)"; "Populations (for example, population dynamics)"; "Entire communities (for example, competition between species for access to resources in an ecosystem or predator-prey relationships)."[19]

The 1992 United Nations Conference drew worldwide attention to ecological sustainability as a matter of concern for everyone. Following the Summit, participating nations developed strategies to meet the decisions taken. For example, Australia's National Strategy based its approaches on a definition of ecologically sustainable development as:

> ... Using, conserving and enhancing the community's resources so that ecological processes, on which life depends, are maintained, and the total quality of life, now and in the future, can be increased.[18]

Unfortunately, the necessary transformational changes that the Summit advised have not eventuated across the world. This has led to a continuation of environmental degradation and an ever-widening gap between the haves and the have nots.[34-37] Greenpeace challenges the current monocultural approach associated with the industrialization of agriculture. It argues that global food commodification and disregard of the ecological, social, and multifunctionality of agriculture will put an end to the supply of food, "threaten the web of life upon which we all depend," and fail to guarantee the survival of 9 billion people on this planet, expect for 2050."[38] Similarly challenging is a 2012 report to the United Nations' Secretary General that states baldly that "business as usual" is not an option. Necessary transformative change should take a holistic approach toward environmental sustainability, inclusive social and economic development, and peace and security. The benefits of globalization are "very unevenly shared" but potentially offer great opportunities if "there is a radical shift toward more sustainable patterns of consumption and production and resource use."[39]

As Shepard foresaw, "ecological thinking requires a kind of vision across boundaries."[40] It is not restricted to the natural environment. It is also concerned with the minimalization or eradication of problems associated with human made environments that cause ill-health to both the natural world and people.

COMMUNITY DEVELOPMENT

Community development is about empowering people to recognize and effect change in their own communities, in response to shared problems and needs. It enables groups within a community and public agencies to work together to improve the quality of community life and government, while promoting social justice, and local, social, economic, cultural, environmental, and political development.[41]

> Community development draws on existing human and material resources in the community to enhance self-help and social support, and to develop flexible systems for strengthening public participation in and direction of health matters.[42]

Methods and approaches are recognized internationally by organizations such as the United Nations, WHO, Organization for Economic Cooperation and Development, World Bank, Council of Europe, and European Union. It was in 1953 that the International Association for Community Development began in the United States. It is currently centered in the United Kingdom and, over that time, a range of approaches have been developed for working within local and disadvantaged communities to mobilize and address issues, such as inequalities in the distribution of wealth, income, and political power.[43] The WHO recognized that "the inextricable links between people and their environment" set the scene for community development to play an important role as part of a "socioecological approach to health."[1]

The idea of community development appreciates that people are social creatures living and doing in the company of others, with survival itself, as well as the promotion of health, being dependent on cooperation within populations, and in accord with the ecosystem:

Health promotion works through concrete and effective community action in setting priorities, making decisions, planning strategies and implementing them to achieve better health. ... At the heart of this process is the empowerment of communities—their ownership and control of their own endeavours and destinies.[1]

It is difficult to assess the health of individuals without also understanding the environment and the health of others within a community, but affluence or poverty plays an important role.[44] The Task Team on the Post-2015 UN Development Agenda propose that the crucial factors that hold back human development and health are the ongoing and persistent inequalities and struggles over scarce resources. These are pivotal to "conflict, hunger, insecurity and violence."[39] Poverty, particularly, exposes people "to greater personal and environmental health risks."[45] They are less well nourished, have less information, and are less able to access health care, resulting in a diminished quality of life. Subsequent illness can further diminish family budgets and savings, reduce educational or work possibilities, and perpetuate poverty. "The poorest of the poor, around the world, have the worst health ... There is a social gradient in health that runs from top to bottom of the socioeconomic spectrum."[45]

Throughout history, the advancement of human progress has disadvantaged many. For example, in the change from agriculture to industry, when large populations resettled into towns, not only unsuited for mass immigration, they also issued forth smoke and fumes that were damaging to human and ecological health. Providing inspiration to current day community developers, Welsh-born Robert Owen (1771-1858), unlike most industrialists of his time, rejected and condemned the de-humanizing effects of industry and capitalism[46-49] and worked energetically toward:

... A society in which individuals shall acquire increased health, strength and intelligence— in which their labour shall be always advantageously directed—and in which they will possess every rational enjoyment.[50]

A brief description of Owen's approach is provided in the Boxed Dialogue 13-1.

In contrast to Owen's inclusive approach to community health, currently decisions, policies, and programs are frequently formulated outside communities with little regard for local occupational, social, economic, or environmental consequences. As a result, many communities have become pawns in a global economy as their environments become production sites for multinational corporations until no longer profitable.[3] Community developers seek to reverse the ill-effect of community roller coaster rides by reinstating local control over development decisions, increasing self-reliance and economic opportunity.

The WHO appeals for community development programs to focus on enhancing "self help and social support, and for developing flexible systems for strengthening public participation and direction in health matters."[51] This requires drawing on already existing human and material resources in combination with "empowerment of communities, their ownership and control of their own endeavours and destinies."[51] The popular phrase "think globally, act locally" applies to this approach, as does Wylie's maxim from approximately 50 years ago—health "is the perfect continuing adjustment of an organism(s) to its (their) environment."[52]

Occupational Eco-sustainable Community Development for Health

The strengthening of community action is one of the five strategies for health promotion prescribed in the Ottawa Charter, which "accepts the community as the essential voice in matters of its health, living conditions, and well-being" and asserts that "empowerment of communities, their ownership, and control of their own endeavours and destinies" are "at the heart" of the community development process.[1] The Bangkok Charter reflects how the global context for health

---

Boxed Dialogue 13-1:
Robert Owen and Environmental Community Development

Robert Owen's mill at New Lanark in Scotland was set in the idyllic Clyde Valley.

An outstanding theorist, Owen (1771-1858) was, essentially, a practical man who addressed many health issues using environmental community development approaches aligned to occupation. He provided education for his workers, their families, and children, and shortened working hours. He improved his workers' immediate environment by adding extra rooms to their one-roomed homes, establishing cooperative buying to reduce costs and improve the range of goods available, and by cleaning and paving the streets. Believing that the essence of communities was created by the nature of their institutions and practices, Owen built a school for the children to attend from the day they could walk by themselves until they started work, and for employees and housewives to attend evening classes. He also built a community center known as the Institute for the Formation of Character where his workers could take part in discussion, entertainment, enjoyment, and leisure.

Owen's concept of community development, health and well-being linked occupation, environment, community, and individual approaches. He was vehement about the need to understand "ourselves, society and nature",[1] and believed that the development of an individual's "entire faculties, senses and propensities" was "for the general advantage of all." Although his approach was basically apolitical, Owen recognized the need to publicize his ideas for the benefit of other communities suffering similar social ills to those he had needed to address in New Lanark. As well he tried to stimulate reform about issues such as child labour and inequities of the poor law.[2,3] Many similar 'Villages of Cooperation' known more commonly as Owenite Communities were established, including at least sixteen in America.[3]

His life and work made obvious the benefits of immediate action to address problems within a community. As well they demonstrate the necessity of raising awareness of social health problems within the population at large, and facilitate sociopolitical understanding. He provides an excellent role model for current day developers of programs aimed towards environmental and community health and development.

1. Owen R. *Works of Robert Owen: Volume 3: Book of the new moral world.* (Pickering Masters Series). London: Pickering & Chatto (Publishers Ltd.); 1993: 156,157.
2. Owen R. *Report to the Committee of the Association for the Relief of the Manufacturing and Labouring Poor.* 1817.
3. Harrison J. Robert Owen and the communities. In: *Robert Owen: Industrialist Reformer, Visionary, 1771-1858.* London, UK: Robert Owen Bicentenary Association; 1971: 27.

---

promotion has changed markedly since 1986. "Some of the critical factors that now influence health are increasing inequalities between and within countries: new patterns of consumption and communication; commercialization, global environmental change, and urbanization."[53] It is often the restrictions imposed by government funding bodies that inhibit the use of community development approaches and maintain a top-down delivery of services.

In line with the WHO directives, an OECD approach to health is defined here as:

The promotion of ecologically sustainable policies and community-wide action to maintain or re-establish healthy relationships between individuals, communities, human societies, other living organisms, environments, habits, and modes of life through participation in health giving and environmentally sustaining occupations that address increasing inequalities between

and within countries: patterns of consumption; urbanization; commercialization, and global environmental change.

This approach combines three complex sets of ideas:

1. The recognition that occupation is inclusive of all that people do; that community occupations reflect and combine the collective occupational strengths and interests of individuals; that this approach can use the skills within a community to address issues of inequalities between and within countries, such as ecologically unhealthy patterns of consumption, urbanization, commercialization, and global environmental change; and can enable sustainable health-giving occupational satisfaction.

2. The conceptual recognition of the need to sustain the environment through a health-giving relationship between all living organisms; their environments, habits, and modes of life; and the powerful effects of people's occupational natures, needs, and behavior on this process.

3. The need for community involvement, exploration, consultation, deliberation, and action to promote self-sustaining occupational development, health, and well-being that is fair and equitable for all.

This holistic, participatory, diverse, and proactive approach is self-sustaining and based on environmental, biological, natural, social, political, health, and occupational sciences that marry human occupation and relationships with environment in the most generic form. The approach accepts that people are part of the natural environment, global economies, and communities. It is inclusive of all levels of the population and is community centered, enabling and empowering development that uses local resources in a way that is ecologically sustaining. It is aimed at promoting global and community health and well-being, reducing disempowerment and ecological degradation and encouraging socioeconomic development in a way that facilitates healthy natural environments, individuals, and societies across the globe. Occupation is a central issue at all levels.

Because it is based on environmental and community analysis, use of local resources, and self-sustaining programs, the approach is in line with new models of population health that have emerged to address health concerns about both people and their environments. For example, Labonte, an international leader of the health promotion movement uses "econology" to describe a union between economy and ecology in theories that integrate health and sustainable development.[54,55] More recently, in respect to the centrality of "the physical environment as a prerequisite of health," he contends that "virtually all environmental markers show deterioration in our life support" and that:

> We need to assess how the economic drivers of globalization are affecting equity in both health opportunities (the determinants of health, or what the Ottawa Charter called the "prerequisites of health") and health outcomes, and at different levels—from the household, to the community, the region, the nation.[56]

It is clear within the WHO's calls for "Health for All" over recent decades that the relationship between community and environment is fundamental to the health and well-being of all people. During that time, concerns about the breakdown of ecological and communal relationships has led to ideology and practical programs that address both environmental and economic sustainability within community development. However, because occupation is most usually viewed as work, and the occupations of collectives outside of work settings are not recognized as emanating from the same source, the links between the occupational nature of people, communities, and environmental concerns have become dislocated.

Such dislocation was not the case when populations were smaller and when their occupations were in line with the natural world. Indeed, many experts consider that, generally, the occupational pursuits of hunter-gatherer communities would not have disturbed the environmental balance. As Lorenz suggested, such cultures "influence their biotope in a way no different from that of animal populations"[57]; Stephenson that hunter-gatherer societies produced "a stable relationship between man and his resources"[58]; and King-Boyes that "in full tribal life, the Aborigines presented an excellent example of a society working in rhythm with its environment."[59] Australia's indigenous people, like many elsewhere, based their oral traditions and religious values on reverence for the land.[60] Such indigenous communities are rapidly becoming extinct, not least because they are dependent on declining natural environments that, in turn, are dependent on the species that inhabit them.

Hunter-gatherer lifestyles, which were followed for several million years and were closely affiliated with all other aspects of the natural world, provided a real test of the potential for engagement in occupations to effectively sustain health and well-being of people, communities, other living creatures, and the environment. Michael Iwama rightly claims that much can be learned from indigenous cultures and from different cosmovisions, such as that held in East Asia.[61] He describes the latter as "arranging deities, nature and humans as inseparable parts of a singular entity, where one's existence is no more important or meaningful than the next entity—be it a tree, a stone, a bird, or another person."[62] Such views differ markedly with the current reality, in which much of humanity is using natural resources "faster than they can regenerate and creating waste such as CO_2 faster than it can be absorbed."[63] This is known as ecological overshoot and, along with humanity's current ecological footprint ("the demand people place upon the natural world" to support present day lifestyles), requires the equivalent of 1.4 planets.[63] Unfortunately, the advancement of affluent economies is based on an "unchallenged traditional assumption that loss is inevitable in the context of advancement of human progress."[64]

In contrast to that assumption, population health expert David Werner argued that the pursuit of world health cannot be separated from "global economics, preservation of ecosystems, and social justice." Unfortunately however, although science, technology, and wisdom have developed sufficiently to permit the development of a more "healthy, humane, and sustainable paradigm," it cannot progress because political will is absent and also perhaps for reasons of personal greed.[65] He pointed out:

> If we are ever to approach "Health for All"—or indeed, to prevent an ecodisaster leading to "Health for No One" we must embark very soon on a radically different model of social development.[65]

To improve the health of communities across the global environment, the importance of understanding and working to improve socioecological-economic and political factors cannot be overstated. That includes proactivity to increase holistic understanding of people as occupational beings as part of the ecology, as distinct from following the mandates of reductionist separationists who study what people do as distinct entities, such as workers, sleepers, consumers of food, physical exercisers, parents, and learners. Although such a study has value, it needs to be enfolded as part of the whole. Simo Algado used the term *occupational ecology* to encompass study of occupation regarded as the "dialogue" between people and their environment. He called for both "awareness of the occupational genocide we are confronting" and proactive occupation "to restore the balance with the natural environment."[61]

Sick environments and communities are, on the whole, the result of human occupations. An obvious example is provided by how people lived and worked according to the conditions imposed by economic and collective occupations at the time of the industrial revolution. The 18th, 19th, and early 20th centuries saw noxious gasses and filth being spewed out over what had been small towns sitting in green landscapes. One of public health's greatest early triumphs was the identification and virtual eradication of some diseases that emanated from sick environments such as those. Industrial complexes, somewhat improved but still injurious to environmental and human health, have moved their locations to less developed parts of the world and continue their unhealthy and deadly practices for "head in the sand" economic policies and gain. For example, development in Thailand that evolved from European priorities caused major socioeconomic and ecological imbalance. Atkinson and Vorratnchaiphan argued that decentralizing power and resources to local authorities and communities could redress the damage, if focused on improved management of the environment for the benefit of local people.[66]

Over the years, community development practitioners working in such environments have been faced with the urgency of empowering disadvantaged people to address both environmental and occupational issues as they strive to survive.[67-70] Community development was widely used in African and Asian colonial administrations after World War II. Local resources and self-sustaining programs stimulated local leadership and facilitated community, social, and economic development and education.[71] In the 1960s, the United States (*National policy: Title II of the Economic Opportunity Act* of 1964) and the United Kingdom adopted community development strategies for use in socially disadvantaged urban areas to stimulate self-help and innovative solutions that were cost-efficient.[72,73] In the 1970s, Australia introduced a Community Health Program that offered a framework for community-based preventive, diagnostic, therapeutic, and rehabilitation services based in local centers and complemented by home care, day care, health education, mental health, and alcohol and drug abuse programs.[74] This resulted in a great variety of community-based services, some, like domiciliary care, with traditional health values, and others that tended to challenge vigorously conventional health ideologies, as some women's health groups did. Perhaps because of these wide-ranging community initiatives, it is common to confuse "health services based in the community" with "community development."

Health services in a community can adopt an environmentally friendly, community development approach by encouraging community consultation as the basis of the service and by being responsive to underlying social and environmental factors that affect health in the long-term. Such an approach is a means of enabling all people to become involved in planning, implementing, questioning, and changing circumstances and occupational opportunities within their own communities so that they are occupationally, economically, socially, and environmentally advantaged. Table 13-2 encapsulates the foundations to this approach.

WHY AN OCCUPATIONAL ECO-SUSTAINABLE COMMUNITY DEVELOPMENT APPROACH IS NECESSARY

Since the 1960s, experts have called for a restructuring of economic goals and societal values, a reformation of resource policies to reflect community interests, a merging of the economic and biological in ecological decision-making, a reduction of population growth and consumption, improved recycling of waste and use of green technologies, and changes to make human activity more sustainable.[36,75-77] The 1970s saw the emergence of Conservation Biology, an interdisciplinary network with alliances between the biological and social sciences that called for conservation action plans to direct research, monitoring, and education programs.[78-80] Occupational scientists could bring valuable insights to the new discipline by advancing consideration of people's occupational interests and pursuits in the context of species and global environmental health.

The problem of maintaining a sustainable ecology against techno-occupational evolution, global population growth, and resource depletion is increasing (Figure 13-1). Curbing those three processes will require fundamental change to assumptions and values about wealth that are at the heart of business relationships that are, themselves, tempered by "decision mechanisms and the natural environment."[81] A fundamental and necessary first step is raising awareness and understanding about those relationships in terms of people's personal health, that of communities, and that of the natural environment.[82]

Some hope for the future is provided by the growth of alternative political parties in Western countries with platforms based on ecological and community needs. Although their policies may not meet with universal approval, their presence, at least, points to an awakening interest in issues that urgently require consideration. A case in point is provided by The Greens/Green Party USA,

Table 13-2		
FOUNDATIONS OF AN OCCUPATIONAL ECO-SUSTAINABLE COMMUNITY DEVELOPMENT APPROACH TO HEALTH		
Basis of Approach	Underlying Beliefs	Underlying Principles
Based on environmental, biological, natural, social, political, and occupational science	Humans as an integral part of the natural world are occupational and social beings.	Health-giving occupational policy and action is integral to community development and ecological sustainability
Aimed at increasing global and community health and well-being by reducing ecological degradation and disempowerment of communities	The health and well-being of the ecology and communities is central to ongoing health for all	Ecological degradation and community disempowerment can be reduced
Applicable to policy makers, populations, communities, and individuals	Community action can lead to healthy socioeconomic policies fostering occupations that sustain the ecology and maintain diversity.	Policy makers, populations, communities, and individuals can act in ways that sustain the ecology while meeting occupational needs
Holistic concept of people as part of the natural environment, global economies, and supportive communities	Communities in diverse socioeconomic systems need to participate in occupations in a manner that sustains the ecology as well as each other	Enablement of occupational diversity through ecologically sustainable community action
Is community centered, enabling, and empowering development that uses local resources and is ecologically sustaining	Devolution of decision making will enable communities to develop in ways that enhance social and environmental health using local resources	Empowerment through community support and relevant occupation is essential to strengthen environmental, community, and social health
Is participatory-diverse, self-sustaining, and inclusive of all levels of the population	Health-giving, safe, satisfying, stimulating, and enjoyable occupational conditions are a global responsibility	Participation in diverse, environmentally friendly, and community developing occupations promote health

which has political values based on ecology, social justice, grassroots democracy, and nonviolence. Since 1984, it has been aiming toward:

> ... An America where decisions are made by the people and not by a few giant corporations: Our environmental goal is a sustainable world where nature and human society co-exist in harmony.[83]

Despite a growing trend to acknowledge environmental concerns, mainstream liberal-democratic policies that uphold individual opportunity over community or environmental issues are seductive. These promote opportunities for individuals to "gain rewards from working hard" within "a system of incentives for merit, productivity and accomplishment," while providing a "minimal floor of compassion" for the many who are in "dire need" or unable to take advantage of such opportunities. Ecological sustainability is not at the forefront of policies, and failure to sufficiently address destruction of communities as a result of multinational corporate activity is common.[84] Pelton suggested that "the ultimate test of any policies and programs must be demonstration of improved outcomes ... [such as] ... reduced violence, drug abuse, mortality rates, child placement rates, child abuse, and homelessness."[85] Most of those unhealthy outcomes have increased in the majority of affluent societies over past decades.

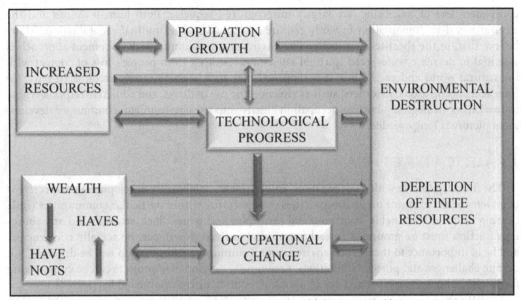

Figure 13-1. Interaction: population/technology/resources/wealth/occupations/the environment.

In terms of the necessity for an occupational focus within this debate, it is important to recognize that what people have done or not done for their own ends has been, over time, a primary force in ecological degradation. Although occupational development has protected people from the discomfort and unhealthy effects of harmful natural phenomena,[86] many of those who live in cities and spend their days "doing" in the "technosphere of human creation"[87] have a loss of connection with ecological reality. Other animals and plants have become regarded and treated as if their only purpose were to serve humans. The widespread practices of replacing natural plants with exotics, hunting and fishing for sport rather than need, and the killing of any animal that dares to attack a human demonstrate this propensity. The successful public health initiatives that condemned animals as the carriers of disease, linked with the hygienic "domesticity cult," separated humans still further from other species. It maintained the human superiority argument and gave permission for material wants to be considered more important than an ecological way of life in which all are dependent on each other. Darwinian theories failed to halt the segregation of people from other species, despite the successful therapeutic use of animals from the 18th century at the York Retreat for the mentally ill to the current day, when researchers are demonstrating substantial health benefits of pets to humans.[88-93] There remain many rules that restrict human-animal partnerships.

David Bellamy, a well-known botanist, has suggested that an occupation-focused approach to ecological sustainability in particular, is one answer to many of the questions posed in this chapter. He explained that:

> For 99% of our existence as a distinct species, the work ethic and everything that went with it held human society together ... the answer is simple, the work ethic must be rekindled by putting people back into the economics of life.[94]

This could be achieved through *environmentally benign tourism* (a term he considers preferable to ecotourism) or compulsory National Heritage Service between school and job and immediately post-retirement.[94] In the long-term, an ecological sustainability model is necessary to maintain the requirements for basic sustenance of life.

The philosophy of humanism is in question here. Humanism has been defined as "any system of thought or action in which human interests, values, and dignity predominate."[95] The drive to "rearrange both the world of Nature and the affairs of men and women so that human life will prosper," despite nature, is humanism gone awry.[96] Spiritual and occupational alienation, and consequent loss of well-being, are largely unrecognized sequelae. Both human doings and the natural world in combination urgently require ecological and attitudinal rehabilitation. Many believe that, in the short-term, a sustainable environment–community development approach is essential to decrease widespread spiritual alienation resulting from people's loss of contact with the natural world and each other. It is supposed that such alienation may account, in part, for increasing occupational disorders, such as violence, the use of drugs, and addictive responsiveness to marketing strategies.[96] Putting occupation clearly into the environment–community development picture is long overdue.

PRACTICAL ACTION

The first step to take with an occupation–environment–community development perspective is to systematically examine occupational issues of importance within particular communities while bearing in mind sustainable environmental principles and issues. Such research and any subsequent action must be grounded in each community's lived experience, be socially constructed, and be of importance to them. Each environment, community, and situation will be different, but despite challenges and possible limitations, community development projects can be empowering for people "who are marginalized due to social, structural, or environmental barriers."[97]

Initially, the process starts as communities identify and explore matters of concern with a view to improve an unsatisfactory situation or to assist occupational development of some kind for the community's future benefit. The ecological issues that could be raised by subsequent actions must be borne in mind. Facilitators or enablers from outside the community could lead the process initially, but, if at all possible, an able community member is preferable. Outside enablers can collaborate as part of the community group assisting in recognizing and valuing each person's particular strengths to community participants. Letting others know of skills that could be used by them is important, particularly if proximity or previous relationships prevent recognition. This will enable as many of the community as possible to feel they are valued members with a capacity to shape action and the outcomes. The kinds of concerns will differ from community to community, but bearing in mind the nature of the approach, they should embrace occupational issues.

For those new to community development and familiar with problems in postindustrial communities, the place to start might be close to home. OECD within affluent nations might be useful with communities of older people who feel marginalized and subsequently restricted in what they are able to do, or if limited social outlets prevent them remaining active and fulfilled. It might be equally useful with communities of parents whose children are autistic, difficult, extremely clever, or dysfunctional in some way. Street kids becoming involved in community development programs might be helped to reestablish in mainstream societies. Migrant groups might comprise another community that could benefit by identification of issues about their circumstances, the restrictions on what they are able to do, or the occupational expectations of their new country. They could also benefit from support as they progress further and then help others through the wisdom gained in the process.

Within developing countries, concerns are often about a lack of the prerequisites of health, such as the getting of food and water; the future of the children; educational and employment opportunities; shelter; and social justice. Social action might take the form of doing with others in like circumstances whatever is required to provide, build, or meet primary health and survival whilst:

- Being energized by the doing and finding meaning, purpose, and satisfaction through meeting community and environmental needs, as well as those of a personal and family nature.
- Belonging to a group of people committed to improving the lot of everyone and finding satisfaction in being able to help others.

- Becoming aware of the growth and development of the community and opportunities for its members, in combination with the gradually renewing health of their environment in a sustainable and valued enterprise.

Initiatives aimed at helping communities develop systems of primary health care that cater to their specific needs, use available resources, and are sustainable are more common in economically disadvantaged countries with poorly developed health services. Such programs may use various approaches, such as the prevention and control of diseases. Although medical personnel might concentrate on interventions such as immunization, others in the community health team might focus on enabling the development of occupational skills to make the most use of available resources, to improve environmental conditions, and to train local health workers. An example of this is provided by a Western-trained group of therapists who worked in Ethiopia in the 1980s and 1990s, when it was so ravaged by civil wars and famine that the economy and environment based on subsistence farming were devastated. An experienced Angolan paramedic explained to the group that how and what therapists from outside the area do is critical.[98] The people were resourceful and were willing and able to help themselves, but they needed support and resources. He advised that initially it is important to find out about the environment and situations people face on a daily basis, how they cope and what they do. Such an approach demands that community developers reflect on their own beliefs, attitudes, and assumptions about life and health, or they may be ineffective or even harmful. In small care centers, this group of therapists found a great need for rehabilitation services that address the long-term future and the means of providing a livelihood, as well as shorter-term intervention that could be shared with family members. They put their efforts into training the surprisingly energetic and young disabled people as rehabilitation workers.[98]

Other examples of where therapists might work with this approach are provided by an occupational therapist experienced in community development initiatives. Rachel Thibeault extends traditional rehabilitation to help reconstruct civil societies in war-torn and disadvantaged communities in hard to reach places. For example, she has worked with communities in the Canadian Arctic, Laos, Nicaragua, Ethiopia, Lebanon, Iraq, Zambia, Haiti, and Sierra Leone toward the reintegration of land-mine victims, AIDS orphans, individuals with leprosy, and earthquake victims. Centered on the principles of sustainable development, community involvement, and social inclusion, her occupation-based action research, frequently undertaken for United Nations agencies, embodies the OECD approach. Thibeault suggested that "to fully develop the potential of occupation in war-torn countries" requires four major steps. These are as follows:

1. The articulation of an intervention model based on the principles developed in the first edition of this text, namely: individual and collective well-being through occupation, "citizen participation, equality and social inclusiveness," "social justice for health care delivery in a context of increasing globalization" and a renewed perspective on societal priorities.[99] These should be coupled with analysis of post-conflict situations and growing evidence from occupational science.

2. The model should partner agencies with similar principles, values, vision, and commitment to social justice.

3. The model should be tested in postwar settings.

4. The model should have as its focus occupation/social justice and sustainable ecology. This should define political advocacy, representation, and action.[99]

Success is more assured if OECD is founded on the strengths of the local people and self-help groups.[100,101] Community members can be encouraged to recognize a particular role they might undertake to shape the direction and process of the project according to those strengths. The exploration can take many forms and be multiple to inform action in a critical way. It can make use of findings from research, individual expertise, and local knowledge, and draw on actual experiences in the community and environment. Focusing the objectives and recognizing issues that lie outside the project or that cannot be controlled are useful strategies. As the process evolves, initial planning might undergo change, according to decisions made by the community collectively and contextually.[102]

Considerable time and commitment may be required for community building through social-ization processes, for developing understanding about power relationships, and for uncover-ing abilities, skills, capacities, and talents. It may also be necessary for community members to explore the following:

- Their specific community in terms of individual and collective occupations, the relationships between the people, and between them and the natural environment.

- Issues of purpose, process, and action and differences between individual and social analyses, about the group process, and about the political nature of social change.[102]

- New sources to inform community action and to develop "reciprocal obligations and expec-tations, increased trust, and perhaps shared norms."[103]

- "The development of relationships across interest lines" to build the community field and "enhance the likelihood that communities will develop innovative approaches to development."[104]

- Understanding of occupation as a mechanism for becoming healthier and experiencing physical, mental, and social well-being through what the community members do to meet the basic prerequisites of health; how they feel about what they do; how it meets social, com-munal, and environmental needs; and how it enables development.

Raising the awareness of the community about doing, being, belonging, and becoming healthy through their occupations is a useful tool in the OECD process. It allows action plans to be devised and developed by the community in response to their needs and in line with available expertise and resources in an environmentally sustaining way. The community may require help with mediation or advocacy; they may need to call on advisors or to seek out extra resources and sup-port to assist in negotiating any necessary occupational change.

Expected outcomes of OECD must be meaningful to the community, be of practical value, and result in change of direct benefit.[102] Sometimes, this may be difficult, but if outcomes can be clearly set out and articulated for all community members, they may be empowered by the realization of what they have done and achieved. Major change will often require feedback and negotiation with outside occupational collectives, such as health or service organizations, environ-mental groups, local authorities, sociopolitical agencies, or media. Former World Bank economist Herman Daly, who espouses an eco-economics approach, argued that "seekers of world health need to enter into a serious dialogue with the leading advocates of healthier paradigms for devel-opment."[105] These include a growing number of unexpected bedfellows in the corporate sector who are beginning to respond to growing community dissatisfaction and concern about the state of the ecology. From the 1980s on, the phrase "think global, act local," has been used at times by multinational corporations, and the words global and local are often united into "glocalization," that refers to the practices of conducting their occupations according to local, global, and environ-mental considerations.[106]

Many of the values of OECD are encapsulated in the "think global, act local" catchphrase, the origin of which has been attributed to many people with differing occupational backgrounds, including Patrick Geddes, a Scottish biologist, philanthropist, town planner, and social activ-ist[107,108]; David Brower, as a slogan for Friends of the Earth[109]; René Dubos in his capacity as advisor to the 1972 United Nations Conference on the Human Environment[110]; and Canadian "futurist" Frank Feather, who chaired a conference on "Thinking Globally, Acting Locally" in 1979.[111] The phrase reflects the all-encompassing nature of OECD and indicates the variety of occupational collectives with whom to form partnerships in the process or who might be support-ive in a variety of ways.

In late 2012, the need to develop healthy built environments was a major theme that emerged at the *6th Australasian Occupational Science Symposium, Occupation for Population Health*.[112] Currently, many population health practitioners are concerned about town planning and urban and rural management and development, which are vital to the health of the environment and expanding or changing the dynamics of communities. Development, it is thought, should aim at stopping suburban sprawl, reducing petrol-driven vehicle dependence,[113] and enhancing livability in town centers through the creation of living streets and walking buses.[114]

Developing such healthy built environments is not without difficulties, and there is a clear need to assess contemporary communities critically and realistically.[115] When doing so, it must be borne in mind that communities are fragile, variable, and characterized by power struggles. Not uncommonly, these may be engendered by "those who seek to maximize growth and profits generated through economic development activities" that are often counter to self-sufficient communities in balance with the local ecosystem.[3] Increasingly, local communities are becoming immersed in larger societies as a result of technological advances in communications and transport that encourage interest in more distant happenings, less involvement in local affairs, and more frequent and distant travel.[116] Although communal doing for the common and individual good has always been part of human activity, in modern societies this has largely become superseded by governmental initiatives that lack a genuine community base. It has been suggested that for some people this has caused a loss of sense of place and the social relationships that depended on the common experience of living and working together.[117] If that is the case, aiming for local decision-making power within sustainable, self-sufficient community development could be an outdated ideal, at least in terms of postindustrial economic-rationalist societies.[118] However, the interest and action generated by the phrase "think globally, act locally" has led many people in such societies to take action within their own communities and cities toward improving the health of the planet by initiatives to protect habitats and the organisms that live within them. Such grassroots efforts are primarily organized by local volunteers and helpers, are true to the spirit of OECD, and should be encouraged by OECD facilitators.

Health giving occupational policy and action should be integral to community development and ecological sustainability rhetoric. However, the limited use of the word occupation, although its meaning is apparent within the WHO health promotion directives, leads to a lack of clarity about how participation in diverse environmentally friendly and community developing occupations can promote health and well-being for both environment and people. Population health practitioners who chose to take an OECD approach need, initially, to enable people to recognize the impact of doing, being, belonging, and becoming through occupation in communal and environmental health terms. Policy makers, populations, businesses, communities, and individuals should consider how they can act in ways that:

- Sustain the ecology while meeting occupational needs
- Reduce ecological degradation and community disempowerment through occupation
- Enable occupational diversity
- Empower people through community support and relevant occupation
- Strengthen environmental, community, social, and occupational health
- Enable and empower appropriate occupations of those who are disadvantaged.

In terms of the latter, by taking a holistic, enabling, participatory, and inclusive approach within a community, it is possible to take action to do something about meeting the needs of people who are at particular disadvantage.[119] A useful approach for health professions new to community development might be community-based rehabilitation (CBR). This is defined as "strategy within community development for the rehabilitation, equalization of opportunity and social integration of all people with disabilities."[120] It is "implemented through the combined efforts of disabled people themselves, their families and communities, and the appropriate health, education, vocational, and social services."[120] Although the principles of sustainable livelihoods and social inclusiveness are central considerations within such programs, issues relating to family and community violence, sexual abuse, and addictions can be recurring problems that also need to be addressed.

Examples of therapists using CBR working in various parts of Africa or in grossly disadvantaged and poor countries were provided earlier in the chapter.[99,102] As in many other communities, CBR has assisted remote and rural First Nation communities in both the Tjalku Warra community and in the "Top End" of Australia to improve conditions and promote independence, healthier lifestyles, and improved quality of life.[121-123] It has also been used in combination with participatory action research for those with acquired brain injury in remote communities:

> A critical element of the project was the employment of a local person in each community to assist with contacts, advising on cultural and community protocols, organization of interviews/meetings, gathering and reviewing of information as well as taking a lead role in assisting in consultations with members of the communities, and actioning the plans made by the communities. The local worker provided a key to successful community engagement and consultation and was evidence of a commitment to this process.[124]

In *Occupational Therapy Without Borders*, Simo Algado and Cordona determined that there is a need to "develop transcultural, holistic, and community-centered interventions" in which therapists work as social activists, fighting for population-focused occupational justice.[125] They describe an occupation-focused community development program over a 6-month period with Mayan Indian families returning to Guatemala after 14 years as refugees in Mexico following the 1978 to 1983 scorched earth campaign in which thousands were murdered or displaced. Children were enabled "to make contact with their Mayan inheritance through legends and stories," and weaving was used as a basis for women's "transgenerational and cultural sharing," as well as for economic reasons. Adolescents were engaged in carpentry that had potential economic and community benefits as well as training as community workers. Elders were assisted to "recover their traditional role as guardians and transferrers of ancient wisdom" through the creation of a Council of Elders and regular meetings between them and adolescents.[125]

The World Federation of Occupational Therapists approved their first position paper on CBR in 2004.[126] Reproting its significance, Kronenberg and Pollard acknowledged:

> ... The worldwide existence of an estimated 600 million people with disabilities, predominantly in the (but not limited to) "developing countries," who with their families and communities are restricted in or denied access to dignified and meaningful participation in daily life. The [WFOT] council recognized the need to develop critical awareness and understanding about these realities, and in response accepted the new and emerging notions of occupational apartheid, occupational deprivation, and occupational justice to guide and inform occupational therapy thinking and action.[127]

However, the occupational perspective should be taken further to maximize opportunities for disadvantaged people in disadvantaged communities whether able or disabled, rich or poor. Exploration of the underlying reasons for disadvantage and how they impact on health and well-being can be undertaken using an OECD approach. This is a suited to increasing awareness about the causes and effects of occupational, communal, and ecological alienation, deprivation, imbalance, and stress, as well as action to support and encourage occupation that increases well-being through meaning, purpose, and social approval.

Numerous initiatives are being undertaken around the world, but more are desperately needed. Some are based at universities. One such is the International Development Community and Environment Department at Clark University, Worcester, MA in the United States. Here, graduate students and faculty undertake collaborative, interdisciplinary research projects that address environment and development issues. One project that involves 18 local organizations aims to encourage leadership among younger members of the community to facilitate positive adolescent mental health and help reduce youth violence, alcohol, tobacco, and other drug use. It has used community-based participatory research to help enforce and strengthen local zoning regulations to reduce tobacco advertising and sales.[128]

Conclusion

Communities of people are part of the natural world and the well-being of both communities and environment are impacted by what they do. Community action can lead to healthy or unhealthy socio-economic-environmental policies by fostering occupations that either do or do not sustain the ecology and maintain diversity. Acceptance of these beliefs requires the provision of environments where health-giving, safe, satisfying, stimulating, and enjoyable occupational conditions prevail across the globe. Communities in diverse socioeconomic systems need to participate in occupations in a manner that sustains the ecology and each other. Devolution of decision making to enable communities to develop in ways that enhance occupational, social, and environmental health using local resources might require redevelopment. To do this requires acceptance of "the community as the essential voice in matters of its health, living conditions and well-being" as well as recognizing "health and its maintenance as a major social investment and challenge, and to address the overall ecological issue of our ways of living."[1]

References

1. World Health Organization, Health and Welfare Canada, Canadian Public Health Association. *Ottawa Charter for Health Promotion*. Ottawa, Canada; 1986:3.
2. Cole D, Davison C, Hanson L, Jackson S, Page A, Lencuch R, Kakuma R. Complementary competencies are needed. *Canadian Journal of Public Health*. 2011;102(5):394-397.
3. Bridger JC, Luloff AE. *Sustainable Community Development: An Interactive Perspective*. 1999. www.cas.nercrd.psu.edu/ Community/Legacy/bridger_intro.htm. Accessed July 10, 2013.
4. Lele S. Sustainable development: a critical review. *World Development*. 1991;19(6):607-621.
5. Korten C. Sustainable development. *World Policy Journal*. 1992;9(1):157-190.
6. Van der Ryn S, Calthorpe P. *Sustainable Communities*. San Francisco, CA: Sierra Club Books; 1986.
7. Kemmis D. *Community and the Politics of Place*. Norman, OK: University of Oklahoma Press; 1990.
8. Fowler EP. Land use in the ecologically sensible city. *Alternatives*. 1991;18(1):26-35.
9. Berry W. *Sex, Economy, Freedom and Community*. New York, NY: Pantheon Books; 1993.
10. Bray PM. The new urbanism: celebrating the city. *Places*. 1993;8(4):56-65.
11. Chamberland, D. The social challenges of sustainable community planning. *Plan Canada*. 1994;July:137-143.
12. Gibbs D. Towards the sustainable city. *Town Planning Review*. 1994;65(1):99-109.
13. Sachs W. Global ecology and the shadow of development. In: Sessions G, ed. *Deep Ecology for the 21st Century*. Boston, MA: Shambhala; 1995.
14. Capon A. Human occupations as determinants of population health: linking perspectives on people, places and planets. *Journal of Occupational Science*. 2014;21(1):9-12.
15. World Commission on Environment and Development. *Our Common Future*. New York: Oxford University Press; 1987:43.
16. United Nations. *Earth Summit: Agenda 21*. United Nations. April 23, 1993.
17. United Nations. *The Johannesburg Plan of Implementation*. World Summit on Sustainable Development. September 2002. http://www.johannesburgsummit.org/html/documents/summit_docs/2309_planfinal.htm. Accessed May 30, 2014.
18. Australian Government. *Ecologically Sustainable Development*. Department of Sustainability, Environment, Water, Population and Communities. Commonwealth of Australia. Last updated: Monday, 06-Jun-2011. http://www.environment.gov.au/about/esd. Accessed March 17, 2013.
19. Ecology. In: Norton AL, ed. *The Hutchinson Dictionary of Ideas*. Oxford, UK: Helicon Publishing Ltd; 1994:162.
20. Lovelock J. *Gaia: A New Look at Life on Earth*. Oxford University Press, Oxford, England; 1979.

21. Lovelock J. *The Ages of Gaia: A Biography of Our Living Earth.* W.W. Norton & Company, Inc., New York; 1988.
22. Lovelock J. *Healing Gaia: Practical Medicine for the Planet.* New York: Harmony Books; 1991.
23. Lovelock J. *Homage to Gaia: The Life of an Independent Scientist.* New York: Oxford University Press; 2000.
24. Lovelock J. *The Revenge of Gaia: Earth's Climate Crisis and the Fate of Humanity.* New York: Basic Books,; 2006.
25. Shepard P, McKinley D, eds. *The Subversive Science, Essays toward an Ecology of Man.* Boston: Houghton Mifflin Company. 1969.
26. Campbell B. *Human Ecology: The Story of our Place in Nature from Prehistory to the Present.* New York: Aldine de Gruyter, 1983.
27. Suzuki D. *The Sacred Balance.* Vancouver: Greystone Books; 2002.
28. Paul Shepard. Biography. http://paulhoweshepard.wordpress.com/bio/. Accessed June 27, 2014.
29. McMichael T. *Human Frontiers, Environments and Disease: Past Patterns, Uncertain Futures.* Cambridge, UK: Cambridge University Press; 2001;21.
30. Shepard P, McKinley D, eds. Introduction: ecology and man - a viewpoint. In: *The Subversive Science, Essays Toward an Ecology of Man.* Boston: Houghton Mifflin Company; 1969.
31. Lander ES, Weinberg RA. Journey to the center of biology. *Science.* 2000;287:1777-1782.
32. The Gaia Hypothesis. *Dr. C's Remarkable Ocean World.* Last updated January 21, 2005. Available at: www.oceansonline.com/gaiaho.htm Accessed February 8, 2006.
33. Ecology Science. *The American Heritage Science Dictionary.* Boston, MA: Houghton Mifflin Harcourt; 2010.
34. Asian NGO Coalition for Agrarian Reform and Rural Development, IRED Asia, People Centred Development Forum. *Economy, Ecology and Spirituality: Toward a Theory and Practice of Sustainability.* 1993.
35. Schroyer T. Research programs from the Other Economic Summit (TOES). *Dialectic Anthroplogy.* 1992;17(4):355-390.
36. MacNeill J. Strategies for sustainable development. *Scientific American.* 1989;261(3):155-165.
37. Bello W. *Dark Victory: The United States, Structural Adjustment, and Global Poverty.* London, England: Pluto (in association with the Institute for Food and Development Policy and Transnational Institute); 1994.
38. Greenpeace. *Agriculture at the Crossroads: Food for Survival.* Available at: Iaastd-rapport-en-anglais.pdf. Accessed June 17, 2013.
39. Report to the Secretary General UN System Task Team on the Post-2015 UN Development Agenda. *Realizing the Future We Want for All: Report to the Secretary General.* New York; June 2012. Available at: Post_2015_UNTTreport.pdf. Accessed March 10, 2013.
40. Shepard P. *Traces of an Omnivore.* Washington, DC: Island Press/Shearwater Books; 1996: xiv.
41. 41. Scottish Community Development Centre. *What is Community Development?* http://www.scdc.org.uk/who/what-is-community-development/. Accessed May 30, 2014.
42. World Health Organization, Health and Welfare Canada, Canadian Public Health Association. *Ottawa Charter for Health Promotion.* Ottawa, Canada; 1986.
43. *International Association for Community Development: A Brief History.* http://www.iacdglobal.org/iacd-brief-history. Accessed May 30, 2014.
44. Bush H, Zvelebil M, eds. *Health in Past Societies: Biocultural Interpretations of Human Skeletal Remains in Archeological Contexts.* Oxford: British Archaeological Reports International Series 567, 1991; 6.
45. World Health Organization. *Poverty.* www.who.int/topics/poverty/en/. Accessed March 15, 2013.
46. Marlo K. cited in Weiss J. *Conservatism in Europe 1770-1945: Traditionalism, Reaction and Counter-Revolution.* London: Thames and Hudson; 1977.
47. Fourier C. *Theory of the Four Movements, 1808* [1968, Oeuvres de Charles Fourier, vol 1 Paris: Editions Anthropos; Le nouveau monde industriel et societaire. 1829. Charles Fourier (1808) 1857 Theory of the Four Movements. ... 1829-1830. Le nouveau monde industriel et sociétaire: Ou invention du procédé ... des manuscrits de Charles Fourier. 4 vols. Paris: Librairie Phalanstérienne.
48. Weiss J. *Conservatism in Europe 1770-1945: Traditionalism, Reaction and Counter-Revolution.* London: Thames and Hudson; 1977:60.
49. Ostergaard G. Proudhon, Pierre-Joseph. In: Bottomore T, ed. *A Dictionary of Marxist Thought.* 2nd ed. Oxford, UK; Blackwell Publishers; 1983:451-452.

50. Owen R. *The Address to the Inhabitants of New Lanark.* The Institute for the Formation of Character. January 1st 1816. In: Owen R. *Works of Robert Owen: Volume 1 (Pickering Masters Series).* London: Pickering & Chatto (Publishers Ltd.); 1993:120-142.

51. World Health Organization, Health and Welfare Canada, Canadian Public Health Association. *Ottawa Charter for Health Promotion.* Ottawa, Canada; 1986:4.

52. Wylie CM. The definition and measurement of health and disease. *Pub Health Rep.* 1970:85:100-104.

53. World Health Organization. *The Bangkok Charter for Health Promotion in a Globalized World.* 2005.

54. Labonte R. Econology: integrating health and sustainable development. Part one: theory and background. *Health Promotion International.* 1991;6(1):49-64.

55. Labonte R. Econology: integrating health and sustainable development. Part two: guiding principles for decision making. *Health Promotion International.* 1991;6(2):147-156.

56. Labonte R. Globalization and health promotion. In: McQueen D, Jones C, eds. *Global Perspectives on Health Promotion Effectiveness.* New York: Springer Science; 2007.

57. Lorenz K. *Civilized Man's Eight Deadly Sins.* Latzke M, trans. London, England: Methuen and Co Ltd; 1974:12-13.

58. Stephenson W. *The Ecological Development of Man.* Sydney, Australia: Angus and Robertson; 1972:94.

59. King-Boyes MJE. *Patterns of Aboriginal Culture: Then and Now.* Sydney, Australia: McGraw-Hill Book Co; 1977:154-155.

60. Andrews M. *The Seven Sisters.* North Melbourne, Australia: Spinifex Press: 2004.

61. Simo Algado S, Estuardo Cardona C. The return of the corn men. In: Kronenberg F, Pollard N, eds. *Occupational Therapy without Borders: Learning from the Spirit of Survivors.* London: Elsevier; 2005;346.

62. Iwama M. Toward culturally relevant epistemologies in occupational therapy. *American Journal of Occupational Therapy.* 2003;57(5):582-587.

63. *What Are The Major Reasons Why We Are Losing So Much Biodiversity?* WFF Global. Available at: http://wwf.panda.org/about_our_earth/biodiversity/threatsto_biodiversity/. Accessed March 16, 2013.

64. Livingston J. *One Cosmic Instant.* Toronto: McClelland Steward; 1973.

65. Werner D. *Health and Equity: Need for a People's Perspective in the Quest for World Health.* Conference: PHC21-Everybody's Business. Almaty, Kazakhstan: 1998:2.

66. Atkinson A, Vorratnchaiphan CP. Urban environmental management in a changing development context: the case of Thailand. *Third World Planning Review.* 1994;16(2):147-169.

67. International Institute for Environment and Development. Whose Eden? Empowering local communities to manage their wildlife resources. *IIED Perspectives.* 1994;13:3-5.

68. Korten DC. *Sustainable Livelihoods: Redefining the Global Social Crisis.* New York, NY: People Centred Development Forum; 1994.

69. Robertson J. *People Centred Development: Principles for a New Civilisation.* New York, NY: People Centred Development Forum; 1994.

70. Vavrousek J. Human values for sustainable living. *Edial. The Network.* The Centre for our Common Future; 1993.

71. Marris P. Community development. In: Kuper A, Kuper J, eds. *The Social Science Encyclopedia.* London, England: Routledge; 1985:137-138.

72. Marris P. *Community Planning and Conception of Change.* London: Routledge; 1982.

73. Marris P, Rein M. *Dilemmas of Social Reform.* 2nd ed. Harmondsworth, England: Penguin; 1974.

74. Milio N. *Making Policy: A Mosaic of Australian Community Health Policy.* Australia: Department of Community Services and Health; 1988.

75. Potter VR. Bioethics, the science of survival. *Perspectives in Biology and Medicine.* 1970;14:127-153.

76. Egger G, Spark R, Lawson J. *Health Promotion Strategies and Methods.* Sydney, Australia: McGraw-Hill; 1990:107.

77. Corson WH. Changing course: an outline of strategies for a sustainable future. *Futures.* 1994;26(2):206-223.

78. Meffe G, Groom M. *Principles of Conservation Biology.* 3rd ed. Sunderland, Mass: Sinauer Associates; 2006.

79. Soule M, Soule ME. What is conservation biology? *BioScience.* American Institute of Biological Sciences. 1986;35(11): 727-734.

80. van Dyke F. *Conservation Biology: Foundations, Concepts, Applications.* 2nd ed. Düsseldorf: Springer Verlag; 2008: 478.

81. Stevens J. Rational decision making in primates: the bounded and the ecological. In: Platt M, Ghazanfar A, eds. *Primate Neuroethology*. Published to Oxford Scholarship Online: February 2010.

82. Stead WE, Stead J. Can humankind change the ecological myth? paradigm shifts necessary for ecologically sustainable business. *Journal of Organizational Change Management*. 1994;7(4):15-31.

83. The Greens/Green Party USA. *Home Page*. Eureka, CA 95502 Available at: www.greenparty.org. Accessed January 3, 2005.

84. Pelton LH. *Doing Justice: Liberalism, Group Constructs, and Individual Realities*. Albany: State University of New York Press; 1999:61.

85. Pelton LH. *Doing Justice: Liberalism, Group Constructs, and Individual Realities*. Albany: State University of New York Press; 1999:93.

86. Ehrenfeld D. *The Arrogance of Humanism*. New York, NY: Oxford University Press; 1981:10.

87. Dubos R. *Only One Earth*. London, England: Doubleday; 1988.

88. Dawn M, Berstein C, Constantin J, Kunkel F, Breuer P, Hanlon R. Animal-assisted therapy at an outpatient pain management clinic. *Pain Medicine*. 2012;13(1):45-57.

89. Vombrock J. Cardiovascular effect of human-pet interventions. *Journal of Behavioural Medicine*. 1988;ii(5):509-517.

90. Hundley J. The use of pet facilitated therapy among the chronically mentally ill. *Journal of Psychosocial Nursing*. 1991;29(6):23-26.

91. Buttner L, Fitzsimmons S, Barba B. Animal-assisted therapy for clients with dementia. *Journal of Gerontological Nursing*. 2011: 37.

92. Chinner T. An exploratory study on the viability and efficacy of a pet facilitated therapy project within a hospice. *Journal of Palliative Care*. 1991;7(4):13-20.

93. Kawamura N, Niiyama M, Niiyama H. Animal-assisted activity: experiences of institutionalized Japanese older adults. *Journal of Psychosocial Nursing and Mental Health Services*. 2009;47(1):41-47.

94. Bellamy DJ. Workaholics anonymous: putting people back into the equation of livelihood. *Journal of Occupational Science: Australia*. 1997;4(3):119-125.

95. Humanism. *Random House Kernerman Webster's College Dictionary*. Available at: http://www.kdictionaries-online.com/DictionaryPage.aspx?ApplicationCode=18#&&DictionaryEntry=humanism&SearchMode=Entry. Accessed June 27, 2014.

96. Southeast Asian contribution to the Earth Charter. *In Our Hands. Southeast Asia Regional Consultation on a People's Agenda for Environmental Sustainable Development: Towards UNCED and Beyond*. SEARCA. Philippines, 1991.

97. Trentham B, Cockburn L. Participatory action research: creating new knowledge and opportunities for occupational engagement. In: Kronenberg F, Pollard N, eds. *Occupational Therapy without Borders: Learning from the Spirit of Survivors*. London: Elsevier Ltd: 2005;440.

98. Personal communication, 2000. Reported in: McDonough S. What's a practitioner to do? challenging environments. In: Crepeau EB, Cohn ES, Boyd Schell BA, eds. *Willard & Spackman's Occupational Therapy*. 10th ed. Philadelphia, PA: Lippincott, Williams & Wilkins; 2003:38.

99. Thibeault R. Occupation and the rebuilding of civic society: notes from the war zone. *Journal of Occupational Science*. 2002;9(1):38-47.

100. McDonough S. What's a practitioner to do? Challenging environments. In: Crepeau EB, Cohn ES, Boyd Schell BA, eds. *Willard & Spackman's Occupational Therapy*. 10th ed. Philadelphia, PA: Lippincott, Williams & Wilkins; 2003.

101. Hobbs E, McDonough S, O'Callaghan A. *Life after Injury*. Penang: Third World Network; 2002.

102. Alary J, Beausoleil J, Guedon M-C, Lariviere C, Mayer R, eds. *Community Care and Participatory Research*. Montreal: Nuage Editions; 1992.

103. Coleman JS. Social capital in the creation of human capital. *American Journal of Sociology*. 1988;94(Supplement):S95-S120.

104. Flora CB, Flora JL. Entrepreneurial social infrastructure: a necessary ingredient. *The Annals of the American Academy of Political and Social Science*. 1993;529(September):45-48.

105. Daly H. *For the Common Good: Redirecting the Economy toward the Community, the Environment and a Sustainable Future*. Boston: Beacon Press. 1989.

106. Sharma C. Emerging dimensions of decentralisation debate in the age of globalisation. *Indian Journal of Federal Studies*. 2009;19(1):47-65.

107. Barash D. *Peace and Conflict*. Thousand Oaks, CA: Sage; 2002:547.

108. Boardman P. *The Worlds of Patrick Geddes: Biologist, Town planner, Re-educator, Peace-warrior*. London: Routledge and Kegan Paul; 1978.

109. David Brower: (obituary). *The Daily Telegraph.* November 8, 2000.

110. Dubos R. The Yale book of quotations. Quoted in: Shapiro F. *Quotes Uncovered: The Real McCoy and Acting Locally Freakonomics.* Blog, 11 March 2010.

111. Keyes R. *The Quote Verifier.* New York, NY: Simon & Schuster; 2006.

112. Thompson S. Healthy built environments supporting everyday occupations: current thinking in urban planning. *Journal of Occupational Science.* 2014;21(1):25-41.

113. Tranter P. Active travel: a cure for the hurry virus. *Journal of Occupational Science.* 2014;21(1):65-76.

114. Coombes P. Town centres, living streets and walking buses: Enhancing liveability. *Occupation for Population Health.* 6th Australasian Occupational Science Symposium: Program and Abstracts. University of Canberra; December 2013.

115. Wilkinson KP. *The Community in Rural America.* Westport, CT: Greenwood Press; 1991.

116. Warren RI. *The Community in America,* 2nd ed. Chicago, IL: Rand McNally and Company; 1972.

117. Meyrowitz J. *No Sense of Place: The Impact of the Electronic Media on Social Behavior.* New York: Oxford University Press; 1986.

118. Bender T. *Community and Social Change in America.* New Brunswick, NJ: Rutgers University Press; 1978.

119. do Rozario L. Keynote address. Purpose, place, pride and productivity: the unique personal and societal contribution of occupation and occupational therapy. *Australian Association of Occupational Therapists 17th Conference Proceedings.* Darwin; 1993.

120. World Health Organization, ILO, UNESCO. *Definition of Community Based Rehabilitation.* Geneva, Switzerland: WHO; 1994.

121. Glynn R. Some perspectives on cross-cultural rehabilitation with remote area Aboriginal people. *Australian Occupational Therapy Journal.* 1993;40(4):159-162.

122. Pondaag B. Working with the Tjalku Warra community: a project report. *The Australian Association of Occupational Therapists 15th Federal Conference.* Sydney, Australia, 1988.

123. Walker V. An occupational therapist's contribution to Aboriginal health worker training. *The Australian Association of Occupational Therapists 15th Federal Conference.* Sydney, Australia, 1988.

124. Gauld S, Smith S, Bowen R. Acquired Brain Injury Outreach Service. Improving community-based rehabilitation for Aboriginal and Torres Strait Islander Queenslanders with acquired brain injury: identification of key dimensions to enhance service suitability. *10th National Rural Health Conference;* Cairns 2009.

125. Simo Algado S, Estuardo Cardona C. The return of the corn men. In: Kronenberg F, Pollard N, eds. *Occupational Therapy without Borders: Learning from the Spirit of Survivors.* London: Elsevier Ltd, 2005;336.

126. World Federation of Occupational Therapists. *Position Statement: Community Based Rehabilitation.* http://www.wfot.org/resourcecentre.aspx. Accessed April 3, 2013.

127. Kronenberg F, Pollard N. Overcoming occupational apartheid: a preliminary exploration of the political nature of occupational therapy. In: Kronenberg F, Simo Algado S, Pollard N, eds. *Occupational Therapy without Borders: Learning from the Spirit of Survivors.* London: Elsevier Ltd, 2005;61-62.

128. *CDP Research Gives Hope.* www.clarku.edu/departments/IDCE/research/. Accessed April 25, 2013.

Theme 14

"Health inequities arise from the societal conditions in which people are born, grow, live, work and age ... Positioning human health and well-being as one of the key features of what constitutes a successful, inclusive and fair society in the 21st century is consistent with our commitment to human rights at national and international levels."

WHO: Rio Political Declaration on Social Determinants of Health, 2011[1]

Chapter 14

AN OCCUPATIONAL JUSTICE
PERSPECTIVE OF HEALTH

This chapter addresses:

- The Concept of Occupational Justice
    - Justice
    - Principles of Social Justice
    - Contemporary Perspectives of Social Justice
- Achieving Social Justice
    - Injustice and Ill Health
- An Occupational Justice Perspective of Health
- The Necessity of an Occupational Justice Perspective of Health
    - Practical Approaches
- Conclusion

The concept of occupational justice was initially aired within a social justice approach to health promotion in the first edition of this book. The concept was developed further in partnership with Elizabeth Townsend, incorporating her previous exploration of justice issues relating to enabling occupation, which were augmented by the thoughts and critique of attendees at international workshops and seminars. Occupational justice has now become accepted as a useful concept within occupational therapy, with a position paper adopted by the World Federation of Occupational Therapists in 2006.[2] Many other voices have joined the discussion, and numerous instances of occupational injustices affecting immigrants, refugees, elderly people, and people with mental and physical health conditions have been documented. Nonetheless, occupational justice remains an aspect of social justice that is largely overlooked. However, much of its substance, while not identified by this nomenclature, is addressed in several clauses of the *United Nations' Universal Declaration of Human Rights* that will be considered later in the chapter.

Wilcock AA, Hocking C.
An Occupational Perspective of Health, Third Edition (pp 390-419).
© 2015 Taylor & Francis Group.

The Concept of Occupational Justice

Occupational justice concerns two complex sets of ideas. First is the conceptual recognition of people's occupational nature as described in this text, which is expressed in individual and collective doing in the context of human life, founded on anatomy and bodily functions, and etched through evolutionary processes.[3,4] In an occupational justice context, occupation is framed as a cornerstone of optimal well-being, and replete with meanings garnered over the centuries that are communally and personally experienced. Second is the concept of justice; a human construction about reciprocity that has been given different emphases in different eras of human history and in diverse cultural contexts.

Although its conceptual basis has not been fully elaborated, discussions of occupational justice are underpinned by a growing awareness that odious and health-depleting occupations are unfairly apportioned across different groups in society and that some groups are excluded from beneficial occupations that support and enhance health. What makes this an issue of justice rather than an unfortunate fact is the serious consequences that occupational injustices have on nations, communities, and individuals. Occupational injustice is not invoked when people occasionally feel stressed or harried, and neither is it an occupational injustice when an individual's aspirations to pleasure, fame, or stellar performance are thwarted by lack of practice or talent or sensible advice to get enough sleep. It is not about getting everything people might want, being insulated from frustration and disappointment, or having to choose between opportunities. By definition, occupational injustice refers to ongoing deprivation or patterns of disruption that jeopardize children's development, create substantive health issues, and reduce individual's lifespan. Occupational injustice has equally serious consequences for society as a whole, undermining social cohesion, a sense of personal safety, and economic well-being. That is, occupational injustices waste human potential, create health burdens and, when perpetuated by entrenched attitudes, institutional racism and the like, plant the seeds of social unrest. The second factor that makes unfair distribution of occupation an issue of justice is that the conditions that give rise to it can be changed; they are not natural or immutable. As with other issues of justice, occupational injustice can be confronted by empowering individuals, communities, and whole countries to improve their material, psychosocial, and political circumstances.

Facing up to occupational injustice means that people have to recognize it. For many, a sense of injustice is heightened when the exclusion or burden is perceived to be deliberately harmful, making it difficult or impossible for people to meet their occupational needs. However, perhaps more commonly, situations of occupational justice are rendered invisible by being part and parcel of longstanding social arrangements that disadvantage those with lower social status and members of minority groups. Occupational justice, then, is concerned with sustainability and the achievement of fair, enabling, and empowering societies. In the sections that follow, the concept of justice is further explored to inform understandings of occupational justice and injustice.

JUSTICE

Benjamin Disraeli, the 19th century British parliamentarian, pronounced "justice is truth in action."[5] The word *action* links justice with doing and perhaps that is apt, because the concept developed in the ancient world to adjudicate disputes over acceptable and unacceptable behavior among people and how they shared resources and possessions.[6] In also linking justice with truth, Disraeli was echoing Aristotle's argument from the 4th century BC that, in the interests of the greater good, an ethical person should exercise truthfulness, compassion, fortitude, and integrity.[7] In identifying these human virtues, Aristotle made an important contribution to ethics, or moral philosophy, which concerns the distinction between right and wrong and the moral consequences of the things people do. Other philosophers have framed ethics in terms of the four principles of equity: justice, beneficence, non-maleficence, and respect for autonomy. Others have championed duty-based ethics or deontology, meaning that people should behave according to a set of beliefs, usually prescribed within a religion.[8]

Justice has many guises, but fundamental to all of them is the principle of ensuring order in social groups. Accordingly, from ancient times, justice encompassed all members of society in the sense that it provided some measure of protection, even to those at lower levels of the social strata who did not enjoy full rights as citizens. Those protections were strengthened over the centuries, firstly by the Stoic's idea of universal justice and later by the rise of Christianity. However, it was Thomas Hobbes, a 17th century philosopher, who championed the idea that humans are equal in nature and all people have certain natural rights. That idea was a profound break from the assumption that had governed human relationships for centuries—that the social order into which people were born was both inviolable and awarded some people power and privilege over others. In recognizing that social hierarchies were constructed rather than natural, and therefore could be redesigned to be more just, Hobbes helped bring about a radical transformation in thinking about justice. In thus freeing people from their ascribed social roles, Hobbes might also be viewed as advancing occupational justice, in opening up the possibility of bettering oneself through education or having some choice over one's vocation.[9]

At a societal level, justice is generally accepted as an ideal set of ethical, moral, and civic principles governing human interaction, which are codified in legal systems within states.[6,10-12] However, depending on the historical and cultural context, values guiding how justice should be dispensed have varied, with Confucian thinking emphasizing the just use of power[7] and Aristotle arguing for impartiality in treating like cases alike.[13] However, Aristotle's principle leaves important questions open to debate, such as how society should respond when bad things are allotted to or befall individuals, which needs are relevant when determining the justice or injustice of a situation, the level to which people should be assisted when injustices are recognized, and what good should come of that assistance. For example, is a fairer distribution of income the desired end point or should societies go so far as to ensure that all people are included and can do things on equal terms?

PRINCIPLES OF SOCIAL JUSTICE

Social justice, in essence, is a societal commitment to implementing the principle of equity. Its particular concern is the origins and consequences of injustices arising from racism, sexism, income inequality, and disability.[14] Importantly, those concerns include the impact of dangerous and grueling occupations on well-being, with slavery, the occupational deprivation of the insane, child labor, and the unsavory living conditions of factory workers being early examples.[15] The three parameters of social justice are how resources, rights, responsibilities, and opportunities in life are distributed ethically; whether people's equal worth and right to meet their basic needs is recognized; and whether unjustified inequities are reduced or eliminated.[16] Depending on how fairly members of different groups are treated, a whole society can be judged to be just or unjust.

Social justice was first named as a concept in 1840 by Sicilian priest Luigi Tamarillo d'Azelglio.[17] However, it was given status by 19th century Utilitarian philosopher and political economist, John Stuart Mill; he propounded belief in an "equitable and compassionate world where difference is understood and valued, and where human dignity, the Earth, our ancestors and future generations are respected."[18] Through the 19th century, two contrasting schools of thought existed in relation to how social justice should be manifested. One was formulated by Herbert Spencer, who coined the expression "survival of the fittest,"[19] often erroneously attributed to the later publication of Darwin's theory of evolution.[20] Spencer emphasized equality in terms of both the freedoms each person is guaranteed and getting one's just deserts, based on the good or harmful consequences of one's actions.[19] Thus, both the burdens accrued by the disadvantaged and privileges that could not be justified by effort or accomplishment would equally be deemed unjust. An alternate view, promulgated by Marx, was that the distribution of societal and material goods should be determined by need.

Both perspectives have been subjected to critique. Giving people what they deserve puts many people at risk of receiving little or nothing because they have nothing to contribute (or do nothing) that society values. Justice based on need addresses that problem but, even if we understood what people need to live a life of dignity and respect, present day societies can afford to more than meet the needs of the disadvantaged while leaving a disproportionate share of wealth, resources, and opportunities in the hands of a privileged minority. Invoking the principle of equality, such that the remaining resources are distributed in equal shares, is unlikely to be successful because those who are most productive or powerful have difficulty accepting the idea that the things they do and their efforts and achievements do not entitle them to a larger share of the rewards.[9]

Social justice was popularized by the Arts and Crafts Movement that flourished from about 1860 into the early 20th century, despite a lack of clarity about rightful beneficiaries. Arts and Crafts ideology had emerged in England as a reaction against the dehumanizing effects of the Industrial Revolution and the profound societal problems associated with it: poverty, overcrowding, child labor, disease, and injury. An additional concern was the imminent loss of crafts skills of the potters, basket makers, weavers, wood workers, stone masons, metal workers, and artisans. They were lauded as using traditional methods, working local materials into beautiful, utilitarian objects. Where creating something by hand was celebrated as "healthy and ennobling labour" that developed workers' creativity and uniqueness, more efficient production-line work was described as servile, soul-destroying, and rendering workers "less than men."[21]

In opposing industrialization, Arts and Crafts proponents championed the values of old fashioned craftsmanship as a mechanism for social change. In the United States, against the backdrop of high unemployment among the floods of European immigrants that were arriving, that communal focus was reinterpreted as individual well-being achieved through self-determination, self-reliance, and economic success.[22] To an extent, the ideology and traditional crafts that the Arts and Crafts Movement promoted live on in occupational therapy, although the profession's roots in social justice have arguably been obscured by individually focused efforts to improve the lot of people with disabilities. Within social justice, the debate about equality of outcomes versus a level of reward commensurate with social status, need, occupational contributions, and effort remains unresolved. People's preferences vary depending on their motives (eg, expedience, self-interest, fairness), and the extent to which they believe it to be possible to achieve valued goals, such as group welfare, productivity, or harmony between different subgroups.[23]

CONTEMPORARY PERSPECTIVES OF SOCIAL JUSTICE

In contemporary western societies, justice means seeking the truth and making impartial, objective judgments based on evidence rather than being swayed by the merits of other arguments, however heartfelt or eloquent. Such determinations of the justice or injustice of a specific social, economic, or political situation are underpinned by the principles of equity and fairness, especially in relation to human rights. In so far as equity implies equal protection from harm or others' unlawful acts, it is a constitutionally protected right enjoyed by citizens of many countries.[8]

Aspirations toward becoming just and equitable societies have served as a powerful philosophical justification for public health advances. That argument is grounded in increasing recognition that disparities in health and longevity are caused by the deprivations associated with lower socioeconomic positions and educational attainment, which jeopardize access to the material requisites of a decent life and participation in decision-making processes. Those impacts are most profound for women and girls, who also experience unequal restrictions on where they can go, ownership and control of material assets, restrictive codes of social conduct, and societal tolerance or reward for sexual violence, all of which restrict access to and participation in occupations outside of the domestic sphere. Among indigenous people, who are the most disenfranchised and marginalized groups in the world, health disparities are also attributable to erosion of culture, loss or denigration of traditional occupations, and dispossession of land. Bringing an equity perspective to health acknowledges both its intrinsic value and "that good health enables people to participate in society, with potentially positive consequences for [a country's] economic performance."[24]

Alongside growing awareness of the relationship between health and equity, the principle of fairness has also been rapidly assimilated into recent philosophical thinking. That trend can be traced back to the early 1970s when American social philosopher John Rawls promoted his theory of justice.[12] Focusing on the opportunities open to people rather than the outcomes achieved, Rawls posited that societies can be viewed as systems in which free and equal individuals cooperate according to moral principles of individual rights, responsibilities, and liberties. Based on the principle of fair equality of opportunity, he argued that whatever their position in society, everyone wants life to be worth living.[12] That demands sufficient effective freedom to pursue one's goals including, by extension, goals to do, be, belong, and become through occupation.

Fairness can also be interpreted to mean the even-handed distribution of goods and services, such as jobs, education, housing, and health care, as well as burdens such as taxes and exposure to hazardous wastes.[25] This perspective is referred to as distributive justice, which is another central tenet of Western understandings of justice and is characteristic of egalitarian societies. According to Rawls, deviations from the ideals of equal liberty for all and fair equality of opportunity are only justifiable if they "level the playing field" to benefit the least advantaged.[12] Referred to as positive discrimination or affirmative action, examples include reserved places in educational programs, targeted scholarships, workplace accommodations, and encouraging job applications from under-represented groups. As such, distributive justice may involve providing preferential services to redress past wrongs against disadvantaged subgroups, when that is deemed necessary or desirable. Because affirmative action and redress are not impartial, such actions can, in themselves, be perceived as unjust.[8] Two further concepts are allied to distributive justice. The first, procedural justice, relates to fair and consistent processes for making decisions, offering an explanation for the specific procedures followed, and treating members of the group in a polite and dignified manner, such as allowing them to have input before decisions are made. The second is interactional justice, or treating individuals in a group fairly.[14] Tara Smith's[26] perspective—that justice is grounded in the personal virtue of respecting and treating others fairly—links the discussion back to Aristotle's 4th century BC idea of justice being the enactment of human virtues.[6] However, what is or is not fair is a subjective judgment and therefore is always open to debate.

In response to mass interest, the social justice imperative for the fair distribution of resources was incorporated into legislation over a relatively short timeframe. For example, in 1994 the British Commission on Social Justice saw its application to the ethical distribution and sharing of resources; recognition of the equal worth of citizens; their equal right to meet basic needs; the diffusion of opportunities and life chances; and the reduction and elimination of unjustified inequalities. Now an accepted part of postmodern societies, social justice is especially related to "the proper division of benefits and burdens within a society or other collective."[27]

The political dimensions of social justice have public and private ramifications. Communities and individuals make decisions about what they need, want, or are obliged to do against a background of governmental or organizational regulations and business decisions. Public policy and funding, and the associated regulation of justice, although largely invisible and unconscious in everyday life, are powerful determinants of what people do and perceive as possible to do, irrespective of individual motivation and energy. That is, policy and funding decisions set the stage for population, subgroup, and individual experiences of justice or injustice.[28] It is when people insist on fairness, respect, shared responsibility in relationships, and equitable opportunities to participate that social justice is enacted through everyday life.[29] However, to resolve the competing claims of different subgroups, more work is needed to understand how people assess whether things are fair or unfair. To inform social change processes and create a more consensual vision of social justice, it will also be necessary to understand better what brings people who benefit from the status quo to a point where they will support changes to established patterns of distribution.[14]

Social psychologists working in this area address the intersection of individuals' objective circumstances, their perceptions about their circumstances, and what they do to obtain a just share of society's goods. One early proposal, Adams' equity theory in 1965, was that perceived injustices engender emotional and psychological reactions, as well as behavioral responses.[30] Subsequent studies support that assumption, providing evidence that those who feel unjustly treated experience distress, dissatisfaction, and anger, and take action to both resolve their emotions and increase the outcomes they receive for their efforts. Equally, in response to feeling over-rewarded for what they do, people have been found to take action to restore equity by increasing their level of input. Folger's 1986 referent cognition theory suggested that when people receive an unfair outcome they compare what actually happened with what might have happened.[31]

People's acceptance or rejection of the outcomes of distributive justice also seems to hinge on how much they know about those outcomes. If little is known, judgments are based on whether individuals felt valued during the process, which signals their inclusion or exclusion from the group. Perceptions of procedural unfairness generate negative attitudes toward the perpetrators of injustice, which threatens compliance with authority figures and their rules. Conversely, perceptions of procedural fairness engender a willingness to comply with requests and, in organizational settings, increased work levels, conscientiously meeting performance expectations, and enhanced courtesy and altruism.[32] Because individuals' evaluations of justice and injustice are sometimes confounded by self-interest and the evaluation of what they deserve, social psychologists are increasingly turning their attention from individual to collective welfare. At that level, distributive justice concerns whether consensual values are upheld and biases suppressed.[14]

Achieving Social Justice

Such concerns bring to light some of the difficulties in truly achieving social justice. Two philosophical perspectives are helpful: Iris Morton Young's justice of difference[33] and economist and philosopher Amartya Sen's capabilities approach.[34] Young's critique of social justice is that it is primarily concerned with distributive justice; that is, the fair allocation of goods and resources across different groups. Young asserts that in focusing on what people have, social justice cannot sufficiently take into account biological or social differences that are based on unequal power relations. Therefore, the pursuit of social justice permits the continued exploitation, marginalization, disempowerment, and alienating experiences of particular groups such as women, people living in poverty, people with disability, or ethnic minorities. Young talks instead about a justice of difference that is congruent with opportunity, empowerment, health, and quality of life. Viewed this way, actions designed to challenge injustice would focus on creating opportunities for people to live, work, play, develop, and age without exploitation or violence.[33] Somewhat similarly, Pelton holds a view of justice that addresses "individual need, circumstances, merit, competence, and responsibility,"[35] even if those individuals are members of a group that is discriminated against. Accordingly, Pelton argues that diversity between people "should be recognized and respected by policies that address the fundamental commonalities of all individuals: their human needs, their right to respect, and their potential to flourish when opportunities to do so are available."[35] In this context, such opportunities encompass opportunities to be, belong, and become through occupation.

Where Young and Pelton are focusing on the outcomes of social justice, Sen's concern is the mechanisms that might bring it into being. From his vantage point of working to resolve real world problems of poverty, famine, and female feticide and infanticide in India and China, Sen is critical of theories of social justice that rely on social institutions cooperating to achieve fairness and equality of opportunity.[34] He argues that Rawls'[12] theory of justice fails to address how institutions would work together or the real position and possibilities of people experiencing injustices. Sen makes the case that a theory of justice must say something about the choices that are actually offered. Equally, it must recognize that applying different principles of justice, such as economic equity, utility, or being entitled to the fruits of one's labor, will generate differing or even incompatible solutions. Furthermore, apparent solutions may be partial or require later revision. However, having diverse inputs to issues of justice can provide functional connections between individual priorities and social policy. Even when possible conclusions conflict, they illuminate possibilities within the situation and inform what might be done to improve things. Sen's capability approach encompasses both opportunities for individuals to pursue what they have reason to value and choices about which opportunities to follow. Although Sen refuses to speculate on what capabilities are most important to human functioning, he has specified that health and education are crucial to their development. The key question when assessing how just a society is, from the perspective of the capabilities approach, is "What is each person able to do and to be?"[34] Those freedoms do justice to the diversity of human positions and interests, which can shift as new information becomes available.

Interpreted from an occupational perspective, the capability approach speaks to access to occupations that are personally and socially valued, and being able to exercise choice about the things one does. Such choices are not open to the 126 million children aged 5 to 17 years that UNICEF reports to be working in hazardous conditions or to the 5.7 million children trapped in bonded labor.[36] For immigrant populations in Norway, Sweden, Belgium, Austria, the Netherlands, Switzerland, and Denmark, who have more than twice the unemployment rate of native-born workers, access to work is tenuous.[37] Well paid work is similarly beyond the reach of the 100 to 200 million Chinese mingong, or farm workers, who have to travel from the rural west to eastern cities to earn around $4 per day in factories and construction sites but cannot integrate, receive medical benefits, or send their children to school there because of China's residence permit system.[38]

INJUSTICE AND ILL-HEALTH

The link Sen drew between health and the capability to do and be opens the door to further elaboration of the relationship between social justice and the social determinants of health and ill-health. A key person informing that initiative is Martha Nussbaum,[39] who teased out the relationship between individuals and their sociopolitical context. She argues that the freedom to do and be rests on both the abilities an individual has developed, such as vocational skills and the confidence to voice an opinion, and real opportunities to deploy those abilities in the political, economic, and social environment. Capability failure comes about in two ways: by being denied opportunities to develop talents and abilities, or by being barred from using them. Socially embedded injustices, such as racial or gender discrimination, are likely to deny individuals' capabilities in both ways, creating barriers to the educational and social opportunities that would have developed skills and knowledge, and creating further barriers to participation in economic, social, and political life. This self-reinforcing cycle of impaired capability development impeding later participation is directly associated with poor health outcomes. For example, literacy rates of 12% to 13% among women in Mali and Afghanistan in 2006, as reported by the World Bank,[40] reflect the lack of educational opportunities for girls; have profound effects on their employment status, income, and living conditions; and substantially reduces the survival rate of their children. As this example illustrates, social and occupational injustices can be both intertwined and intergenerational.

To make any progress, Nussbaum believes that the capabilities that are most important to human functioning must be identified. Without that knowledge, she asks, how can societies determine which capabilities are worth developing and who needs most help? Which should a minimally just society support and nurture? Invoking the concept of a life worthy of human dignity, Nussbaum contends that some capabilities are necessities—the universal entitlements required for human dignity and a minimally decent life.[39] Topping Nussbaum's list of central capabilities are achieving a normal lifespan, as opposed to dying prematurely from an avoidable illness or injury; bodily health and integrity, including reproductive choice and freedom from violent assault; and further down the list, being free of extreme fear and anxiety. Such capabilities are implicit within the prerequisites for health and relate to what people do to attain them. Other capabilities align with doing, being, belonging, and becoming through participation in education, the arts, and recreation; having attachments to people and things; reflection; and affiliation with others. In sum, Nussbaum's philosophically derived vision of social justice is implicitly occupational and rests on a health and well-being agenda.

That three-way linkage between social justice, occupation, and well-being has a long history among social institutions and activists concerned with the well-being of disadvantaged groups. As described in earlier editions of this text, monasteries in feudal Europe demonstrated their appreciation of human need by initiating the first health and social welfare services for the masses.[15] In a context where science and medicine became subordinate to religious dogma, monks believed that labor and "morally good" occupations were essential to physical and spiritual health and considered it their duty to take in "the poor, the oppressed, the sinners, and the sick," promising them both "healing and redemption."[41] John Howard (1726-1790), an Enlightenment philanthropist, also drew attention to the link between occupation and health in raising public awareness of the horrors and injustices taking place in prisons and hospitals throughout Europe. He noted that the poverty of occupations available to patients meant they were often discharged "very unfit to work, or the common mode of living."[42] Howard brought about prison reform in Britain by contrasting the good health of convicts provided with ventilation, water supply, cleanliness, wholesome food, and a "proper degree of labor," with the abuses, lack of occupation, and ill-health of convicts in other prisons.[42]

Appreciation of occupation's healing power is also evident in psychiatry's moral treatment era, as mentioned in earlier chapters. For example, when 19th century psychiatrist WAF Browne instituted a new treatment program at Montrose Lunatic Asylum in Scotland in 1837, he based it on "justice, benevolence, and occupation."[43] Prior to 1815, lunatics had been kept chained in cages and dungeons, provided with insufficient food and clothing, force fed, exhibited to the public, and suffered death and injury at the hands of their keepers. In Browne's program, there was a graduation of employment, structured to "be easy and well performed, and so apportioned that it may suit the tastes and powers of each laborer." The asylum was a hive of industry, with inmates "anxious to be engaged and toiling incessantly" because they understood how being occupied lessened their pain and disagreeable thoughts, earned the praise of others and self-respect, and gave them a good night's sleep. Perhaps most important, Browne conveyed his approach to the asylum managers in a series of lectures, so that they too could appreciate the place of occupation in enhancing well-being. The common thread across these accounts is that the changes instituted in monasteries, prisons, and lunatic asylums were directed toward meeting people's occupational needs and natures, and recognizing those as not just health issues, but also as a matter of justice. Capitalizing on different opportunities and resources, these initiatives enabled participation in occupation for individuals and whole populations that were in need. Furthermore, in changing both policy and common practice, the perpetuation of injustice was interrupted.

Notwithstanding that social history and the prominence Sen[34] and Nussbaum[39] give to health, social philosophers have typically disavowed any relationship between justice and health. For example, John Rawls believed health was a matter of luck and a natural good constitution. Apparently because he did not recognize that social influences directly or indirectly produce health, Rawls considered it to be outside the scope of social justice.[12] Venkatapuram strenuously opposes such a position, pointing to the social determinants of longevity, mental and physical functioning, and illness. The capability to be healthy, he asserts, is as fundamental as the right to life, recognition of the equal moral worth and dignity of every individual, and the freedom to determine, pursue, and revise one's life plan. Therefore, when assessing how just or unjust the political, legal, economic, cultural, educational, and religious arrangements are within a society,

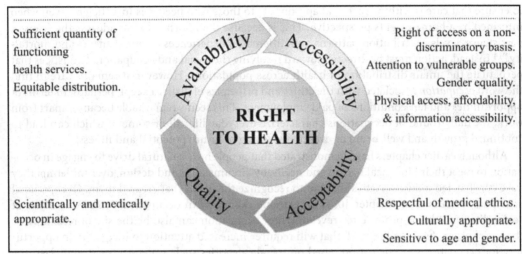

Sufficient quantity of functioning health services. Equitable distribution.

Availability

Accessibility

RIGHT TO HEALTH

Quality

Acceptability

Right of access on a non-discriminatory basis. Attention to vulnerable groups. Gender equality. Physical access, affordability, & information accessibility.

Scientifically and medically appropriate.

Respectful of medical ethics. Culturally appropriate. Sensitive to age and gender.

Figure 14-1. A health care services perspective of the right to health.

consideration must be given to people's capability to be healthy. Although not denying the role of biological endowments, personal behavior, and the physical environment, he is adamant that social arrangements that determine, constrain, or influence the distribution of preventable impairments or premature death are the preserve of social justice. The force behind his argument, consistent with the occupational perspective presented in this text, is that "most everything in a person's life is contingent on health."[44]

Irrespective of the philosophical debate, the reciprocal relationship of health and justice is well embedded in United Nations and WHO documents published over the past two decades, which cite human dignity, equality, equity, and a duty to protect the most vulnerable.[45] For example, principles of equity and distributive justice underpinned the WHO's goal to achieve "health for all by the year 2000."[46,47] That ambitious target was based on closing "the gap between the 'haves' and 'have nots'" to achieve "more equitable distribution of health resources within and among countries, including preferential allocation to those in greatest social need so that the health system adequately covers all the population."[46] Heightened awareness of the justice issues in health is being promoted through documents coauthored by the Office of the UN High Commissioner for Human Rights and the WHO, which explicitly address health as a human right to be protected under the *International Covenant on Economic, Social and Cultural Rights*.[48] Over time, the WHO has become increasingly forceful in its assertion that addressing the social determinants of health is an issue of justice, such that "a society, rich or poor, can be judged by … how fairly health is distributed across the social spectrum."[49] Health is held to be a fundamental right, and the key to enabling communities to lift themselves out of poverty.[50] A rights-based approach to health promotion is also evident in WHO documents addressing racial intolerance and ending the social exclusion experienced by many people with disabilities.[51,52]

Accordingly, equity and distributive justice are identified as important ethical principles guiding population health measures.[8] However, in many contexts, the human right to health continues to be narrowly interpreted as equity of access to healthcare services, irrespective of cultural, ethnic, or social status. Even when couched under the more encompassing rubric of availability, accessibility, acceptability, and quality (Figure 14-1), the right to health is frequently positioned in relation to reforming health services rather than from a population health or occupational perspective. That medically oriented view was cited in a WHO tool developed and piloted by teams in Uganda, Yemen, and Zambia to assess the coherence of health sector policy in relation to gender equality.[53]

There is clearly a need to draw attention to the ways that medical knowledge and health service practices are gender, age, or culturally biased and exclude some groups. However, health reforms to ensure that care is within reach and appropriate to those who need it is insufficient, even when informed by a human rights perspective. This is because the reforms do not address the "causes, persistence, levels, distribution patterns and differential experiences of impairments and mortality."[44] Instead, action must be directed toward resolving the social and occupational injustices that perpetuate the unfair distribution of health across populations. However, it remains rare to find the word *occupation* associated with the ethics and principles of justice except, perhaps, in terms of opportunities and fair conditions of paid employment. This seems remarkable because, apart from work, the daily round of occupations characterize everyday life, all or some of which can lead to continued growth and well-being or eventual stunting of future potential and illness.

Although earlier chapters have demonstrated that people have a natural drive to engage in occupation to meet their biological nature and needs, by circumstance and design, over millennia they have constructed unjust societies that fail to recognize the needs that created them. Occupational apartheid, discussed in Chapter 10, is an extreme example. An occupation-centered analysis of social difference holds promise for revealing how occupation can also be the site of resistance to the social order. As Angell argued, that will require "increased attention to inequality in opportunity for occupational participation based on social categories such as gender, race, and class; the development of occupation-centered analyses; and the movement from individualistic to contextual approaches which consider all occupation to be inherently intersubjective."[54]

Unless the occupational nature and needs of people are recognized in occupationally just policies, the majority of the world's population will fail to flourish. This is already the case. Although some people find meaning and well-being through what they do, the majority are relegated to a life in which they are unable to meet the occupational challenges of their environments to obtain the prerequisites of survival, quite apart from achieving their being or becoming needs. Without occupational justice, people across the world experience inequities that touch the very essence of human life.

An Occupational Justice Perspective of Health

An occupational perspective of justice has many commonalities with social justice. Indeed, some argue that it is but a subset of the better-known concept. Occupational justice can thus be described as concerning what people need, want, and are obliged to do in their relationships and everyday lives, as part of a broader social justice that addresses social relations and conditions of living (Table 14-1). Like social justice, occupational justice rests on the concept of equity, which implies equal protection for all members of society from harms relating to both participation in and exclusion from occupation. Equity also presumes equitable access to occupation, the places where occupations occur, the prerequisite resources, and the benefits and burdens derived from occupation. In this sense, occupational justice is a distributive justice that is concerned with fair distribution and the sharing of opportunities, choices, and freedoms to participate in and share the outcomes of occupation, including satisfaction, enjoyment, and the development of individual capabilities and social capital. The fair and proper division of opportunities, resources, privileges, rights, and responsibilities includes access to life's prerequisites and an expectation of supporting and empowering disadvantaged subgroups to participate. Equity, fairness, and empowerment do not call for all people to be able to do exactly the same things. Rather, occupational justice is a justice of difference.[55a] It recognizes people's equal worth, dignity, and need for occupation, irrespective of differing capabilities and knowledge, skills, competence, and experiences of participating. As a justice of difference, occupational justice enables the prerequisites of life to be obtained according to needs, and acknowledges the differing meanings derived from participation.

Like social justice, an occupational perspective of justice is universal. It occurs when all people are valued for what they do; their occupational capacities, performance, and goals; and their contribution to communal and societal endeavors. Occupationally just societies assure members of

Table 14-1		
COMPARING SOCIAL AND OCCUPATIONAL JUSTICE		
Characteristic	Social Justice	Occupational Justice
Focus	The human rights, responsibilities, and dignity of people from all social classes, with particular reference to subgroups that are most vulnerable	All people's rights to "participate to their potential and... exert control over what they do everyday[55a] to meet survival, developmental, belonging, and spiritual needs
World View	Laws, policies, regulations, and media images that promote nondiscriminatory social relationships Fair processes to address injustices Poverty reduction strategies	Laws, policies, regulations, economic, and professional practices, media images, and other factors governing what people can do, want to do, and imagine as being possible to do that support well-being and reaching potential
Educational focus	Human rights education for respect, tolerance, and recognition[92]	Human rights education to promote critical consciousness of causes of occupational injustices, and critical action to document injustices and work collaboratively with those experiencing occupational injustice to analyze, plan, and evaluate effective responses[55b]
Still to be determined	What a socially just society ought to support and nurture Who most needs help How to create consensual vision of social justice How people assess whether things are fair or unfair, in order to resolve competing claims How to get people who benefit from the status quo to accept changes to established pattern of distribution	Which occupations societies and individuals have reason to value What pattern of occupation optimally supports health Whether justice is achieved through equity of access to occupation or equitable distribution of its risks and burdens and benefits Whether the distribution of occupations is fair Who most needs help The level and kind of assistance that ought to be available Mechanisms to create societal consensus about occupational justice
Projected outcome	Human rights upheld Human dignity affirmed and valued Opportunities for all people to live, work, and play without exploitation or violence Reduced disparities in conditions of living Justice of difference: Diversity is recognized and respected Distributive justice: Fair and equitable allocation of goods and resources across different groups, biases suppressed Sustainable and peaceful future	Occupational rights upheld Enablement of participation and choice Reduced participation restrictions, including universal design[2] Reduction in circumstances that require some to do too much while others have too little to do Not being coerced or forced to participate in degrading, illegal, or dangerous occupations[2] Greater equity across groups to choose and participate to their potential in necessary, obligatory, and meaningful occupations[55a] People with disability supported to participate Enhanced societal and individual well-being Inclusive society

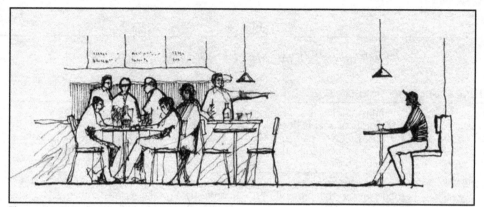

Figure 14-2. Exclusion from social premises that restrict entry according to ethnicity. (© Trevor Bywater 2013. Used with permission.)

every subgroup or community of opportunities to meet their own and each other's survival, developmental, belonging, and spiritual needs through occupations that recognize their strengths.[22] Occupational justice is challenged when external barriers unfairly prevent some people and advantage others in meeting their basic requirements, demonstrating their capacities and abilities, expressing themselves, developing their potential, or experiencing well-being through what they do. Occupational injustice concerns encompass those groups excluded from or marginalized within the social framework, as well as those excluded by hegemonic understandings of the occupations available and valuable for specific subgroups.

Occupational injustices are evident when economic policy and societal structures result in some people having an unhealthy mix of occupations, including some having too much to do while others have too little. That situation is associated with unequal power relations and established social and institutional structures and functions that exploit, marginalize, disempower, restrict, alienate, and inflict physical, psychological, and spiritual harm on people. These injustices become visible when participation is devalued, barred or prohibited, disrupted, confined or segregated, or creates illness and injury for some groups of people more than others.[56] Occupational injustices might be localized, such as children in economically deprived neighborhoods lacking safe places to play; culturally based, such as women and girls being excluded from sports because of norms of femininity,[57] or people of any age group not being permitted to spend social time in premises that restrict entry according to ethnicity (Figure 14-2); or global, such as people employed in sweatshops to provide cheap clothing to affluent, off-shore markets. Experiencing occupational injustices, as with social injustices, can be interpreted as exclusion from the greater society, which generates emotional reactions, as well as behavioral responses that might ameliorate or worsen the situation and its consequences.

Occupational injustice is a human rights issue when unjustified inequalities in people's access to occupation are present, with long-term deleterious consequences. Occupational justice is served by reducing or eliminating inequalities, such that people's capabilities to participate in society, experience well-being, and live a life with human dignity and respect are protected. One example would be the population level interventions promoted by the United Nations and WHO, targeted toward lifting people out of poverty and the occupational deprivation that brings. Another example might be the appropriate enablement of individuals living with disability,[58] a focus supported in affluent nations by legislation, technology, financial resources, research findings, and the efforts of professions such as occupational therapy.

Positioning occupational justice as bridging societal and health concerns also situates it as relating to people's sociocultural, civil, and political circumstances. In the extreme, occupational justice includes freedom from being coerced or forced to participate in degrading, illegal, or dangerous occupations.[2] However, also like social justice, occupational justice leaves open to debate how to determine whether the distribution of occupations is fair, which occupations societies and individuals have reason to value, who most needs help, the level and type of assistance that ought to be available, and whether justice is achieved through equity of access to occupation or equitable distribution of its risks, burdens, and benefits. Mechanisms to create consensus about occupational justice have not, so far, been identified.

In contrast to social justice, which readily identifies the groups subject to injustice as those who are materially disadvantaged by poverty or discrimination, occupational injustice might impact groups at all levels of society and at different life stages. Occupational justice and injustice are produced by the broad social conditions and structures that shape daily life. In low-income societies, the intertwined network of structural conditions perhaps most liable to bring about both occupational injustices and health inequities, are poverty and its associated gender discrimination,[59] vulnerability to avoidable and treatable health conditions and high HIV/AIDS rates, and disempowerment and social exclusion.[60] In addition, frequently evident are lack of universal access to education and unfavorable economic conditions, including free trade agreements, exploitation by multinational corporations, and lacking or ineffective workplace safety measures. In high-income societies, occupational injustice is perhaps most visible in relation to the availability of, access to, and remuneration for paid work, which are impacted by factors including economic restructuring and recessions; structural unemployment; gender-based pay disparities; education that fails to meet individual capacities and interests, and leads to dropouts and eventual reliance on social services; lack of practical and financial assistance with workplace accommodations; failure to recognize immigrants' credentials and prior work experience;[61] and legislation restricting or removing asylum seekers' and undocumented migrants' access to employment.[62-64] As discussed in Chapter 10, such factors can create situations of occupational deprivation. Additional systemic factors that create occupational injustice are homelessness,[65] urban sprawl, failure to implement universal design, and lack of or ineffective antidiscrimination legislation.

In any country, having a disability or chronic health condition is associated with exclusion from everyday occupations, education, and employment opportunities, which is increasingly understood as a human rights concern,[66] as well as being an occupational injustice. Equally, minority groups, immigrants,[67] and groups that have been forcibly or socially segregated are more likely to experience social and occupational injustices. In addition, being internally displaced by war or civil unrest, large-scale projects to develop national infrastructure, natural disasters, nuclear accidents, or changing climactic conditions are also associated with occupational injustice where local, societal, and international aid responses fail to reestablish safe living conditions and the housing, sanitation, education, employment, social, and healthcare infrastructure for all those affected. Degradation and depletion of natural resources, such as fisheries and forests, are also associated with occupational injustice when alternate employment options are not available. On top of these influences, in countries with a history of colonization, the loss of language and culture, displacement from ancestral lands, institutional racism, and negative stereotyping of the indigenous population are human rights issues that affect health[68] and create additional layers of occupational injustice.

Although not subject to social injustices, people in affluent circumstances might also experience narrowed opportunity and demand for occupation that undermines their health and ability to achieve their potential because they, too, are conditioned to lifestyles and cultural norms that fail to meet their basic needs. Illustrating that point, Crawford, a motorbike mechanic and philosopher, argued that in spurning manual work in favor of the financial security of white collar work, America's youth are being channeled away from intellectually engaging vocations that provide a sense of agency, competence, usefulness, and creativity.[69] Equally, even among well-heeled seniors, the right to participate in meaningful occupations might be jeopardized by barriers in the built environment, societal attitudes that devalue their expertise and opinions, health policies that position them as an economic burden, and an assumption of caregiving rather than enablement in residential facilities. **Considering all the above, we define an occupational justice approach to health as the promotion of just socioeconomic and political conditions to increase population and political awareness, resources, and opportunity for people to be, belong and become healthy through engagement in occupations that meet the prerequisites of health and each person's and community's different natures, capacities, and needs.**

One difficulty with such definitions is determining exactly what is required to achieve justice. Clearly, occupational justice does not mean that each person receives, as a right, opportunities to participate in every occupation in which he or she might wish to engage. Equally, lost opportunities and barriers to occupation, however appealing or health enhancing that activity might be, do not necessarily have ill-health consequences. Given that, which and how many opportunities and resources might people reasonably expect? What is a prerequisite, and what a luxury? Nussbaum's 10 central capabilities for a minimally dignified life, mentioned earlier, offer some guidance.[39] Although needing to be interpreted in context, her work provides a basis for determining the parameters for justice that societies ought to ensure for their citizens. Equally, because each capability is implicitly occupational, her capabilities can be read from the perspective of an occupational justice perspective of population health (Table 14-2). Thus interpreted, Nussbaum's capabilities give a sense of the range and extent of engagement in occupation necessary to preserve a minimal level of health, and the manner in which health risks must be averted to support engagement in occupation.

Bringing these perspectives together, the foundations of an occupational justice approach to health can be identified. Accepting the notion of enablement of occupational potential as paramount for healthy populations and individuals is a first principle. Enablement presupposes empowerment through occupation. At an experiential level, that might be expressed as being decisive, assertive, or confident to share thoughts, make suggestions, and ask questions. Being empowered might also be felt as having drive, purpose, or motivation; having a choice or direction for future actions; having a positive identity; having a sense of confidence; or as being happy or content. The ongoing societal failure to enact occupational justice at this level is experienced by those who are excluded from typical patterns of occupation as a loss of self-value and of being valued by others, as occupational deprivation and imbalance, and as unrealized capabilities to contribute to society. Such losses cut to the heart of their humanity.[70]

At a structural level, empowerment means questioning the economic, legislative, corporate, educational, or cultural determinants that grant or allow some, but not other, people to have power, privilege, and control and identifying how that is achieved, who is expected to comply, and what is the cost of noncompliance. Empowerment is achieved through power sharing, collaboration, and partnership to challenge determinants such as the gender- and race-based division of labor, caste, and class structures; relegation of low status unpaid care and domestic work to women, at the expense of other occupations suited to their interests and abilities; discrimination against minority groups and people with disabilities; federal and state regulations, trade deals, corporate, and managerial practices; professional protectionism; corruption and war; and cultural imperialism that generates occupational injustices.[71]

As the work of institutional ethnographers reveals, if progress toward the enablement of a minimally decent life for all is to be achieved, empowerment processes must reach into the laws, policies, processes, procedures, and other texts that govern commerce, employment, education, housing, hospitalization, incarceration, and other forms of institutional living, as well as societal responses to homelessness.[70] Underpinning all such moves to promote occupational justice is acceptance of the principle of diversity, and that a more socially inclusive valuing of participation in many types of doing is called for, whether that performance fits with normative expectations or not. Inequities in opportunities for participation in diverse occupations for health and well-being can be reduced, but to achieve that, both a justice of distribution and a justice of difference will be required (Table 14-3).

Table 14-2

AN OCCUPATIONAL PERSPECTIVE OF NUSSBAUM'S CENTRAL CAPABILITIES FOR A MINIMALLY DIGNIFIED LIFE

Central Capability	Nussbaum's Definition[39]	Occupational Perspective
Life	Normal lifespan, not so reduced as to be not worth living	Survival occupations, preserving health by exercising capacities, sufficient health to engage in occupation
Bodily health	Good health, adequate nutrition, adequate shelter	Health promoting balance of occupations; cultivation, procurement, preparation, and consumption of adequate nutritious food and clean water; construction of adequate shelter
Bodily integrity	Being able to move from place to place, free from violent assault; sexual satisfaction; choice about reproduction	Safe travel between occupations; safe, consensual sexual satisfaction; child-rearing occupations
Senses, imagination, and thought	Informed and cultivated by education, including literacy, numeracy, experiencing, enjoying, and producing arts, music, religion, freedom of expression	Becoming through educational occupations; use and development of innate skills; engagement in culturally meaningful artistic occupations, self expression through occupation and occupational choices
Emotions	Attachments to people and things; experiencing love, longing, anger, grief, gratitude, not being blighted by fear and anxiety	Belonging and being through occupation; experiencing competence and satisfaction; not being forced into anxiety-provoking, dangerous, or degrading occupations
Practical reason	Being able to understand what is good and engage in critical reflection to plan one's life	Being able to understand the consequences of occupations; learning through doing; recognizing occupational possibilities and potential
Affiliation	Living with and toward others, showing concern for others, interacting with others, being able to imagine the situation of another	Social and intimate occupations; coordination of occupations with others; co-occupation; care occupations; belonging through doing
Other species	Playing, laughing, enjoying recreational activities	Childhood play and playfulness; enjoyable recreations
Play	Playing, laughing, enjoying recreational activities	Childhood play and playfulness; enjoyable recreations
Control over one's environment	Participating in political choices that govern one's life, right to participate in politics; property ownership and property rights; right to employment and mutual recognition with other workers; freedom from unwarranted search and seizure	Freedom to participate in civic and political occupations; access to safe, meaningful work, reasonable workplace accommodations; opportunities to do, be, belong, and become; opportunities to realize one's occupational potential

Table 14-3		
FOUNDATIONS OF AN OCCUPATIONAL JUSTICE APPROACH TO HEALTH		
Basis of Approach	*Underlying Beliefs*	*Underlying Principles*
Applicable to populations, communities, and individuals	Humans are occupational beings	Occupational opportunities as a human right
Aimed at reducing inequities in the experience of health/ill health	Participation is a determinant of health and well-being	Inequities in opportunities for participation can be reduced
Based on social, political, and occupational science	People need to participate in occupations as autonomous beings in diverse socioeconomic systems	Both justice of distribution and justice of difference required
Holistic concept of people within natural and constructed environments	Participation is interdependent and contextual	Enablement of occupational potential for populations and individuals
Person-centered, enabling, and empowering	Coordinated action leads to health and social policies that foster justice	Empowerment through occupation
Participatory, diverse, and inclusive	Safe, satisfying, stimulating, and enjoyable occupational conditions are a global responsibility	Diversity and inclusivity of occupational participation

The Necessity of an Occupational Justice Perspective of Health

Over the past 30 years particularly, public health practitioners have concentrated their efforts on issues of social justice, usually prompted by or in line with United Nations and WHO directives. Indeed, it is they who lead much of the action toward those directives. However, they have not sufficiently addressed the injustices caused by the lack of recognition of the holistic occupational nature and needs of people and the relationship of those to health. Occupational therapists also have an implicit concern with social justice and occupational justice as part of their philosophical base but have failed to recognize or to act sufficiently on injustices of all kinds. Townsend has suggested that occupational therapists need to become conscious of how "the social vision which forms the foundation of occupational therapy" is "narrowed to comply with dominant community, managerial, and medical approaches."[72] She advances the idea that "enabling people to participate as valued members of society despite diverse or limited potential" is central within the vision, explaining that justice usually depends on processes that recognize, approve, celebrate, and provide meaningful experiences. The governance of injustice is through laws, rules and regulations, policies, procedures, penalties, disincentives, disempowerment, mistreatment, exclusion, and domination.[73] However, messages about social expectations, justice, and injustice to populations are conveyed mainly through informal rather than formal ways, such as via cultural materials, telecommunications, films, and websites.[74,75]

The basis of an occupational justice perspective of health is that, currently, there are inequities in the experience of health and of ill-health in all populations around the globe because of a lack of awareness or policies to enable people to establish occupational patterns supportive of health and relevant to particular groups and individuals. The lack of awareness, the policies, and the inequities all need to be recognized and addressed. An occupational justice perspective of population health fits well with the WHO directives in that it is person-centered, enabling, and empowering and encourages participatory, diverse, inclusive, and shared advantage. The personal and population consequences of occupational injustice are not discrete. They are the foundations of illness, or of health and well-being, for individuals, groups, communities, and countries. At stake is not only the reduction of illness or disability, which may be outcomes of people participating in occupation to obtain the prerequisites of health, but also the promotion of physical, mental, social, and spiritual well-being. That is dependent on the ability, opportunity, and meaningfulness of living, working, and playing in safe, supportive, inclusive communities in accord with the WHO 1986 mandate[76] and its follow-up "Health for All in the 21st Century."[77] This mandate touches on one of the difficulties of health systems and approaches controlled by medical science. Medical science places social health largely outside its boundaries, thus separating it from physical and mental health. Yet, people are social and occupational beings whose doings are embedded in the social values, rules, and constraints of different cultures and populations and in the nature of their physical environment, and the social and occupational doing has healthy or unhealthy outcomes.[78]

Following the lead of the WHO, tackling occupational injustices necessitates a human rights approach that attends to human dignity, gender issues, equality, and freedom from discrimination. That approach is underpinned by the United Nations' 1948 Universal Declaration of Human Rights, which, "to promote social progress and better standards of life in larger freedom," asserts the "equal and inalienable rights of all members of the human family."[79] In terms of occupations, the declaration directly addresses governance, work, rest and leisure, home life, education, cultural life, and duties in the community. Importantly, it also speaks to freedom from slavery, and the conditions and context of occupation, addressing concerns such as freedom of movement between different activities, privacy, ownership of resources, marriage, and access to information (Table 14-4). Informed by these provisions and cross-referenced to documents such as a national Bill of Rights or the American Constitution, issues such as being dependent on others to get from place to place, a lack of privacy for self-care tasks, and the restriction of association often associated with residential care settings can be analyzed in terms of human and occupational injustices.[80]

At issue is the capability of all people to engage in a health-sustaining balance of occupations and to be, belong, and become through occupation. Guided by social philosophers, such as Sen,[34] Nussbaum,[39] and Venkatapuram,[44] occupational justice is concerned with having the freedom to lead a minimally decent life. That implies having a core set of capabilities, sufficient material requisites to sustain life and health, control over one's pattern and range of occupations, participation in decision-making processes, and a political voice.[24] It also requires knowledge of the relationship between occupation and health, so that the changes that are negotiated are effective.

Elaboration of an occupational justice perspective has included various attempts to articulate the nature and scope of occupational rights. For example, in 2006 the World Federation of Occupational Therapists adopted a position statement incorporating seven principles that elaborated on both occupational rights and the circumstances that breach those rights (Boxed Dialogue 14-1).[2] Later refinements are narrowing toward four succinct claims:

- Right 1: Participation in a range of occupations for health, development and social inclusion.
- Right 2: Making choices and sharing decision-making power in daily life.
- Right 3: To experience meaning and enrichment in one's occupations.
- Right 4: To receive fair privileges for diverse participation in occupations.[71,81,82]

From her vantage point of participation in community-based rehabilitation with populations in the Middle East, the High Arctic, Central America, and South Africa, Rachel Thibeault proposed that to protect these rights, change agents such as external aid agencies and government bodies must account for the impact their actions have on the web of occupations that sustain the livelihoods and cultural imperatives of the target community. She asserted that working with local people is crucial to gaining access to real-life experience and information, sharing power, and

Table 14-4

OCCUPATIONAL FOCUS WITHIN THE UNIVERSAL DECLARATION OF HUMAN RIGHTS[79]

The Equal and Inalienable Rights of All Members of the Human Family to:	
Article 4	Not be held in slavery or servitude
Article 12	Not be subjected to arbitrary interference with his privacy, family, home, or correspondence
Article 13	Freedom of movement (such as between occupations)
Article 16	With full consent, marry and to found a family
Article 17	Own property alone as well as in association with others and not arbitrarily deprived of his property
Article 18	Manifest his religion or belief in teaching, practice, worship, and observance
Article 19	Hold opinions without interference and to seek, receive, and impart information and ideas through any media
Article 20	Peaceful assembly and association
Article 21	Take part in the government of his country, directly or through freely chosen representatives
Article 22	Social security ... in accordance with the organization and resources of each State, of the economic, social, and cultural rights indispensable for his dignity and the free development of his personality
Article 23	Work, to free choice of employment, to just and favorable conditions of work and to protection against unemployment and to equal pay for equal work
	Just and favorable remuneration ensuring for himself and his family an existence worthy of human dignity, and supplemented, if necessary, by other means of social protection
Article 24	Rest and leisure, including reasonable limitation of working hours and periodic holidays with pay
Article 25	A standard of living adequate for the health and well-being of himself and of his family, including food, clothing, housing, and medical care and necessary social services, and the right to security in the event of unemployment, sickness, disability, widowhood, old age, or other lack of livelihood in circumstances beyond his control
Article 26	Education ... directed to the full development of the human personality and to the strengthening of respect for human rights and fundamental freedoms
Article 27	Participate in the cultural life of the community, to enjoy the arts and to share in scientific advancement and its benefits
Article 29	Duties to the community in which alone the free and full development of his personality is possible

building local competence, capacity, and leadership. That is achieved by mindful respect of the strengths, dignity, and power residing in the community, irrespective of the need for assistance.[82] Avoidance of images of poverty and disadvantage is necessary, however effective for fund-raising purposes, because such negative images convey the message that people are helpless, passive, without resources, and unable to cope.[82]

Based on personal experience of the devastating, albeit unintended, ill-effects that aid provision can generate, Thibeault also holds that honoring a community's occupational rights means that aid agencies must closely examine their own values and motives, to reduce the risk of imposing their biases and assumptions on aid recipients. It also demands that the initial inquiry and subsequent planning, implementation, and evaluation are performed with communities to ensure that partnerships are fair and do not displace local workers, and that outcomes are sustainable. To that

---

Boxed Dialogue 14-1:
World Federation of Occupation Therapists Position Statement: Human Rights

Introduction

The World Federation of Occupational Therapists (WFOT) endorses the United Nations Declaration of Human Rights. The purpose of this position paper is to state the WFOT position on human rights in relation to human occupation and participation.

Principles

- *People have the right to participate in a range of occupations that enable them to flourish, fulfill their potential, and experience satisfaction in a way consistent with their culture and beliefs.*

- *People have the right to be supported to participate in occupation and through engaging in occupation, to be included and valued as members of their family, community, and society.*

- *People have the right to choose for themselves to be free of pressure, force, or coercion; in participating in occupations that may threaten safety, survival, or health and those occupations that are dehumanizing, degrading, or illegal.*

- *The right to occupation encompasses civic, educative, productive, social, creative, spiritual, and restorative occupations. The expression of the human right to occupation will take different forms in different places, because occupations are shaped by their cultural, societal, and geographic context.*

- *At a societal level, the human right to occupation is underpinned by the valuing of each person's diverse contribution to the valued and meaningful occupations of the society, and is ensured by equitable access to participation in occupation, regardless of difference.*

- *Abuses of the right to occupation may take the form of economic, social, or physical exclusion, through attitudinal or physical barriers, or through control of access to necessary knowledge, skills, resources, or venues where occupation takes place.*

- *Global conditions that threaten the right to occupation include poverty, disease, social discrimination, displacement, natural and manmade disasters, and armed conflict. In addition, the right to occupation is subject to cultural beliefs and customs, local circumstances, and institutional power and practices.*

Reprinted with permission from World Federation of Occupational Therapists' 2006 Position Statement: Human Rights.[2]

---

end, tactful, collaborative exploration of possibilities is needed to bring forth their stifled dreams and enhance the scope of occupational possibilities in ways that respect the local talents, tastes, and culture. Hearing all of the voices in a community is imperative, with particular reference to women, who typically accumulate occupational responsibilities and schedules far in excess of those of men. By adopting an occupational lens, the existing webs of occupations and inter-relationships will be brought into sharper focus, revealing issues of occupational deprivation, exploitation and alienation. Mechanisms that both maintain and threaten the equilibrium of existing patterns of occupation and protect equitable social participation must also be brought to light.[82]

Weaving these ideas together, occupational justice approach to health implies that practitioners will develop interventions aimed at and leading to equitable opportunity and resources that enable all people to survive and develop through what they do. It is a necessary approach because its substance is largely overlooked. If appreciated at all, the occupational needs and natures of people as a health issue are given lip service and despite the efforts of health professions aimed at people's doings, there is scant acknowledgement of their contribution. For example, occupational therapy

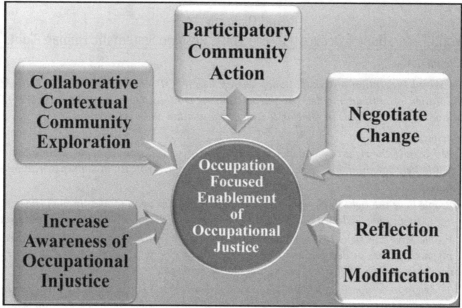

Figure 14-3. Occupation-focused enablement of occupational justice.

has been described as a neglected or invisible profession.[83,84] Survival is dependent on occupation, and meaning and potential are embedded in what people do as both connectedness with communities and as expressions of personal capabilities and spirituality. Ensuring ways for people to engage in survival and meaningful occupations is a practical means through which health, community, and personal transformation becomes possible. Such transformation requires action for it to be recognized politically and organizationally, and practitioners taking this approach would need to direct their efforts to that end, as well as toward survival, health, well-being, and happiness for populations and individuals.

PRACTICAL APPROACHES

To overturn occupational injustices demands action that challenges international relations and trade agreements, domestic norms and policies, economic structures, institutional and corporate practices, societal attitudes, and activities that create and perpetuate them. Initially, action is needed to raise awareness of the occupational injustices that exist in all societies, as well as the embedded attitudes and mechanisms that render such injustices invisible, acceptable, inevitable, or seemingly beyond resolution. It is not until the impact of occupational injustice is exposed, along with its costs in relation to social cohesion, stability, and mutual support, that societies will commit resources to finding and implementing solutions (Figure 14-3). Exploring the extent, effect, and ramifications of occupational injustices will require contextualized, collaborative community action (ie, action that is sensitive to the context, and led by or in partnership with people of that context). Attention must be focused on the conditions in which people live, learn, work, love, grow, and age and on the most vulnerable groups: "indigenous and tribal populations; national, ethnic, religious and linguistic minorities; internally displaced persons; refugees; immigrants and migrants; the elderly; persons with disabilities; prisoners; economically disadvantaged or otherwise marginalized and/or vulnerable groups."[85]

History is replete with examples of well-meaning community development and aid initiatives that failed to deliver sustainable outcomes. Indeed, many have done more harm than good, including some with an occupational justice agenda. One illustrative example is Thibeault's[82] account of a foreign aid project involving U.S. university students providing second-hand wheelchairs and helping construct a school, clinic, and bridge for a Nicaraguan village. The students' pride in their accomplishments demonstrated their ignorance of other outcomes: that they had taken the jobs of local construction workers, compounded existing health risks, and destroyed a business that employed people with disabilities. Although acknowledging that locally developed initiatives are not guaranteed to satisfy all of the diverse needs and interests of a community, participatory community approaches have the advantage of bringing local knowledge and networks to a project.

Incorporating members of the community into the process of exploring the need, planning, and implementation holds promise for engaging with the various stakeholders to navigate a path between their divergent views about what can and should be done, which needs have priority, and what occupations will be effective in creating the conditions for occupational justice. Local experts are also likely to be better equipped than outsiders to identify an effective point of entry to begin to introduce change, and to have a sense of the community's existing occupational capital (the skills, capacities, and knowledge of individuals and groups that might be called on). In addition, local expertise can be helpful in determining the occupational capital that projects should seek to develop and how such skills, knowledge, and capacities might cascade to support ongoing development, or be passed on to other members of the community.[86] Equally, those who have first-hand experience of occupational injustice will bring invaluable understanding to reflections on progress made and necessary modifications to the plan.

An example of how increasing public awareness can lead to social action to halt an occupational injustice comes from early 20th century America. To expose the hazardous work conditions and stark poverty of child workers in America, Lewis Wickes Hine (1874-1940) left his job as a teacher in 1908 to become the photographer for the National Child Labor Committee (NCLC). Believing that an education was a better way out of poverty, the NCLC enlisted Hine's photojournalism to lobby for federal laws to regulate child labor and raise public awareness of the need to police existing state regulations.[87] Although best remembered for his images of men working on the Empire State building, astride girders hundreds of feet up in the air, Hine spent a decade traveling the country documenting children working as cotton pickers, farm laborers, breaker boys in coal mines, factory hands, laborers in glass works, spinners in cotton mills, newsies (newspaper boys), shrimp pickers, oyster shuckers, restaurant workers, street vendors, bootblacks (shoe-shine boys) and garbage scavengers. The captions on his untouched-up photographs record the names, ages, role, employer, and state in which children as young as 3 and 4 years worked to help support their families. Many were the children of European immigrants who came to the United States in search of a better life. Most were illiterate, and worked 8 to 10 hour days, including shift work. Hine documented how some of them started work at 3:30 or 4:00 a.m., cramming more than 7 hours of work into the time before and after school.[88] In commemoration of his work, the NCLC established the Lewis Hine Award to recognized people who help children and youth.[89]

Despite its proud history in addressing human rights, the United States is one of only three countries, along with Somalia and South Sudan, that has not ratified the *Convention on the Rights of the Child* that was adopted by the United Nations in 1989.[90] As mentioned in Chapter 12, the Convention has at its roots Eglantyne Jebb's 1923 draft declaration of the *Rights of the Child*,[91] the *Universal Declaration of Human Rights*, and an earlier UN *Declaration of the Rights of the Child* in 1959 that provided a statement of general principles but was not legally binding.[92] These special rights were created because of the physical and mental immaturity of children, which makes them vulnerable to decisions and actions taken by adults, and to being viewed collectively rather than as individuals with needs and rights. The basic principles of the Convention bring together civil, political, social, economic, and cultural rights of the child in a holistic way. Relevant to achieving occupational justice, it calls for their right to the following:

- Survival—"including nutrition, shelter, an adequate standard of living"
- Development—so that children "reach their full potential," including education, play, leisure, and cultural activities

- Protection from all forms of abuse, neglect, and exploitation
- Participation, including enablement of active roles in "decisions affecting their own lives, in their communities and societies in preparation for responsible adulthood."[90]

Realizing the centrality of public awareness to protecting people's civic, political, economic, social, cultural, and, by inference, occupational rights, in December 2011 the United Nations' General Assembly[93] adopted a resolution asserting that "respect for and observance of all human rights … concerns all parts of society." The resolution declares that everyone has the "right to know, seek, and receive information about all human rights and fundamental freedoms" and that it is essential to incorporate human rights training into all levels of education, from preschool to higher education. In thus empowering people to contribute to and promote a universal culture of human rights, the aim is to prevent violations and abuses and eradicate "all forms of discrimination, racism, stereotyping and incitement to hatred, and the harmful attitudes and prejudices that underlie them." Underpinning that goal are three principles: respect, tolerance, and recognition.[93] Tolerance is perhaps the central concept, encompassing ideas about "permission" for minority groups to live according to their convictions; coexistence and tolerance to avoid conflict; respect and mutual acknowledgement between groups; and appreciating others' way of life as a valuable contribution to society.[94] Such principles are enacted, in the first instance by delivering human rights education that respects the rights of both educators and learners, using language and methods suited to the specific needs and conditions of the target group.[95]

As with education for human rights, education for occupational justice is a process of developing learners' knowledge, attitudes, values, skills, and behaviors. Borrowing from the thoughts of Tibbitts et al on human rights competencies, that knowledge ranges from the dimensions of occupational rights and the mechanisms in place to protect them, to the linkage between local, national, and global abuses of people's occupational rights. Acting to promote and protect occupational rights calls on empathy in the face of suffering, motivation, and commitment to act when rights are violated. In turn, that requires skills in using the language of occupational rights, recognizing violations, analyzing power relations, and planning effective strategies to raise awareness and empower and influence others.[96]

In searching for ways to apply these ideas in practice, the necessary starting point is often to help people become aware of their assumptions, biases, values, and privileges. From that vantage point, they can shift their gaze to others and the conditions that create and perpetuate occupational injustice. This process of raising critical consciousness is more effective using small group discussions than open forums such as lectures or presentations, because they provide a safer context for honest dialogue. This is particularly so when people are considering controversial issues or unfamiliar perspectives, identities, and scenarios.[97] Introducing accounts of occupational injustice through storytelling is, perhaps, the most effective method. However trite, there is truth in the idea that "whoever tells the stories, defines the culture."[98] First-person narratives, in particular, are powerful because they engage people at experiential, cognitive, and affective levels. One example is of sharing stories of compassionate rebels—those ordinary citizens who encountered injustices, responded with, "That's not fair," and were energized to take action. Such stories bring to light injustices that others are genuinely unaware of, or routinely overlook, opening up the possibility of creating a more just society and helping people to get in touch with their own capacity for compassionate rebellion.[99]

Beyond fostering awareness of occupational injustices, educational approaches seek to promote critical action. This might range from documenting instances of occupational injustice, the factors that give rise to them, and their consequences, to collaborating with others to develop and implement plans to promote justice and participation. Whiteford and Townsend's *Participatory Occupational Justice Framework* provides a stepwise process to guide such initiatives using an occupation-based approach.[56] Examples of critical action include assisting disenfranchised groups to increase public awareness of their inequitable occupational load or the barriers that hinder participation in occupation. Helping people tell their own story in a public forum is perhaps a more confronting way to bear witness to injustice, in that audiences can no longer sustain a position of not knowing. For example, Horghagen and Josephsson[100] documented their collaboration with asylum seekers in Norway to develop a theater production that spoke of their lives and the occupational deprivation they endured.

For those who actively engage in addressing occupational injustices through occupation-based approaches, Thibeault's description of her seven-step community-building process is instructive.[82] Spanning needs assessment, mobilization, implementation, monitoring, and maintenance phases, it uses occupations that are carefully selected to foster self-discovery, dignity, solidarity, collective inquiry, and the development of people who can become leaders within the community. The process is grounded in a strengths-based, client-centered approach, and draws on the facilitators' willingness to bring their power to the service of vulnerable communities by building networks and helping them to see and move toward new horizons. The process generally unfolds over 7 to 10 years, starting with step 1: befriending the community. This bonding process, achieved through sharing occupations of significance to that community, cultivates relationships, trust, and collective memories. Important here is that the outsider joins in, learning the local ways, building a sense of belonging, and, in being prepared to demonstrate a lack of expertise, grace, and skill in executing the tasks others perform with ease, signals an equal footing, and that each will learn from the other.

Step 2 is directed toward discovery of the implicit power differentials and most vulnerable members within the community, and establishing the basis for communication as the project unfolds. Nonthreatening collective occupations, such as an informal shared meal, create a safe space to get to know each other and grow closer. That groundwork sets the scene for the development of a communication charter, which is Thibeault's term for an agreed communication plan to address the most likely points of conflict. Gender equity, and the fair distribution of workload and resources are predictable concerns. In keeping with the occupational focus, interactive methods such as role play are used to identify such concerns and the means of responding to them. Step 3 is to uncover the core values, and occupational methods, such as visiting people's workplaces and homes, used to collect stories about daily life and see firsthand what community members do. Richer insights and enhanced communication spring from this validation of people's everyday realities.[82]

Step 4 focuses on equality, specifically the dignity accrued from participation in occupations that have higher status, earn respect, and demonstrate a sense of responsibility and trustworthiness. Equally, the unfair occupational burden shouldered by women and people with disabilities, who are relegated the task of looking after the sick, the orphans, and the elderly, are also brought to light. Gradually and gently, vulnerable members of the community are eased into occupations with higher prestige and local customs are modified to ease the burden of care. Achieving that kind of cultural shift needs the support of positive leaders from within the community who are closely aligned with those affected by the existing occupational arrangements. Step 5 is identifying these people. The approach is pragmatic—what have aspiring leaders done to benefit the community? How can they be supported to become effective advocates? Will their successes be attributed to the group for which they act?[82]

In step 6, there is a subtle shift in the occupations instigated in step 2. Where the goal at step 2 was in building cohesion, step 6 focuses on collaborative community building occupations are intended to build the group's solidarity, identity, or network. To build solidarity, shared occupations that serve the community and mobilize goodwill are undertaken, such as creating a community garden or working with a play group to admit children with disabilities. Identity building activities are about reaching out to other communities, individuals in positions of influence, or causes. That might revolve around showcasing their cultural traditions to others, or lobbying a politician about a matter of shared concern. Once a sense of cohesion is established, communities will be able to move on to the next phase of building their network. Members of the community might enlist their own networks to support activities of benefit to others, such as hosting a social event that will help them form connections with a similar group. Step 7 is about sustainability. By this stage, the community will be mobilized as a cohesive group that can set goals, plan projects, discuss issues, and continue to do things that will sustain a sense of cohesion. Critical questions will include the future of the occupations that have been introduced, whether unrealistic expectations have been raised and how that might be dealt with, and how existing projects can be evaluated so that the community can continue to learn from its experiences. The final stage, and perhaps the hardest, is to leave as a friend rather than a hero; as one who shared a journey, not a savior.[82]

Not all occupation-based community building ventures arise as planned interventions. The original concept behind Men's Sheds, an Australian grass roots initiative from the 1990s, was that a man with a shed equipped with power and hand tools would open it up to other men. In creating opportunities for purposeful occupation, Men's Sheds counter the deprivation experienced by those older men who, after redundancy, ill-health, or retirement, find themselves devoid of things to do. Viewed from an occupational perspective, Men's Sheds replace the structure, social contact, and sense of purpose previously derived from work, while also providing respite from the feminized environment of domestic life. By 2010, there were approximately 500 Men's Sheds associations in Australia, with more being established in New Zealand and Ireland. Men's Sheds are now recognized as a public health initiative in the Australian National Male Health Policy and the Victoria and New South Wales' state plans for men's well-being.[101] That success can be understood in its Australian context, where backyard sheds are a quintessentially male environment within which "blokes" tinker with personal or shared projects and enjoy the company of men with similar skills and interests. Promoted as "more than a place to do woodwork," Men's Sheds are filled with familiar sights, sounds, materials, and tasks. In that context, the skills built up over a lifetime are valued and new skills learned. Having things to do in a shed is about feeling competent, useful, and busy and, perhaps more importantly, having a place to be "shoulder to shoulder" with other men.

Many of the men who join the Men's Shed movement face multiple issues, including social isolation, unemployment, being separated from their spouse, and aging. These are the men who are most difficult to engage through conventional health initiatives, which means that messages about healthy lifestyles, seeking help for depression, having health checks, and recognizing the symptoms of potentially life threatening conditions do not reach them. Perhaps the most important health issue is suicide, which is the 10th leading cause of death for men in Australia. Rates peak for men aged 35 to 45 years and then drop off before increasing steeply in men in their retirement years. The highest rates are in men aged 85 years and older (28.2 per 100,000 in 2009, down from a peak of 46.4 in 2000).[102] There has been some success in taking health messages out to Men's Sheds, where understanding the preference for hands-on, practical learning styles is key to getting the message across. However, perhaps more convincing is research showing that, with their occupational focus, Men's Sheds "achieve positive health, happiness and well-being outcomes for men who participate, as well as for their partners, families and communities."[103] In addition, Men's Shed projects have been used as tailored interventions for older men living with dementia, both in the community and in residential care settings, and to provide safe "yarning spaces" for male Aboriginal and Torres Strait Islanders dealing with anxiety and depression.[104]

Conclusion

Occupational justice can be viewed as a derivative of social justice specifically concerned with people's right to engage in a sufficient variety and amount of occupation to support development, health, and well-being. That is, fair opportunities to do, be, belong, and become what people have the potential to be and the absence of avoidable harm from occupational alienation, deprivation, imbalance, stress, or apartheid. In the 2011 Rio *Political Declaration on Social Determinants of Health*,[1] the WHO declared that human health and well-being are a key feature of successful, inclusive and fair societies. Equally, health and well-being are the most significant outcomes of societal arrangements that apportion occupation according to need and with due concern for enabling vulnerable members of society to engage in a health-promoting array of daily occupations. Like social justice, occupational justice demands that attention be paid to people's dignity and to their differences, given the diversity of cultures, economies, and potential. Finally, just as social justice is grounded in relationships, working for justice in occupation demands collaborative action to raise public awareness of occupational injustices and carry through the community development initiatives that will bring about an occupationally just and inclusive societies.

References

1. World Health Organization. *Rio Political Declaration on Social Determinants of Health*. Rio de Janeiro, Brazil, 21 October 2011. Available at: http://www.who.int/sdhconference/declaration/Rio_political_declaration.pdf
2. World Federation of Occupational Therapists. *Position Paper: Human Rights*. 2006. Available from http://www.wfot.org/ResourceCentre.aspx
3. Ellerin BE. The culinary origins of human occupation: part 1 (motor and process skills). *Journal of Occupational Science*. doi:10.1080/14427591.2013.775916
4. Ellerin BE. The culinary origins of human occupation: part 2 (communication and interaction skills). *Journal of Occupational Science*. doi:10.1080/14427591.2013.775917.
5. Disraeli B. *"Agricultural Distress" Speech in the House of Commons*. London, UK: 11th February, 1851. http://www.bartleby.com/73/952.html
6. Irani KD, Silver M, eds. *Social Justice in the Ancient World*. Westport, CT: Greenwood Press; 1995.
7. Saul JR. *The Unconscious Civilization*. Ringwood, Australia: Penguin; 1997.
8. Last JM, ed. *A Dictionary of Public Health*. Oxford, UK: Oxford University Press; 2012. Retrieved from http://www.oxfordreference.com
9. Johnston D. *A Brief History of Justice*. Chichester, West Sussex: Wiley-Blackwell; 2011.
10. Habermas J. *The Philosophical Discourse of Modernity: Twelve Lectures*. (Trans. F. Lawrence). Cambridge, MA: MIT Press; 1995.
11. Pitkin HF. Justice: on relating public and private. *Political Theory*. 1981;9:327-352.
12. Rawls J. *A Theory of Justice*. Cambridge, MA: Belknap Press of Harvard University Press; 1971.
13. Justice. *Encyclopaedia Britannica*; 2013. http://www.britannica.com
14. Hegtvedt KA. "Social Justice, Theories of." Ritzer, G (ed). *Blackwell Encyclopedia of Sociology*. Blackwell Publishing; 2007. Blackwell Reference Online; http://www.sociologyencyclopedia.com/subscriber/tocnode.html?id=g9781405124331_chunk_g978140512433125_ss1-156
15. Wilcock AA. *Occupation for Health. Volume 1: A Journey from Self Health to Prescription*. London: British Association and College of Occupational Therapy; 2001.
16. Commission on Social Justice. *Social Justice: Strategies for National Renewal*. London, UK: Vintage; 1994.
17. *Definitions of Social Justice on the Web*. www.aworldconnected.org. August 2005.
18. Mill JS. *Utilitarianism*. London; 1863. Reprinted from Fraser's Magazine, 1861.
19. Weinstein D. Herbert Spencer. *Stanford Encyclopedia of Philosophy*; 2012. Retrieved from http://plato.stanford.edu/entries/spencer/
20. Darwin C. *The Descent of Man*. Amherst, NY: Prometheus Books; 1998. First published 1871.
21. Ruskin J. *The Stones of Venice*. Volume II. In K Clark, ed, Ruskin Today. London: John Muray; 1964:282-283. Original work published 1853.
22. Wilcock AA, Townsend EA. Occupational justice. In: Boyt Schell BA, Gillen G, Scaffa ME, eds, *Willard and Spackman's Occupational Therapy*, 12th ed. Philadelphia, PA: Wolters Kluwer Lippincott Williams & Wilkins; 2014:541-552.
23. Leventhal GS, Karuza Jr. J, Fry WR. Beyond fairness: a theory of allocation preferences. In: Mikula G, ed. *Justice and Social Interaction*. New York: Plenum; 1980:167-218.
24. Commission on Social Determinants of Health. *Interim Statement: Achieving Health Equity: From Root Causes to Fair Outcomes*. Geneva: Commission on Social Determinants of Health: 2007: 14.
25. Norton AL, ed. Justice. In: *The Hutchinson Dictionary of Ideas*. Oxford, UK: Helicon Publishing Ltd; 1994.
26. Smith T. Justice as a personal virtue. *Social Theory and Practice*. 1999;25:361-384.

27. Geras N. Justice. In: Bottomore T, ed. *A Dictionary of Marxist Thought*. 2nd ed. Oxford, UK: Blackwell; 1991:275.

28. Townsend EA, Wilcock AA. Occupational justice. In: Christiansen CH, Townsend EA, eds. *Introduction to Occupation: The Art and Science of Living*. Upper Saddle River, NJ: Pearson Education Inc; 2004.

29. Marshall G, Swift A, Roberts S. Social justice. In: *Against the Odds? Social Class and Social Justice in Industrial Societies*. Oxford: Clarendon Press; 1997.

30. Adams JS. Inequity in social exchange. *Advances in Experimental Social Psychology*. 1965;2:267-299.

31. Folger R. Rethinking equity theory: a referent cognition model. In: Bierhoff H, Cohen RL, Greenberg J, eds. *Justice in Social Relations*. New York: Plenum; 1986:145-163.

32. van den Bos K, Lind AE, Wilke HAM. The psychology of procedural and distributive justice viewed from the perspective of fairness heuristic theory. In: Cropanzano R, ed. *Justice in the Workplace: From Theory to Practice, Vol. 2*. Mahwah, NJ: Erlbaum; 2001:49-66.

33. Young IM. *Justice and the Politics of Difference*. Princeton, NJ: Princeton University Press; 1990.

34. Sen A. *The Idea of Justice*. Cambridge: The Belknap Press; 2009.

35. Pelton LH. *Doing Justice: Liberalism, Group Constructs, and Individual Realities*. Albany: State University of New York Press; 1999: 218.

36. United Nations Children's Fund (UNICEF). *Child Protection Information Sheets*. New York, NY: UNICEF; no date.

37. *OECD Factbook 2013: Economic, Environmental and Social Statstics*. Migration and Unemployment. http://www.oecd-ilibrary.org/sites/factbook-2013-en/01/02/04/index.html;jsessionid=1rkfl5vtcew6x.x-oecd-live-01?contentType=/ns/Chapter,/ns/StatisticalPublication&itemId=/content/chapter/factbook-2013-9-n&containerItemId=/content/serial/18147364&accessItemIds=&mimeType=text/html.

38. Reuters. *FACTBOX-Key Facts about China's Millions of Migrant Workers*. Beijing: Reuters: Sunday February 11, 2007.

39. Nussbaum MC. *Creating Capabilities: The Human Development Approach*. Cambridge: The Belknap Press; 2011.

40. World Bank. *World Development Indicators 2006*. Washington, DC: World Bank: 2006.

41. Marti-Ibañez F, ed. *Henry E. Sigerist on the History of Medicine*. New York: MD Publications Inc.; 1960:7-8.

42. Howard J. *An Account of the Principle Lazarettos in Europe; with Various Papers Relative to the Plague: Together with Further Observations on Some Foreign Prisons and Hospitals; and Additional Remarks on the Present State of Those in Great Britain and Ireland*. Warrington: Printed by William Eyres; 1789:140-142.

43. Browne WAF. *What Asylums Were, Are, and Ought to Be*. Edinburgh: Adam and Charles Black; 1837:229-230.

44. Venkatapuram S. *Health Justice: An Argument from the Capabilities Approach*. Cambridge, UK: Polity; 2011:7.

45. United Nations General Assembly. *United Nations Millennium Declaration* (A/RES/55/2); 2000:1.

46. World Health Organization. *Formulating Strategies for Health for All by the Year 2000*. Geneva: WHO; 1979.

47. World Health Organization. *Global Strategy for Health for All by the Year 2000*. Geneva: WHO; 1981. Available at: http://whqlibdoc.who.int/publications/9241800038.pdf

48. United Nations High Commissioner for Human Rights and World Health Organization. *The Right to Health. Fact Sheet No. 31*. Geneva: Author; 2008.

49. World Health Organization. (2008). *Closing the Gap in a Generation: Health Equity through Action on the Social Determinants of Health*. Geneva: WHO; 2008:i.

50. United Nations High Commissioner for Human Rights and World Health Organization. *Human Rights, Health and Poverty Reduction Strategies*. Geneva: Author; 2008. http://www.who.int/hhr/activities/publications/en/

51. World Health Organization. *WHO's Contribution to the World Conference against Racism, Racial Discrimination, Xenophobia and Related Intolerance: Health and Freedom from Discrimination*. Geneva: Author; 2001.

52. World Health Organization. *World Report on Disability*. Geneva: 2011. Retrieved from www.who.int/disabilities/world_report/2011/report/en/. Accessed October 29, 2012.

53. WHO and UN: Human Rights. *Human Rights and Gender Equality in Health Sector Strategies: How to Assess Policy Coherence.* 2011. Available at http://www.who.int/gender/documents/human_rights_tool/en/index.html

54. Angell AM. Occupation-centred analysis of social difference: contributions to a socially responsive occupational science. *Journal of Occupational Science.* 2012;1-12. doi:10.1080/1427591.2012.711230.

55a. Nilsson I, Townsend E. Occupational justice: bridging theory and practice. *Scandinavian Journal of Occupational Therapy.* 2010;17:57-63. doi:10.3109/11038120903287182.

55b. Hocking C, Merritt B, Patterson M, Thibeault R. WFOT International Advisory Group: Human rights. Educating occupational therapists [Poster]. *Canadian Occupational Therapy Conference*, Saskatoon, Canada; 2011. Available from http://www.wfot.org/ResourceCentre.aspx. Accessed November 5, 2013.

56. Whiteford G, Townsend E. Participatory Occupational Justice Framework (POJF 2010): enabling occupational participation and inclusion. In: Kronenberg F, Pollard N, Sakellariou D, eds, *Occupational Therapies without Borders. Vol. 2: Towards an Ecology of Occupation-based Practices.* Edinburgh, UK: Churchill Livingstone Elsevier; 2011: 65-84.

57. Kirk D. *Empowering Girs and Women through Physical Education and Sport: Advocacy Brief.* Bangkok: United Nations Educational, Scientific and Cultural Organization; 2012.

58. College of Occupational Therapists. *Making the Connections: Delivering Better Services for Wales.* London, UK: Author; 2005.

59. World Health Organization. *Human Rights and Gender Inequality in Health.* Geneva: WHO; 2011.

60. United Nations High Commissioner for Human Rights and World Health Organization. *Human Rights, Health and Poverty Reduction Strategies.* Geneva: Author; 2008:74. http://www.who.int/hhr/activities/publications/en/.

61. Mpofu C, & Hocking C. "Not made here": occupational deprivation of non-English speaking background immigrant doctors and dentists in New Zealand. *Journal of Occupational Science.* 2013;20:131-145. doi:10.1080/14427591.2012.729500

62. Bailliard AL. Laying low: fear and injustice for Latino Migrants to Smalltown, USA. *Journal of Occupational Science.* 2013;1-15. doi:10.1080/14427591.2013.799114

63. Burchett N, Matheson R. The need for belonging: the impact of restrictions on working on the well-being of an asylum seeker. *Journal of Occupational Science.* 2010;17:85-91. doi:10.1080/14427591.2010.9686679

64. Morville A-L, Erlandsson L-K. The experience of occupational deprivation in an asylum centre: the narratives of three men. *Journal of Occupational Science.* 2013;20:212-223. doi:10.1080/14427591.2010.9686679

65. Thomas Y, Gray M, McGinty A. Homelessness and the right to occupation and inclusion. *World Federation of Occupational Therapists Bulletin.* 2010;62:19-25.

66. World Health Organization. *World Report on Disability;* 2011: p. xxi. Retrieved from www.who.int/disabilities/world_report/2011/report/en/. Accessed October 29, 2012.

67. World Health Organization. International Migration, Health & Human Rights. *Health and Human Rights Publication Series, Issue no. 4.* Geneva: Author; 2003.

68. World Health Organization. *Health and Human Rights: Indigenous People's Right to Health.* WHO; 2012. Retrieved from http://www.who.int/hhr/activities/indigenous_peoples/en/

69. Crawford MB. *Shop Class as Soulcraft: An Inquiry into the Value of Work.* London, UK: Penguin; 2010.

70. Townsend EA. Boundaries and bridges to adult mental health: critical occupational and capabilities perspectives of justice. *Journal of Occupational Science.* 2012;19(1):8-24. doi:10.1080/14427591.2011.639723

71. Stadnyk RL, Townsend EA, Wilcock AA. Occupational justice. In: Christiansen CH, Townsend EA, eds. *Introduction to Occupation: The Art and Science of Living (2nd edition).* Upper Saddle River, NJ: Pearson Education Inc; 2009; 329-358.

72. Townsend E. *Muriel Driver Memorial Lecture: Occupational Therapy's Social Vision.* Canadian Journal of Occupational Therapy. 1993;60(4):174-184.

73. Townsend E. *Good Intentions Overruled.* Toronto: University of Toronto Press; 1998.

74. Giddens A. *Modernity and Self Identity: Self and Society in the Late Modern Age.* Stanford, CA: Stanford University Press; 1991.

75. Smith DE. *Texts, Facts and Femininity: Exploring the Relations of Ruling.* New York: Routlege; 1990.

76. World Health Organization, Health and Welfare Canada, Canadian Public Health Association. *Ottawa Charter for Health Promotion.* Ottawa, Canada. 1986.

77. World Health Organization. *Jakarta Declaration on Leading Health Promotion into the 21st Century.* 4th International Conference on Health Promotion, Jakarta, Indonesia, 21-25th July, 1997.

78. Doyal L, Gough I. *A Theory of Human Need.* Houndmills, Hampshire: Macmillan; 1991.

79. Office of the High Commission of Human Rights. *Universal Declaration of Human Rights.* United Nations Department of Public Information: 1948. http://www.un.org/en/documents/udhr/.

80. McIntyre J. Wheelchirs; A human rights issue or a mere mobility device? personal reflections of an occupational therapist. *South Africal Journal of Occupational Therapy.* 2010:40(1); 27-31.

81. Townsend EA, Wilcock AA. occupational justice and client-centred practice; a dialogue in progress. *Canadian Journal of Occupational Therapy.* 2004;71:75-87.

82. Thibeault R. Occupational justice's intents and impacts: from personal choices to community consequences. In: Cutchin MP, Dickie VA, eds. *Transactional Perspectives on Occupation.* Dordrecht: Springer; 2013; 245-256.

83. Blom Cooper L. *An Emerging Profession in Health Care.* Report of a Commission of Inquiry 1989. London, UK: Duckworth; 1990.

84. Bockhoven JS. Occupational therapy: A neglected source of community rehumanization. In: *Moral Treatment in Community Health Care.* New York, NY: Springer Publishing Co, Inc; 1972.

85. World Health Organization. *Health & Human Rights Publication Series, Issue No. 1: 25 Questions & Answers on Health & Human Rights.* Geneva: World Health Orgnization; 2002: 16. http://www.who.int/hhr/activities/publications/en/.

86. Frank G. Twenty-first century pragmatism and social justice: problematic situations and occupational reconstructions in post-civil war guatemala. In: Cutchin MP, Dickie VA, eds. *Transactional Perspectives on Occupation.* Dordrecht: Springer; 2013; 229-255.

87. *Lewis Hine.* Wikipedia: 2013. http://en.wikipedia.org/wiki/Lewis_Hine. Accessed July 6, 2013.

88. Evans B. *The Photos that Changed America's Child Labor Laws: Harrowing Images of Children as Young as Three Forced to do Back-breaking Work in Fields, Factories and Mines.* Mail Online: 8 April 2013. http://www.dailymail.co.uk/news/article-2305630/Lewis-Hine-Harrowing-images-child-labourers-children-young-forced-breaking-work-fields-factories-mines.html.

89. Jay. *The Reel Foto: Lewis Hine: The Littlest Laborers.* May 6, 2011. http://reelfoto.blogspot.co.nz/2011/05/lewis-hine-littlest-laborers.html. Accessed July 6, 2013.

90. United Nations. *Convention on the Rights of the Child.* New York: United Nations;1989. http://treaties.un.org/Pages/ViewDetails.aspx?mtdsg_no=IV-11&chapter=4&lang=en

91. Save the Children Norway. *History.* No date. Available at: http://www.scnorway.ru/eng/history/.

92. United Nations. *Declaration of the Rights of the Child.* Adopted by UN General Assembly Resolution 1386 (XIV) of 10 December 1959. Available at: http://www.un.org/cyberschoolbus/humanrights/resources/child.asp .

93. United Nations. *Declaration on Human Rights Education and Training.* A/RES/66/137. Official Records of the General Assembly, Sixty-sixth Session, Supplement No. 53 (A/66/53), chap. I. 2011. http://www.un.org/Docs/asp/ws.asp?m=A/RES/66/137.

94. Knauth T. *Tolerance: A Key Concept for Dealing with Cultural and Religious Diversity.* http://www.theewc.org/uploads/files/State%20of%20the%20Art_Knauth_alt.pdf.

95. UNESCO. (2011). *Contemporary Issues in Human Rights Education.* Paris, France: Author.

96. Tibbitts F, van Driel C, Sganga P, Kirchschlager P, Sinclair M. *Human Right Education Core Competencies for Young Adults and Adult Learners.* 2009. ftibbitts@hrea.org.

97. Kumagai AK, Lypson ML. Beyond cultural competence: critical consciousness, social justice, and multicultural education. *Academic Medicine.* 2009:84(5);597-603.

98. Daloz LAP. Transformative learning for the common good. In: Mezirow J, ed. *Learning as Transformation: Critical Perspectives on a Theory in Progress.* San Francisco, CA: Jossey-Bass; 2000; 103-124.

99. Janke R. *Growing Communities for Peace.* The Beyond September 11 Project. http://www.hrusa.org/september/activities/storytelling.htm.

100. Horghagen S, Josephsson S. Theatre as liberation, collaboration and relationship for asylum seekers. *Journal of Occupational Science.* 2010;17(3);168-176. doi:10.1080/14427591.2010.9686691

101. *Australian Men's Shed Association: Shoulder to Shoulder. Research.* 2011. http://www.mensshed.org/research/.aspx.

102. Australian Bureau of Statistics. *Suicides.* Canberra: Author; 2013. http://www.abs.gov.au/ausstats/abs@.nsf/Lookup/by+Subject/4125.0~Jan+2012~Main+Features~Suicides~3240.

103. Golding B, Brown M, Foley A, Harvey J, Gleeson L. *Men's Sheds in Australia: Learning through Community Contexts.* Adelaide: National Centre for Vocational Education Research; 2007:6. http://www.ncver.edu.au/publications/1780.html.

104.   Bulman J, Hayes R. Yarning spaces: dealing with depression and anxiety among Aboriginal and Torres Strait Islander males the 'proper way'. *The CAPA Quarterly (Journal of the Counsellors and Psychotherapists Association of NSW)*. 2010:1;24-28.

Theme 15

"A few largely preventable risk factors account for most of the world's disease burden. This reflects a significant change in diet habits and physical activity levels worldwide as a result of industrialization, urbanization, economic development, and increasing food market globalization."

WHO: Global Strategy on Diet, Physical Activity, and Health, 2004[1]

Chapter 15

OCCUPATION IN ILLNESS PREVENTION

This chapter addresses:
- Preventing Illness
- Occupation as a Means to Prevent Illness
  - Foundation Initiatives
  - Recent Considerations
- Occupation-Focused Prevention of Illness and Disability
  - Is Occupation-Focused Prevention of Illness and Disability Necessary?
  - Poverty Is a Great Threat
  - Urbanization
  - Increased Drug Abuse and Civil and Domestic Violence
  - Decrease of Physical Occupations
  - Approaches to Occupation-Focused Prevention of Illness and Disability
- Occupation-Focused Prevention of Illness and Disability: Collective Occupations Across the Sleep-Wake Continuum
- Conclusion

The third perspective to be considered is concerned with occupation-focused prevention of illness and disability (OPID), which is defined here as **the application of medical, epidemiological, behavioral, social, and occupational science to prolong quality of life for all people by preventing physiological, psychological, social, and occupational illness, accidents and disability through occupation-focused advocacy, mediation and programs to enable people to do, be, belong and become according to their natural health needs.**

An OPID approach is necessary because the piecemeal nature of current lines of attack recognize either the inter-relationship of individual, familial, economic, communal, corporate, or political occupations with illness and disability, or the impact and combined effects on health of what people do. A much broader understanding of occupational illness is required. Occupational illness may manifest in a medically recognized disorder and may require occupational resolution rather than, or as well as, a medical prescription.

Wilcock AA, Hocking C.
An Occupational Perspective of Health, Third Edition (pp 420-449).
© 2015 Taylor & Francis Group.

Occupation as a means of illness prevention often appears to be disregarded, despite the many sources of information that make it clear that ill-health and disability could be reduced, and in some cases prevented, according to what people do or do not do. The misuse of tobacco and alcohol is perhaps an exception and is a prime example of social occupations that are well recognized as a problem within population health. In addition, some aspects of paid employment and the effects of a lack of physical exercise have been specifically targeted as causes of illness. However, there is scant recognition that how people feel about what they do is a primary factor in the adoption of occupations that can be life threatening. In addition, not much interest is shown in the combined health effects or illness potentials of specific or combined active and rest occupations across each day over the lifespan.

Common understanding of occupation's effects on health is skewed toward the exploration of physical illness that is a prime focus of mainstream medicine. Despite being a medical specialty and attempts to alter the stigma attached to mental illness, occupational illness remains sidelined, whereas social illness is largely considered the domain of politics. Perhaps because of the enormity of the task, concerted efforts to research the effects of national policies on social issues from this holistic occupation for health perspective have not been realized. There is also little appreciation or research that considers the total repertoire of people's doing in terms of healthy or unhealthy outcomes, and holistic study of combined physical, mental, and social illness is rare.

No known studies have addressed preventing illness and disability in terms of all the things that people want, need, or have to do, occasionally or day by day, across the 24-hour cycle and a lifetime; what such doing means to them as individuals, family, or community members; or the physical, mental, and social health outcomes. The concept is complex, but unless it is addressed more thoroughly, any current occupation-specific preventive approaches would be incomplete, even though they may be beneficial in some respects. In addition, and increasing the complexity, is the fact that little attention has been paid to collective, political, or corporate occupations of an economic nature that directly determine, to a large extent, the everyday occupations of individuals and communities.

Preventing Illness

A simple definition of prevention is "the action of stopping something from happening or arising."[2] Disease prevention is the name given to action usually emanating from the health sector about risk factors and risk behaviors.[3] It is commonly referred to as preventive medicine. In affluent countries, preventive medicine can be addressed by specialized authorities at national, state, or local levels based on research or in response to an emergency. It is often performed by general medical practitioners who use population-based studies as a foundation for advice or prescriptions to protect individuals against disease agents, and for early diagnosis and retardation of disability and illness. In developing countries, it is best known for methods such as immunization, vaccination, and screening, as well as for social initiatives like quarantine, improved sanitation, and encouragement of breastfeeding, particularly where food is scarce and nutrition is poor. Preventive medicine is, in itself, the rationale and basis of a variety of individual, collective, corporate, and political occupations, and is extremely complex.

One way to illustrate the complexity in a manner that is true to the notion of physical, mental, and social health is to consider a range of organizations that are committed to preventing some aspect of living deemed counterproductive to personal, community, or world health. Organizations include those aimed at:

- Prevention of illness such as cancer, HIV/AIDS, sexually transmitted disease, tuberculosis, obesity-related disorders, noncommunicable disorders, and mental illness.
- Prevention of work-related illness or accidents.

- Prevention of behaviors, such as suicide, drug, alcohol, or other substance abuse.
- Prevention of school drop outs, bullying, and cruelty to or abuse of children.
- Prevention of teen pregnancies or child sex abuse.
- Prevention of family, sexual, and youth violence, juvenile delinquency, or gang behavior.
- Prevention of poverty.
- Prevention of terrorism.
- Prevention of pollution and ecological degradation.

Many of those address occupational aspects of ill-health or physical, mental, and social disability; however, an occupation-focused perspective extends lines of attack. It would single out aspects to be considered or addressed as part of the total intervention package that otherwise might easily be overlooked.

To illustrate this complexity, the public health concerns about cigarette smoking can be considered briefly. Rather than researching why individuals might find it necessary or comforting to take up the habit in the first place, approaches to stop it have concentrated on shocking people about the health hazards. Questions about what other forms of occupation it replaces, supplements, or enhances are disregarded. Peer pressure, the greed of multinational tobacco companies, and advertising are often blamed, and rightly so, but to take a more holistic stance from an occupational perspective requires consideration of what basic needs are fulfilled by taking it up; what occupational needs are not met to make it necessary or possible to ignore the many and various warnings; a teasing out of what cigarette smoking replaces in terms of habits of past millennia; and whether there could be changes in social, political, and economic pressures on tobacco entrepreneurs or on lifestyle and occupation across the board, that would reduce the incidence. Lorenz's[4] useful question about behavior in general can be applied to smoking in particular—what does smoking have to do with survival? Restated: Can the origins of behavior that have similar traits, benefits, or challenges to smoking be traced, and what purpose did they serve? Alternatively, are there occupations that appear to reduce the incidence of smoking or that are so appealing that they replace the habit? Armed with such knowledge, strategies to reduce the incidence of smoking might be more wide-ranging or effective.

Preventive approaches generally take for granted a medical science explanation of the cause of disease and the mechanisms for prevention, notwithstanding the holistic philosophy of the "new public health" movement[5] or the Ottawa or Bangkok Charters[6,7] and Jakarta Declaration.[8] Erroneously, many view preventive medicine as synonymous with "health promotion."[9] This misconception has a historic foundation when, understandably, the two ideas were frequently linked. An example of such entwining is provided by Last when writing of preventive initiatives aimed at noncommunicable diseases, the hazards of paid employment, "smoking cessation, reduced alcohol use, nutrition, exercise, stress reduction, and control of violent behavior" and describes them as aspects of "more effective health promotion programs."[10] Last considers that, despite different intervention strategies, public health practitioners across disciplines, such as health educators, industrial hygienists, and sanitary engineers, share a common reliance on epidemiology to uncover physiological causes of illness and disease. The most fundamental purpose of epidemiology is to "supply information, and ways to interpret it, for the diagnosis and measurement of the health problems of the population."[11]

Epidemiologist's interest in socially and economically productive lives tends to concentrate on specific known social habits and how they affect physical and mental states of health, reflecting the pervasiveness of the medical view of prevention. Despite a stated commitment to social health, it is the prevention of illness through epidemiological research aimed at "early preclinical factors" that is the most influential aspect of public health in affluent societies, and the one that attracts the most resources. Despite the emergence of social medicine that occasionally extends to how people work or play in different cultures, the pursuit of a medically defined, disease-free state is the idea that prevails and attracts funding. Noncommunicable diseases and cancer are major problems that, although often reflecting changes in what people do, are a major concern of medically focused interventions that attract public funding.

Because prevention appears a less immediate need than treatment of an existing problem, it is often overlooked, put aside, and forgotten despite the life-saving and remedial successes of early public health initiatives. Sir William Osler (1849-1919) claimed there is no doubt:

> ... that it was in the field of prevention of disease that modern medicine attained its greatest achievements. Our life is no longer shortened by diseases such as leprosy, plague, smallpox, and rabies. Our life expectation is about twice as long as it was half a century ago.[12]

However, the outcome of potentially health-threatening behavior does not necessarily disappear when it is overlooked. With the WHO calling for partnerships to make better health a reality for all people, it might be timely to reawaken the "preventive" potential of occupation. As McKeown pointed out, noncommunicable diseases are a response to "conditions that have arisen in the last few centuries" acting on a genetic constitution suited to the lifestyles of at least 100,000 years ago, some of which have occurred on a large scale only from the last century:

> Living conditions have changed profoundly since industrialization, in ways that might be expected to prejudice both physical and mental health: increased size and density of populations; transfer from rural to urban life; reduction of fibre and increase of fat, sugar and salt in the diet; increased use of tobacco, alcohol and illicit drugs; reduction of physical exercise; changes in patterns of reproduction, with fewer and later pregnancies.[13]

An OPID approach would address the prevention of physical, mental, and social illness and disability at primary, secondary, and tertiary levels by focusing on occupational causation or intervention strategies. In that way, it would continue the historic origins of public health whose approaches were remarkably successful, particularly when attentive to work-related occupational disorders, and sometimes to the composite effect of people's regular activities.

Occupation as a Means to Prevent Illness

Usually, in the current day, many aspects of occupational dysfunction remain the domain of social planners and economic policy but are sometimes linked with health. In 1988, the Australian Commonwealth Department of Community Services and Health provided evidence of the links in a brief summary of the WHO's unsuccessful but still valid appeal for "Health for all by the year 2000":

> In addition to the availability of suitable health services at a cost the country can afford, ... member states will continue to consider obstacles to health such as ignorance, malnutrition, poor housing, unemployment, and contaminated drinking water just as important as other considerations such as the lack of nurses and doctors, drugs, vaccines, or hospital beds.[14]

FOUNDATION INITIATIVES

The story of how the preventive movement began provides an understanding of how changing the occupational status quo can effectively reduce illness and disability. It was the emerging industrial economy that led Lettsom, a late 18th century British medical reformer, to warn how ignorance and filthy, overcrowded slums that housed workers created ideal conditions for epidemics to occur. Pollution, lack of water, poor sanitation, and waste disposal coupled with uninformed occupations of personal and population hygiene led to regular outbreaks of cholera in plague proportions. His warning led to an Act of Parliament empowering parishes to levy a rate for maintenance, with the subsequence emergence of civic occupations such as street cleaning and refuse disposal.[15]

Boxed Dialogue 15-1:
Robert Owen's Views on an Occupation-Centred Preventive Approach to Illness

...members of the medical profession know that the health of society is not to be obtained or maintained by medicines;- that it is far better, far more easy, and far wiser, to adopt substantive measures to prevent disease of the body or mind, than to allow substantive measures to remain continually to generate causes to produce physical and mental disorders.

Owen R. Works of Robert Owen: Volume 3: Book of the New Moral World. (Pickering Masters Series). London, England: Pickering & Chatto Publishers Ltd; 1993:156.

...the prevention of disease will be obtained only when arrangements shall be formed, to well educate, physiologically, every man, woman, and child, so as to enable them to understand their own physical and mental nature; in order that they may learn to exercise, at the proper period of life, all their natural faculties, propensities and powers, up to the point of temperance; neither falling short, nor exceeding in any of them, or discontent and disease must necessarily follow.

Owen R. Paper: Dedicated to the Governments of Great Britain, Austria, Russia, France, Prussia and the United States of America. London, England. New Lanark Conservation; 1841.

Eighteenth and 19th century social reformers were dominant forces in early illness prevention. Industrialist Robert Owen recommended "the discovery of the means, and the adoption of the practice, to prevent disease of body and mind." He believed that "disease is not the natural state of man," and that what people do is integral to health or illness.[16] Preempting ideas about occupational alienation, imbalance, deprivation, and boredom, he suggested that in a "perfect" world "the physical sciences" would render unnecessary "all severe, unhealthy, or even unpleasant labour" and "idleness and uselessness will be unknown."[17] Boxed Dialogue 15-1 provides some insights into Owen's views on an occupation-centered preventive approach to illness.

However, it was lawyer and politician Sir Edwin Chadwick who led the social reform that resulted in the emergence of public health in Britain. His *Report on the Sanitary Condition of the Labouring Population of Great Britain* made clear that plentiful supplies of clean drinking water and underground drainage were necessary in urban environments.[18] His interest in public health also encompassed planning healthy home environments, the provision of public recreation grounds, and the conditions in which children worked.[19] In 1848, a public health act was passed, in which issues such as water, drainage, disposal of rubbish, slaughterhouses, poisonous fumes, and suspect food establishments were addressed. Those ongoing concerns of public health are deemed to have led to a decrease in morbidity and mortality statistics that overshadow significantly those attributable to modern medicine.[15,20]

It has been described in previous chapters how, prior to the industrial revolution, children learned adult skills, roles, and traditions from their parents as an integral aspect of family life and economy. Industry radically transformed their occupations, as they endured long and often harsh working conditions that were not universally condemned. Even some doctors failed to understand fully the occupational needs of children, physician Edward Holme denying the harmful effects of long hours of labor, and surgeon Thomas Wilson seeing no necessity to permit recreation.[21] In 1832, physician and social reformer Thomas Southwood-Smith along with Chadwick and economist, Thomas Tooke, sent a questionnaire on the health of employed children to medical practitioners in the heartland of industrial development as part of a parliamentary commission.[22] The Factory Act of 1833 incorporated the findings of the commission, including clauses that children younger than 9 years were not permitted to work in textile mills, and if younger than 13 years, they could not work at night or for more than 8 hours per day. In addition, children were to be subject to medical inspection and to receive a minimum of 2 hours schooling each working day.[16]

Southwood-Smith's *Report on the Physical Causes of Sickness and Mortality to Which the Poor are Particularly Exposed* identified safety hazards and illnesses resulting from industrial and mining occupations. They included respiratory problems, accidents from unprotected machinery, and the dangers of fatigue and monotony.[21] His report addressed the conditions of employment, such as hours, wages, meal-breaks, clothing, holidays, and the incidence and type of accidents and health issues. In the mines, women and children as young as 6 years were employed underground for 10 to 12 hours per day. Conditions were often socially, mentally, and physically brutal. Continuous damp led many to suffer rheumatism and appear old and worn beyond their years. Southwood-Smith's medical evidence was tabled in a parliamentary report, unique because it was graphically illustrated and told how the work produced fatigue, extraordinary muscular development, stunted growth, crippled gait, and skin disorders. The report provided an unequivocal link between occupation and ill-health, and shocked the nation. Despite clamorous opposition from mine-owners, public outrage led to the 1842 *Act to Prohibit the Employment of Women and Girls in Mines and Collieries, and to Regulate the Employment of Boys.*[16,22]

Since that time, safety in the workplace has been the predominant aspect of occupation to be considered in terms of prevention. In Canada for example, the Ontario Factories Act was passed as early as 1884, establishing a system of inspection to ensure safety and health standards in factories; in 1917, nineteen safety associations amalgamated to form the Industrial Accident Prevention Associations; in 1932, an Employment and Social Insurance Act and a Minimum Wage Act were passed, and workers were limited to a 44 to 48 hour working week; in the 1950s, safety films and training courses were being offered, and approximately 1.5 million pieces of literature on workplace health and safety were published; 1964 saw the role of the work safety associations change to education rather than inspection; and 1975 saw an emphasis on injury prevention.[23]

The favored preventive approaches based on occupational, social, and environmental engineering that grew in affluent societies were largely outside medicine but perhaps had a medical officer in charge. As epidemiological research advanced, the focus began to change; more medically trained health workers became interested, and the nature of prevention focused more on internal physiology and the detection of factors that might lead to epidemics of both infectious and other diseases. The overall combined effects of occupations to prevent illness have yet to be addressed.

RECENT CONSIDERATIONS

A major mission of the WHO is preventing and combating illness through both medical and social engineering, especially in developing countries such as in Africa, South America, and an expanded Europe.[24] The WHO directs and coordinates health initiatives within the United Nations system. Health is a shared responsibility, with WHO providing "collective defense against transnational threats " and "leadership on global health matters, shaping the health research agenda, setting norms and standards, articulating evidence-based policy options, providing technical support to countries, and monitoring and assessing health trends.[25] By its publications, declarations, and charters, the WHO, most importantly, suggests ways forward and challenges those involved in population health to think and act outside the medical square.

Meeting that challenge, the United Kingdom's National Institute for Health and Care Excellence (NICE) has developed an "emerging conceptual framework for public health."[26] This recognizes that "it is the social and population vectors working in tandem with the environmental and organizational vectors which accounts for the patterning of disease." To illustrate, they provide an example of an outbreak of a diarrheal infection following flooding of houses built on a flood plain:

> *The epidemiology of the outbreak showed that the residents who contracted infections were mainly from routine and manual occupations, and were living in cheaper housing areas. This outbreak had its immediate infective root in the bacteria in the sewage floating in the*

flood water. This is an interactive example of exposure to an environmental hazard—the bacteria—caused by the meteorological activity and the human activity in building houses on the flood plain.[26]

There is another explanation to that outcome concerning the social processes of different groups competing for scarce resources, linked to the decision by local authorities and builders, leading to cheaper housing being built in higher flood risk areas:

This is a subset of a broader patterning of social life which arises as a consequence of the billions and billions of individual thoughts and actions which, despite their apparent randomness at individual level, produce contours or patterns socially.[26]

The concept of OPID is one way to make it more possible to identify occupational risk factors to health and well-being as subsets of commercial and social life. This can be achieved by considering already completed research undertaken with other rationales. Studies from education and sociopolitical fields, such as that provided above, are often relevant, as well as what is reported in health, medical, and preventive medicine literature. Within epidemiological research, a connection between occupation and health began to be considered seriously approximately half a century ago. Douglas Gordon, a medically trained pioneer of social medicine, argued that there are "associations between much of this human behavior and human health and disease." He suggested that the practice of social medicine includes coming to understand the motives, values, social organizations, and structures of different cultures, as well as the "philosophies and essential mysteries of human behaviors insofar as these affect health."[27] Similar interest was manifest in other health professions, such as occupational therapists, at about the same time.

Much earlier, in 1921, psychiatrist Adolf Meyer had put into words his philosophical stance on the new health profession of occupational therapy, as has already been noted. His concept reflected ideas about occupation as a means to prevent illness while, at the same time, promoting health. He claimed that occupation requires people's active interaction with the environment and reality in a way that maintains and balances them, because the mind and body work in unison. He recognized that activity in tune with natural rhythms has a positive effect on human functioning, and that there is a need to strive for balance in the various types of occupation.[28] Occupational therapists, as a whole, did not immediately respond to the preventive aspects of his message, despite some interest evident in Canada as early as 1934. Le Vesconte suggested then, that in combination with social workers, occupational therapists should be involved in social and economic reorganization toward the prevention of illness; however the suggestion got lost in the medicalization of professional offerings and did not reemerge until the 1960s and 1970s.[29,30]

In the 1960s, Wilma West proposed that occupational therapists should:

- Function as "health agent[s] [rather than therapists] with responsibility to help ensure normal growth and development"
- Encourage occupation focused programs aimed toward "maintaining optimum health rather than ... intermittent treatment of acute disease and disability"
- Consider more fully, and in a "new mold," the "socio-economic and cultural as well as biological causes of disease and dysfunction"
- Develop a health model of practice with the assumption that health care would be as concerned with prevention as with rehabilitation
- Find more effective methods to enhance and enrich development of physical, mental, emotional, social, and vocational abilities
- Make a "timely translation" from a "long time focus on activities of daily living for the disabled to advocacy of the balanced regimen of age appropriate, work play activities for man in the predisease/disability phase"
- Revisit their underlying philosophy and facilitate a "broader application of existing knowledge about the effects of activity, or its absence, on health."[31-34a]

Table 15-1

OCCUPATIONAL THERAPY: PREVENTION PARADIGMS OF THE '60s AND '70s

Therapist	Proposal
Florence Cromwell[34b]	Specialize in human behavior in ordinary environments where patients live, work, and play
	Think about the global trend toward preventive rather than curative programs, about world health care, and about searching for more universal systems of care
	Consider how different nations combat the problems facing them
Wiemer R. (nee Brunyate)[34c]	Play an increasing "vital, distinct, and elsewhere unattainable" role in "restorative, preventive, and maintenance health" in both medicine and civic life
	Commit to "health protection and health maintenance as well as to health restoration and rehabilitation"
	Occupation within preventive medicine deals "with the quality of life and interdependence of people, ... to limit health problems and stress arising from them"
	Occupational therapy has a "natural vested interest" in preventive health, but has not found its "appropriate place within it" and needs to take a more active role in community and preventive health[34d]
Walker L[34e]	The "emerging model of occupational therapy" is concerned "with the well community and the maintenance of health and prevention of deficits, diseases, and disabilities"
	Take on the role of consultant in the development of programs for the well community that address home, maternal, and child health care, community guidance, school systems, and chronic disease care
Anne Mosey[34f]	Health needs are "inherent human requirements that must be met for an individual to experience a sense of physical, psychological, and social well-being"
Judy Grosman[34g,34h]	Preventive health care takes place in physical, psychosocial, and sociocultural environments, within the community at schools, health centers, or housing developments and demands collaborative efforts to develop community resources, natural support systems, and natural caretakers
	As part of multidisciplinary teams, "the value of occupation in maintaining health and preventing disability" should be widely spread
Geraldine Finn[34i]	Develop a model of practice addressing the issue of the significance of occupation to human life
	As primary prevention is directed toward an understanding of both the relationship between the basic structural elements of society and health and of what keeps people in a state of health, occupational therapists should make their contribution with a greater understanding of the effects of occupation on health
Gail Fidler[34j]	Health is the ability to carry out activities that are essential for developmentally appropriate self-maintenance and meeting intrinsic needs according to the social context.
American Occupational Therapy Association[34k]	"Human beings are able to influence their physical and mental health and their social and physical environment through purposeful activity"
	"Occupational therapy is based on the belief that purposeful activity (occupation) ... may be used to prevent and mediate dysfunction."
	"The Philosophical Base of Occupational Therapy"

Table 15-1 provides other examples of the preventive paradigm that emerged in the 1960s and 1970s.

Occupational therapists' interest in the prevention of ill-health, perhaps like that of other disciplines, emerged at that time for several reasons. Brown suggested that these include advances in technology, an escalation of health care costs, a general increase of health care knowledge leading

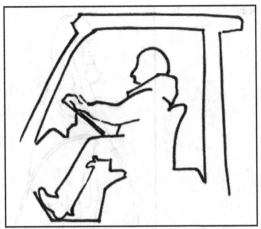

Figure 15-1. Heavy vehicles demand attention to workplace ergonomics. (© Carol Spencer 2012, otspencer@adam.com.au. Used with permission.)

to the dominant role of physicians being challenged, and a societal reaction against the complexities of modern medicine toward simpler, more natural remedies.[35] Johnson cited growing dissatisfaction with medicine and perceived dehumanization in the medical care system as important factors, along with increasing recognition of ways in which the world was being polluted.[36]

For the few committed to work outside the clinical field, the attainment of well-being took over from prevention as a way forward. Ongoing interventions have included education for back injury prevention and management in the work place,[37,38] assessment and monitoring of work methods, and advice on the adaptation of heavy vehicles and equipment being used in the mining industry in geographically hostile environments (Figure 15-1).[39] At a recent symposium, discussion covered not only rehabilitation needs and plan development for people with disabilities to gain and maintain employment, but also the prevention of work injury; the assessment of workers, work environment and performance; and workplace modifications, manual handling, injury risk management, psychosocial hazards in the workplace, work-related stress, and workplace bullying.[40] Beyond the workplace, a variety of other occupational therapy interventions to prevent particular illness and disability have continued to emerge, with the most currently favored concern being home safety programs to prevent falls among older people.[41-43] By breaking the cycle of inactivity and sedentary lifestyles that increase the risk of falling, recipients are enabled to engage in roles as "community dwellers, family members, friends, workers, leisure devotees, or volunteers."[44] A variety of strategies for children have included attention to safe transportation for those with physical handicaps[45] and community outreach programs using play and group process for preschool-aged children at risk of developing disorders of mental health (Figure 15-2).[46]

Occupation-Focused Prevention of Illness and Disability

OPID is aimed at reducing the experience of physical, mental, social, and occupational illness by occupational means and is applicable to individuals, communities, collectives, and populations (Table 15-2 provides an overview.). The foundation belief of this approach is that people are occupational beings and that much illness can be prevented, naturally, through what people do day by day throughout life. Through informed and wise choice of occupation, people can influence the state of their own and others' health, reduce illness and disability directly or indirectly, and meet biological needs and potentials across the 24-hour active-rest continuum throughout life. Occupations known to lead to illness should be replaced by illness-preventing occupations

Figure 15-2. Water play to prevent disorders of mental health by promoting confidence, fun, and learning. (© Carol Spencer 2012, otspencer@adam.com.au. Used with permission.)

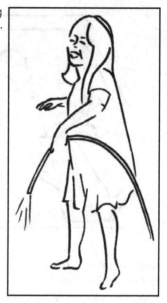

that are socio-culturally valued and afford individual and collective meaning and purpose. For occupations to be illness preventive, they need to provide opportunity for growth and development according to human biological capacity; meet the prerequisites and the physiological requirements for physical, mental, and social exercise; and result in the well-working of each human organism as a whole.

This approach looks to implement the WHO's objectives for preventing disease and reducing disability by increasing awareness and understanding that occupation can affect health in either a negative or positive way. It recognizes that all the prerequisites for health are related in some way to people's occupations. For example, poverty, often described as the greatest threat to health, has a primary relationship with occupational opportunities to attain the requirements for life itself. Other WHO occupation related health threats include the increase in "sedentary behavior," "drug abuse, and civil and domestic violence," and demographic trends toward urbanization and globalization.[47] Increasingly, physical, mental, social, and occupational health can be compromised by transnational factors that effect what people do or do not do, such as:

> … The global economy, financial markets and trade, wide access to media and communications technology, and environmental degradation as a result of the irresponsible use of resources. These changes shape people's values, their lifestyles throughout the lifespan, and living conditions across the world.[48]

The underlying principle of OPID is that occupation needs to be understood as a collective whole in the prevention of illness. Although there is general appreciation that physical, mental, and social illness can result from interactive causes, the collective picture of all that people do—the sum of the parts—is seldom recognized, investigated, or attended to. Perhaps the collective whole is too large and the societal structure of occupation too complex to grapple with. However, it is important to find out how complex political, corporate, and collective structural factors of occupation affect what people do to meet basic requirements, the meaning they find, and the opportunity to meet biological potential. Effects appear to be vastly different for the majority as opposed to the affluent minority who thrive.

The chance for all people to be free of illness because of opportunities for engagement in occupations is unequal. In no societal structure are everyone's different capacities recognized equally or even as positive factors; occupational chances are not given equally; and potential is not recognized equally. The oft-quoted saying that anyone could be president of the United States may

Table 15-2

FOUNDATIONS OF AN OCCUPATIONAL FOCUSED APPROACH TO PREVENTION OF ILLNESS AND DISABILITY

Basis of Approach	Underlying Beliefs	Underlying Principles
Applicable to populations, communities, and individuals	Humans are occupational beings, natural health is attained and maintained and illness prevented through doing	Occupation should be both a source of health and an impediment to illness
Aimed at reducing the experience of physical, mental, social, and occupational illness	Physical, mental, social, and occupational illness can be impeded and reduced	Physical, mental, social, and occupational illnesses result from many interactive causes
Based on medical, epidemiological, behavioral, social, and occupational science	Research should be holistic and reductionist. Information about physical, mental, social, and occupational illness should be inclusive of all that people do.	Limited attention to selectivity to particular types of research slows down the process of understanding and ignores people's interactive physiology
People influence the state of their health through what they do	People need information about how what they do affects physical, mental, and social health and illness	Information about the social and occupational nature of illness is as important as physical and mental factors
Is informative, can be reductionist and/or holistic	Integration of research findings from various fields will assist policies and action to reduce illness	Quantitative, qualitative, and critical research needs to be integrated and disseminated
Is diverse, addressing many different and interactive causes of illness	Prevention of physical, mental, social, and occupational illness is a global responsibility	Diversity and inclusiveness of preventive research and action

be true in theory, but the chance for it to happen is very unequal. It is only those who manage to exercise the range of their particular physical, mental and social abilities and thrive in existing and particular societal structures who are occupationally advantaged in an ongoing way. That implies that some people are more likely than others to experience illness because of their occupations. Getting the balance right for as many people as possible would be a desirable outcome of OPID.

The call for "the creation of new partnerships for health" proposed in the *Jakarta Declaration* provides the opportunity to those who recognize the connection between occupation and health to come together "on an equal footing" to help everyone address inequities.[48] The boundaries that exist between public and private sectors and organizations throughout the world require breaching, because cooperation is essential for new forms of action to develop that address emerging threats to health. This may be achieved through research, through promoting social responsibility to reduce illness and disability, through protecting environments, and through helping to increase awareness of unhealthy aspects of occupation in all facets of personal and communal life in an equitable and just way.[49] Increasing awareness within the population at large would be a valuable starting place. Encouraging sociopolitical processes and policies to consider occupational health effects of legislation in a much broader way is essential in the longer term and will not be achieved without a gradual increase of understanding of the relationship between illness and the composite effects of individual and collective occupations.

Social and occupational illnesses do not necessarily manifest in medically defined mind or body ailments. Such illnesses can be evident in maladaptive behaviors, stress, frustration, boredom, and aggression, as discussed in the third section of this book, and in some cases can be early identifying factors in later medical diagnosis or lead to death though suicide. OPID can utilize epidemiological and other quantitative and qualitative tools to explore the holistic, interactive, and complex nature of human doings and their relationship to illness and disability. Combined approaches can use both a wide occupational lens and a reductionist focus and are necessary for various reasons, such as recognition by the medical research authorities and granting bodies, reduction of bias, as well as a rounded exploration of people's aspirations and potential. Because this new branch of learning has not yet gathered together an appropriate mix of interdisciplinary interest, its research is particularly vulnerable to neglect. Table 15-3 outlines contrasting research paradigms.

Is Occupation-Focused Prevention of Illness and Disability Necessary?

Approximately 35 years ago, the *Declaration of Alma Ata* asserted that "primary health care includes at least: education about the prevailing health problems and the methods of preventing and controlling them..."[50] Currently:

Chronic diseases are now the major cause of death and disability worldwide. Noncommunicable conditions, including cardiovascular diseases (CVD), diabetes, obesity, cancer and respiratory diseases, now account for 59% of the 57 million deaths annually and 46% of the global burden of disease.[1]

The WHO and others in the population health fraternity have also recognized that, as was the case in the 19th century, policies to improve a population's social experience and environment could be more important than improving individual health using medicine.[51] The greatest benefits could be achieved by "investing in policies that promote sustainable development, protect the environment, promote equity, and tackle the social gradient of health."[51] Occupation-focused interventions need to be developed along those lines. These might be as varied as reducing inequalities in child development and education, improving the quality of life of older people,[52-54] improving parenting, improving recreational opportunities, reducing consumption of fossil fuel by encouraging walking or cycling,[55-60] or persuading politicians to adopt innovative population occupation based policies.

Urgent preventive measures that could respond to an OPID approach are required for mental health problems and the high prevalence of noncommunicable diseases, as the number of elderly people increases in all parts of the world.[8] The impact of illness or premature death can also be associated with ongoing, unresolved stress from occupational imbalance, deprivation, or alienation that may result from paid employment, corporate occupations, or sociopolitical initiatives. Those can be risk factors in themselves or result in the development of health risk behaviors. In turn, they may lead to early, preclinical health disorders, such as boredom; burnout; depression; decreased fitness, brain, or liver function; increased blood pressure; changes in sleep patterns, body weight, and emotional state; and, ultimately, to disease, disability, or death. Intervention programs that address the occupational issues related to the early cause of the disorder are required.

It has already been noted that national priorities and policies, the type of economy, and cultural values determine occupational risk factors and behaviors, such as overcrowding, loneliness, substance abuse, lack of opportunity to develop potential, imbalance between diet and activity, and ecological breakdown. To make the occupation connection clear, four examples will be discussed according to population health priorities.

Poverty Is a Great Threat

Historically, occupation has been the way people obtain the basic prerequisites. The past decades have been marked by global poverty and debt crises around the world, including the newly

Table 15-3

CONTRASTING RESEARCH PARADIGMS THAT COULD INFORM OCCUPATION-FOCUSED PREVENTION OF ILLNESS AND DISABILITY

	Quantitative	Qualitative	Critical
Nature	Reductionist Positivist Predetermined structure	Holistic Interpretive Flexible as ideas emerge	Embedded in society Interactive, participatory Flexible and dynamic
Purpose	Test hypotheses Test empirical observation Measure Discover laws Generalize	Explore Understand subjective realities Discover meanings	Uncover inequity Facilitate social action
Values	Value free Objective	Value bound Subjective	Value laden Cannot be value free
Examples of research methods for occupation-focused prevention of illness and disability	Cohort, case control, and cross sectional studies Vital, health, and population statistics Measurement of biorhythms, biomechanics, etc Surveys and questionnaires Time-use diaries Experience sampling	Questionnaires Time-use diaries Experience sampling In-depth interview Focus groups Field observation	Quantitative data Questionnaires Time-use diaries Experience sampling In-depth interview Focus groups Field observation Critical praxis Self reflection History of ideas

industrialized countries of Southeast Asia and the Far East, those of the former Soviet block, and in Western Europe and North America. There have been famines in sub-Saharan Africa, South Asia, and parts of Latin America. In developing countries, Eastern Europe, and the Balkans, a resurgence of infectious diseases has been rife. Health services and schools have closed.[61] Although natural disasters can account for some of the present experience of poverty, much more can be laid at the doors of political and multicorporate occupational initiatives, will and greed. It is, as the Jakarta Declaration argues, "the global economy, financial markets and trade" that shape "living conditions across the world," as well as the occupations and values of people.[8] Environments and other living things have become less healthy, degraded by what a handful of humans with money and power have done and continue to do in pursuit of more money and power.

Lack of work occupation often leads to poverty, which is accompanied by hunger, disease, and illiteracy, as well as by addiction, violence, and depression, as in the case of many Arctic Inuit communities.[62] People with disabilities are another group who often experience poverty beyond the norm. This is particularly the case in developing countries where prejudicial attitudes are common and access to education and employment is limited. For example, they are often excluded from opportunities to develop farming skills—a basic means of livelihood for many.[63] People without a means of livelihood are doubly disadvantaged as they are, largely, restricted in engaging in other activities because they lack resources to access or continue participation or to cover costs involved.

Lack of a range of occupations limits the use of capacities and skills and reduces physical, mental, and social exercise potential, increasing susceptibility to illness. Poverty is more than lack of income. The poor have described it as ill-being. This includes experiences such as living and working in risky, unhealthy, or polluted environments and being, belonging, and becoming experiences, such as bad feelings about self, loneliness, powerlessness, voicelessness, anxiety and fear for the future, as well as more obvious experiences of poverty, such as lack of food, work, money, shelter, and clothing.[64]

URBANIZATION

For people with outgoing natures, the chance to meet others with like interests and to share occupational pursuits appears to be increased by urban living. Although, intuitively, cities appear to be less healthy places to live in than rural environments, doing things, becoming fulfilled, and being with others is so important that those left behind in rural communities can experience occupational deprivation. However, there is a downside, and in many places the centralization of big business and paid employment leads to population masses without any sense of community where countless people experience feelings of isolation, loneliness, boredom, and alienation. It is easier to be unknown and remain so in a crowded city than in a smaller community where people's capacities and interests are more readily observed. There are fewer places to walk in safety and fresh air, the pace of life is faster, and demands on attention are more frequent.

In rural communities, the opportunities for people to live out their lives with the diverse advantages of modern amenities and services are reducing. Services are centered in large urban settings or, increasingly, moved off-shore. The demands on local government escalate in line with the legislative requirements in urban centers, where there are more residents to pay for the services. The bureaucracy, of necessity, increases while essential services and occupational opportunities decrease. When local government can no longer exist financially, centralization follows. Support facilities continue to decline, yet more occupational deprivation occurs and illness follows. Childcare, education, recreation, sporting, communal, commercial, and employment opportunities dwindle, and older people are left with decreasing support from diminishing family, social, health, or public service facilities or activities in which they can participate. For many, active aging is reduced to domestic and garden chores, and suicide rates amongst old and young are a matter of concern.

For people living outside urban centers, long and tiring travel is an ongoing and increasing necessity as rural services are closed down. Road accidents are a major concern. These concerns, as well as suicide are becoming common for rural youth, as often, the most obvious form of local recreation is alcohol, "burn-ups," and "going to town." Earlier and simpler ways to spend free time in the country, such as walking, swimming, fishing, and other nature-based occupations are frequently discouraged in childhood as unsafe and so are underdeveloped and become outside the regular occupations of the majority, are not "deemed cool" for an electronically focused youth culture, and are dependent on a type of personal occupational enterprise that is reducing as rules and regulations increase across the board to an unhealthy point. Depression, not surprisingly, is increasing for all ages.[65] The need for urban and rural occupation-focused community redevelopment is a growing and critical need.

INCREASED DRUG ABUSE AND CIVIL AND DOMESTIC VIOLENCE

Substance abuse and violence are unhealthy occupational behaviors. They are learned occupations drawing on or copying activity observed within families, community, and media, and are encouraged as a means of participating and sharing with others. The young appear particularly at risk, and the age at which some develop aggressive behavior or start becoming "a user" is early.

Exposure, particularly to other young people "doing their own thing," apparently having fun, getting their own way, and growing up through what appears to be risky and adventurous, can appear exciting, with other risk-taking occupations such as driving recklessly, substance abuse, and bullying, almost appearing to have taken over earlier puberty rites of passage. For some young people, perhaps of an adventurous or rebellious nature or those who are more easily led, and particularly for those whom education systems and processes fail, such occupations provide a means of forgetting failure and a way of hitting back at established norms.

Sometimes it is changes in sociocultural, community, and family occupations that lead to boredom and loss of direction for the young. Modern adult occupational conduct can result in overprotection of the young from the realities of living, and in communities where there are increasing numbers of both parents working, problems with child care, boredom, and teenage freedoms may be a factor. Overprotection might also be a factor in disguising the need for young people to develop responsible doing to meet life's needs, dangers, and potentials. Currently, for many, this appears to have resulted in decreased attention being given to learning of adult self-care behavior, future "survival" activity, and personal responsibility. Health problems can occur when there appears to be not enough "to do" that holds meaning or purpose for them or there may be an imbalance of too much or too little responsibility in what they are expected to do or to become. In addition, frequent media coverage of substance abuse and of incidents of aggression appears to glorify ill-doing.

These unhealthy methods of doing, being, belonging, and becoming have multiple causes, but not least can be blamed on decreasing opportunities for people to learn about looking after themselves in practical ways and their responsibilities to the community and to others. The ever-increasing size of collectives of people may have played some part in the growth of the use of legal or illicit drugs and of civil and domestic violence. Engagement in pleasurable doings is becoming more expensive and elitist as it becomes tied to material artifacts like the right shoes, clothes and tools, specialty venues, and making money. Such exclusion can lead some people to seek other forms of self-expression through things such as fundamentalism. Others experience boredom, self-depreciation, envy, and ennui, which can be magnified if social welfare support becomes preferable to unwanted types of paid employment. Getting back at "the system," at "the establishment," at those closest, or at those who are different is a maladaptive form of occupation that increases as socioeconomic policies fail to recognize the range of people's doing, being, belonging, and becoming as basic health needs. Those examples, of course, oversimplify the complex matter of the search for self-worth, meaning, and purpose that are essential elements of preventive occupations.

DECREASE OF PHYSICAL OCCUPATIONS

Physical doing has altered throughout time as a result of accelerating changes in societies across the world. On the whole, most people in postmodern cultures are no longer required to undertake either sustained or substantial physical exercise through what they do. They undertake it at will rather than for necessity. This contrasts markedly with the situation that existed until fairly recently:

> Vigorous physical activity was part of everyday life for most people, at home, at work, and in transit between them. Even as recently as 1850, human muscles provided up to one-third of the energy used by workshops, factories, and farms. Today the figure is less than 1%; the human body is becoming redundant as a source of energy in the workplace [with physical activity having become] largely a recreational option rather than a survival necessity.[66]

Few people in affluent societies would run or walk for several hours every day, as early humans did and as some in hunter-gathering or agricultural economies still do. This lack of physical activity is despite considerable media exposure to the claims that exercise of sufficient vigor and regularity is protective of cardiovascular disease and conducive to general well-being. Commonly accepted standards about what a protective level of fitness entails varies from a mixture of regular daily physical activity[1] to vigorous, repetitive, rhythmic activity, such as walking, running, swimming, or cycling, for at least 20 minutes for 3 to 4 times per week.[67] In Britain, the United States, and Australia, by the 1990s less than half the adult population met that standard, with women less likely at that time to engage in physical activity than men.[68-71] This continues to be the case today.[1] Physical inactivity remains a major concern because it declines with age from as early as adolescence and many studies have found differences between groups not only according to age and gender but also according to ethnicity, sociocultural status, education, and employment.[1,72-75]

Because "the study of physical activity as it relates to health is in its infancy" and has used different criteria to define, describe, or quantify its many variations, it has proved difficult to estimate and measure in the past.[76] In 2004, the WHO reported that "most data was available for leisure time activity, with less direct data available on occupational (paid employment) activity, and little direct data available for activity related to transport and domestic tasks."[77] That report indicates how occupation is not viewed as a holistic factor but as individual, and perhaps, unrelated components. A dearth of longitudinal population-level research has resulted in the relationships between socioenvironmental factors and preventable illness being poorly understood. An example of one attempt to overcome such difficulties is a 2013 study of aspects of obesity. Archer et al used national time-use data collected over a 45-year period from 1965 of women aged between 19 to 64 years. Their objective was to examine trends in household time allocation (inclusive of food preparation, post-meal cleaning activities, clothing maintenance, and general housework) in relation to household management energy expenditure (calculated using body weights from national surveys and metabolic equivalents). They found a large and significant decrease in the time allocated to household occupations and a 25% reallocation of time from active to sedentary pastimes, such as watching television. The changes have, beyond doubt, contributed to the increasing prevalence of obesity in women during the past 5 decades and subsequent illness.[78]

Just as occupation is divided in a reductionist way, in many respects the phrase "physical activity" maintains the myth that physical, mental, and social health can be separated, despite many of the WHO directives substantiating the interaction between them. This could be strengthened if the word occupation was used to include collectives of active-rest activities across 24 hours. That could replace or include physical activity, suggesting that preventive benefits can be gained from work, domestic chores, play, and leisure pursuits, all of which are occupations with social and mental attributes, as well as physical.

An overload of sedentary occupation (or physical inactivity) contributes significantly to the global burden of chronic disease "estimated to cause 2 million deaths worldwide annually." Throughout the world "about 10-16% of cases each of breast cancer, colon cancers, and diabetes, and about 22% of ischemic heart disease" result from sedentariness.[1] It is as strong a risk factor as increased blood pressure, smoking, and high levels of cholesterol, and adults who are inactive are twice as likely to die from cardiovascular disease than those who are very active.[79] Sedentariness cannot be adequately assessed without a 24-hour view over time.

The protective effect of vigorous activity is part of the occupation/survival-based health mechanism of biological evolution. The protective effects have been found to include strengthening of heart muscle,[80,81] increased production of protective HDL cholesterol,[82,83] reduction in triglycerides,[76] reduced blood pressure,[1,84,85] improved glucose metabolism,[1,86] increased resting metabolic rate, maintenance of weight loss,[1,87] and reduction of fibrin stickiness (and therefore the formation of blood clots).[88] Apart from cardiovascular disease, several studies have shown a protective effect against osteoporosis, some cancers,[89] anxiety, and depression.[1,90] Additional benefits result from the way it discourages substance abuse, "helps reduce violence, enhances functional capacity and promotes social interaction and integration," and "interacts positively with strategies to improve diet."[1]

The WHO *Global Strategy on Diet, Physical Activity and Health* provides the following facts:

- "Appropriate regular physical activity is a major component in preventing the growing global burden of chronic disease."

- "At least 60% of the global population fails to achieve the minimum recommendation of 30 minutes moderate intensity physical activity daily."
- "The risk of getting a cardiovascular disease increases by 1.5 times in people who do not follow minimum physical activity recommendations."
- "Inactivity greatly contributes to medical costs—by an estimated $75 billion in the USA in 2000 alone."
- "Increasing physical activity is a societal, not just an individual problem, and demands a population-based, multi-sectoral, multi-disciplinary, and culturally relevant approach."[1]

Those four examples, poverty, urbanization, drug abuse, and civil and domestic violence, and the decrease of physical occupations, provide some indication of where to begin tackling the enormous task of preventing physical, mental, social, and occupational illness. People need information about how the things they do can prevent illness or disability, and the importance to health of being, belonging, and becoming through what they do. Integration and extensive promulgation of research from various fields has the potential to assist both policy development and personal and community action to reduce illness, and requires multimedia attention. Prevention of physical, mental, social, and occupational illness is a global responsibility, and not just the responsibility of medical science alone. Broad-minded watchdogs are probably required to make this begin to happen.

APPROACHES TO OCCUPATION-FOCUSED PREVENTION OF ILLNESS AND DISABILITY

The terms *primary, secondary,* and *tertiary prevention* are used to differentiate different stages of the preventive process:
- Primary prevention is about preventing the occurrence of illness or injury
- Secondary prevention is about early detection or arrest
- Tertiary prevention is about the reduction of chronicity or possible relapse.

This chapter mainly addresses the primary prevention of illness, disability, and premature death for both populations and individuals at risk because of what they do or do not do. Focusing on what people do, how they feel about what they do, how it enables them to belong, and whether they are able to use their particular capacities in ways that allow them to grow toward potential is central in the prevention of illness.

That this claim is understood and promoted by the WHO is clear. However, as suggested earlier, because the concept of occupation as a whole entity is not currently recognized by the WHO or the population health fraternity, the understanding is fragmented. Current ways of considering parts of occupation as factors in illness rather than whole phenomena means that they are less obvious, easy to overlook, and that causative confounding factors may be missed. The fragmentation is relatively short lived in terms of human existence, being in accord with sociocultural patterns that emerged with industrialization. Time and motion science broke up the occupational process into meaningless parts as it looked for the fastest, most successful, and economical ways of manufacturing things. The processes effectively reduced people to objects, equivalent to machines. Action is needed to reverse the lingering ill-effects of fragmenting occupation:
- Into physical, mental or social categories
- So that the continuum of sleep and wake activity is considered separately.
- So that paid employment is not given greater payment and attention than work done in the home
- So that leisure is not studied apart from work.

- So that self-care is not taken for granted for all but the very young, the very old, and people with disabilities.
- So that education is not separated from families and community life
- So that recommendations about healthy behavior are less medicalized
- To limit the power of corporate activity that drives much of current day occupational form, function, and opportunity
- So that political action becomes less remote from real life.

The fragmentation of occupation into different categories such as those provided has some value, despite making it difficult to appreciate or take into account the interactive nature of physiology, health, and occupation that crosses numerous domains. It allows researchers opportunities for greater depth of understanding particular components, that need then to be applied to the whole. Research and action that takes into account a holistic picture of people's occupations across the sleep-wake continuum could provide different answers and potential outcomes that are overlooked in present day societal structures. Prevention through occupation approaches that cross existing reductionist disciplinary boundaries might be more difficult but research, reflection on, and action from its outcomes could enable people to equate more easily what they do in their everyday lives to prevention of illness.

Preventing illness and disability through advice about what people should do or not do was a lynchpin of medical practice for about 2000 years, as part of the ancient rules of health. Such intervention needs reactivating from both an individual and a population point of view. That should be based on close scrutiny of the occupational nature and needs of people in differing environments according to modern explanations of health and illness, similar in some ways to inquiry into the social nature of illness. Maddi, for example, in a discussion about stress mastery in Friedman's *Personality and Disease* explains how playing sports can be relaxing because "one is using the mind and body the way they were intended to be used in fighting or running away" in response to the fight or flight reaction.[91]

The major difference of an OPID approach is that it makes clear the interaction between illness and different aspects of what people do, while addressing the occupational determinants as a whole rather than as parts. OPID would focus debate and raise awareness and action toward preventing people from being ill or experiencing disability or premature death using occupation as the medium of intervention. A starting point could be primary exploration of occupational patterns within a community or population or by individuals. In consultation and participation, action could include mediation, advocacy, and negotiation toward further exploration, awareness raising, and action. The process could continue monitoring and affecting change toward preventing illness caused or worsened by occupation (Figure 15-3).

Clearly, not all occupational risk factors have been established nor have they been considered in a holistic way. Other possibilities and the underlying determinants of risk factors need to be studied with rigor, and methods of implementing change require ongoing scrutiny, as is the case for other illness prevention initiatives. For preventive occupation initiatives to be valued and resourced by population health authorities, it is necessary to more effectively publicize the linkages between engagement in occupation and illness. Because of the preoccupation with medically defined risk factors of illness, the most respected population health disciplines, as well as the media, effectively ignore many research studies focusing on occupational elements. Even major Harvard studies, such as that by Glass et al about the positive effects of social and productive occupation on mortality rates in older Americans,[92] do not seem to have effected wide scale changes in policy or emphasis. More studies that replicate and support those findings and others of similar magnitude are required.

Although calling for more holistic research on the range of occupations that together are effective in reducing ill-health or disability, OPID recognizes that a "few, largely preventable, risk factors account for most of the world's disease burden" as the WHO maintains.[1] This is increasingly

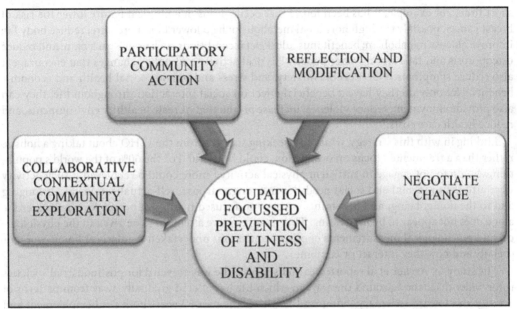

Figure 15-3. Occupation-focused prevention of illness and disability.

so in both developing and postindustrial nations. As people changed their predominant occupations from hunting and gathering to agriculture, to industry, and to highly technical computerized lifestyles, significant changes to diet, substance use, and physical, mental, and social activity have also occurred. An example illustrating a small part of the complex jigsaw is provided by McCrady and Levine's exploration of the association between sedentariness and obesity. They examined people's inactivity within sedentary jobs and during leisure time and found that more sitting and less walking or standing time occurred in working rather than leisure days. They suggest "a need to develop approaches to free people from their chairs and render them more active."[93] That requires vigilance and potential ongoing change as technology evolves and occupational and social structures crumble and redevelop in different and possibly unhealthy ways.

Economic and sociopolitical structures are in a state of constant ever-increasing change. This demands both vigilance and ongoing research, as the changes tend to encroach more and more on what people do naturally to maintain their health and prevent illness. For example, as the world becomes increasingly urbanized, occupations have changed dramatically, and urbanization has been found to be associated with obesity, diabetes, hypertension, and cardiovascular disease. When Levine et al compared daily habitual physical activity and non-activity between rural and urban dwellers in Jamaica and North America, they found that urbanization is associated with low levels of daily activity and non-exercise activity thermogenesis (NEAT).[94] This is one of many studies that support the close links between health and illness, shelter, and occupation. However, to effectively alter the impact of detrimental changes will require radical measures, a redirection of many corporate and political occupation, and major efforts toward promulgating information to the world at large.

Although requiring a more holistic approach, a focus on known and largely preventable occupational risk factors makes sense alongside efforts that generate greater understanding of how the combination of occupations can generate illness and disability. Sustained behavioral interventions have already been shown to be effective in reducing global behavioral risk factors associated with poor diet, reduced physical activity, substance abuse, and health. The WHO has adopted a broad-ranging Global Strategy[1] based on scientific validation that moderating those known, largely preventable risk factors has a major impact on chronic diseases in a relatively short time. For example, it has been found that occupations of a physical nature lower the risk of breast cancer, possibly through hormonal metabolism; help lower blood pressure; reduce body fat; improve glucose metabolism; benefit musculoskeletal conditions such as low back pain; and reduce osteoporosis and falls among older people. Physical activity and policy changes that encourage it also reduce symptoms of depression, anxiety, and stress and provide social health and economic benefits. Not only do they have a beneficial effect on social interaction throughout life, they can also provide enjoyment, reduce violence, increase productivity, create healthier environments, and reduce health care costs.[1]

Linking in with this strategy, while also seeking support from the WHO about taking a holistic rather than a fragmented focus on occupation, could be useful. For the 60% of the world's population who do to not engage in sufficient physical activity,[1] more could be achieved if such activity were attuned to mental and social needs for meaning, purpose, self-actualization, and belonging and to the doing, being, and becoming, occupation-focused natures of people for whom exercise alone does not appear to be motivating. This requires more attention to be given to the physiological and psychological measurements of other occupations undertaken regularly at home, work, or socially and how they interact or combine.

The study by Archer et al reported earlier suggests the way forward for postindustrial societies is for wider discussion around the ways in which life has altered gradually away from patterns of activity and toward sedentary living, and how over the past 50 years both paid employment and housework have changed considerably.[78] Their data clearly shows that increasing the amount of time spent around the home doing an activity that demands movement and greater energy expenditure is necessary. In line with those findings, and because appliances currently used in the home are more efficient, lighter, and easier to use than in previous eras, householders are being advised to routinely keep track of time spent in active or passive occupations, to reduce sitting time and increase non-sitting work activities.[95,96] Such advice requires wider dissemination, and application to the whole range of people's occupations. This should follow an evaluation of the combination of passive or active occupations people pursue regularly. Similar findings emerged from James Levine's studies on what he calls "Sitting Disease," or NEAT mentioned earlier.[97] In *Move a Little, Lose a Lot*, he estimates it is the 1500 to 2000 unexpended calories that are no longer used in daily lives that have led to the increasing problem of obesity in postindustrial communities.[98] The metabolic burn of daily life through what people do has altered dramatically. He recommends major changes in how people go about their everyday occupations, reprogramming themselves to become "movers" and reducing sitting times dramatically through changing office layouts, television viewing, and computing habits; walking more or climbing stairs; using motorized transport or escalators less; and generally "spending two hours more everyday just doings things."[99]

Occupation-focused programs reflecting "just doing things" and the "Move for Health" WHO strategy for all people to increase regular physical activity are valuable because they are inclusive of all leisure, play, work, domestic, and travel activities.[1] In line with this, education and advice should continue to support physical activity programs in schools and communities, as well as encouraging regular walking, and being vigilant about what is sold in school cafeterias and fast food outlets, because exercise and consumption are closely linked. Every available opportunity should be taken to provide information about the dangers of poor eating habits, the impact of smoking or alcohol abuse, and their effect on physical, mental, or social occupations.

However, it appears that too much exercise can be as detrimental to health as too little, and can lead to atrophy of body tissue and organs. As outlined in Chapter 10, over-exercising has been linked to the overproduction of free radicals, which could be linked with many lifestyle disorders and even sudden death during exercise.[100,101] Athletes experiencing some form of breakdown of health at the time of major competition is not uncommon. Evidence about the cause of pathophysiology of what is sometimes called overtraining syndrome is limited, but it has been suggested that the stress of training can cause depression and decreased immune function.[102] Moderate, rather than strenuous, exercise is now often recommended. That recommendation fits in well with aiming toward occupational balance.

The WHO perspective recognizes that increasing the level of "physical activity is not merely about individual behavior. Multi-sectoral policies and initiatives are needed to create environments that help people to be physically active."[1] It recommends such policies and initiatives be population-based and involve both public and private stakeholders. Policy makers, urban planners, and local governments concerned with health, sport, education, transport, culture, and recreation should be supportive and encourage relevant "physical activity in all life settings."[1]

Despite a common misconception, exercise and sport are not the only way to prevent illness, although extremely valuable for those who find pleasure and purpose in participation. Because of the value given to such forms of exercise, some people to whom it does not appeal may become stressed or more inactive, and fall victim to noncommunicable diseases. Fashionable, societal, cultural, or political directions or pressures make it possible for people to lack awareness of how particular talents or capacities outside exercise parameters can be used in ways that are health-giving and satisfactory in the longer term. Indeed, there is some evidence that the majority of people fail to associate their chosen life's occupations with their health.[103]

Recognizing and providing programs based on occupational interests to enable people to recognize the links between what they do and their health is a primary requirement. Programs that include sociopolitical activism should aim at linking people's activity and rest continuums in ways that enable them to become more active, food aware, and satisfied without excessive or destructive use of tobacco, alcohol, or other drugs. Every major legislative change should include information about the occupation-health nexus and requirements to prevent future illness and disability.

Healthy diets have been at the forefront of health education campaigns for many years and appear to be heeded by those who are health conscious. They are heard but not accessed efficiently by many others—those who diet for the sake of fashion rather than health; those with poor skills in terms of acquiring or preparing food; those who experience food insecurity or whose lifestyles are unbalanced or dependent on copying food behavior to belong to a particular set; or those who are occupationally alienated, deprived, depressed, or unhappy in other ways. It is important to address the underlying occupational problems, as well as those primarily concerned with what people consume. Varied approaches are necessary to learn practical food skills and strategies to assist in understanding the relationship between occupation demands and calorie intake in very down to earth and practical ways.

The WHO recommends "a 'Life Course' approach to eating and physical activity that begins with pre-pregnancy, includes breast feeding, and extends to old age" and argues for multifaceted, multi-institutional approaches because:

> The evidence (of behavioral interventions in reducing the rates of CVD, cancers and diabetes in populations have been well-proven in countries such as Finland, Japan and Singapore) is overwhelming that prevention is possible when sustained actions are directed both at individuals and families, as well as the broader social, economic and cultural determinants of [noncommunicable diseases].[1]

A life course approach is commensurate with OPID's holistic line of attack. Both need to consider the combined effects of what people do across the daily and occasional active-rest and life continuum in combination with political, social, and corporate directives. Both need to design action to prevent illness while effecting change in attitudes for individuals and the population at large.

With that in mind, it is useful to consider strategies aimed at changing unhealthy environments and conditions. An example provided by the Behavioral Health Services Division of the U.S. Department of Health to reduce substance use and abuse advises:

- "The creation or strengthening of regulations and normal population behaviors"
- "An active process to prevent alcohol, tobacco and other drug use

- Addressing "the personal, physical and social well-being of individuals and families not in need of treatment services" and those deemed to be at risk in the future
- Primary, secondary, and tertiary prevention to integrate strategies targeting the general population, those at average to high risk, and those already "using."[104]

Health is more likely to be maintained if individuals have the skills and resources to cope effectively with the diversity of life's challenges.[105] Patterns of doing acquired early in life establish the foundation for health or illness, are often maintained unconsciously, and are difficult to overturn. To reduce the continuance of unhealthy patterns, it appears important to assist individuals and populations as a whole to advocate for the development of structures and ways of life that enable a greater number of people to become active and involved in occupations from childhood that:

- Fulfill occupational natures and needs rather than being "add-on" requirements.
- Provide for basic requirements.
- Provide meaning, purpose, and a sense of belonging.
- Provide opportunities to develop and grow.

Current global initiatives and national occupational structures in developing and affluent countries alike differ significantly from the occupational freedoms of earlier times. Some commercial or entrepreneurial activities, along with some communal rules and regulations, even if originally intended to reduce the incidence of illness or to improve safety or equitable lifestyles, have altered the freedom of people to follow their inbuilt health needs in natural ways that provide for different natures and capacities. Modern expectations, as well as commerce or regulations, can segregate people according to what they do, and judge or reward those who succeed in particular, but not necessarily healthier ways.

Grass root programs where people with similar natures and occupational needs have a chance to meet and develop with the support of like-minded others is a suggested starting point. Although that can occur naturally for those who recognize their interests and capacities and live in a place where such connection is feasible, it is not available everywhere or possible for everyone. Bringing potentially like-minded people together might be a useful strategy. Another might be action specifically targeting vulnerable adolescents and people with health problems that can be carried through into later life.[106]

The ancient health rules provided the basis for daily health maintenance regimes for people of different trades and callings. Different routines were advised for particular interests, duties, or skills. For example, Ramazzini provided information to scholars of when and what to eat, when to work at scholarly activity, when to take physical exercise each day, and when to rest:

> The Professors of Learning ought therefore to pursue the Study of Wisdom with Moderation and Conduct, and not be so eager upon the Improvement of their Mind, as to neglect the Body: they ought to keep an even balance, so that the Soul, and the Body may like Landlord and Guest observe the due Measures of Hospitality, and do Mutual Offices, and not trample one another under Foot.[107]

Currently, occupational research in affluent societies tends to focus on employment, and although that, in itself, points to numerous health concerns, even those are seldom addressed fully or applied to potential problems across any worker's day-night continuum. No recent research has considered whether there are different requirements for different occupations, and what happens outside designated work-time is largely forgotten except for the new mandates to exercise regularly. Neither is there a general understanding of the day-night occupation continuum in health terms, although some experts might hold very specific views.

In countries were poverty is rife, occupation-based programs might need to center on skills to increase access to particular prerequisites of health. Practical programs to help people with food production or preparation on a small, personal scale, as well as a community or population scale, could be useful in some situations. Shelter building, clothing manufacture, first-aid information, or information on ways to maintain a rudimentary education when disaster occurs might be other useful occupational programs that could snowball into community-based action should the need arise. This can be particularly important for people with disabilities who may have been excluded from learning such skills. If poverty is a result of war or conflict, the prevention of further social illness and reduction of physical and mental illness might include communal occupations that meet the people's needs for belonging and building trust. Thibeault tells how home building in war-torn Sierra Leone assisted community members to gradually come together again after having been on different sides in the conflict.[108]

Rewarding occupation,[109] relaxation techniques,[110] and learning to cope with stress can provide resistance to stress-related disorders that appear to lead to other forms of illness. Fear of stress-related illness and of litigation has prompted many programs aimed at risk reduction. Antonovsky, following Selye's lead, asked the important question of not whether stress is bad for health, but for whom and under what conditions is it good or bad.[111,112] Successful coping with stressors requires some experience of stress, and, indeed, moderate stress that augments the functional capacities of all systems is necessary for maintaining positive health and vitality, as well as providing a reserve against extreme stress. "Heart attacks are not the result of shoveling snow or running for a train, ...they are the product of a lifetime of not doing things like shoveling snow or running for a train."[113]

Other types of occupation-focused prevention could assist population groups to address political structural change. Well-established occupational institutions, such as the division of labor and the effects of the rampant growth of technology in daily living, could be subjected to investigation. Considering illness from the perspective of occupational imbalance, deprivation, alienation, and a lack of opportunities to develop potential, as well as boredom, burnout, or sleep disturbance would be other useful ways to explore prevention of illness with an occupational lens. That may well include identification of occupational factors that lead to:

- Stress related and mental illness, or lack of learning to cope with stress.
- Ineffective parenting, child exploitation or deprivation, and food abuse.
- Child cruelty/abuse, family/sexual violence, juvenile delinquency, or teen pregnancies.
- Bullying and people abuse (women, children, elders, disabled, ethnic or religious groups).
- School dropout, street-living, suicide, aggression, or substance abuse.
- Work related alienation, dissatisfaction, illness or accidents, welfare fraud.
- Exclusion from work or chosen occupations that ensure active aging.
- Terrorism or gang behavior.
- Pollution or ecological degradation.

OCCUPATION-FOCUSED PREVENTION OF ILLNESS AND DISABILITY: COLLECTIVE OCCUPATIONS ACROSS THE SLEEP-WAKE CONTINUUM

As OPID has to be aimed at finding the overall effects of people's occupations across the sleep-wake continuum as a potential cause of illness, time-use studies might be useful to highlight communal and policy changes that are needed to reduce barriers to occupational participation.[114] In *Time Use: A Report of the Canadian Index of Wellbeing*, Brooker and Hyman took a gendered, life-stage approach because of differing time use patterns and challenges between men, women, and age groups. They found that a substantial proportion of children and adolescents do not participate in organized extracurricular activities, that average screen time was increasing, and that "the proportion of teenagers eating family meals at home" has decreased. Those negative trends go alongside "increasing proportions of adults working non-standard hours, providing care to seniors and experiencing high levels of time pressure." Women reported more time pressure than men, and a higher proportion provided time consuming care to seniors. Also concerning is the significant number of retirees who do not engage in active leisure occupations.[115] They suggest that:

> *National trends may mask the Time Use patterns among population subgroups. Canadians marginalized by race, ethnicity, religion, socioeconomic status, disability, gender, sexual orientation and language proficiency, etc, experience systemic barriers to social and economic opportunity that directly influence their Time Use patterns and indirectly impact on their exposure to health risks and participation in health enhancing activities.[115]*

Some 20 years earlier, social epidemiologists, Bird and Fremont also noted differences in men's and women's activities in relation to illness. They hypothesized that although women live longer, they experience more sickness than men because of occupational and social role variance. Those include the combined effects of:

- Less paid work and lower remuneration
- More time expended in household labor
- More time expended in child care and helping others
- Fewer hours of leisure and sleep
- Mostly holding less "highly rewarding roles" than men.

They concluded that women would experience better health than men if gender roles were more alike because, when gender differences are controlled, being a man is associated with poorer health than being a woman.[116]

Conclusion

The probability of more radical changes in occupation as the century progresses holds potentially serious health consequences. Dubos' warning that people's biological inheritance only enables adaptation up to a point and that chronic disease states develop over time[117] are an precursor of Maslow's concerns that the rapidity of the changing world called for "a different kind of human being ... who is comfortable with change"[118] because the huge acceleration in technology could lead to death for those unable to adapt. The WHO expresses similar concerns associated with socio-ecological change, calling for a "systematic assessment of the health impact of a rapidly changing environment, particularly in areas of technology, work, energy production, and urbanization."[6] Unfortunately, the concerns are real and are made more so by the culturally constructed global community. It appears that the 21st century is beginning to uncover some of the connections between people's doings and illness, and an occupation-focused preventive approach is called for to help people to understand the connections and to overcome them. The theme of this chapter suggests that prevention of much illness is possible because it is mainly preventable risk factors that cause "most of the world's disease burden."

It has been argued in this chapter that people's health maintaining occupations across the 24-hour rest-activity cycle have changed because of "industrialization, urbanization, economic development and increasing food market globalization" and will continue to change and affect health in a detrimental way unless effectively researched and widely promulgated.[1] The health and illness outcomes of corporate and political occupations particularly require ongoing investigation in terms of their impact on the occupations of individuals and subsequent health in both the developing and developed world. In retrospect, occupational behavior can be seen as central to changes in morbidity and mortality. This has been recognized (although not described in the same way) by the WHO and noted public health researchers such as Dubos,[119] McKeown,[120] and McMichael.[121] Even those authorities do not draw together the occupational inferences in a holistic way that provides the different and potentially useful way of looking at the evidence provided here.

References

1. World Health Organization. *Global Strategy on Diet, Physical Activity and Health. Chronic Disease Information Sheets.* World Health Organization Documents and Publications: 2004. Available at: http://www.who.int/topics/physical_activity/en/. Accessed December 15, 2005.

2. Prevention. *Oxford Dictionaries.* http://www.oxforddictionaries.com/definition/english/prevention. Accessed June 6, 2014.

3. Nutbeam D. Health promotion glossary. *Health Promotion International.* 1998; 13(4): 349-64.

4. Lorenz K. *The Waning of Humaneness.* Boston, Mass: Little, Brown and Co; 1987.

5. Ashton J, Seymour H. *The New Public Health: The Liverpool Experience.* Milton Keynes: Open University Press; 1988.

6. World Health Organization, Health and Welfare Canada, Canadian Public Health Association. *Ottawa Charter for Health Promotion.* Ottawa, Canada: 1986.

7. World Health Organization.*The Bangkok Charter for Health Promotion in a Globalized World.* 2005.

8. World Health Organization. *Jakarta Declaration on Leading Health Promotion into the 21st Century.* 1998.

9. Hetzel BS, McMichael T. *L S Factor: Lifestyle and Health.* Ringwood, Victoria: Penguin; 1987:186-187.

10. Last JM, ed. *Public Health and Preventive Medicine.* East Norwalk, Conn: Appleton and Lange; 1987:4.

11. Last JM, ed. *Public Health and Preventive Medicine.* East Norwalk, Conn: Appleton and Lange; 1987: 6.

12. Sigerist HE. *On the History of Medicine.* Marti-Ibañez F, ed. New York: MD Publications; 1960:16.

13. McKeown T. *The Origins of Human Disease.* Oxford, UK: Basil Blackwell, 1988:154.

14. Commonwealth Department of Community Services and Health. *World Health Organization: A Brief Summary of its Work. (Clause 24).* Canberra: Australian Government Publishing Service; 1988:10.

15. Porter R. *Disease, Medicine and Society in England 1550-1860.* Basingstoke and London: MacMillan Education; 1987.

16. Wilcock AA. *Occupation for Health. Volume 1. A Journey from Self Health to Prescription.* London: British College of Occupational Therapists; 2001.

17. Owen, R. *Paper: Dedicated to the Governments of Great Britain, Austria, Russia, France, Prussia and the United States of America.* London: New Lanark Conservation; 1841.

18. Chadwick E. *Report on the Sanitary Condition of the Labouring Population of Great Britain.* Edinburgh: Edinburgh University Press; 1965. Original work published 1842.

19. MacDonald EM. *World-wide Conquests of Disabilities: The History, Development and Present Functions of the Remedial Services.* London: Bailliere Tindall; 1981:88-89.

20. Girling DA, ed. *New Age Encyclopedia, Vol. 6.* London: Bay Books; 1983:150.

21. Guy Rev Dr JR. *Compassion and the Art of the Possible: Dr. Southwood Smith as Social Reformer and Public Health Pioneer.* Octavia Hill Memorial Lecture. December 1993. Cambridgeshire: Octavia Hill Society & The Birthplace Museum Trust; 1996.

22. Poynter F. *Thomas Southwood Smith-the Man (1788-1861).* London: Wellcome Historical Medical Library; 1961. http://pubmedcentralcanada.ca/picrender.cgi?accid=PMC1896581&blobtype=pdf. Accessed May 30, 2014.

23. The Industrial Accident Prevention Associations (IAPA). *90 Years of Workplace Health and Safety History at IAPA.* 2008-2010. http://www.iapa.ca/Main/about_iapa/ninety_history.aspx. Accessed April 18, 2013.

24. Personal communication. Dr Erio Ziglio: Head, European Office for Investment for Health and Development, World Health Organization; Edinburgh:10th June 2005.

25. World Health Organization. *About WHO.* http://www.who.int/about/en/. Accessed May 30, 2014.

26. UK NICE. *A Conceptual Framework for Public Health.* 2008. http:/www.sciencedirect.com/science/article/pii/S0033350608002795#. Accessed October 2, 2013.

27. Gordon D. *Health, Sickness and Society: Theoretical Concepts in Social and Preventive Medicine.* St. Lucia, Queensland: University of Queensland Press; 1976:5.

28. Meyer A. The philosophy of occupation therapy. *American Journal of Occupational Therapy.* 1977;31:639-642. (First presented to the National Society for the Promotion of Occupational Therapy in 1921 and published 1922.)

29. Le Vesconte HP. The place of occupational therapy in social work planning. *Canadian Journal of Occupational Therapy.* 1934;2:13-16.

30. Le Vesconte HP. Expanding fields of occupational therapy. *Canadian Journal of Occupational Therapy.* 1935;3:4-12.

31. West W. The occupational therapists changing responsibilities to the community. *American Journal of Occupational Therapy.* 1967;21:312.

32. West W. The 1967 Eleanor Clarke Slagle Lecture. Professional responsibility in times of change. *American Journal of Occupational Therapy.* 1968;XXII(1):9-15.

33. West W. The growing importance of prevention. *American Journal of Occupational Therapy.* 1969;23:223-231.

34a. West W. The emerging health model of occupational therapy practice. *Proceedings of the 5th International Congress of the WFOT.* Zurich: WFOT; 1970.

34b. Cromwell FS. Our challenges in the seventies. Occupational therapy today—tomorrow. *Proceedings of the 5th International Congress.* Zurich, 1970:232-238.

34c. Brunyate R. After fifty years, what stature do we hold. *American Journal of Occupational Therapy.* 1967;21:262-267.

34d. Wiemer R. Some concepts of prevention as an aspect of community health. *American Journal of Occupational Therapy.* 1972;26:1-9.

34e. Walker L. Occupational therapy in the well community. *American Journal of Occupational Therapy.* 1971;25;345-347.

34f. Mosey AC. Meeting health needs. *American Journal of Occupational Therapy.* 1973;27:14-17.

34g. Grosman J. Preventive health care and community programming. *American Journal of Occupational Therapy.* 1977;31(6):351-354.

34h. Grossman J. A prevention model for occupational therapy. *American Journal of Occupational Therapy.* 1991; 45(1):33-41.

34i. Finn GL. Update of Eleanor Clarke Slagle Lecture: the occupational therapist in prevention programs. *American Journal of Occupational Therapy.* 1977;31(10):658-659.

34j. Fidler GS, Fidler JW. Doing and becoming: purposeful action and self actualisation. *American Journal of Occupational Therapy.* 1978;32:305-310.

34k. American Occupational Therapy Association. AOTA Representative Assembly minutes. *American Journal of Occupational Therapy.* 1979;33:780-813.

35. Brown KM. Wellness: past visions, future roles. In: Cromwell FS, ed. *Sociocultural Implications in Treatment Planning in Occupational Therapy.* New York, NY: Haworth Press; 1987.

36. Johnson JA. *Wellness: A Context for Living.* Thorofare, NJ: SLACK; 1986.

37. Arvier R, Bell A. Back injury management and prevention in the New South Wales coal mining industry. *The Australian Association of Occupational Therapists 15th Federal Conference.* Sydney, Australia: OT Australia; 1988.

38. Schwartz RK. Cognition and learning in industrial accident injury prevention: an occupational therapy perspective. In: Johnson JA, Jaffe E, eds. Health promotive and preventive programs: models of occupational therapy practice. *Occupational Therapy in Health Care.* 1989;6(1):67-85.

39. Rudge MA. Occupational therapy in the underground mining industry. *The Australian Association of Occupational Therapist's 15th Federal Conference.* Sydney, Australia; OT Australia; 1988.

40. Occupational Therapy Australia. *The Spectrum of Work Practice: Prevention to Participation.* Work Symposium. Brisbane, 31 May & 1 June 2013. Available at: http://www.otaus.com.au/conference-information. Accessed July 17, 2013.

41. Deily J. Home safety program for older adults. In: Johnson JA, Jaffe E, eds. Health promotive and preventive programs: models of occupational therapy practice. *Occupational Therapy in Health Care.* 1989;6(1):113-124.

42. South Australian State Program. *Falls Prevention Program for the Elderly.* Noarlunga Community Health Service, South Australia. 1992.

43. Reducing Falls: Examples of local and national collaborative falls prevention strategies. *Occupational Therapy News.* October 2005;13(10):22-25.

44. Toto P. *Occupational Therapy and Prevention of Falls.* The American Occupational Therapy Association: Living Life to its Fullest. 2012. Available at: www.aota.org/Consumers/Professionals/WhatisOT/PA/Facts/39478.aspx. Accessed June 2, 2013.

45. Stout JD. Occupational therapists' involvement in safe transportation for the handicapped. In: Johnson JA, Jaffe E, eds. Health promotive and preventive programs: models of occupational therapy practice. *Occupational Therapy in Health Care.* 1989;6(1):45-56.

46. Olson L, Heanery C, Soppas-Hoffman B. Parent-child activity group treatment in preventive psychiatry. In: Johnson JA, Jaffe E, eds. Health promotive and preventive programs: models of occupational therapy practice. *Occupational Therapy in Health Care.* 1989;6(1):29-43.

47. World Health Organization. *Jakarta Declaration on Leading Health Promotion into the 21st Century.* 1998:2.

48. World Health Organization. *Jakarta Declaration on Leading Health Promotion into the 21st Century.* 1998:3.

49. World Health Organization. *Jakarta Declaration on Leading Health Promotion into the 21st Century.* 1998:4.

50. World Health Organization. *The Declaration of Alma Ata. International Conference on Primary Health Care.* Alma Ata, USSR: WHO; 1978.

51. Richards T. News extra: social policy more important for health than medicines, conference told. *British Medical Journal.* 1999;319:1592.

52. Bassuk SS, Glass TA, Berkman LF. Social disengagement and incident cognitive decline in community dwelling elderly persons. *Annals of Internal Medicine.* 1999;131(3):165-173.

53. Iwarsson S, Isacsson A, Persson D, Scherston B. Occupation and survival: a 25-year follow-up study of an aging population. *American Journal of Occupational Therapy.* 1998;52:65-70.

54. Rudman D, Cook J, Polatakjo H. Understanding the potential of occupation: a qualitative exploration of senior's perspectives on activity. *American Journal of Occupational Therapy.* 1997;51:640-650.

55. Evans R. Doctors –get on your bikes. *British Medical Journal.* Available at: bmj.com. Accessed March 31, 2000 (full text).

56. Mason B. Prescribed cycling. *British Medical Journal.* Available at: bmj.com. Accessed April 2, 2000 (full text).

57. Xavier G. Bicycle use is even more important to poor countries. *British Medical Journal.* Available at: bmj.com. Accessed April 2, 2000 (full text).

58. Wardlaw M. Of steel and skulls. *British Medical Journal.* Available at: bmj.com, 17 Apr 2000 (full text).

59. Chiheb Z. Why do school children cycle on the continent, but not in the UK? *British Medical Journal.* Available at: bmj.com. Accessed May 14, 2000 (full text).

60. Wardlaw M. Segregating cyclists is not the answer. *British Medical Journal.* Available at: bmj.com. Accessed May 19, 2000 (full text).

61. Chossudovsky M. Global poverty in the late 20th century [Electronic version]. *Journal of International Affairs.* 1998;52:293-311.

62. Thibeault, R. Fostering healing through occupation: the case of the Canadian Inuit. *Journal of Occupational Science.* 2002:9;153-158.

63. Yeoman S. Occupation and disability: a role for occupational therapists in developing countries. *British Journal of Occupational Therapy.* 1998:61;523-527.

64. *Listen to the Voices.* Available at: http://www.worldbank.org/poverty/voices/listen-findings.htm. Accessed June 2, 2014.

65. Probst JC, Laditka S, Moore CG, Harun N, Paige Powell M. *Depression in Rural Populations: Prevalence, Effects on Life Quality, and Treatment seeking Behavior.* Rockville, Maryland: Office of Rural Health Policy, US Government of Health and Rural Services; 2005.

66. Hetzel BS, McMichael T. *L S Factor: Lifestyle and Health.* Ringwood, Victoria: Penguin; 1987:186.

67. American College of Sports Medicine. *Guidelines for Exercise Testing and Prescription.* 4th ed. Philadelphia, PA: Lea and Febiger; 1991.

68. Hetzel BS, McMichael T. *L S Factor: Lifestyle and Health.* Ringwood, Victoria: Penguin; 1987.

69. Caspersen CJ, Christensen GM, Pollard RA. Status of the 1990 physical fitness and exercise objectives—evidence from NHIS 1985. *Public Health Reports.* 1986.

70. Blaxter M. *Health and Lifestyles.* London, England: Tavistock/Routledge; 1990.

71. Clee J. *Unpublished study.* University of South Australia; 1991.

72. Gilliam TB, Freedson PS, Geenen DL, Shahraray B. Physical activity patterns determined by heart rate monitoring in 6-7 year-old children. *Medicine and Science in Sports and Exercise.* 1981;13:65-67.

73. Stephens T, Jacob DR, White CC. A descriptive epidemiology of leisure time physical activity. *Public Health Reports.* 1985;100:147-158.

74. Shea S, Basche CE, Lantigua R, Weschler H. The Washington Heights-Inwood healthy heart program: a third generation community-based cardiovascular disease prevention program in a disadvantaged urban setting. *Preventive Medicine.* 1991;21:201-217.

75. King AC, Blair SN, Bild DE, et al. Determinants of physical activity and interventions in adults. *Medicine and Science in Sports and Exercise.* 1992;24:S221-S237.

76. Kaplan RM, Sallis JF, Patterson TL. *Health and Human Behavior.* New York, NY: McGraw-Hill Inc; 1993:350.

77. World Health Organization. *Global Strategy on Diet, Physical Activity and Health. Chronic Disease Information Sheets.* World Health Organization Documents and Publications: 2004:1. Available at: http://www.who.int/topics/physical_activity/en/. Accesed December 7, 2005.

78. Archer E, Shook R, Thomas D, Church T, Katzmarzyk P, et al. 45-Year trends in women's use of time and household management energy expenditure. *PLoS ONE.* 2013:8(2);e56620. doi:10.1371/journal.pone.0056620

79. Powell KE, Thompson PD, Caspersen CJ, Kendrick JS. Physical activity and the incidence of coronary heart disease. *Annual Review of Public Health.* 1987;8:253-287.

80. Blair SN, Kohl HW, Paffenbarger RS, Clark DG, Cooper KH, Gibbons LW. Physical fitness and all-cause mortality: a prospective study of healthy men and women. *Journal of the American Medical Association.* 1989;262:2395-2401.

81. Ekelund LG, Haskell WL, Johnson JL, Whaley FS, Criqui MH, Sheps DS. Physical fitness as a predictor of cardiovascular mortality in asymptomatic North American men. *New England Journal of Medicine.* 1988;319:1379-1384.

82. Haskell WL. Exercise induced changes in plasma lipids and lipoproteins. *Preventive Medicine.* 1984;13:23-36.

83. Wood PD, Haskell WL, Blair SN, et al. Increased exercise level and plasma lipoprotein concentrations: a one-year randomised study in sedentary middle-aged men. *Metabolism.* 1983;32:31-39.

84. Hicky N, Mulcahy R, Bourke GJ, Graham I, Wilson-Davis K. Study of coronary risk factors relating to physical activity in 15,171 men. *British Medical Journal.* 1975;5982:507-509.

85. Siegel WC, Blumenthal JA. The role of exercise in the prevention and treatment of hypertension. *Annals of Behavioural Medicine.* 1991;13:23-30.

86. Vranic M, Wasserman D. Exercise, fitness and diabetes. In: Bouchard C, Shephard RJ, Stephens T, Sutton JR, McPherson GD, eds. *Exercise, Fitness and Health: A Consensus of Current Knowledge.* Champaign, Ill: Human Kinetics; 1990:467-490.

87. Epstein LH, Wing RR, Thompson JK, Griffin W. Attendance and fitness in aerobic exercise: the effects of contract and lottery procedures. *Behavior Modification.* 1980;4:465-479.

88. Haskell WL, Leon AS, Caspersen CJ, et al. Cardiovascular benefits and assessment of physical activity and fitness in adults. *Medicine and Science in Sports and Exercise.* 1992;24:S201-S220.

89. Calabrese LH. Exercise, immunity, cancer and infection. In: Bouchard C, Shephard RJ, Stephens T, Sutton JR, McPherson GD, eds. *Exercise, Fitness and Health: A Consensus of Current Knowledge.* Champaign, Ill: Human Kinetics; 1990:567-579.

90. Stephens T. Physical activity and mental health in the United States and Canada: evidence from 4 population surveys. *Preventive Medicine.* 1988;17:35-47.

91. Maddi SR. Issues and interventions in stress mastery. In: Friedman HS, ed. *Personality and Disease.* New York, NY: John Wiley and Sons; 1990:132.

92. Glass TA, de Leon CM, Marottoli RA, Berkman LF. Population based study of social and productive activities as predictors of survival among elderly Americans. *British Medical Journal.* 1999:319:478-483.

93. McCrady S, Levine J. Sedentariness at work: how much do we really sit? *Obesity (Silver Spring).* 2009;17(11):2103-2105. doi:10.1038/oby.2009.117.

94. Levine J, McCrady S, Boyne S, Smith J, Cargile K, Forrester T. Non-exercise physical activity in agricultural and urban people. *Urban Studies.* 2011;48(11);2417-2427.

95. Rebel J. It sounds sexist, but women doing less housework than in the 1960s may be related to the obesity epidemic: study 2013. *National Post, a Division of Postmedia Network Inc.* Available at: http://life.nationalpost.com. Accessed April 9, 2013.

96. Reynolds G. What housework has to do with waistlines. *The New York Times.* February 27, 2013. http://well.blogs.nytimes.com/2013/02/27/what-housework-has-to-do-with-waistlines. Accessed April 9, 2013.

97. McCrady-Spitzer S, Levine J. Nonexercise activity thermogenesis: a way forward to treat the worldwide obesity epidemic. *Surgery for Obesity and Related Diseases.* 2012;8(5):501-506. doi:10.1016/j.soard.2012.08.001

98. Levine J. *New N.E.A.T. Science Reveals How to Be Thinner, Happier, and Smarter.* NewYork, NY; Crown Archetype: 2009.

99. Billings-Coleman L. *Standing Up to Sitting Down Disease: Dr James Levine.* ProBonoPress. Available at: www.probonopress.org/?p=01002. Accessed May 2, 2013.

100. Cooper K. *Dr Kenneth Cooper's Antioxidant Revolution.* Melbourne, Australia: Bookman; 1994.

101. Siscovick DS, Weiss NS, Fletcher RH, Lasky T. The incidence of primary cardiac arrest during vigorous exercise. *New England Journal of Medicine.* 1984;311:874-877.

102. Budgett R. Overtraining syndrome. *British Journal of Sports Medicine.* 1990;24(4):231-236.

103. Wilcock AA, et al. *Retrospective Study of Elderly Peoples' Perceptions of the Relationship Between Their Lifes' Occupations and Health.* Unpublished material, University of South Australia, 1990.

104. US Department of Health and Human Services. *Behavioral Health Services Division. Prevention Definition.* Available at: 176_DOHpreventiondefinition.pdf. Accessed December 14, 2005.

105. Eisler RM. Promoting health through interpersonal skills development. In: Mattarazzo JD, Weiss SM, Herd JA, Miller NE, Weiss SM, eds. *Behavioural Health: A Handbook of Health Enhancement and Disease Prevention.* New York, NY: John Wiley and Sons; 1984.

106. Viner RM, Barker M. Young people's health: the need for action. *British Medical Journal.* 2005;330:901-903.

107. Ramazzini B. *A Treatise of the Diseases of Tradesmen (etc).* London: Printed for Andre Bell et al; 1705:273.

108. Thibeault R. Occupation and the rebuilding of cival society: Notes from the war zone. *Journal of Occupational Science.* 2002;9(1);38-47.

109. Hazuda H. Women's employment status and their risks for chronic disease. Colloquium presentation, University of Texas School of Public Health, Houston. Reported in: Justice B. *Who Gets Sick: Thinking and Health.* Houston, Texas: Peak Press; 1987.

110. Pelletier KR. *Mind as Healer, Mind as Slayer.* New York, NY: Delta; 1977.

111. Antonovsky A. The sense of coherence as a determinant of health. In: Matarazzo JD, ed., *Behavior Health: A Handbook of Health Enhancement and Disease Prevention.* New York, John Wiley & Sons; 1984.

112. Selye, H. The general adaptation syndrome and the diseases of adaptation. *Journal of Clinical Endocrinology.* 1946;6:117.

113. Klump TG. How much exercise to avoid heart attacks? *Medical Times.* 1976;4(104):64-74.

114. Xu L, Gauthier A, Strohschein L. Why are some children left out? factors barring children from participating in extracurricular activities. *Canadian Studies in Population.* 2009;36(3-4):325-345.

115. Brooker A, Hyman I. *Time Use: A Report of the Canadian Index of Wellbeing.* Waterloo, Ontario; Canadian Index of Well-Being and University of Waterloo: 2010.

116. Bird C, Fremont A. Gender, time use, and health. *Journal of Health and Social Behavior.* 1991;32(June):114-129.

117. Dubos R. Changing patterns of disease. In: Brown RG, Whyte HM, eds. *Medical Practice and the Community: Proceedings of a Conference Convened by the Australian National University, Canberra.* Canberra: Australian National University Press; 1968:59.

118. Maslow A. *The Farther Reaches of Human Nature.* New York, NY: Viking Press; 1971.

119. Dubos R, ed. *Mirage of Health: Utopias, Progress and Biological Change.* New York, NY: Harper and Row; 1959.

120. McKeown T. *The Origins of Human Disease.* Oxford, UK: Basil Blackwell;1988.

121. McMichael T. *Human Frontiers, Environments and Disease: Past Patterns, Uncertain Futures.* Cambridge UK: Cambridge University Press; 2001.

Theme 16

"The role of the health sector must move increasingly in a health promotion direction, beyond its responsibility for providing clinical and curative services."

WHO: Ottawa Charter for Health Promotion, 1986[1]

Chapter 16

OCCUPATION, HEALTH, AND WELL-BEING

This chapter addresses:
- The Urgency of Health Promotion
- Concepts of Health Promotion and Well-Being
  - Health Promotion
  - Well-Being and Wellness
- Occupation to Promote Health and Well-Being
  - Health Promotion Is the Process of Enabling People to Increase Control over, and to Improve, Their Health
  - Health Is a Resource for Everyday Life, Not the Objective of Living
  - Health Is a Positive Concept Emphasizing Social and Personal Resources, as Well as Physical Capacities
  - Health Promotion Is Not Just the Responsibility of the Health Sector, but Goes Beyond Healthy Lifestyles to Well-Being
  - An Individual or Group Must Be Able to Identify and Realize Aspirations, to Satisfy Needs, to Change or Cope with the Environment
- Why Is an Occupation to Promote Health and Well-Being Approach Necessary?
- Occupation Focussed Health Promotion
  - Well Doing, Being, Belonging, and Becoming
    - How People Obtain the Requirements for Living
    - Social Determinants
    - Occupational Behavior Develops Early
    - Education Is a Primary Concern
    - Practical Based Programs
    - Active Aging
    - Function
    - Meaning, Purpose, and Choice
    - Tertiary and Quaternary Approaches

Wilcock AA, Hocking C.
An Occupational Perspective of Health, Third Edition (pp 450-480).
© 2015 Taylor & Francis Group.

➢ Environment
- Occupation Toward WHO Health for All Objectives Across the Globe
- Conclusion

Occupation is a natural phenomenon fundamental to the health of humans. Exploring the concept as doing, being, belonging, and becoming has touched on how it entwines with health and well-being. Until fairly recently, what humans did naturally to survive and maintain health was concerned with obtaining the prerequisites of life. For many, that remains the case today despite major changes in occupational patterns. In other parts of the world and over millennia, rules to achieve and maintain health were established based on observation of occupational patterns, the environment and communal structure, the differing natures of people, where and how they lived, and what they did. During the past century, when modern medicine evolved, earlier rules were largely disregarded without due consideration that some might have worth. As a result, in the period of limbo while medical science grew apace, there was a lack of direction about how to promote health and well-being.

The establishment of the WHO began to alter that loss of direction, and for more than half a century it has provided the modern world with guidance to improve the experience of health. Some of that guidance has been directed to political administrations throughout the world, but pressure from multinational corporations or technologically driven economic and medical policies led to more basic understandings being largely neglected. Ecological degradation, poverty, and illness for millions, and reliance on a "live now, reverse the consequences later" cult has been the result. Priorities for health promotion in the 21st century, therefore, include the pursuit of "policies and practices that":

> ... *Avoid harming the health of individuals; protect the environment, and ensure sustainable use of resources; restrict production of and trade in inherently harmful goods and substances such as tobacco and armaments, as well as discourage unhealthy marketing practices; safeguard both the citizen in the marketplace and the individual in the workplace; and include equity-focused health impact assessments as an integral part of policy development.*[2]

The Urgency of Health Promotion

The evidence and experience accumulated from the WHO global congresses on health promotion, from Ottawa onwards, points to its importance as "an integrative, cost-effective strategy" essential for dealing with emerging concerns. *The Ottawa Charter*[1] remains the WHO's primary authority on the promotion of health, having been ratified and extended at subsequent world health promotion congresses with focus toward the globalized world emerging in the *Bangkok Charter*.[3] That health promotion is a matter of urgency was identified specifically at the 7th congress in Nairobi. Delegates recognized financial crises that threaten the viability of national economies; global warming, and climate change; and threats to security that pose unprecedented threats to health. Urgent attention was seen as necessary to overcome "a sense of shared uncertainty for communities around the world"[4] that took its toll on human life. At the time of writing this text, the congress held in 2013 addressed the idea of *Health in All Policies*. Its working definition as follows:

> *Health in All Policies is a systemic and sustained approach to taking into account the impacts of public policies on health determinants and health systems across sectors, at the levels the decisions are made, in political, legislative and administrative processes, in order to realize health-related rights and to improve accountability for population health and health equity.*[5]

The *Health in All Policies* approach is aimed at providing "the framework for all activities in society, including those of private households, the private sector and civil society" so that all sectors are enabled to realize gains in health, well-being, and development.[5] It is imperative that political, corporate, and communal authorities recognize and act on the breadth and depth of occupational issues that affect health and well-being, but it is also important that individuals are enabled to appreciate what they can do for themselves. As the political message gets stronger, there is a tendency for the more immediately applicable messages of the *Ottawa Charter* to get lost, particularly as individual health interventions continue to remain in the medical/preventive domain. The politicizing of health promotion messages, too, falls far short of the required action, in part because experts tend to consider phenomena through single-disciplinary lenses rather than holistically.[2-8]

Concepts of Health Promotion and Well-Being

Population health embraces approaches to promote health, as well as prevent illness, despite some ideological difference between the concepts. Currently, the latter is founded on the largely medically focused disease orientation, whereas health promotion follows a more holistic approach that incorporates well-being, [9] recognizing the necessity for all people "to satisfy needs" and to "identify and realize aspirations."[10] The closeness of fit between the promotion of health and the prevention of illness is clear when the different levels of the approach, given in health promotion texts, are listed and compared with those for prevention in the previous chapter:[9,11]

- Primary—for the general population: inclusive of averting health damaging behavior and illness
- Secondary—for people who have already experienced health damage: to effect behavior change or retard progression
- Tertiary—for people with chronic diseases or disability
- Quaternary—for the terminally ill.

HEALTH PROMOTION

The term *health promotion* was coined in the 1970s,[12] with its emergence being linked not only with preventive medicine, but also with health education, social medicine and social health, the women's movement, community development, and other "participatory" population health approaches.[9,13-15] The 1986 *Ottawa Charter* was the catalyst for the idea becoming widely embraced, but not everyone approved the resulting declaration. There are those who castigate the *Ottawa Charter* for being too general, resulting, it is believed, in it being meaningless.[16] Reflecting that criticism, Cribb and Duncan claimed that its purpose is vague and elusive with significant ethical dilemmas, but are clear that promoting health is a political activity.[17] In a similar mode, Tones maintained that promoting health is public health's radical, militant component.[18] It is, without a doubt, more than that, with some of the *Ottawa Charter's* apparent simplicity making it accessible to all people, its generality a result of the fact that it speaks to many different disciplines and enablement and empowerment is inclusive of individuals and the wider community. Those particular advantages can only be effective if there is equality in the consideration of different ways of viewing the issues. That is potentially difficult, as the following differences in health approaches from diverse disciplines illustrate:

Medicine and public health—Epidemiology and disease prevention[19]
Social sciences—Social determinants and empowerment[20,21]

Environmental sciences—Ecological sustainability and global health

Political science—Economic equity and development

Occupational science—Occupational determinants and enablement

Occupational therapy—Restorative occupations and functional well-being

The *Ottawa* and *Bangkok Charters* set as foundations for health that all people need to meet the basic requirements of life through:

- The opportunities available
- The sociopolitical and economic constraints and liberties of situations that enable or control what they do
- The environmental factors that impact on what they can do
- Policies and partnerships that empower communities at the center of global and national developments
- Health being the central aspect of development.

As the *Bangkok Charter* explains, health promotion "reaches out to people and organizations critical to the achievement of health," including governments, civil society, international organizations, and private and public health sectors.[3] This is because promoting physical, mental, and social health and well-being is applicable across the globe to populations and communities, as well as individuals, and is an integrated, multi-professional, and holistic approach using overlapping strategies.[22] It is complementary to and informed by medical science but is based to a greater extent on behavioral, social, and environmental sciences, encompassing health education, community development, empowerment and justice, prevention, economics, and politics.[23,24]

WELL-BEING AND WELLNESS

The terms *well-being* and *wellness* were explored in the Chapter 1, but because they are central to health promotion, they are briefly reconsidered here. The WHO has described well-being in various ways since the word was included in its definition of health approximately 70 years ago. The definition triggered useful debate and controversy, especially with the inclusion of two words: social and well-being. The first of those has enabled a valuable social model of health to emerge, despite being separated from the other two in most health and medical research and care. That is even the case currently, when the social health problem of poverty is critical in terms of population health. The second controversial word (well-being) continues to provide another trigger for debate in the medical fraternity. The WHO describes how:

> Well-being is a general term encompassing the total universe of human life domains including physical, mental and social aspects (education, employment, environment, etc), that make up what can be called a "good life."[25]

Well-being is certainly a complex phenomenon, generating research across time and cultures in a variety of fields and viewed from different perspectives. Major foci have included inquiry about the place of pleasure and happiness, full functioning, optimal experience, meaning, and self-realization.[26] Apart from psychologists' and social scientists' attention, there has been an apparent increase of interest in how to facilitate the experience of feeling well. It has been associated with a growth of alternative health services, such as acupuncture, reflexology, herbalism, homeopathy, naturopathy, massage, aromatherapy, and relaxation therapy, for those unhappy with the range of solutions provided by conventional medicine. The more holistic notions of traditional Asian philosophies have been influential. This has increased acknowledgment that well-being is related to spiritual, social, and behavioral factors, such as where and how people live, what they believe, their rest, relaxation, and self-care practices, and the balance of work with other activities they pursue, including a noticeable fascination in all manner of sport.[27-29]

Wellness is sometimes used interchangeably with well-being. Definitions of wellness hold appeal and have the potential for empowering and enabling people outside the medical profession who embrace ideas such as holism, finding meaning, the search for philosophies of living, and "state of being."[30,31] Outside the medical field, in America particularly, a wellness approach has also been adopted on many industrial, business, and corporate work sites.[32-35] It is used as a marketing tool[36] and has become a business offering in its own right,[37] with courses available on becoming a "wellness trainer."[38] In this corporate context, Opatz has defined health promotion in wellness terms as "systematic efforts by an organization to enhance the wellness of its members through education, behavior change, and cultural support."[39]

The wellness movement that emerged in the early 1960s along with exploration of alternative lifestyles[40,41] also embraces occupation-focused values such as:

- "An optimal or ideal condition toward which to strive"[42]
- "A context for living"[43]
- "A lifestyle … to reach optimal potential"[44]
- "A state of mental and physical balance and fitness."[45]

The wellness model follows the humanist tradition of personal growth ideologies and the development of self-esteem, performance, roles, and quality of life skills. It is an approach suited to all people, including those who are physically, mentally, socially, or occupationally disadvantaged. It has been found that:

- Despite appearances "a person can be living a process of wellness and yet be physically handicapped, aged, scared in the face of challenge, in pain, imperfect …"[30]
- Facilitating the wellness process is particularly useful "when people are under varying degrees of stress or illness" and "lose their appreciation for life's purpose and meaning"[30]
- Diseases or symptoms may, in fact, be "the body-mind's attempt to solve a problem."[46]

The wellness model can be a useful adjunct to conventional medicine[47] to counteract the trend toward increasingly restricted acute care with a focus on high technology, which is expensive and expects a passive, rather than participatory, attitude from consumers.

Seeking ways to improve well-being is not new. In 20th century Australia, both mainstream medical authorities and peripheral therapies have displayed interest,[48-50] and in America, Halbert Dunn worked tirelessly toward maximizing the potential of individuals according to environmental possibilities.[51] Wellness tends to address an individual as distinct from communal state, but embraces multidimensional concepts. Those include balance; work, play, and rest; nutrition; and use of physical, psychological, intellectual, and spiritual capacities within self, environment, and culture.[52] According to Dossey and Guzzetta, the wellness health model assumes that all people are searching for answers about the life process, meaning, and purpose; that every individual has innate capacities for healing, nurture, self-reflection, taking risks, and for making change toward wellness; and that health is also about individuals being able to live according to their beliefs.[30] Bill Hettler, one of the co-founders of the U.S. National Wellness Institute, described wellness as "an active process through which individuals become aware of and make choices toward a more successful existence."[53] He called for people to "balance the six dimensions of life," namely social, intellectual, spiritual, physical, emotional, and occupational (applied in this case to work).[54] Those ideas imply that well-being is multidimensional, bringing together the physical, mental, and social aspects of life. All of the dimensions touch on or are central to the holistic nature of occupation described here.

With the term "functioning meaningfully," the ESRC Research Group on Well-being in Developing Countries (WeD), introduced in the first chapter, recognizes, at least in part, the place of occupation in well-being. It proposes that well-being is multidimensional and context specific and includes a state of feeling well, as well as a process of "functioning meaningfully."[55] It can be equated with wealth, happiness, or goal satisfaction but is also linked with having resources, capabilities, and opportunities to achieve goals. They describe the reverse of well-being as ill-being, which is associated with material poverty, unhappiness, unfulfilled goals, and compromise:

> Poor people may have to sacrifice education or food to obtain health care, sacrifice longer-term autonomy to alleviate short-term insecurity, sacrifice peace of mind to survive and thrive in unpredictable modernity or sacrifice short-term happiness to secure longer-term satisfaction.[55]

Well-being, rather than wellness, is used repeatedly by the WHO and appears to be in more common usage in many countries, whereas wellness is often applied to popular, fashionable, or naturopathic aspects rather than mainstream health. Therefore, well-being is the chosen terminology here, although it is accepted that the terms are largely interchangeable.

Occupation to Promote Health and Well-Being

The Ottawa Charter description of health promotion is a useful starting place:

> Health promotion is the process of enabling people to increase control over, and to improve, their health. To reach a state of complete physical, mental and social well-being, an individual or group must be able to identify and realize aspirations, to satisfy needs, and to change or cope with the environment. Health is, therefore, seen as a resource for everyday life, not the objective of living. Health is a positive concept emphasizing social and personal resources, as well as physical capacities. Therefore, health promotion is not just the responsibility of the health sector, but goes beyond healthy lifestyles to well-being.[1]

This description is recognizably occupation-focused and clearly identifies important issues to promote population health that are widely acknowledged.

Ideology recognizing the personal and societal benefits of interaction between occupation and positive health has early origins. Industrialist Robert Owen, whose ideas have been touched on in earlier parts of the book, espoused some 200 years ago that "individuals should be placed, through life, within those external arrangements that will ensure the most happiness, physically, mentally, and morally; ... and the greatest practical benefit to the whole of society."[56] Other examples of his health promotion explanations are in Boxed Dialogue 16-1.

With others of like mind who knew and respected Owen's work, 19th century public health pioneer physician Thomas Southwood-Smith held as his creed the "promotion of human longevity and happiness." He argued that there is "a close connection between happiness and longevity...to add enjoyment, is to lengthen life," and that it is, in fact, "pleasurable consciousness which constitutes the feeling of health."[57] He considered the development of capacities through doing was both a source of pleasure and a means of prolonging life (Boxed Dialogue 16-2).[58,59]

The ideas advanced by Owen,[56] Southwood-Smith, and others held some similarity to the utilitarian doctrine of happiness attributed to Jeremy Bentham. He proposed that "nature has placed mankind under the governance of two sovereign masters, pain and pleasure. It is for them alone to point out what we ought to do."[60] Pain and pleasure could be measured according to duration and intensity. Utilitarian philosophers speak of ill-being to capture the negative aspects of individuals' lives.[61] Such 19th century views were, to some extent, a response to the health horrors that industrialization brought and the comparison between the lives of rich industrialists with that of the laboring poor.

In many parts of the world today, utilitarians could observe equally horrific consequences. In developing countries, they could witness people starving, with no way to meet their basic requirements, partially because of the greed of multinational corporations, self-seeking economic policies, and environmental mismanagement, or they might look at the health effects on the people of war-torn countries and following acts of terrorism. In affluent postindustrial nations, they could

---

Boxed Dialogue 16-1:
Robert Owen's Occupation-Focused Vision of Health Promotion

Is it not in the interest of the human race that everyone should be so taught, and placed, that he would find his highest enjoyment to arise from the continued practice of doing all in his power to promote the well-being, and happiness, of every man, woman, and child, without regard to their class, sect, party, country, or color?"

When society shall be based on true principles, it will not permit any of its members to be thus made small and imperfect parts of what man might be more easily made to become. It will perceive the great importance of training infants from birth, to become full-formed men or women, having every portion of their nature duly cultivated and regularly exercised.

It will discover that man has not been created to attain the full excellence and happiness of his nature, until all his faculties, senses and propensities, shall be well cultivated, and society shall be so constructed that all of them, in each individual, shall be temperately exercised, and their powers continued and increased by such exercise, until arrested by natural old age.

It is in the highest interest of all the human race, to which there cannot be a single exception; 1st. That the entire faculties, senses and propensities, should be well cultivated, and at all times duly or temperately exercised, according to the physical and mental strength and capacity of the individual; in order that whatever may be done by each, should be performed in the best manner for the general advantage of all.

Owen R. Works of Robert Owen: Volume 3: Book of the New Moral World. *(Pickering Masters Series). London, England: Pickering & Chatto (Publishers Ltd.);1993:156.*

Boxed Dialogue 16-2:
Southwood-Smith's Occupation-Focused Vision of Health Promotion

... pleasure resulting from action of the organs is conducive to their complete development, and thereby to the increase of capacity for affording enjoyment; ... but also... to the perpetuation of their action, and consequently to the maintenance of life; it follows not only that enjoyment is the end of life, but that it is the means by which life is prolonged. ... It is interwoven with the thread of existence; it is secured in and by the actions that build up and that support the very frame-work, the material instrument of our being.

Organs of sense, intellectual faculties, social affections, moral powers, are superadded endowments of a successively higher order: at the same time they are the instruments of enjoyment of a nature progressively more and more exquisite.

Any attempt to exalt the animal life beyond what is compatible with the healthy state of the organic, instead of accomplishing that end, only produces bodily disease. Any attempt to extend the selfish principle beyond what is compatible with the perfection of the selfish, instead of accomplishing the end in view, only produces mental disease...

Southwood-Smith T. The Philosophy of health; or an exposition of the physical and mental constitution of man, with a view to the promotion of human longevity and happiness. Vol 1.
London, England. Charles Knight; 1836:75,81-82,85,92.

---

observe children and adolescents living in the streets; lethargy, over-indulgence, and substance abuse rife in many and various walks of life; and not uncommonly, violence and riots. The lean and the fat live side by side, the blitzed and the bored, and the alienated and the complacent, with all experiencing less than optimal health because of many factors, but one of which is a lack of appreciation of the health-promoting effects of occupation. The concept of a balance of occupations across the sleep-wake continuum and a variety throughout days and weeks to exercise a range of capacities; to meet the basic requirements for health; to provide meaning, purpose, satisfaction, and belonging; and to encourage potentialities, appears poorly understood by the majority who seek get rich quick schemes toward personal gratification and lazy luxury. However, despite the critiques of the general nature of its health promotion directives, the WHO appears to appreciate that most people have a need for income through what they do and that all humans require satisfaction, meaning, caring and sharing relationships, challenge, and growth.

Health promotion cannot be achieved without basic requirements being met by what people are able to do and facilitated by global, national, local, or family agendas. As part of what people do, the importance of being is recognized in terms of an individual's spiritual quest for meaning, purpose, and mental and spiritual well-being; belonging is recognized as part of effective communities, caring for others, and receiving and providing social support; and becoming is recognized because "an individual or group must be able to identify and to realize aspirations."[1] The importance of the doing, being, belonging, and becoming aspects of health and well-being are central within other WHO directives, such as those addressing Active Aging[62] or Mental Health,[63] as well as charters, declarations, or recommendations from subsequent health promotion congresses.

People can improve their health and lengthen their life through occupation when it is oriented toward maximizing potential within a range of environments; enhances feelings of satisfaction; provides meaning, purpose, and belonging; and meets basic health needs.[64,65] At the same time, it is understood that health is not the objective of living but rather an outcome, and is an invaluable resource for people in everyday life in doing what is necessary or chosen to do in many different and interactive ways. The emerging science of occupation has begun to explore not only if but how people influence the state of their health through what they do and how, why, with whom, and where they do it.[66,67] Figure 16-1 demonstrates that those ideas are clearly compatible with the occupational science perspective taken here, encapsulating people's doing, being, belonging, and becoming activities individually and across populations and communities within and as part of a global context.

Conceptually, occupation to promote health and well-being (OPHW) encompasses the living relationship between cellular and global, biological and sociocultural, and microscopic and macroscopic factors. What people do, singularly or collectively, affects health and well-being:

- On an individual basis through the integrative systems of the organism
- On a social level through shared, corporate, and sociopolitical activity, as well as continuously changing occupational technology
- On a global level through occupational development affecting natural resources and ecosystems.

The three are inextricably linked. This implies that practitioners focusing on promoting the health-giving relationship of occupation have to consider or explore all levels.

The promotion of health through occupation is more than lifestyles based on known health behaviors that form the thrust of current initiatives. It is possible to improve health and well-being by maximizing opportunities and maintaining or developing environments to meet the differing and equally valuable occupational capacities of people. That requires extensive population health research, with an occupational focus on individual, familial, communal, corporate, and political opportunities and outcomes, followed by action. Understanding at the highest level needs to be increased. Because OPHW holds the central belief that people are occupational beings and that occupation should be a source of health as nature intended, it also maintains that health and well-being through occupation should be a primary focus of governments, health professions, and others across the globe (Table 16-1). An extensive dispersion of WHO directives and what they mean

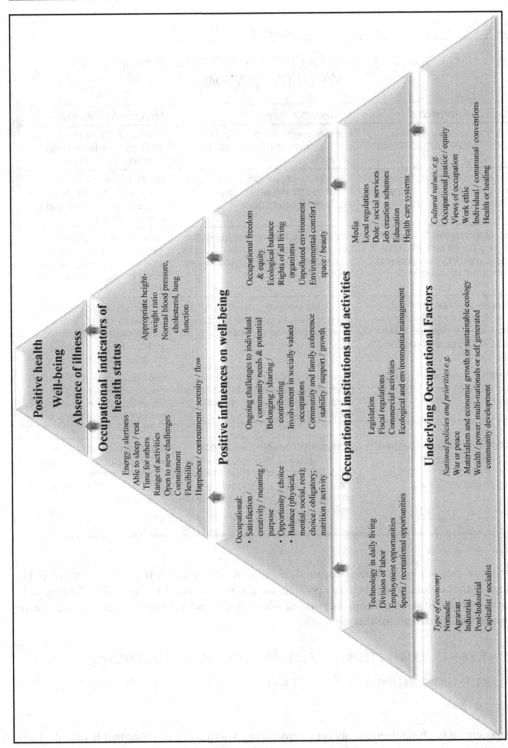

Positive health

Well-being

Absence of illness

Occupational indicators of health status

Energy / alertness
Able to sleep / rest
Time for others
Range of activities
Open to new challenges
Commitment
Flexibility
Happiness / contentment / serenity / flow

Appropriate height-
weight ratio
Normal blood pressure,
cholesterol, lung
function

Positive influences on well-being

Occupational:
• Satisfaction /
creativity / meaning /
purpose
• Opportunity / choice
• Balance (physical,
mental, social, rest);
choice / obligatory;
nutrition / activity

Ongoing challenges to individual
/ community needs & potential
Belonging / sharing /
contributing
Involvement in socially valued
occupations
Community and family coherence
/ stability / support / growth

Occupational freedom
& equity
Ecological balance
Rights of all living
organisms
Unpolluted environment
Environmental comfort /
space / beauty

Occupational institutions and activities

Technology in daily living
Division of labor
Employment opportunities
Sports / recreational opportunities

Legislation
Fiscal regulations
Commercial activities
Ecological and environmental management

Media
Local regulations
Dole / social services
Job creation schemes
Education
Health care systems

Underlying Occupational Factors

Type of economy
Nomadic
Agrarian
Industrial
Post-Industrial
Capitalist / socialist

National policies and priorities e.g.
War or peace
Materialism and economic growth or sustainable ecology
Wealth / power: multi-nationals or self generated
community development

Cultural values, e.g.
Occupational justice / equity
Views of occupation
Work ethic
Individual / communal conventions
Health or healing

Figure 16-1. WHO directives and prerequisites for health link with occupation.

Table 16-1

FOUNDATIONS OF AN OCCUPATION TO PROMOTE HEALTH AND WELL-BEING APPROACH

Basis of Approach	Underlying Beliefs	Underlying Principals
Applicable to populations, communities, and individuals	Humans are occupational beings, and occupation should be a source of health	Natural health can be attained, maintained, and improved through doing
Aimed at promoting physical, mental, social, and occupational health and well-being	Physical, mental, social, and occupational health and well-being can be improved for all people	Health promotion is the process of enabling people to increase control over, and to improve, their health
An integrated method of functioning based on behavioral, social, medical, environmental, and occupational science	Research and information about the promotion of physical, mental, social, and occupational well-being should be inclusive and holistic	Socioeconomic, political, and medical decisions affect the promotion of health and well-being through what people do
People can improve the state of their health through what they do when it is oriented toward maximizing potential within environments	Health is a positive concept emphasizing social and personal resources, as well as physical capacities	Individuals or groups must be able to identify and realize aspirations, to satisfy needs, and to change or cope with the environment
Health is a resource for everyday life, not the objective of living.	People need information and assistance about what they should do to reach a state of physical, mental, and social well-being	Wide dispersion of World Health Organization directives will assist achievement of health for all in the 21st century
Is holistic and diverse addressing many different and interactive ways to promote health and well-being	Promotion of health goes beyond healthy lifestyles to physical, mental, social, and occupational well-being across the globe and should be a primary focus of governments, health professions, and others	Action across various fields will enable positive interventions to promote individual and community health and well-being

in terms of people's occupation is required to promote action across the wide variety of public sectors. If that occurs, it will be more possible for the promotion of health and well-being to be given more than lip service within socio-economic-political decision making. The Ottawa Charter provides basic guidelines for this approach.

HEALTH PROMOTION IS THE PROCESS OF ENABLING PEOPLE TO INCREASE CONTROL OVER, AND TO IMPROVE, THEIR HEALTH[1]

Enablement is a fundamental concept in promoting health and well-being that is valued widely. For example, it has been adopted by occupational therapists as an essential principle of practice, combined with participatory, client-centered approaches.[68-72] It is linked in the Ottawa Charter with advocacy and mediation.[1] Health promotion practitioners combine the three in empowerment, claiming this as the key philosophical tenet and guiding principle.[9,23,73] It provides the link between facilitating choice and action, and increasing control over ways to improve health.[74]

Empowerment is also evident in occupational therapy literature, despite the rhetoric of a profession that, on the whole, is unpracticed in sociopolitical debate and largely dominated by medical values.[75-79] Townsend and Landry[80] claim that:

> *Awareness of the need to shape environments to enhance occupational performance locates occupational therapists' practice implicitly and sometimes explicitly in the work of enabling, empowerment and justice.*

HEALTH IS A RESOURCE FOR EVERYDAY LIFE, NOT THE OBJECTIVE OF LIVING[1]

People's doing, being, belonging, and becoming is a primary concern and health is a biproduct. Health can be a reason to engage and continue an occupation, but the actual doing to meet other life needs may not consciously hold health outcomes to the fore. In most instances, a varied and full occupational lifestyle that encompasses regular, adequate, and timely active and rest components will coincidentally maintain and improve health if it enables people:

- To meet life needs
- To be creative and adventurous physically, mentally, and socially
- To explore emotions, personal need, and environmental adaptation without undue disruption
- To experience meaningful and supportive relationships that enable a sense of belonging
- To experience sufficient physical, intellectual, spiritual, and social challenges to stimulate neuronal physiology, balanced by timely relaxation and adequate sleep
- To experience a sense of timelessness and "higher-order meaning" interwoven with time for simply "being" or reflection on "becoming."[81,82]

A lifestyle with such ingredients will not prevent all illness, disability, or untimely death, but there is increasing evidence that, coupled with modern medical approaches, they contribute to positive health. The contribution is greater if occupation is varied.

Some occupations maintain and enhance joint stability and range, muscle tone, body size, cardiovascular fitness, and respiratory capacity. Others are a kind of "brain food." They stimulate interest, give meaning to living, and do not under- or overstress people so they are able to meet reasonable demands, accept responsibility, plan ahead, respond to problems, and establish realistic goals.[83] Yet others are integral to mental and social determinants of health, and occur when people feel comfortable about themselves and with others; when they interact and fulfill needs to belong and to give and receive love; when they balance challenges and relaxation; and when the society and environment in which they live allows and values such activity.[84] As has been the case through millennia, it is purposeful, meaningful, and fulfilling occupations that maintain homeostasis and sustain health by connecting people and keeping body parts and the mind functioning efficiently. Those, coupled with sufficient rest and relaxation to prevent overuse and allow time for repair are requirements of regular health schedules. This is evidenced by the number of older people who lead active lives pursuing a wide range of occupations. They tend to feel better, to require less medical attention, and to live longer than those who are isolated and sedentary.[64,85,86]

HEALTH IS A POSITIVE CONCEPT EMPHASIZING SOCIAL AND PERSONAL RESOURCES, AS WELL AS PHYSICAL CAPACITIES[1]

Social and personal health and well-being is dependent on satisfying and stimulating relationships, experienced through a range of shared, supporting, or complementary occupations and roles (Figure 16-2). Doyal and Gough go so far as to suggest "to be denied the capacity for

Figure 16-2. Physical and mental benefits are gained through shared activity. (© Carol Spencer 2012, otspencer@adam.com.au. Used with permission.)

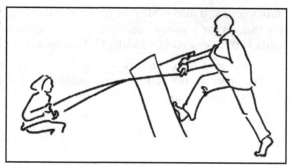

potentially successful social participation is to be denied one's humanity."[87] It is the need for social connectedness that causes people to embrace causes and occupations that may be unhealthy in other ways. Excessive drinking bouts common to young adults in affluent countries, or rioting and war-making, are obvious examples. Occupations that have the most obvious beneficial effects on health are those that utilize personal strengths and resources; that people feel good about; that they know make others feel good; that perhaps endow them with some kind of social status; and that enable them to have the freedom to effectively use personal capacities in combination with activities that are socially sanctioned, approved, and valued, even if only by a subculture.[88]

HEALTH PROMOTION IS NOT JUST THE RESPONSIBILITY OF THE HEALTH SECTOR, BUT GOES BEYOND HEALTHY LIFESTYLES TO WELL-BEING[1]

Health promotion is a complex issue within public health and mainstream medicine and, because it entails more that preventing illness or disability, has become the province of many other organizations and vocational groups.[89] This is appropriate but has the disadvantage that only pockets of communities are served. Concerted efforts that are necessary are almost beyond what is possible unless integrated into some sort of health framework that enables coordination and encourages appropriate extension of activities.

The United Kingdom's NICE conceptual framework for public health attempts such integration, recognizing that positive and negative causal pathways cross physical, biological, social, economic, political, and psychological boundaries (Table 16-2).[90] In this, both individual and population patterns of positive health are recognized as having biological and social mechanisms that are causal and interactive: a person's state of health at any one time reflects their hereditary, biological structure, and the microbiological environment; the immediate physical, social, psychological, and emotional environment; and the consequences of social, organizational, population, and environmental, as well as occupational behavior. That makes for complexity, individual difference, and variability. It results in health outcome predictions being difficult at an individual level, although possible at group and population levels. Both life-course sociology and epidemiology demonstrate clearly that throughout life, the human organism accumulates benefits, as well as insults, similar to "a health profit and loss account." A life-course approach demonstrates that:

> ... At critical points on life's journey, which are very highly socially patterned, benefits and insults can be greatly magnified, past insults can be canceled out, and new benefits can come into play. It is also clear that these changes may be self-reinforcing, producing and reproducing patterns of health advantage and disadvantage. Those critical points on life's journey are like gateways, or forks in the road, setting in train patterns that may endure and have long-lasting effects.[90]

Table 16-2
A CONCEPTUAL FRAMEWORK (UK NATIONAL INSTITUTE FOR HEALTH AND CARE EXCELLENCE)[90]

Message

1. There are social, economic, psychological, and biomedical determinants of health and disease
2. Determinants impact on individuals to produce individual-level pathology, but also produce highly patterned health differences in populations that reflect inequalities in society
3. Determinants have discernible causal pathways
4. Causal pathways help to identify ways to prevent and ameliorate disease
5. There are causal pathways for the promotion of health
6. Positive and negative causal pathways cross physical, social, economic, political, and psychological boundaries

Apart from the United Kingdom, in some parts of the world, regional and local governments have become important players in developing infrastructures to improve the health and well-being for members of their communities. In Australia, Health Partnership Agreements and strategic policy reforms are in place to strengthen municipal planning in population health and to reduce the financial burden in health care. The Geelong Regional Alliance provides an example. Its discussion paper, *Health and Well-Being Planning 2013-2017*, in line with the changing public health emphasis on population rather than individuals, seeks to query and challenge communal understandings and to develop intervention or action toward building a healthier society by reducing population inequalities. Key elements of the planning framework include the "adoption of a whole systems approach embedding plans across the broader municipal landscape; collaborative planning with broad community consultation;" and "encouraging cross sectoral action."[91]

The growing interest of local government is encouraging, as a 2008 report from Canada's Public Policy Forum discussed. This report argues that "none of us can achieve the big goals we set for ourselves without the help of others … especially … in the pursuit of societal goals." Action and discussion are necessary: "Governments, stakeholders, communities and citizens need to have a real dialogue where they listen, learn and then act, together."[92] Well-being is frequently equated to quality of life, which has been identified as the degree to which a person enjoys life's possibilities. The Ontario Social Development Council describes quality of life as the "product of interplay among social, health, economic, and environmental conditions which affect human and social development." It claims the purpose of quality of life indexes is to monitor people's living and working conditions to focus attention on community action to improve health.[93] The Quality of Life Research Unit at the University of Toronto recognizes three major domains similar to how doing, being, belonging, and becoming within occupation were described earlier. The first domain is inclusive of personal identity and personal physical, psychological, and spiritual factors and equates with being. The second domain includes personal fit within the physical, social, and community environment and equates with belonging. The third domain includes engagement in purposeful activities to meet personal needs and goals including those of a practical, leisure, and growth nature and equates with doing and becoming.[94] Quality of life has also been addressed in many occupational therapy publications focusing on such issues as living circumstances, empowerment, hope, motivation, meaning, satisfaction, happiness, socializing, expanding horizons, and promoting health.[68,95-97] With such an apparent degree of interest in the topic, it is timely to develop supportive and proactive partnerships across disciplines, communities, interest groups,

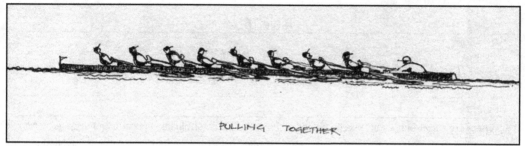

Figure 16-3. Realizing individual and community aspirations through a team occupation that exercises body, mind, and spirit. (© Trevor Bywater 2013. Used with permission.)

and concerned individuals to promote health and increase well-being in many differing spheres, especially because environmental and social conditions are major contributors to illness:

> ... It is disingenuous, however, to talk about getting enough sleep while disregarding the economic pressures on tens of millions of people, which compel them to moonlight or work extra shifts; to talk about eating well but say nothing of the powerful advertising industry; to talk of not smoking and drinking moderately yet be blind to the manifold social stressors that lead people to use smoking and drinking as maladaptive coping responses.[98]

OPHW encompasses more than the achievement of individual goals. If that were the only criterion, it would be as narrow as a biomechanical approach that only considers physical factors.[99] A health and well-being perspective calls for greater understanding of all people's occupational needs from the attaining of the prerequisites of life to the opportunities within populations around the globe to be able to realize individual and community aspirations that exercise body, mind, spirit, and social capacities in a way that is healthy for the earth itself (Figure 16-3). That understanding needs to be articulated and reflected in the range of organizations that legislate activity within populations and for individuals, and to be recognized in all health professional agendas. Occupational therapy would appear to be an appropriate profession to work with OPHW, yet it is poorly recognized as a potential resource, leading to a tendency for the profession's members to take a narrow, medicalized position rather than a broad stance based on how occupation and health interact across the population. However, a 1976 definition of health provided by the American Occupational Therapy Association[100] reflects a broader understanding, describing health as:

> ... biological, social, and emotional well-being whereby an individual is capable and able to perform those tasks or activities which are important or necessary to him to promote or maintain a sense of well-being. The individual state of health is influenced by forces such as heredity, behavior, physical environment, and the economic and social system in which he lives.

AN INDIVIDUAL OR GROUP MUST BE ABLE TO IDENTIFY AND REALIZE ASPIRATIONS, TO SATISFY NEEDS, TO CHANGE OR COPE WITH THE ENVIRONMENT[1]

Earlier chapters addressing doing, being, belonging, and becoming explored this theme in many ways. Satisfying needs, coping with the environment, and realizing aspirations are integral to health and well-being; this is achieved through occupation at an individual level and determined by familial, communal, corporate, political, and environmental occupations and actions.

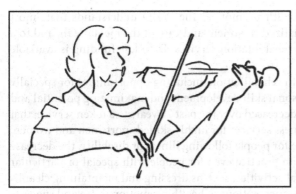

Figure 16-4. Mental well-being through encouragement of a special skill (violin). (© Carol Spencer 2012, otspencer@adam.com.au. Used with permission)

Why Is an Occupation to Promote Health and Well-Being Approach Necessary?

The WHO premise that health is not the objective of living, and that "good health is a major resource for social, economic and personal development and an important dimension of quality of life" is at the core of this approach.[1] Ornstein and Sobel's surmise that the principal function of the human brain is to maintain health appears to have largely "escaped the attention of the mainstream of medical practice and psychological thought." They suggest medicine has largely regarded "the body as a mindless machine" and that psychology has been restricted by "a view that the main purpose of the human brain is to produce rational thought. Never mind that the … neuron [does] not for the most part, serve thought or reason."[101] Integrative notions of health have not been assimilated well into mainstream health care practices.[102-106] The older dualism of body versus mind or the modern one of body-mind versus socioenvironmental are contrary to the holistic notion of health and occupation resulting from all parts of brain and body working in harmony within social, natural, or human-made environments.

Currently, particularly in affluent parts of the world, reliance on medicine to put right illness appears the easy solution, yet it is very expensive. Technological advances keep the costs escalating, and the demand for medical miracles to right the wrongs of unhealthy lifestyles is not abating. Suffering could be substantially reduced if all professional health encounters and community endeavors reinforced health promotion messages and if people recognized the part played by everyday occupations in their experience of health and well-being. Incorporating health promotion into the everyday doing, being, belonging, and becoming occupations of life is an obvious way forward as a means to meet survival, health, and well-being requirements. It is the positive and the negative aspects that need explicating to the world at large. This would be an ongoing project, because the issues will change as natural, sociopolitical, corporate, technological, cultural, familial, and spiritual environments change.

Some of the immediate issues to be overcome are poverty and reducing the risks of infectious diseases, noncommunicable diseases, and mental illness through positive and health-enhancing activity. There is a pressing and fundamental need to find ways for people everywhere to meet the requirements of survival and positive health through what they do in ways that address their other biological needs. For example:

> *...mental health promotion [is] an umbrella term that covers a variety of strategies, all aimed at having a positive effect on mental health well-being in general. The encouragement of individual resources and skills [such as music, art or sport; Figure 16-4], and improvements in the socio-economic environment are among the strategies used.[107]*

Despite recognizing the need for mental health promotion, the WHO understands that "most health care resources are spent on the specialized treatment and care of the mentally ill, and to a lesser extent on community treatment and rehabilitation services. Even less funding is available for promoting mental health."[107]

Tertiary health promotion concerned with rehabilitation, including opportunities for specially trained health professions to assist with personal skill development and maximizing potential and quality of life using actual occupations, has decreased over the past 20 years to a token service; that is except for very personal and extensive fitness services for highly skilled sportsmen and women. Once an extension of conventional medicine for people following illness or disability, the decrease points to serious neglect of health promotion practice even for people with special or particular needs, except, perhaps to assist with personal activities, such as dressing and maintaining cleanliness. A 2003 study of occupational therapists' perceptions of health promotion in Ireland suggests that limited resources in terms of time, staff, and funding are the major perceived barrier.[108] As longevity increases, more elderly are living alone. Loneliness, isolation, and sedentary lifestyles are likely to become increasingly widespread problems as the age of death is put on hold.[109] Loneliness is characterized by feelings of being disconnected, not belonging, and isolation. "The strength of social isolation as a risk factor is comparable to obesity, sedentary lifestyles and possibly even smoking,"[110] requiring specific investigations about the determinants of social support, networks, and activities that are required to prevent dependency in old age.[111] Active aging policies build on such knowledge and concerns.[62,112]

The WHO accepted that:

> *The essence of Fries's tenets, that chronic diseases and physical decline 'originate in early life, develop insidiously' and can be prevented, as well as his vision—rejecting conventional predictions of an ever more feeble older populace—now lie at the heart of today's approach to NCDs, aging and health with its focus on the life course, health promotion, and 'active aging.'*[113]

The compression of morbidity predicted by Fries[114] in 1980 has begun to take effect, leading McMurdo to argue that it is "the undreamed of improvements in average life expectancy that have thrust aging to the forefront of attention." He suggests "laying to rest the pervasive misconception that all the ills of old age are 'just old age' would represent a major breakthrough for health care of older people."[115] Although it is now predicted that lifestyle improvements will enable more people in affluent countries to reach age 100 years, the insidious development of noncommunicable diseases in developing and new industrial regions is increasing.[65]

Occupation-Focused Health Promotion

Occupation-focused health promotion is dependent on how people obtain the requirements for living; social determinants, acceptance, and equity issues; occupational behavior that develops from the earliest age; family and close community activities, education, and work opportunities; being able to function; finding meaning, purpose, and choice; practical based programs; tertiary and quaternary approaches; and environmental issues. It also depends on people realizing that what they do affects their health, well-being, longevity, and life course and that it affects others.

The Jakarta Declaration identified five health promotion priorities for the 21st century: the advancement of social responsibility for health; an increase in investments for health development; an expansion of partnerships for health promotion; an increase in empowerment of individuals and communities; and the building and safeguarding of health promotion infrastructures.[2] Aimed at those priorities, the OPHW would not only focus on what, how, why, and with whom people engage in the doings of ordinary life, it needs to explore aspects of occupation within communities, populations, corporate, and political organizations and social infrastructures. Raising awareness

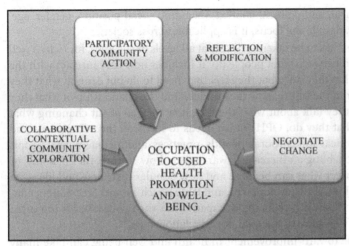

Figure 16-5. Occupation-focused health promotion and well-being.

about the health and social benefits of meeting people's need to engage in occupations that provide for basic requirements, improve health, and reduce personal and financial costs, would empower action. Action would utilize occupations to exercise particular capacities and potential and enable growth, development, and a sense of belonging as members of a community (Figure 16-5).

The exploration of health and well-being through occupation (often described in terms such as time-use or activity) is in its infancy, but is ongoing in various parts of the world, with Canada being a leader in the field. Researchers for the Canadian Index of Wellbeing have examined associations between identified time use indicators with those of health and well-being. They used an age and life stage approach and identified a need for policies and programs that promote time spent in health-enhancing activities to address social level factors in workplaces, communities, and schools.[116] The Wellbeing in Developing Countries (WeD) center at the University of Bath, mentioned in the first chapter, began as a major multicountry, interdisciplinary study.[55] That approach considers three interlinked aspects of life, described as material, relational, and subjective, that all relate to aspects of doing, being, belonging, and becoming:

1. The material is concerned with people's bodies, the physical environment, and "what people have or do not have," such as food and shelter
2. The relational is about action, referring to "what people do or cannot do" with the material, as well as the rules, practices, power, and connections between people that affect action and social interaction
3. The subjective relates to "what people think or feel" about their situation, and the "cultural values, ideologies and beliefs" that affect what they do.[55]

Well-being, the study argues, poses questions about what is good for individuals, communities, and societies. Accordingly, intervention needs to relate to local understanding of well-being, and to be positive, holistic, and person-centered:

> Being positive places the emphasis on what people have, can do or hope for; rather than seeing people and places in terms of their problems, deficiencies, or what they lack.

> Being holistic gives a rounded understanding of quality of life that sets conventional material indicators in the context of other things that matter to people.

> Being person-centered recognises the importance of social and personal relationships and people's own perceptions, including the way these are shaped by culture, values, and meaning.[118]

The WeD approach focuses specifically on poorer people's strengths rather than needs, capabilities and entitlements, culture and meaning, and personal and social relationships, while bearing in mind the historical, geographical, and cultural context, including social position, gender, age, ethnicity, caste, or class; however, despite the focus, it is applicable across societies.

The OPHW focus is similar and has to be taken seriously at all levels of societies, for rich as well as poor, because of the interaction between what people do. It includes how they interact with the world and with others through what they do; what they feel they need to do but cannot; what they value and would like to do now or in the future; how they understand the relationship of what they do with their health status; how they talk about what they do; how they go about changing what they do; or feeling good about what they do. OPHW also needs to focus on the occupations and influence of social structures, political and corporate worlds, practices, and media on what people do or do not do. It would aim at enabling an increased awareness of how culture, the economy, or political ideologies or activities affect what can be done and how popular discourse and ideas act on notions about occupational values, skill development, and issues, such as work, recreation, education, play, or power. Changing the health-reducing occupations of such collectives is too often overlooked as a given, particularly because of unequal power relationships.

To enable and empower people toward improvement in health and well-being can take many forms. It might include coaching, encouraging, facilitating, guiding, listening, prompting, or reflecting.[119] It might involve mass media campaigns or action to highlight issues of legislative or corporate decisions that disempower or disenable. It might include health education campaigns aimed at possible health outcomes associated with occupational change. Counseling or group programs might be used, along with community development or self-help initiatives aimed at personal development. The approach could require the learning of new skills or new ways of doing. It would also require skill building programs to empower action and enable participants to communicate effectively, to research and explore the background to perceived problems, to make decisions, to follow through with their ideas, and to practice new ways of doing to meet personal and communal being, belonging, and becoming needs.

WELL DOING, BEING, BELONGING, AND BECOMING

Because this text has used the terms *doing, being, belonging,* and *becoming* to explore the idea of an occupational perspective of health, it is appropriate to use the same terms at the conclusion to bring the ideas full circle.

How People Obtain the Requirements for Living

Over the longer term, as the previous chapter illustrated, a lack of necessity to do can lead to social, mental, and physical illness that, in turn, can lead to disorders in communities. Except in emergencies, what people do to acquire the necessities of life must meet their biological needs and exercise at least some of their particular capacities. This implies that people need to be more aware of their skills and capacities than is the case for most currently. The concept may appear as common sense and current practice, but that is far from the case. Many people do not know themselves well; education may not be available or may not interest them because it fails to tap into their capacities; and inappropriate employment may be sought because in affluent countries it is trendy, well-paid, and carries status. In both affluent and developing countries, limited opportunities can mean that any vacant job has to be taken because it may be the only kind available. Whilst a lack of employment creates health disasters in the developing world, in social welfare states it can also be disastrous to health in the longer term. To some unemployment may appear more attractive than working, especially if jobs do not pay well, are socially unpopular, or if self-knowledge is limited, longer-term reduction in morbidity and mortality is a distinct possibility.

Social Determinants

Social and equity issues may make self-knowledge and occupational development particularly difficult for some people. Programs to increase people's understanding of the occupation, social determinants, and health relationship are required, particularly for those who are severely marginalized, such as "refugees, disaster victims, the socially alienated, the mentally disabled, the very old and infirm, abused children and women, and the poor."[63]

Occupational Behavior Develops Early

The origins of physical inactivity and increasingly sedentary lifestyles can be traced from childhood. Poulsen and Ziviani[119] argued that profiling the multidimensional occupation patterns of children requires "a broad understanding of the complex, interrelated contextual, interpersonal, intrapersonal and temporal aspects of occupational performance." They provided a conceptual framework for advice on the optimal balance between physically active and sedentary pursuits that underpins physical and mental health.[119] The WHO's international program to stimulate mother-infant interaction is another avenue that could be utilized to improve the emotional, social, cognitive, and physical development of children. This is particularly suitable for those whose living conditions are stressful and socially impoverished.[120]

Education Is a Primary Concern

The WHO calls for the establishment of child-friendly schools aimed at promoting sound psychosocial environments that encourage tolerance and equality. It recommends that schools should facilitate:

- "Active involvement and cooperation"
- "Education which responds to the reality of the children's lives"
- "Establishment of connections between school and family life"
- "Creativity as well as academic abilities"
- Self-esteem and self-confidence
- Healthy social and emotional development
- Supportive and nurturing environments that avoid or do not tolerate bullying.[63]

The WHO curriculum was developed to enable the growth of sound and positive mental health, including "problem-solving, critical thinking, communication, interpersonal skills, empathy, and methods to cope with emotions."[63] A combination of occupation-based initiatives and the WHO's life skills curriculum could utilize any or all of those recommendations for people of any age. Those past school age who, for whatever reason, were deprived of the chance to learn and develop capacities are in need of assistance.

Practical Based Programs

These are valuable for those who want to develop particular skills, such as how to maintain a home, build shelter, store clean water, grow food, or learn to cook. It appears that in affluent countries, food preparation skills have been lost to many of the younger generations. This appears more so amongst those less affluent, and those who are ethnic minorities in an unfamiliar environment,[121,122] and can be linked to noncommunicable diseases[123] and to social exclusion.[124] In situations such as this, health promotion action could address the specific needs of the group by encouraging productive home gardening; increasing marketing skills, awareness of food types, and sources within communities; providing group access to occupational programs that includes information about healthy eating; and undertaking a group investigation of food production sources.[125] Enlisting support of private and community organizations and government agencies for and in programs of this nature can be empowering. Mediating or advocating on behalf of an action research community to such effect could be the role suited to health professional participants.

Active Aging

The WHO's Active Aging policy guidelines are fundamental to health promotion and well-being. They provide direction for action with and for all older people to:

- Realize physical, social, and mental potential
- Participate in communities
- Participate in economic, cultural, spiritual, and civic affairs
- Be assured of adequate protection, security, and care when necessary.[62]

Decline is not necessarily a part of normal aging but occurs if there is a lessening in activity and participation. Because of the ageist orientation of postindustrial societies, support for when the health of older people declines is given more attention than the provision of doing, being, belonging, and becoming opportunities within normal life. Numerous studies have demonstrated the benefits of having active lifestyles with other likeminded individuals, which provides participants with meaning, purpose, and continued development.[64,67,126-129] There is a great need within communities throughout the world to promote continuing good health for older people by enabling and extending social support networks and leisure opportunities.[130,131] Programs in which older people empower and assist younger people in many spheres will be particularly effective for both provider and receiver. It is useful for population health practitioners to bear in mind Wilson's view of working with older people as a "privilege of recognizing, respecting and integrating the richness and individuality of a person's longer lifespan."[132]

Function

The word *function* is used by the WHO in the ICF as an active descriptive term that encompasses the necessary doings of daily life.[25] Active function depends on adequate sleep and rest.[133] Greiner et al described the physical, mental, and social domains of function, including activity-exercise, roles-relationships, cognition-perception, self-perception-self-concept, and coping-stress tolerance. They explained "functioning is integral to health" and loss of function may be a sign of ill health.[134] Function, in those terms, is as close in meaning to occupation as doing, being, becoming, and belonging.

Meaning, Purpose, and Choice

Coupled with control,[135,136] meaning, purpose, and choice are fundamental to self-worth,[137]quality of life, and well-being.[138] They are integral to people's doing, being, becoming, and belonging, which are positive attributes to health or negative attributes when lacking.[139] Research indicates that when people "are given an opportunity to gain personal meaning from everyday activities, when their sense of optimism is renewed, and where they believe that there is choice and control in their lives," it is possible to avert depression.[137,140] It is a sad indictment of the affluent world that the negative effects of what, how, and why people do must be partly to blame for the incidence of depression reaching epidemic proportions.[141] It is also clear that economic, material, and educational advantages alone are insufficient to ensure health and well-being. Action to promote health needs to facilitate people's positive capacities and discard the negative while ensuring that social and natural environments are maintained or enhanced. Programs focusing on population understanding of occupation's association with health and well-being outcomes could be useful. A range of studies support such action,[142-145] not least to counteract deficit-based services, a lack of voice, and communication barriers.[146] Common themes in the capabilities framework developed by Sen[147] might prove useful. They include the relationship between social barriers and individual limitations, the importance of autonomy, the value of freedom, and dissatisfaction with income as measures of well-being.[148,149]

Tertiary and Quaternary Approaches

Programs toward health promotion and quality of life for people with chronic diseases, disabilities, or terminal illnesses require support mechanisms that provide people with opportunities to make choices, to enable them to set their own goals, and to make life more meaningful.[150,151] Enabling terminally ill people to self-actualize or to accomplish long-held dreams is a health-promoting initiative that may stimulate community action and support. So, too, would programs extended into the community for those with chronic disorders or noncommunicable diseases who are unable to access regular offerings. While that would call for support and resources in addition to the norm, opportunities might be rife given the overwhelming acceptance, at present, of the significance of physical activity and diet in medical, economic, and humanitarian terms. Focusing on health promotion rather than independence will provide benefits for the latter because, as Geller and Warren maintained, "both rehabilitation and healing are meant to enhance all aspects of well-being, restore integrity to a person, and facilitate the creation of meaning."[152] Health promotion and well-being are rights of all people, enabling responsible and healthy lifestyle choices that match personalities, capacities, needs, meaning, and challenge with environmental factors and independent of personal circumstances.[153-156]

Environment

Environmental issues are an essential, yet often forgotten aspect of health initiatives, with benefits derived from people's interaction with the natural world. Theories, hypotheses, and experimental evidence demonstrate positive effects on human health, such as a lessening of the physiological effects of stress on the autonomic nervous system.[157] The most celebrated early hospitals for the treatment of tuberculosis were situated in beautiful and isolated natural environments, and patients often lived and slept in outdoor rooms. There are current moves to reincorporate the natural world into the design of settings where medicine is practiced because the impact of the built environment in lessening or aggravating feelings of dis-ease, known as sick building syndrome,[158] is acknowledged. New-age architecture is responsive to health and quality of life needs in similar fashion, while tackling the necessity for urban rather than rural growth as the world's population grows.[159] The development of "lifetime homes," flexible to meet people's changing needs throughout the lifespan, and "smart homes" that incorporate assistive technology are recognized as a way forward.[160]

Occupation Toward WHO "Health for All" Objectives Across the Globe

The ideas about occupation and health that have been explored sustain the view that there are not only "occupational indicators of health and wellness," but also three distinct categories of underlying factors that can negatively and positively influence occupation and subsequently health. These are:

1. The type of economy, such as nomadic, agrarian, industrial, postindustrial, capitalist, or socialist
2. National policies and priorities, such as toward war or peace, economic growth, sustainable ecology, wealth and power of multinational corporations, or self-generated community development
3. Dominant cultural values about ideas such as spiritual beliefs or matters of social justice and equity as they relate to occupation, how different aspects of occupation are perceived, the work ethic, individualistic or communal conventions, and respect for health or healing.

Figure 16-6 encapsulates the concept of how these underlying factors give rise to particular occupational institutions and activities in any given society. For example, the type of economy has a direct influence on the amount and type of technology in daily living; how labor is divided between classes, genders, and age groups; and employment opportunities. National priorities have direct influence on legislative and fiscal institutions that provide rules by which people live, commercial and material activities, and management of the environment and the ecology. Cultural values will affect the media, local regulations, social services, job creation schemes, education, and

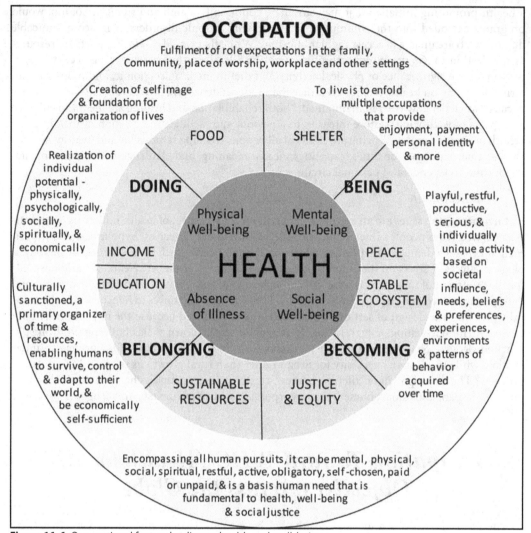

Figure 16-6. Occupational factors leading to health and well-being.

health care systems. These activities and institutions can be positive influences on community, family, or individual health by providing equitable opportunity to develop potential, creativity, and balanced use of capacities; to experience satisfaction, meaning and purpose, stability and support, and belonging and sharing; and being able to contribute in a way that is socially valued, yet maintains natural resources and recognizes the rights of all living organisms. The effects of the underlying factors may not be the same for all communities or for all individuals. For example, although to the green lobby, ecological sustainability appears to be the healthy way for all to survive, to power-broking corporations and politicians, the opposite may be conducive to their well-being. Occupational indicators of health and well-being include energy and alertness, a range of activities, flexibility, interest, contentment, commitment, the ability to relax and sleep, time for others, openness to new challenges, and minimal absenteeism from obligatory tasks.

The health promoting and well-being directions recognized within the WHO policies over the past 30 years have increasingly espoused the importance of what people do without identifying occupation in a holistic way that encompasses doing, being, belonging, and becoming across the day-night continuum. Instead, policy documents such as those addressing social determinants of health or active aging have included aspects of occupation, but without the benefits a total picture might add to policy and program development. Such a total picture would have to include how people experience and feel about what they do; how the day-night, active-rest continuum encompasses meaning, as well as the prerequisites of survival; and that the interactive nature of being, belonging, and becoming are part of and increase the known benefits of physical activity. It is critical to make clear to the WHO and other health, political, community, and corporate organizations the need to address their own and the population's occupational nature and needs.

It is timely to act now, but to create a new profession to specialize in occupation-focused policies and initiatives would waste existing expertize. Time-use researchers are an underused resource whose work complements and extends the understanding of population health. Public health and occupational health and safety practitioners could take a more holistic focus with a broader appreciation of occupation less bounded by or limited to paid employment. Occupational therapists would need to embrace total population concerns, as well as those of sick or disabled individuals, and be prepared to take action toward challenging underlying sociopolitical and ecological issues. All health practitioners require a greater understanding of the positive and negative health outcomes of occupation as an environmental, population, social, communal, and individual fact of life. All would be required to understand and accept the nature of dysfunction, such as war, under- or over-employment, and poverty as occupational and social domains of concern equal importance to physical and mental illness. All would need to take on board the WHO health promotion directives since Alma Ata, into the *Ottawa Charter* and beyond.

In the WHO health promotion rhetoric, health is indivisibly connected to people's doing, being, belonging, and becoming but many of the occupational elements have been labeled according to current disciplinary foci and understandings, so the combined effects have not been uncovered. It remains debatable whether existing disciplines will make such changes. It is negligent not to recognize the 24-hour per day nature of factors that make up occupation and relate to health outcomes, and not to accept responsibility for research and action in this domain. However, it appears to be a major problem for existing disciplines to articulate and follow a direction different from their own dominant paradigms. A leading Australian social commentator suggests that although in current society there is a "need to encourage new ideas, dissident views, debates, and critics," those who argue have had "to speak the same language and work from similar sets of assumptions to those in power."[161]

Conclusion

Physiological systems support and necessitate occupation to such an extent that the need to do is natural, and so much a part of being human that it has not been recognized as an entity worthy of study. Perhaps its value has been obscured because it is the natural means to survive, prevent illness, minimize disability, and achieve health and well-being. The division of occupation as needs and conditions altered by evolution, the endowment of specific aspects with particular value, and cultural diversity, reduced the ability to recognize it as a whole and continually increased its complexity. To complicate matters further, occupation is also susceptible to and developed according to environmental demands. As a result of those external variables, coupled with each person's different occupational nature, no two people have the same occupational capacities, potential needs, or experiences. Therefore, health promotion through occupation is essential but difficult to operationalize.

Through their daily occupations, health promotion becomes everyone's business. As the *Ottawa Charter*[1] postulates, health promotion (as health itself) is "a positive concept emphasizing social and personal resources, as well as physical capacities." Therefore, it is not only "the responsibility of the health sector, but goes beyond healthy life-styles to well-being."[1] The *Bangkok Charter*[3] builds on those ideas, explaining new critical factors that influence health inequalities between and within countries, new patterns of communication and consumption, urbanization, commercialization, and global environmental changes. Further challenges that make the attainment of health and well-being difficult include the "rapid and often adverse social, economic and demographic changes" that affect occupational determinants such as "working conditions, learning environments, family patterns, and the culture and social fabric of communities."[3]

Despite the variability, six major functions of occupation form a 3-way link with survival, health, and well-being. These functions enable individuals and collectives of people to try to:

- Attain the prerequisites of survival and health
- Maintain safety from predators and environmental hazards while preserving the interactive and diverse nature of the world's ecosystem
- Exercise personal physical, mental, and social capacities
- Find meaning, purpose, choice, satisfaction, and self and community growth through doing
- Experience a sense of belonging through shared occupations
- Develop and create inclusive societies that recognize the importance to health of people's occupations, so that both individuals and the species will flourish.

Human occupations shape culture and the environment and are, in turn, shaped by culture and environments. It is important to subject economic evolution to an occupational perspective because of the variability between people and cultures over time. People's potential for new and different pursuits, for exploring ways of making their lives easier and giving themselves time for chosen occupations, has led to a situation in which the products and results of doing have assumed a greater importance than natural human need or the health and survival of the ecosystem on which people depend. In addition, the physical and mental effort demanded of necessary occupations for people in advanced economies has reduced and has not, in the majority of cases, been replaced by other activities of equal value to maintain and enhance health. As the theme of this chapter claims, "The role of the health sector must move increasingly in a health promotion direction, beyond its responsibility for providing clinical and curative services."[1] As it is important not to overlook the health-promoting properties of all that people "do", it is vital to increase understanding of how collective occupations are central to maintaining and improving the health of individuals and populations. This demands people of differing disciplines coming together to effect change.

References

1. World Health Organization, Health and Welfare Canada, Canadian Public Health Association. *Ottawa Charter for Health Promotion*. Ottawa, Canada; 1986.
2. World Health Organization. *Jakarta Declaration on Leading Health Promotion into the 21st Century*. 1998.
3. World Health Organization. *The Bangkok Charter for Health Promotion in a Globalized World*. The Sixth International Conference on Health Promotion. Bangkok: WHO; 2005.
4. World Health Organization. *7th Global Conference on Health Promotion*. Nairobi, Kenya; October 2009.
5. World Health Organization. *Health in all Policies*. 8th Global Conference on Health Promotion. Helsinki: WHO; 2013.
6. World Health Organization. *Adelaide Recommendations on Healthy Public Policy*. 2nd International Conference on Health Promotion. Adelaide, Australia; 1988: 5-6.
7. World Health Organization. *3rd International Conference on Health Promotion*. Sundsvall, Sweden: WHO; 1991.
8. World Health Organization. *Mexico Ministerial Statement for the Promotion of Health*. 5th International Conference on Health Promotion. Health Promotion: Bridging the Equity Gap. Mexico City, June 5th, 2000.
9. Scriven A, ed. *Health Promoting Practice: The Contribution of Nurses and Allied Health Professionals*. Basingstoke, UK: Palgrave Macmillan; 2005.

10. World Health Organization, Health and Welfare Canada, Canadian Public Health Association. *Ottawa Charter for Health Promotion*. Ottawa, Canada; 1986:2.

11. Ewles L, Simnett I. *Promoting Health: A Practical Guide*. Edinburgh, UK: Bailliere Tindall; 2003:29.

12. Lalonde M. *A New Perspective on the Health of Canadians*. Ottawa: Information Canada; 1974.

13. Green LW, Frankish JC. Health promotion, health education and disease prevention. In: Koop CE, Pearson CE, Schwarz MR, eds. *Critical Issues in Global Health*. San-Francisco: Jossey Bass; 2002.

14. Nutbeam D. Foreword. In: Bunton R, MacDonald G, eds. *Health Promotion: Disciplines, Diversity and Development*. 2nd ed. London, UK: Routledge; 2002.

15. Scriven A, Garman S, eds. *Promoting Health: Global Issues and Perspectives*. Basingstoke, UK: Palgrave Macmillan; 2005.

16. Seedhouse D. *Health Promotion: Philosophy, Prejudice and Practice*. 2nd ed. Chichester, UK: Wiley; 2004:28-32.

17. Cribb A, Duncan P. *Health Promotion and Professional Ethics*. Oxford, UK: Blackwell Science; 2002.

18. Tones K. Health promotion: the empowerment imperative. In: Scriven A, Orme J, eds. *Health Promotion: Professional Perspective*. Basingstoke, UK: Palgrave Macmillan; 2001.

19. Department of Health. *The Report of the Chief Medical Officer's Project to Strengthen the Public Health Function*. London, UK: The Stationers Office; 2001.

20. Mittelmark M. Global health promotion: challenges and opportunities. In: Scriven A, Garman S, eds. *Promoting Health: Global Issues and Perspectives*. Basingstoke, UK: Palgrave Macmillan; 2005.

21. Laverack G. *Health Promotion Practice: Power and Empowerment*. London, UK: Sage; 2004.

22. Tannahill A. What is health promotion. *Health Education Journal*. 1985;44:167-168.

23. Jones L. Promoting health: everybody's business? In: Katz J, Peberdy A, Douglas J, eds. *Promoting Health: Knowledge and Practice*. Basingstoke, UK: Macmillan; 2000:1-17.

24. Katz J, Peberdy A, Douglas J, eds. *Promoting Health: Knowledge and Practice*. Basingstoke, UK: Macmillan; 2000.

25. World Health Organization. *International Classification of Functioning, Disability and Health*. Geneva, Switzerland: WHO; 2001.

26. Ryan R, Deci E. On happiness and human potentials: a review of research on hedonic and eudaimonic well-being. *Annual Review of Psychology*. 2001;(52):141-166.

27. Hetzel BS, McMichael T. *L S Factor: Lifesyle and Health*. Ringwood, Victoria: Penguin; 1987.

28. Iwama M. Occupation as a cross-cultural construct. In: Whiteford GE, Wright-St Clair V, eds. *Occupation and Practice in Context*. Sydney: Elsevier/Churchill Livingstone; 2005.

29. Iwama M. In: Kronenberg F, Simo Algado S, Pollard N. *Occupational Therapy without Borders: Learning from the Spirit of Survivors*. London: Elsevier Ltd, 2005.

30. Dossey BM, Guzzetta CE. Wellness, values clarification and motivation. In: Dossey BM, Keegan L, Kolkmier LG, Guzzetta CE. *Holistic Health Promotion. A Guide for Practice*. Rockville, MD: Aspen Publishers; 1989:69-70.

31. Johnson J. Wellness and occupational therapy. *American Journal of Occupational Therapy*. 1986;40(11):753-758.

32. Zechetmayr M. Wellness programs and employee assistance programs in industry. *Arena Review*. 1986;10(1):28-42.

33. Conrad P. Wellness in the workplace: potentials and pitfalls of worksite health promotion. *Milbank Quarterly*. 1987;65(2):255-275.

34. Conrad P, Walsh DC. The new corporate health ethic: lifestyle and the social control of work. *International Journal of Health Services*. 1992;22(1):89-111.

35. Walsh DC, Jennings SE, Mangione T, Merrigan DM. Health promotion versus health protection? employees' perceptions and concerns. *Journal of Public Health Policy*. 1991;12(2):148-164.

36. Melaleuca: *The Wellness Company*. Available at: http://www.articlesbase.com/mlm-articles/melaleuca-inc-melaleuca-the-wellness-company-3527421.html?utm_source=google&utm_medium=cpc&utm_campaign=ab_paid_12&gclid=CL-xjfznk78CFZd6vQodBlcA5A. Accessed June 20, 2014.

37. National Exercise and Sports Trainers Association. *Corporate Fitness and Trainers Programs*. 2006. Available at: http://www.ideafit.com/organization/nesta. Accessed June 20, 2014.

38. The Mayo Clinic. *Wellness Coach Training (Minnesota)*. http://www.mayo.edu/mshs/careers/wellness-coach/wellness-coaching-training-minnesota. Accessed June 21, 2014.

39. Opatz JP. *A Primer of Health Promotion: Creating Healthy Organizational Cultures*. Washington, DC: Oryn Publications; 1985:7.

40. Neville R. *Play Power*. London, England: Cape; 1970.

41. Roszak T. *The Making of a Counter Culture*. New York, NY: Doubleday; 1969.

42. Reed KL, Sanderson SN. *Concepts of Occupational Therapy*. Baltimore: Williams & Wilkins; 1980:92.

43. Johnson JA. Wellness: Its myths, realities and potential for occupational therapy. *Occupational Therapy in Health Care*. 1985; 2(2):117-138.

44. White VK. Promoting health and wellness: A theme for the eighties. *American Journal of Occupational Therapy*. 1986; 40(11):743-748.

45. Thomas TL, ed. *Taber's Cyclopedic Medical Dictionary*. 18th ed. Philadelphia: F.A. Davis; 1997:2110.

46. Ryan RS, Travis JW. *The Wellness Workbook*. Calif: Ten Speed Press; 1981:xv.

47. Levenstein S. Wellness, health, Antonovsky. *Advances*. 1994;10(3):26-29.

48. Roe M. *Nine Australian Progressives: Vitalism in Bourgeois Social Thought 1890-1960*. Australia: University of Queensland Press; 1984.

49. Cilento R. *Blueprint for the Health of a Nation*. Sydney, Australia: Scotow Press; 1944.

50. Powles J. Professional hygienists and the health of the nation. In: Macleod J, ed. *The Commonwealth of Science*. Melbourne, Australia: Oxford University Press; 1988.

51. Dunn H. *High Level Wellness*. Arlington, VA: RW Beatty; 1954.

52. Howard RB. Wellness: obtainable goal or impossible dream. *Post Graduate Medicine*. 1983;73(1):15-19.

53. Hettler W. Wellness—the lifetime goal of a university experience. In: Matarazzo JD, et al, eds. *Behavioural Health. A Handbook of Health Enhancement and Disease Prevention*. New York, NY: John Wiley and Sons; 1990:1117.

54. Travis JW, Ryan SR. *The Wellness Workbook: How to Achieve Enduring Health and Vitality*. 3rd ed. New York: Ten Speed Press; 2004.

55. ESRC Research Group on Wellbeing in Developing Countries (WeD). *Research Statement*. Available at: http://www.welldev.org.uk/research/aims.htm. Accessed May 30, 2014.

56. Owen R. *Twenty Questions to the Human Race: Dedicated to the Governments of Great Britain, Austria, Russia, France, Prussia and the United States of America*. London; 1841. (New Lanark Conservation)

57. Southwood-Smith T. *The Philosophy of Health; or an Exposition of the Physical and Mental Constitution of Man, with a View to the Promotion of Human Longevity and Happiness*. Volume 1. London: Charles Knight; 1836:101.

58. Southwood-Smith T. *The Philosophy of Health; or an Exposition of the Physical and Mental Constitution of Man, with a View to the Promotion of Human Longevity and Happiness*. Volume 1. London: Charles Knight. 1836:92.

59. Wilcock AA. *Occupation for Health. Volume 1. A Journey from Self Health to Prescription*. London: British College of Occupational Therapists; 2001.

60. Bentham J. (1789) *An Introduction to the Principles of Morals and Legislation*. Burns J, Hart HLA, eds. Oxford, UK: Clarendon Press; 1996:1.

61. Crisp R. Well-being. *Stanford Dictionary of Philosophy*. http://plato.stanford.edu/contents.html#w. Accessed January 9, 2006.

62. World Health Organization. *Active Aging: A Policy Framework*. Geneva: WHO; 2002. WHO/NMH/NPH/02.8.

63. World Health Organization. *Mental Health: Strengthening Our Response*. Fact sheet N°220. Updated April 2014. http://www.who.int/mediacentre/factsheets/fs220/en/. Accessed June 24, 2014.

64. Glass TA, de Leon CM, Marottoli RA, Berkman LF. Population based study of social and productive activities as predictors of survival among elderly Americans. *British Medical Journal*. 1999:319:478-483.

65. Kalache A, Aboderin I, Hoskins I. Compression of morbidity and active aging: key priorities for public health policy in the 21st century. *Bulletin of the World Health Organization*. Geneva: World Health Organization. http://www.scielosp.org/scielo.php?script=sci_arttext&pid=S0042-96862002000300011. Accessed June 25, 2012.

66. Wilcock A. The occupational brain: A theory of human nature. *Journal of Occupational Science Australia*. 1995;2(1):68-73.

67. Clark F, Azen SP, Zemke R, Jackson J, Carlson M, Mandel D, et al. Occupational therapy for independent older adults: a randomised controlled trial. *Journal of the American Medical Association*. 1997:22/29:1321-1326.

68. Townsend, EA, Polatajko HJ. *Enabling Occupation II: Advancing an Occupational Therapy Vision for Health, Well-being, & Justice through Occupation*. Ottawa: CAOT Publications; 2013.

69. Letts L, Rigby P, Stewart D, eds. *Using Environments to Enable Occupational Performance*. Thorofare, NJ: Slack Inc; 2003.

70. Law M. Distinguished Scholar Lecture: Participation in the occupations of everyday life. *American Journal of Occupational Therapy.* 2002;56:640-649.

71. Law M, Baum CM, Baptiste S. *Occupation Based Practice: Fostering Performance and Participation.* Thorofare, NJ: Slack Inc; 2002.

72. Sumsion T. Promoting health through client centred occupational therapy practice. In: Scriven A, ed. *Health Promoting Practice: The Contribution of Nurses and Allied Health Professionals.* Basingstoke, UK: Palgrave Macmillan; 2005.

73. 73. Society of Health Education and Promotion Specialists. Health promotion in transition, paper 5: principles and philosophy. Birmingham, UK: SHEPS; 2002. In: Scriven A, ed. *Health Promoting Practice: The Contribution of Nurses and Allied Health Professionals.* Basingstoke, UK: Palgrave Macmillan; 2005.

74. Labonte R. Foreword. In: Laverack G, ed. *Health Promoting Practice: Power and Empowerment.* London, UK: Sage; 2004.

75. Corring D, Cook J. Client-centred care means that I am a valued human being. *Canadian Journal of Occupational Therapy.* 1999;66(2):71-82.

76. Honey A. Empowerment versus power: consumer participation in mental health services. *Occupational Therapy International.* 1999:6(4):257-276.

77. College of Occupational Therapists. *COT Strategy: From Interface to Integration.* London, UK: COT: 2002.

78. Madill H, Townsend E, Schultz P. Implementing a health promotion strategy in occupational therapy and practice. *Canadian Journal of Occupational Therapy.* 1989;56(2):67-72.

79. Letts L, Fraser B, Finlayson M, Walls J. *For the Health of It! Occupational Therapy within a Health Promotion Framework.* Toronto, Ontario: CAOT Publications; 1996.

80. Townsend E, Landry J. Interventions in a societal context: enabling participation. In: Christiansen CH, Baum CM, eds. *Occupational Therapy Performance, Participation, and Well-being.* Thorofare, NJ: Slack Inc; 2005:507.

81. do Rozario L. Ritual, meaning and transcendence: the role of occupation in modern life. *Journal of Occupational Science: Australia.* 1994;1(3):46-53

82. Rappaport R. *Ecology, Meaning, and Religion.* Richmond, VA: North Atlantic Books; 1979.

83. Payne WA, Hahn DB. *Understanding Your Health.* 4th ed. St. Louis, MO: Mosby; 1995:26.

84. Wilcock AA, et al. *Retrospective Study of Elderly People's Perceptions of the Relationship Between Their Lifes' Occupations and Health.* Unpublished material, University of South Australia, 1990.

85. Ciechanowski P, Wagner E, Schmaling K, Schwartz S, Williams B, Diehr P, Kulzer J, Gray S, Collier C, LoGerfo L. Community–integrated home-based depression treatment in older adults: A randomised controlled trial. *JAMA.* 2004;291:1569-1577.

86. Cacioppo J. Biological costs of social stress in the elderly. Paper given at the American Psychological Association. Washington, D.C. 2000. (Reported in: *The University of Chicago Chronicle.* 2000;19(20)).

87. Doyal L, Gough I. *A Theory of Human Need.* Houndmills, Hampshire: Macmillan; 1991:36-37,172,184.

88. Maguire G. An exploratory study of the relationship of valued activities to the life satisfaction of elderly persons. *Occupational Therapy Journal of Research.* 1983;3:164-171.

89. Kelly M. Mapping the life world: a future research priority for public health. In: Killoran A, Swann C, Kelly M, eds. *Public Health Evidence: Tackling Health Inequalities.* Oxford University Press, Oxford; 2006: 553-574.

90. *UK NICE: A Conceptual Framework for Public Health.* 2008. http:/www.sciencedirect.com/science/article/pii/s0033350608002795#. Accessed April 14, 2012.

91. *G21: Geelong Regional Alliance: Health and Wellbeing Planning 2013-2017.* www.geelongaustralia.com.au/.../documents/8d04097afe4f0e2-City%20. Accessed June 20, 2014.

92. Canada's Public Policy Forum. *It's More Than Talk: Final Report of the New Brunswick Public Engagement Initiative.* Ottawa, Canada: Canada's Public Policy Forum; 2008. https://www.ppforum.ca/sites/default/files/final_report_public_engagement_eng.pdf. Accessed June 20, 2014.

93. Shookner M. *The Quality of Life in Ontario.* Ontario Social Development Council; 1997. Available at: http://cdcquinte.com/Resources/Quality%20of%20Life-1997.pdf. Accessed June 24, 2014.

94. Quality of Life Research Unit. University of Toronto. *Notes on "Quality of Life."* Available at http://www.utoronto.ca/qol/about_us.htm (accessed November 5, 2005).

95. Christiansen CH, Baum C, eds. *Occupational Therapy: Enabling Function and Well-being.* 2nd ed. Throfare, NJ: Slack Inc: 1997.

96. Punwar AJ, Peloquin SM, eds. *Occupational Therapy: Principles and Practice.* 3rd ed. Philadelphia: Lippincott Williiams and Wilkins; 2000.

97. Stein F, Roose B. *Pocket Guide to Treatment in Occupational Therapy.* San Diego, CA: Singular Publishing Co; 2000.

98. Antonovsky A. The sense of coherence as a determinant of health. In: Matarazzo JD, et al, eds. *Behavioural Health: A Handbook of Health Enhancement and Disease Prevention.* New York, NY: John Wiley and Sons; 1990:124.

99. Boddy J, ed. *Health: Perspectives and Practices.* New Zealand: The Dunmore Press; 1985:48.

100. American Occupational Therapy Association. Glossary: essentials for an approved program for the occupational therapy assistant. *American Journal of Occupational Therapy.* 1976;30:262.

101. Ornstein R, Sobel D. *The Healing Brain: A Radical New Approach to Health Care.* London, England: Macmillan; 1988:11-12.

102. Rosi EL. *The Psychobiology of Mind-Body Healing.* New York, NY: WW Norton and Co, Inc; 1986.

103. Pert C. The wisdom of receptors: neuropeptides, the emotions, and bodymind. *Advances.* 1986;3(3):8-16.

104. Dossey B. The psychophysiology of bodymind healing. In: Dossey B, et al, eds. *Holistic Health Promotion: A Guide for Practice.* Rockville, MD: Aspen Publishers; 1989.

105. Emeth EV, Greenhut JH. *The Wholeness Handbook: Care of Body, Mind and Spirit for Optimal Health.* New York, NY: The Continuum Publishing Co; 1991.

106. Pelletier KR. *Sound Mind, Sound Body.* New York, NY: Simon and Schuster; 1994.

107. World Health Organization. *What is Mental Health?* Available at: www who.int/features/qa/62/en/. Accessed June 24, 2014.

108. Flannery G, Barry M. An exploration of occupational therapists' perceptions of health promotion. *The Irish Journal of Occupational Therapy.* 2003;Winter:33-41.

109. British Geriatrics Society. *Health Promotion and Preventive Care.* (March, 2005). Available at: http://www.bgs.org.uk/index.php/topresources/publicationfind/goodpractice/362-healthpromotion. Accessed June 20, 2012.

110. Harms B. (News Office). New research reveals how loneliness can undermine health. *The University of Chicago Chronicle.* 2000;19(20):17.

111. Stoddart H, Sharp D, Harvey I. Letters: Social networks are important in preventing dependency in old age. *British Medical Journal.* 2000;320:1277.

112. United Nations. *Global Issues: Aging.* Available at: http://www.un.org/en/globalissues/aging/. Accessed June 23, 2014.

113. World Health Organization. Health and aging: A discussion paper. Geneva: World Health Organization; 2001. Unpublished document WHO/NMH/HPS/01.1. In: Kalache A, Aboderin I, Hoskins I. Compression of morbidity and active aging: key priorities for public health policy in the 21st century. *Bulletin of the World Health Organization.* Geneva: World Health Organization. http://www.scielosp.org/scielo.php?pid=0042-968620020003&script=sci_issuetoc. Accessed June 20, 2014.

114. Fries JF. Aging, natural death, and the compression of morbidity. *New England Journal of Medicine.* 1980;303:130-135.

115. McMurdo MET. A healthy old age: realistic or futile goal? *British Medical Journal.* 2000;321:1149-1151.

116. Brooker A-S, Hyman I. Time Use: A Report of the Canadian Index of Wellbeing (CIW). Waterloo, Canada: University of Waterloo; 2010. www.uwaterloo.ca. Accessed June 29, 2014.

117. Wellbeing in Developing Countries (WeD): ESRC Research Group. *Wellbeing Research in Developing Countries: Our Approach to Wellbeing.* University of Bath. http://www.welldev.org.uk. Accessed May 30, 2014.

118. Townsend E, Landry J. Interventions in a societal context: Enabling participation. In: Christiansen CH, Baum CM, eds. *Occupational therapy Performance, Participation, and Well-being.* Thorofare, NJ: Slack Inc; 2005.

119. Poulsen AA, Ziviani, JM. Health enhancing physical activity: factors influencing engagement patterns in children. *Australian Occupational Therapy Journal.* 2004; 51(2):69-79.

120. World Health Organization. *Improving Mother-infant Interaction to Promote Better Psychosocial Development in Children.* http://www.who.int/mental_health/media/en/29.pdf. Accessed June 19, 2014.

121. Scott P, Verne J, Fox C. Promoting better nutrition: the role of dieticians. In: Scriven A, ed. *Health Promoting Practice: The Contribution of Nurses and Allied Health Professionals.* Basingstoke, UK: Palgrave Macmillan; 2005.

122. Lang T, Raynor G, eds. *Why Health is the Key to the Future of Food and Farming*. London, UK: UK Public Health Association, Chartered Institute of Environmental Health, Faculty of Public Health Medicine, National Heart Forum and Health Development Agency; 2002.

123. James WPT, Nelson M, Ralph A, Leather S. Socioeconomic determinants of health: the contribution of nutrition to inequalities in health. *British Medical Journal*. 1997;314:1545-1548.

124. Leather S. *The Making of Modern Malnutrition: An Overview of Food Poverty in the UK*. London, UK: Caroline Walker Society; 1996.

125. Department of Health. *Towards a Food and Health Action Plan: Discussion Paper*. London, UK: Department of Health; 2004.

126. Yaffe K, Barnes D, Nevitt M, Lui L, Covinsky R. A prospective study of physical activity and cognitive decline in elderly women. *Archives of Internal Medicine*. 2001;161(14):1703-1708.

127. McIntyre A, Bryant W. Activity and participation. In McIntyre A, Atwal A, eds. *Occupational Therapy for Older People*. Oxford, UK: Blackwell Publishing; 2005.

128. Mather AS, Rodriguez C, Guthrie MF, McHarg AM, Reid IC, McMurdo MET. Effects of exercise on depressive symptoms in older adults with poorly responsive depressive disorder. *British Journal of Psychiatry*. 2002;180:411-415.

129. Manson JE, Greenland P, La Croix AZ, et al. Walking compared with vigorous exercise for the prevention of cardiovascular events in women. *New England Journal of Medicine*. 2002;347(10):716-725.

130. Mayers CA. The Casson Memorial Lecture 2000: Reflect on the past to shape the future. *British Journal of Occupational Therapy*. 2000;63(8):358-366.

131. Reynolds F, Kee HL. The social context of older people. In: McIntyre A, Atwal A, eds. *Occupational Therapy for Older People*. Oxford, UK: Blackwell Publishing; 2005.

132. Wilson L. Activity and participation: Part 2. In; In McIntyre A, Atwal A, eds. *Occupational Therapy for Older People*. Oxford, UK: Blackwell Publishing; 2005.

133. Labyak S. Sleep and circadian schedule disorders. *Nursing Clinics of North America*. 2002;37(4):599-610

134. Greiner PA, Fain JA, Edelman CL. Health defined: objectives for promotion and prevention. In: Edelman CL, Mandle CL, eds. *Health Promotion throughout the Lifespan*. 5th ed. Mosby: St Louis; 2002:6.

135. Hammell KW. Using qualitative evidence to inform theories of occupation. In: Hammell KW, Carpenter C, eds. *Qualitative Research in Evidence-based Rehabilitation*. Edinburgh: Churchill Livingstone; 2004.

136. Hammell KW. Dimensions of meaning in the occupations of daily life. *Canadian Journal of Occupational Therapy*. 2004;71(5):296-305.

137. Somner KL, Baumeister RF. The construction of meaning from life events. In: Wong PT, Fry PS, eds. *The Human Quest for Meaning*. Mahwah, NJ: Erlbaum; 1998.

138. Plahuta JM, McCulloch BJ, Kasarshis EJ, Ross MA, Walter RA, McDonald ER. Amyotrophic lateral sclerosis and hopelessness: psychosocial factors. *Social Science and Medicine*. 2002;55:2131-2140.

139. Canadian Association of Occupational Therapists. *Enabling Occupation. An Occupational Therapy Perspective*. Rev. ed. Ottawa, ON: CAOT Publications ACE; 2002.

140. Christiansen C. Defining lives: occupation as identity: an essay on competence, coherence, and the creation of meaning. Eleanor Clarke Slagle lecture. *American Journal of Occupational Therapy*. 1999;53:547-558.

141. Murray CJL, Lopez AD. *The Global Burden of Disease*. Geneva: WHO; 1996.

142. Rask K, Astedt-Kurki P, Paavilainen E, Laippala P. Adolescent subjective well-being and family dynamics. *Scandinavian Journal of Caring Science*. 2003;17(2);129-138.

143. Gunnarsdottir S, Bjornsdottir K. Health promotion in the workplace: the perspective of unskilled workers in a hospital setting. *Scandinavian Journal of Caring Science*. 2003;17(1);66-73.

144. Guinn B, Vincent V. Select physical activity determinants in independent-living elderly. *Activity, Adaptation, Aging*. 2002;26(4):17-26.

145. Messias DK, De-Jong MK, Mcloughlin K. Being involved and making a difference: empowerment and well-being among women living in poverty. *Journal of Holistic Nursing*. 2005;2391:70-88.

146. Sheehy K, Nind M, Emotional well-being for all: mental health and people with profound and multiple learning disabilities. *British Journal of Learning Disabilities*. 2005;33(1):34-38.

147. Sen A. *Commodities and Capabilities*. Oxford, Oxford University Press; 1985.

148. Burchardt T. Capabilities and disability; the capabilities framework and the social model of disability. *Disabilit-Society*. 2004;19(7):735-751.

149. Sen A. Capability and well-being. In: Nussbaum M, Sen A, eds. *The Quality of Life*. New York: Oxford Clarendon Press; 1993:30-53.

150. Menon S. Toward a model of psychological health empowerment: implications for health care in multicultural communities. *Nurse Education Today*. 2002;22:28-39.

151. Sinclair K. World connected: the international context of professional practice. In: Whiteford GE, Wright-St Clair V, eds. *Occupation and Practice in Context*. Sydney: Elsevier/Churchill Livingstone; 2005.

152. Geller G, Warren LR. Toward an optimal healing environment in pediatric rehabilitation. *Journal of Alternat-Complement –Med*. 2004;10(Suppl):S179-192.

153. Christiansen CH, Townsend EA, eds. *Occupation: The Art and Science of Living*. Upper Saddle River, NJ: Prentice Hall; 2004.

154. Callahan D. *False Hope*. New York, NY: Simon & Schuster; 1998.

155. Csiksentmihalyi M. *Flow: The Psychology of Optimal Experience*. New York, NY: Harper and Row; 1990.

156. Christiansen CH, Little BR, Backman C. Personal projects: A useful approach to the study of occupation. *American Journal of Occupational Therapy*. 1998;52(6):439-446.

157. Irvine KN Warber SL. Greening healthcare: practicing as if the natural environment really mattered. *Alternative Ther Health Med*. 2002;8(5):76-83.

158. Government of South Australia. *Sick Building Syndrome*. Adelaide: Safe Work SA; 2007. http://www.safework.sa.gov.au/show_page.jsp?id=2315. Accessed July 15, 2013.

159. Thompson S. Healthy built environments – supporting everyday occupations. *6th Australasian Occupational Science Symposium: Program and Abstracts*. University of Canberra; December 2012.

160. Atwel A, Farrow A, Sivell-Muller M. Environmental impacts, products and technology. In: McIntyre A, Atwal A, eds. *Occupational Therapy for Older People*. Oxford, UK: Blackwell Publishing; 2005.

161. Cox E. A truly civil society: lecture 1: broadening the views. *The 1995 Boyer Lectures*. Australia: Radio National Transcripts; November, 1995.

Printed in the United States
by Baker & Taylor Publisher Services

Printed in the United States
by Baker & Taylor Publisher Services